Diagnostic Imaging in Ophthalmology

Diagnostic Imaging in Ophthalmology

Edited by
CARLOS F. GONZALEZ
MELVIN H. BECKER
JOSEPH C. FLANAGAN

With 326 Illustrations in 785 Parts

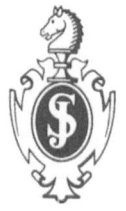

Springer-Verlag New York Berlin Heidelberg Tokyo

Carlos F. Gonzalez, M.D.
Professor of Radiology, Thomas Jefferson University Hospital, Philadelphia, Pennsylvania 19107, USA

Melvin H. Becker, M.D.
Professor of Radiology, New York University Medical Center, New York, New York 10021, USA

Joseph C. Flanagan, M.D.
Professor of Ophthalmology, Thomas Jefferson University, Wills Eye Hospital, Philadelphia, Pennsylvania 19107, USA

Library of Congress Cataloging in Publication Data
Main entry under title:
Diagnostic imaging in ophthalmology.
  Bibliography: p.
  Includes index.
  1. Eye—Diseases and defects—Diagnosis. 2. Imaging
systems in medicine. I. Gonzalez, Carlos F., 1935–
II. Becker, Melvin H. III. Flanagan, Joseph C.
[DNLM: 1. Eye Diseases—diagnosis. 2. Nuclear Magnetic
Resonance—diagnostic use. 3. Orbital Diseases—
diagnosis. 4. Tomography, X-Ray Computed. 5. Ultrasonic
Diagnosis. WW 143 D536]
RE76.D53 1985   617.7'0757   85–8063

© 1986 by Springer-Verlag New York Inc.
Softcover reprint of the hardcover 1st edition 1986

Typeset by Kingsport Press, Kingsport, Tennessee.

9 8 7 6 5 4 3 2 1

ISBN-13: 978-1-4613-8577-6   e-ISBN-13: 978-1-4613-8575-2
DOI: 10.1007/978-1-4613-8575-2

Preface

This book has been written for radiologists, ophthalmologists, neurologists, neurosurgeons, plastic surgeons, and others interested in the evaluation of disorders with ophthalmologic signs and symptoms. It is designed to provide recent knowledge in this area derived from ultrasonography, computed tomography (CT), and magnetic resonance imaging (MRI).

In the past decade, the advent of ultrasonography, computed tomography, and more recently magnetic resonance imaging has provided diagnostic images of the eye, orbit, and brain in a fashion that had been a dream of many prior to the development of these techniques. These newer modes of diagnosis have replaced some previous techniques, such as nuclear medicine imaging and, to some degree, vascular studies and orbitography.

There are three sections to this book. The first section is a discussion of the imaging techniques. The second is devoted to the role of these imaging methods in the evaluation of ophthalmic disorders. The last section, dealing with radiotherapy for ophthalmologic tumors, is included because the current imaging techniques are needed for treatment planning.

We wish to thank the many people who have assisted us in preparing this manuscript. Among these are many librarians, secretaries, trainees, and photographers. We are especially indebted to artist Peter Clark for his illustrations and to Mr. Martin Leibovici, Associate Curator of New York University Medical School and Director of Health Sciences Library of Goldwater Memorial Hospital, New York City.

Also, we wish to thank our families for their help and patience.

Carlos F. Gonzalez
Melvin H. Becker
Joseph C. Flanagan

Contents

1 Plain Film Radiography and Polytomography of the Orbit
Vijay M. Rao and Carlos F. Gonzalez   1

2 Computed Tomography of the Orbit   *Robert G. Peyster*   19

3 Computed Tomography Scanning in the Evaluation of Ocular
Motility Disorders   *Mahmood F. Mafee and Marilyn T. Miller*   43

4 Ultrasonography of the Eye and Orbit   *Richard L. Dallow*   55

5 Investigation of the Orbit by Contrast Techniques
Carlos F. Gonzalez   71

6 The Lacrimal Drainage System   *Melvin H. Becker*   81

7 Foreign Body Localization   *Melvin II. Becker*   93

8 Magnetic Resonance Imaging (MRI) of the Eye and Orbit
David F. Sobel, Ivan F. Moseley, and Michael Brant-Zawadzki   99

9 Congenital Abnormalities   *Melvin H. Becker and
Joseph G. McCarthy*   115

10 Evaluation of Exophthalmos and Thyroid Ophthalmopathy
Thaddeus S. Nowinski and Joseph C. Flanagan   189

11 Orbital Tumors   *Mark C. Ruchman, Mary A. Stefanyszyn,
Joseph C. Flanagan, Carlos F. Gonzalez, and Melvin H. Becker*   201

12 Lesions Involving the Visual Pathways   *Carlos F. Gonzalez,
Edward W. Gerner, Gary DeFilipp, and Melvin H. Becker*   239

13 Computed Tomography Assessment of Paraorbital Pathology
*Mahmood F. Mafee, Glen D. Dobben, and
Galdino E. Valvassori*   281

14 Computed Tomography in Evaluation of the Orbits in Patients
with Basal and Squamous-Cell Tumors of the Face
Hossein Firooznia and Cornelia Golimbu   303

15 Infection of the Orbit   *K. Jack Momose*   307

16 Orbital Trauma   *Joseph A. Mauriello, Jr., Carlos F. Gonzalez,*
    Charles B. Grossman, and Joseph C. Flanagan   323

17 Radiation Therapy for Malignant Intraocular Tumors
    Luther W. Brady, Jr., Jerry A. Shields, James J. Augsburger,
    John L. Day, Arnold M. Markoe, Joseph R. Castro, and
    Herman D. Swit   343

    Index   359

Contributors

James J. Augsburger, M.D.
Associate Clinical Professor of Ophthalmology, Thomas Jefferson University, Wills Eye Hospital, Philadelphia, Pennsylvania

Melvin H. Becker, M.D.
Professor of Radiology, New York University Medical Center, New York, New York

Luther W. Brady, Jr., M.D.
Chairman and Professor, Department of Radiation Therapy, Hahnemann University, Philadelphia, Pennsylvania

Michael Brant-Zawadzki, M.D.
Associate Professor of Radiology, University of California at San Francisco, San Francisco, California

Joseph R. Castro, M.D.
Professor of Radiation Oncology, University of California at San Francisco, San Francisco, California

Richard L. Dallow, M.D.
Assistant Clinical Professor of Ophthalmology, Harvard Medical School, Boston, Massachusetts

John L. Day, Ph.D.
Professor of Radiation Oncology and Nuclear Medicine, Hahnemann University, Philadelphia, Pennsylvania

Gary DeFilipp, M.D.
Assistant Professor of Radiology, Temple University Hospital, Philadelphia, Pennsylvania

Glen D. Dobben, M.D.
Professor of Radiology, University of Illinois Hospital, Chicago, Illinois

Hossein Firooznia, M.D.
Professor of Clinical Radiology, New York University School of Medicine, New York, New York

Joseph C. Flanagan, M.D.
Professor of Ophthalmology, Thomas Jefferson University, Wills Eye Hospital, Philadelphia, Pennsylvania

Edward W. Gerner, M.D.
Assistant Professor of Ophthalmology and Neurology, Thomas Jefferson University Hospital, Wills Eye Hospital, Philadelphia, Pennsylvania

Cornelia Golimbu, M.D.
Clinical Associate Professor of Radiology, New York University School of Medicine, New York, New York

Carlos F. Gonzalez, M.D.
Professor of Radiology, Thomas Jefferson University Hospital, Philadelphia, Pennsylvania

Charles B. Grossman, M.D.
Department of Radiology, Methodist Hospital Graduate Medical Center, Indianapolis, Indiana

Joseph G. McCarthy, M.D.
Lawrence D. Bell Professor of Plastic Surgery, New York University Medical Center, New York, New York

Mahmood F. Mafee, M.D.
Associate Professor of Radiology, Eye and Ear Infirmary, University of Illinois Hospital, Chicago, Illinois

Arnold M. Markoe, M.D., Sc.D.
Assistant Professor of Radiation Oncology and Nuclear Medicine, Hahnemann University, Philadelphia, Pennsylvania

Joseph A. Mauriello, Jr., M.D.
Assistant Professor of Ophthalmology, Director of Oculoplastics, University of Medicine and Dentistry of New Jersey/New Jersey Medical School, Newark, New Jersey

Marilyn T. Miller, M.D.
Associate Professor of Ophthalmology, Eye and Ear Infirmary, University of Illinois Hospital, Chicago, Illinois

K. Jack Momose, M.D.
Professor of Radiology, Massachusetts General Hospital, Boston, Massachusetts

Ivan F. Moseley, F.R.C.R.
Visiting Professor, Department of Radiology, University of California at San Francisco, California

Thaddeus S. Nowinsky, M.D.
Instructor, Thomas Jefferson University, Wills Eye Hospital, Philadelphia, Pennsylvania

Robert G. Peyster, M.D.
Associate Professor of Radiology, Neurology, and Neurosurgery, Hahnemann University, Philadelphia, Pennsylvania

Vijay M. Rao, M.D.
Associate Professor of Radiology, Thomas Jefferson University Hospital, Philadelphia, Pennsylvania

Mark C. Ruchman, M.D.
Associate Attending in Ophthalmology, Waterbury Hospital Health Center, St. Mary's Hospital, Waterbury, Connecticut

Jerry A. Shields, M.D.
Professor of Ophthalmology, Thomas Jefferson University, Wills Eye Hospital, Philadelphia, Pennsylvania

David F. Sobel, M.D.
Assistant Professor of Radiology, University of California at San Francisco, San Francisco, California

Mary A. Stefanyszyn, M.D.
Clinical Assistant, Department of Oculoplastics, Wills Eye Hospital, Philadelphia,
Pennsylvania

Herman D. Swit, Ph.D.
Chairman and Professor, Department of Radiation Medicine, Harvard University,
Massachusetts General Hospital, Boston, Massachusetts

Galdino E. Valvassori, M.D.
Professor of Radiology and Otolaryngology, University of Illinois Hospital, Chicago,
Illinois

1
Plain Film Radiography and Polytomography of the Orbit

Vijay M. Rao and Carlos F. Gonzalez

Diagnostic imaging technologies are becoming of increasing value in the evaluation of ophthalmologic patients. These techniques include routine radiographic studies, tomographic radiography, computed tomography (CT), ultrasound imaging, and magnetic resonance imaging (MRI). To understand and evaluate these studies, a knowledge of orbital anatomy is vital.

Anatomy

The orbit is pyramid-shaped, being wide anteriorly and gradually narrowing posteriorly. The central axis of each bony orbit lies approximately at 25° to the sagittal plane, but the axis of the globe itself is parallel to the sagittal plane. Seven different bones contribute to the formation of the bony orbit: the frontal, ethmoid, maxillary, sphenoid, palatine, lacrimal, and zygomatic bones. The anterior aspect of the orbital roof is formed by the orbital plate of the frontal bone separating it from the frontal sinus. The posterior portion of the orbital roof is composed of the lesser wing of the sphenoid, which separates the orbit from the anterior cranial fossa. The lateral wall is comprised of the orbital process of the zygomatic bone anteriorly and the greater wing of the sphenoid posteriorly. Along the superolateral aspect of the orbit lies the fossa for the lacrimal gland, behind the zygomatic process of the frontal bone. The medial wall of the orbit is formed by the frontal process of the maxilla, lacrimal bone, orbital plate of the ethmoid, and the body of the sphenoid from front to back. Anteriorly along the medial wall lies the deep groove lodging the lacrimal sac. The floor of the orbit is formed by the orbital plate of the

maxilla, the orbital surface of the zygomatic bone, and the palatine bone (Fig. 1.1).

The superior orbital fissure is the biggest opening between the orbit and middle cranial fossa. It lies between the lesser wing of the sphenoid (forming the roof of the orbit) and the greater sphenoid wing (forming the lateral orbital wall). It is separated from the optic canal by a bony strut connecting the lesser sphenoid wing with the body of the sphenoid. The superior orbital fissure is comma-shaped, and it can show marked variations in size and shape. The third, fourth, and sixth cranial nerves, the ophthalmic division of the fifth cranial nerve, the superior ophthalmic vein, and branches of the lacrimal and middle meningeal arteries all pass through this fissure.

The inferior orbital fissure lies between the lateral wall formed by the greater sphenoid wing and the floor of the orbit. The inferior ophthalmic vein, the sphenopalatine branches of the internal maxillary artery, and several nerves all pass through the fissure from the orbit into the sphenopalatine and infratemporal fossa.

The optic canal is a passage in the sphenoid bone through which the optic nerve, optic nerve sheath, sleeve of the subarachnoid space surrounding the sheath, and ophthalmic artery all pass from the middle cranial fossa to the orbital apex. The roof of the optic canal is formed by the lesser wing of the sphenoid. The floor and lateral walls are formed by the optic strut, and the medial wall is formed by the body of the sphenoid wing. The shape of the optic canal changes from the cranial to the orbital end. The cranial end is oval with the longest axis in the transverse plane, the central portion is circular, and the orbital end is oval with the longest axis in the vertical plane. The average diameters (adult) are 4.5 mm × 6 mm; 5 mm;

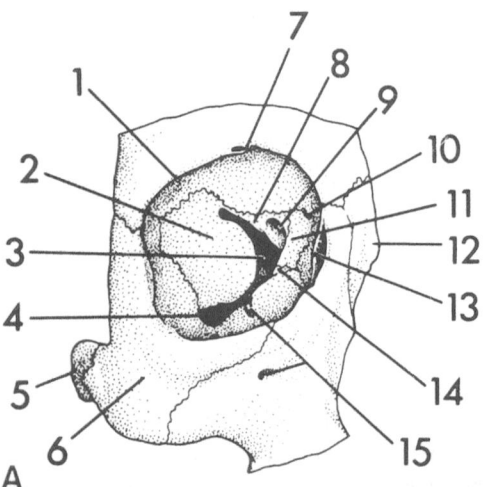

Figure 1.1. Anatomy of the orbit. **A.** (1) Supraorbital margin; (2) Greater wing of sphenoid; (3) Superior orbital fissure; (4) Inferior orbital fissure; (5) Zygoma; (6) Zygomatic bone; (7) Supraorbital notch; (8) Lesser wing of sphenoid; (9) Optic canal; (10) Anterior ethmoidal foramen; (11) Orbital plate of ethmoid; (12) Nasal bone; (13) Posterior lacrimal crest; (14) Orbital process of palatine bone; (15) Infraorbital groove and foramen.

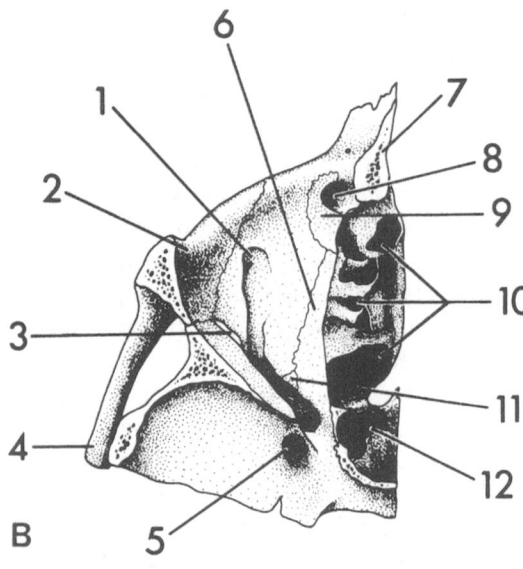

Figure 1.1 B. (1) Infraorbital groove, leading into canal; (2) Zygomatic bone; (3) Inferior orbital fissure; (4) Zygoma; (5) Foramen rotundum; (6) Orbital plate of ethmoid; (7) Frontal process of maxilla; (8) Nasolacrimal canal; (9) Lacrimal bone; (10) Ethmoidal sinuses; (11) Palatine bone, orbital process; (12) Sphenoidal sinus.

and 5 mm × 6 mm at the cranial, mid, and orbital portions, respectively. The roof of the canal is 8–10 mm long, while the floor and lateral walls are 6–8 mm long.

The orbits are usually symmetric, with differences of 2 mm in diameter or more being significant. The average diameters of the orbital opening are: height, 3.5 cm; width 4 cm; and depth 4 cm. The volume measure is about 30 cc.

Routine Examination of the Orbit

The routine examination of the orbit usually should include the following radiographs:

1. Caldwell projection (posteroanterior projection)
2. Water's projection
3. Lateral projection
4. Rhese projection (oblique projection) to show the optic foramina

Additional radiographs that may be needed include:

5. Submento-vertex projection (base view)
6. Towne's projection
7. Bucket-handle view of the zygoma for trauma

Caldwell Projection

The head is positioned in the posteroanterior position, and the central ray is directed 23° caudad to the canthomeatal line. The central beam enters at a point approximately 3 cm superior to the external occipital protuberance and exits at the glabella (Fig. 1.2).

The Caldwell projection is a very useful radiograph in evaluation of the orbits. The petrous pyramids are projected below the orbit. The structures that are visualized include lateral, medial, and superior margins of the orbits, the oblique line (innominate line), and the superior orbital fissure bordered by the lesser and greater sphenoid wings. The oblique line (innominate line or sphenoorbital line) has been described by several authors as a projection of the temporal surface of the greater sphenoid wing. Anatomically, it is a projection of the portion of the squamozygomatic surface of

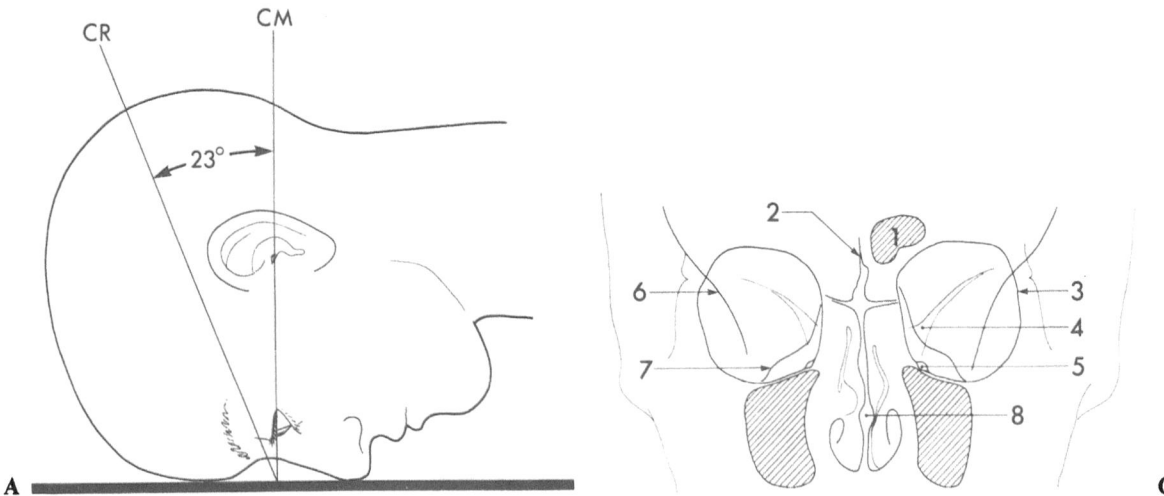

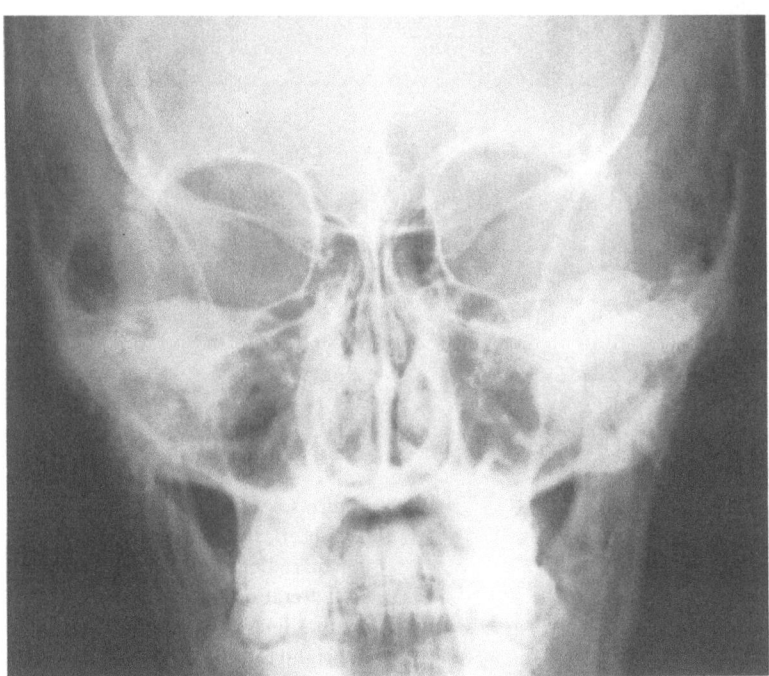

Figure 1.2 A. Caldwell projection, positioning. Central ray (CR), canthomeatal line (CM). B. Radiograph. C. Line drawing of radiograph. (1) Frontal sinus; (2) Crista galli; (3) Lateral orbital margin (orbital process of zygoma); (4) Superior orbital fissure; (5) Foramen rotundum; (6) Orbital oblique line; (7) Posterior aspect of orbital floor; (8) Nasal septum.

the sphenoid bone, which is articulated with the squama of temporal bone posteriorly and zygomatic bone anteriorly. The infraorbital foramina can sometimes be seen along the inferior orbital margin. The superior orbital fissure is best visualized in this projection. Tomographic section in this projection may be necessary for better evaluation. In addition to the orbital structures, the frontal and ethmoid sinuses, planum sphenoidale, and floor of the sella turcica are demonstrated.

Water's Projection

The head is extended in such a way that the canthomeatal line forms an angle of 40° with the table top. The midsagittal plane of the skull and the central ray are perpendicular to the film. The central ray exits at the nasal spine (Fig. 1.3).

The orbital floor and inferior orbital rim are well visualized. The anterior portion of the orbital floor, which is the rim of the orbit, projects at a

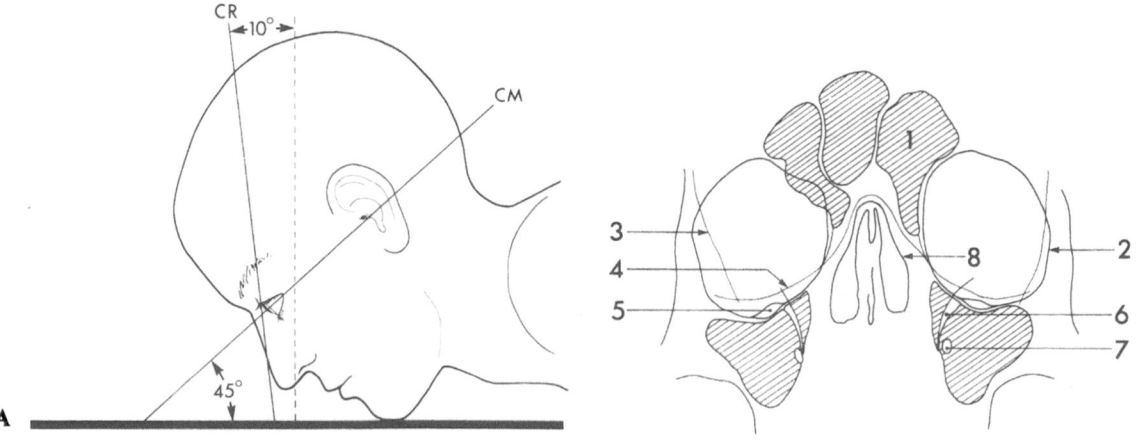

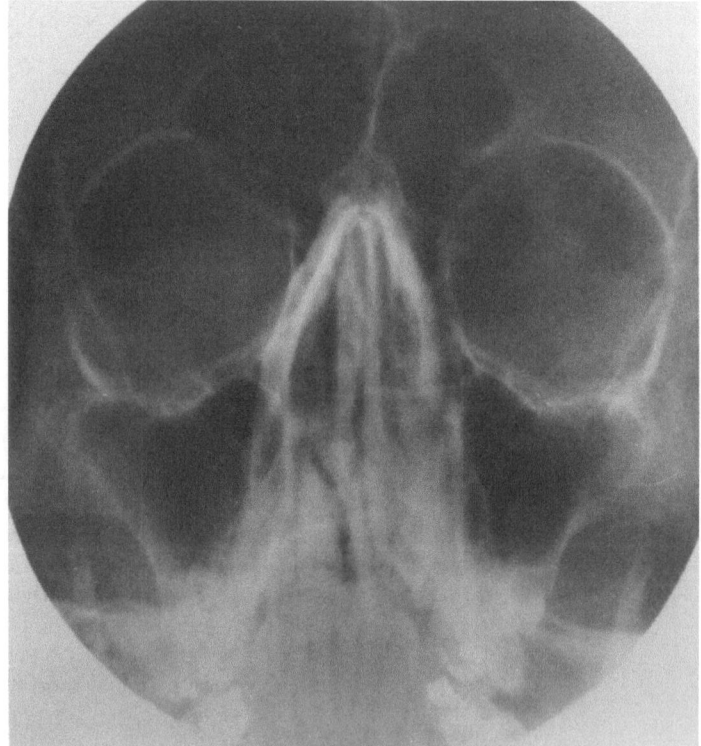

Figure 1.3 A. Water's projection, positioning. **B.** Radiograph. **C.** Line drawing of radiograph. (1) Frontal sinus; (2) Lateral orbital margin; (3) Orbital oblique line; (4) Orbital floor; (5) Infraorbital foramen; (6) Superior orbital fissure; (7) Foramen rotundum; (8) Nasal bone.

slightly higher level than the more posterior portion of the orbital floor. The distance between these two lines should be bilaterally symmetric. The medial and lateral orbital walls are well visualized. Caution is advised in evaluating the superior aspect of the orbital margins adjacent to the frontal sinus, since this area may be indistinct due to angulation. This view is particularly helpful in evaluating or-

bital blow-out fractures and the maxillary antrum. The infraorbital foramen is seen along the inferior orbital rim.

Lateral View

The head is positioned so that the midsagittal plane is parallel to the film. The central ray is perpen-

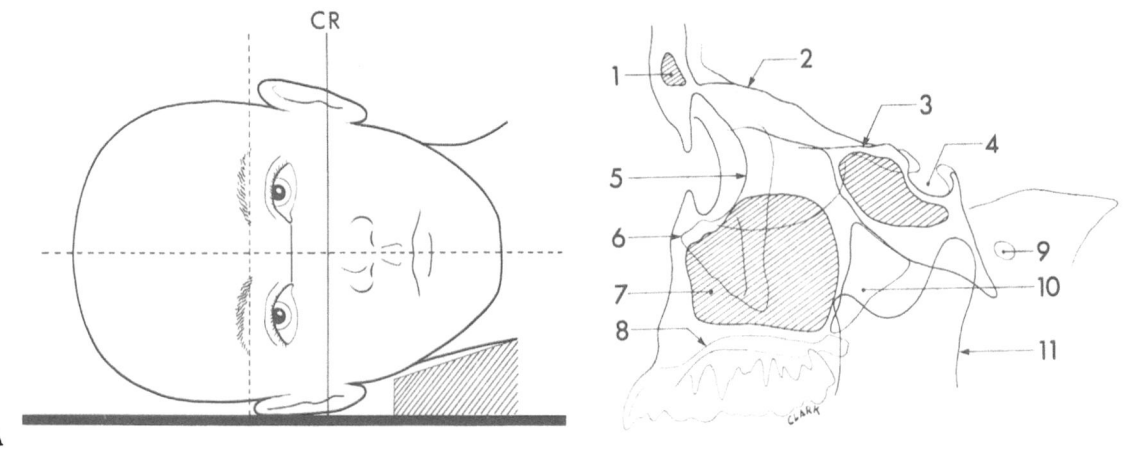

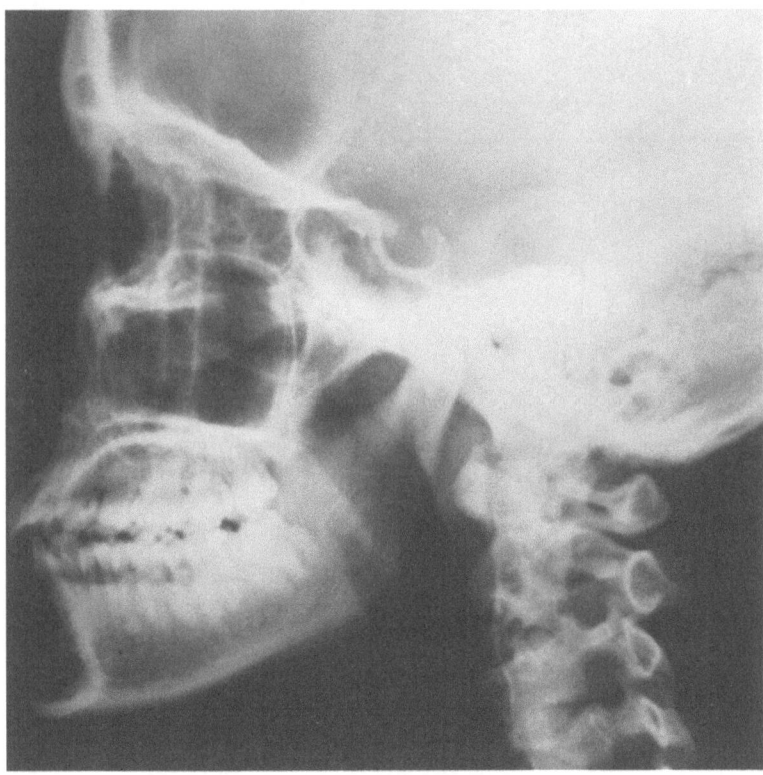

Figure 1.4 A. Lateral projection, positioning. B. Radiograph. C. Line drawing of radiograph. (1) Frontal sinus; (2) Orbital roof; (3) Planum sphenoidale; (4) Sella turcica; (5) Lateral orbital margin (orbital process of zygoma); (6) Zygoma; (7) Maxillary sinus; (8) Hard palate; (9) External auditory meatus; (10) Pterygoid plate; (11) Mandible.

dicular to the film. The central ray enters the skull 2 cm anteriorly and above the external auditory canal (Fig. 1.4).

The two orbits are superimposed. The roof of the orbits can be seen, with evidence of brain convolutions. Ethmoid air cells obscure the orbital detail. The region of the cribriform plate is identified by tracing the planum sphenoidale anteriorly.

Other structures of importance that are well demonstrated include the sella turcica, planum sphenoidale, clivus, and sphenoid sinus.

Rhese View (Optic Canal View)

This projection is obtained in a posteroanterior position with the patient's head rotated 40° to

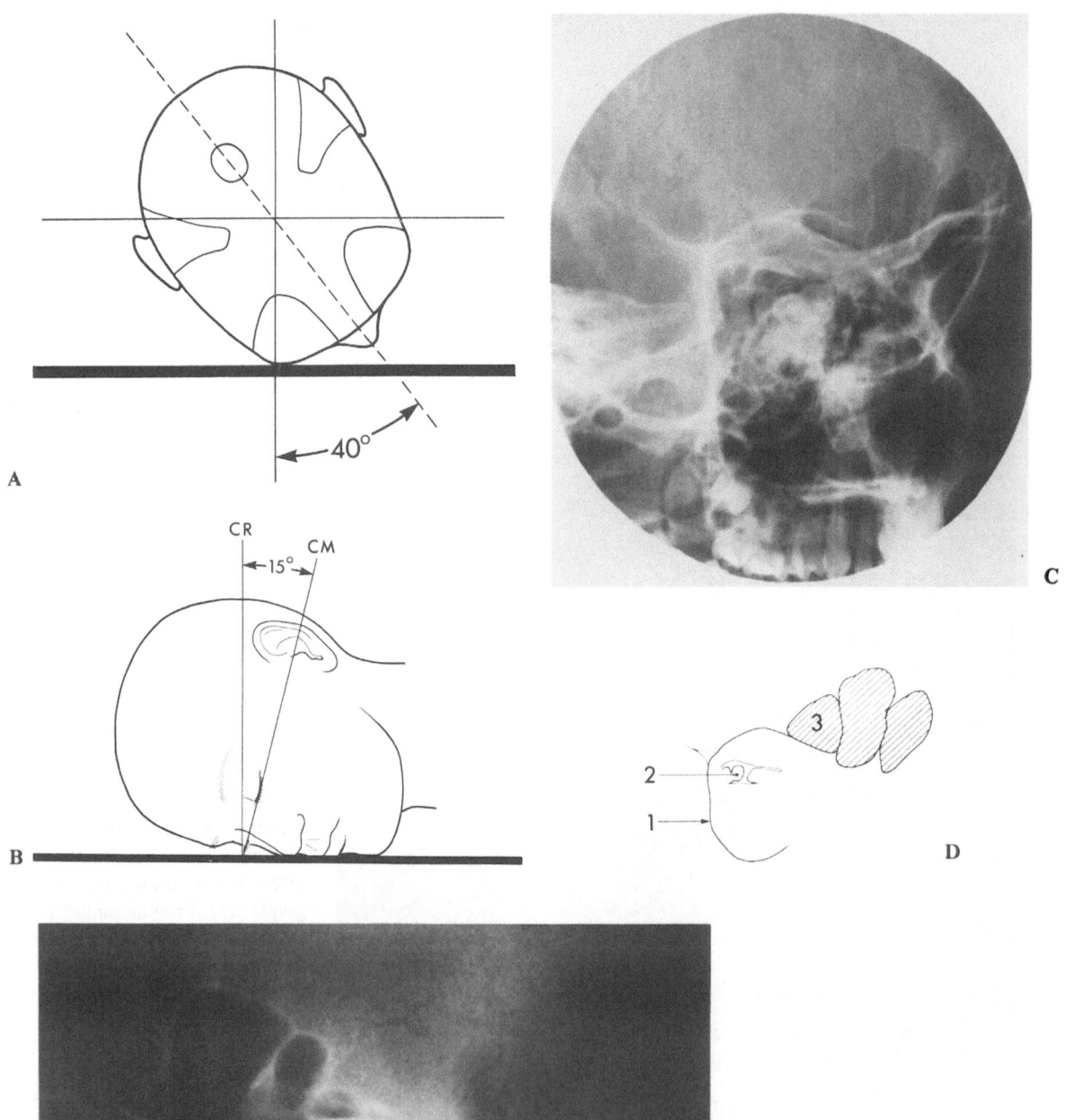

Figure 1.5 A, B. Optic canal view, positioning. Canthomeatal line (CM) C. Radiograph. D. Line drawing of radiograph. (1) Lateral orbital margin; (2) Optic canal; (3) Frontal sinus; E. Pneumatization of the anterior clinoid-simulating optic foramen.

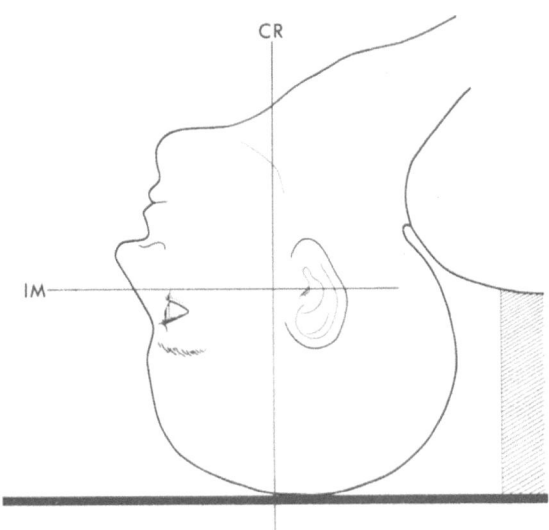

A

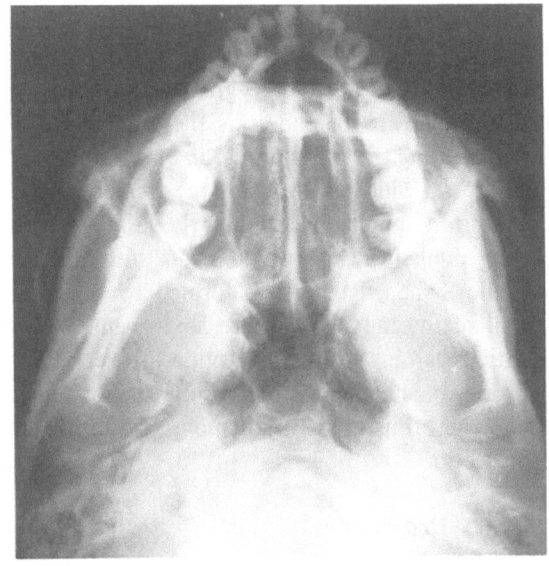

B

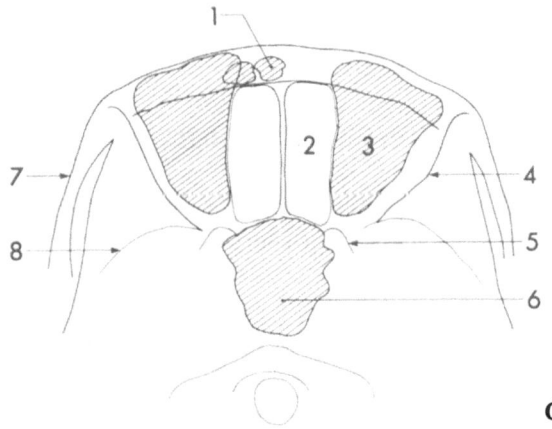

C

Figure 1.6 A. Submento-vertex (base) projection, positioning. Infraorbitomeatal line (IM). **B.** Radiograph. **C.** Line drawing of radiograph omitting the mandible. (1) Frontal sinus; (2) Ethmoid sinus; (3) Maxillary sinus; (4) Lateral orbital wall; (5) Pterygoid plate; (6) Sphenoid sinus; (7) Zygomatic arch; (8) Anterior wall of middle cranial fossa.

the contralateral side. The head is extended so that the canthomeatal line (CM) forms an angle of 15°–20° with the central ray (Fig. 1.5).

The orbital ends of the optic canals are well visualized and should be symmetric. Commonly found normal variants of the optic canal include the keyhole anomaly that occurs as a result of an absence of the floor at the cranial opening of the canal and the "figure eight" optic canal, which is due to a separate canal for the ophthalmic artery. Pneumatization of the optic strut or the anterior

clinoids also can create the appearance of two canals (see Fig. 1.5E).

Base or Axial Projection

The central ray is perpendicular to the film. The head is positioned such that the infraorbitomeatal line is parallel to the film and enters the skull in the midline midway between the mandibular angles (Fig. 1.6). For optimal visualization of the anterior fossa and optic canals, the extension of the head must be maximal.

The posterolateral wall of the orbit formed by the orbital surface of the greater sphenoid wing is well shown. Behind it is the curvilinear line representing the anterior margin of the middle cranial fossa, which is formed by the greater sphenoid wing in its outer third and by the lesser sphenoid wing along its medial two-thirds. A third landmark is the S-shaped bony line formed by the lateral wall of the maxillary sinus. Tomograms of both optic foramina in this projection are very useful. Processes affecting the base of the skull extending into the orbits are easily demonstrated using this projection.

Other Projections

The Towne's projection is occasionally used to visualize the inferior orbital fissure. The Buckethandle view of the zygoma is used in trauma involving this area.

Multidirectional Tomography

Plain film examination of the orbits is limited in its value because of the superimposition of the various facial and cranial structures. Complex motion tomography is especially valuable when seeking orbital or sinus fractures, expansile or erosive bony lesions secondary to benign or malignant tumors, and inflammatory conditions. The recent introduction of CT scanning has reduced the indications for plain tomographic examination. A tomographic study visualizes the bone structures in a section plane. For studying orbits, tomographic sections in straight anteroposterior and lateral projections are usually adequate. In specific evaluation of optic canals, tomography in oblique and axial projections are necessary.

Figures 1.7, 1.8, and 1.9 demonstrate the anteroposterior multidirectional tomograms at different levels proceeding from the anterior to posterior plane. Note that the orbits are rounded and closer together anteriorly. The orbital margins are well visualized. Figure 1.7 shows the crista galli and the region of the cribiform plate. In cases where the cribriform plate is the region of interest, 2-mm sections should be obtained through that area. Otherwise, routine 5-mm sections are usually adequate. Evaluation of the frontal, maxillary, ethmoid, and sphenoid sinuses cannot be overemphasized while looking for the etiology of orbital pathology. On the posterior section (Fig. 1.9), the superior orbital fissure and foramen rotundum are adequately visualized. Also, the shape of the orbit changes, and it is quadrangular posteriorly. The pterygoid plates and vomer are well visualized.

Lateral tomography (Figs. 1.10, 1.11, and 1.12) demonstrates the structures visualized in the lateral projection proceeding from the lateral to medial direction. The orbital roof, floor, and apex are well visualized. This projection is excellent for visualization of the pterygopalatine fossa.

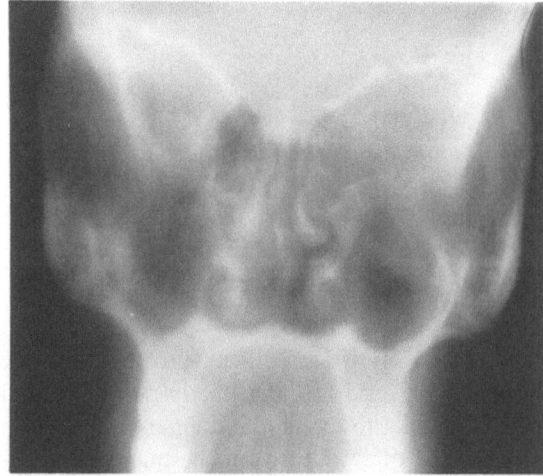
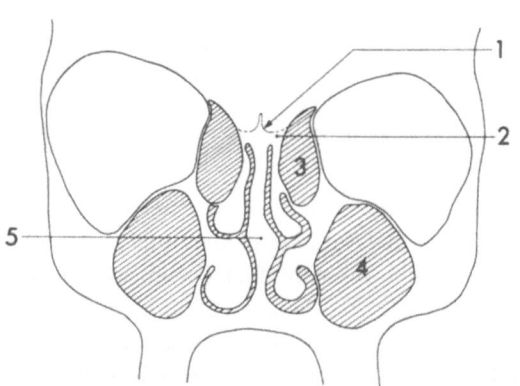

A   B

Figure 1.7 A. Tomogram in anteroposterior (*AP*) projection. **B.** Line drawing of radiograph. (1) Crista galli; (2) Cribiform plate; (3) Anterior ethmoid air cells; (4) Maxillary sinus; (5) Nasal septum.

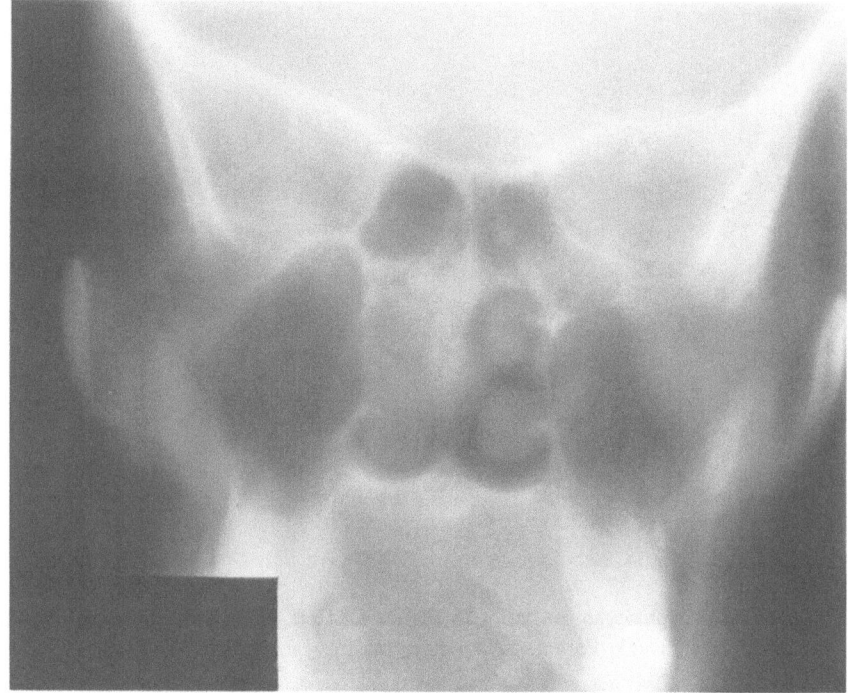

A

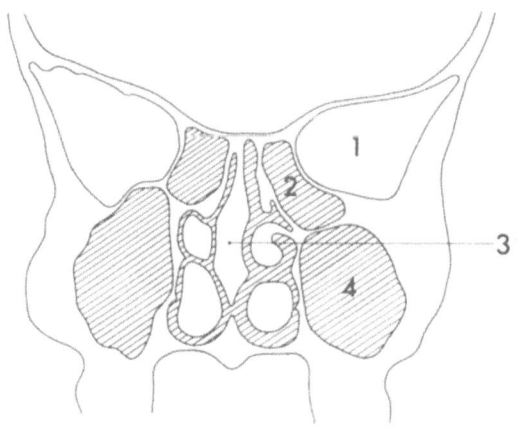

B

Figure 1.8 A. Tomogram in AP projection—section plane posterior to Figure 1.7A. **B.** Line drawing of radiograph. (1) Orbit; (2) Posterior ethmoid cells; (3) Nasal septum; (4) Maxillary sinus.

Tomography of the Optic Canals

Tomographic sections of the optic canals can be obtained along the long axis in the submento-vertex (base) position (Fig. 1.13) or along the transverse axis in the oblique projection (Figs. 1.14, 1.15, and 1.16). In the base position, both canals are visualized throughout their length. This projection may be difficult to obtain in older patients who have trouble extending their heads. The oblique projection is better tolerated, and both canals have to be imaged separately. The sections should be obtained at 1–2-mm intervals, as the shape of the canal changes in its course from the cranial to the orbital end. The optic canal is oval toward the cranial end, with its longest diameter being horizontal (Fig. 1.14). The optic canal is round in its midportion (Fig. 1.15), and the longest axis is vertical near the orbital end (Fig. 1.16). Comparison of the two sides is essential. The optic canal should be symmetric, with differences of even 2 mm raising concern.

Lists of the differential diagnostic possibilities corresponding to pathologic changes in the orbit follows in Tables 1.1 to 1.11.*

---

* The 11 tables have been duplicated with minor modifications from *Gamuts in Radiology* with Dr. Benjamin Felson's permission.

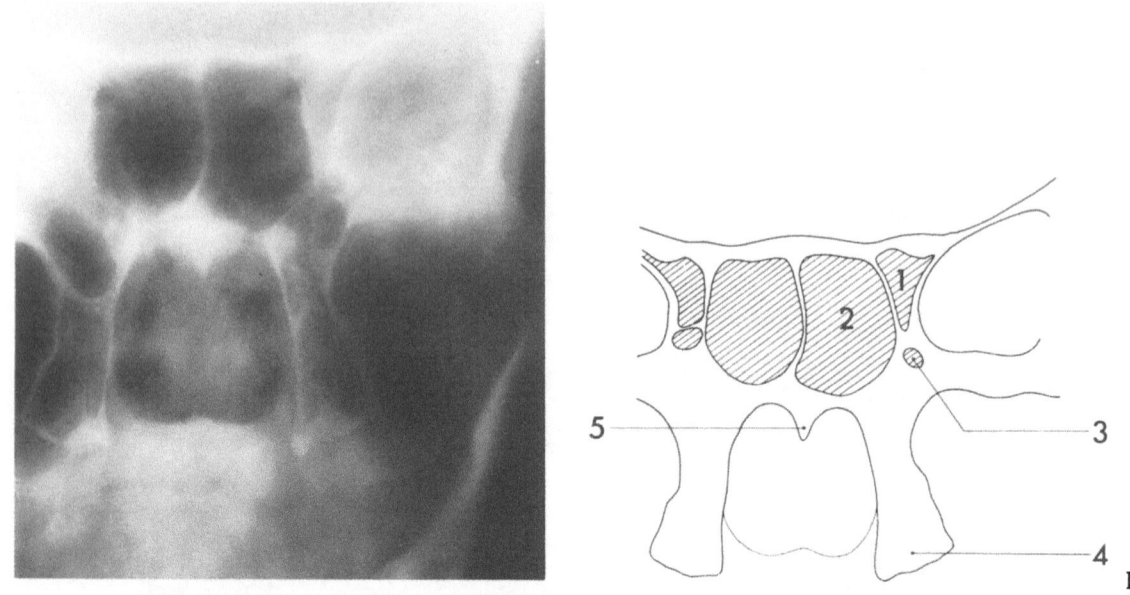

Figure 1.9 A. Anteroposterior tomogram posterior to Figure 1.8A. **B.** Line drawing of radiograph. (1) Superior orbital fissure; (2) Sphenoid sinus; (3) Foramen rotundum; (4) Pterygoid plate; (5) Vomer.

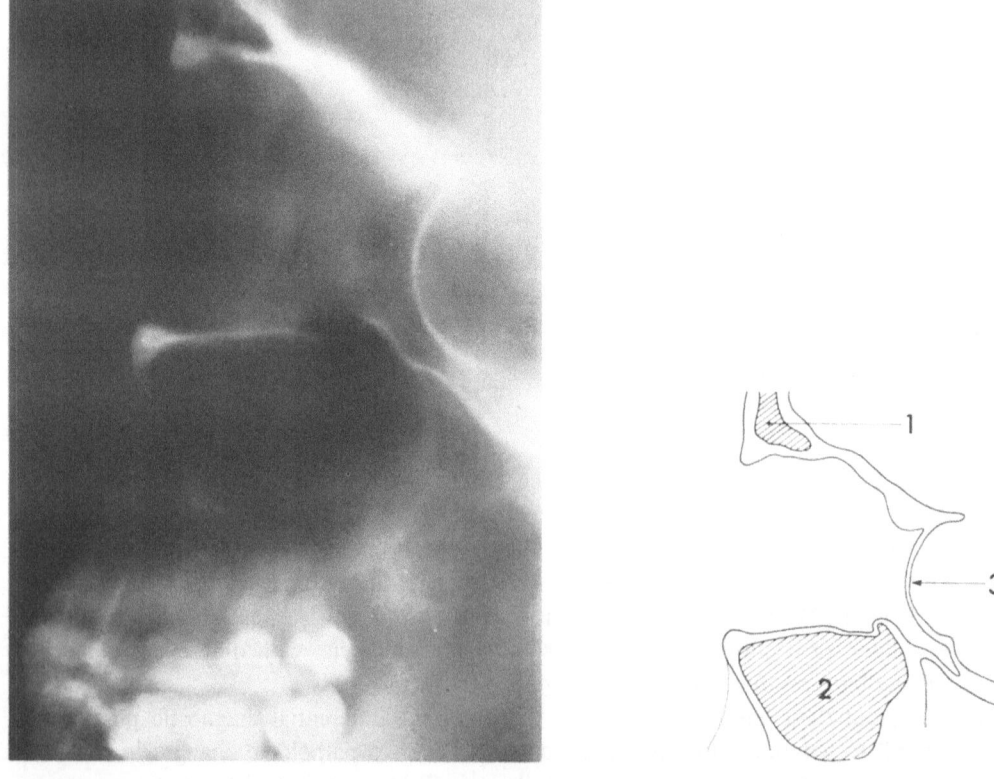

Figure 1.10 A. Lateral tomogram. **B.** Line drawing of radiograph. (1) Frontal sinus; (2) Maxillary sinus; (3) Greater sphenoid wing.

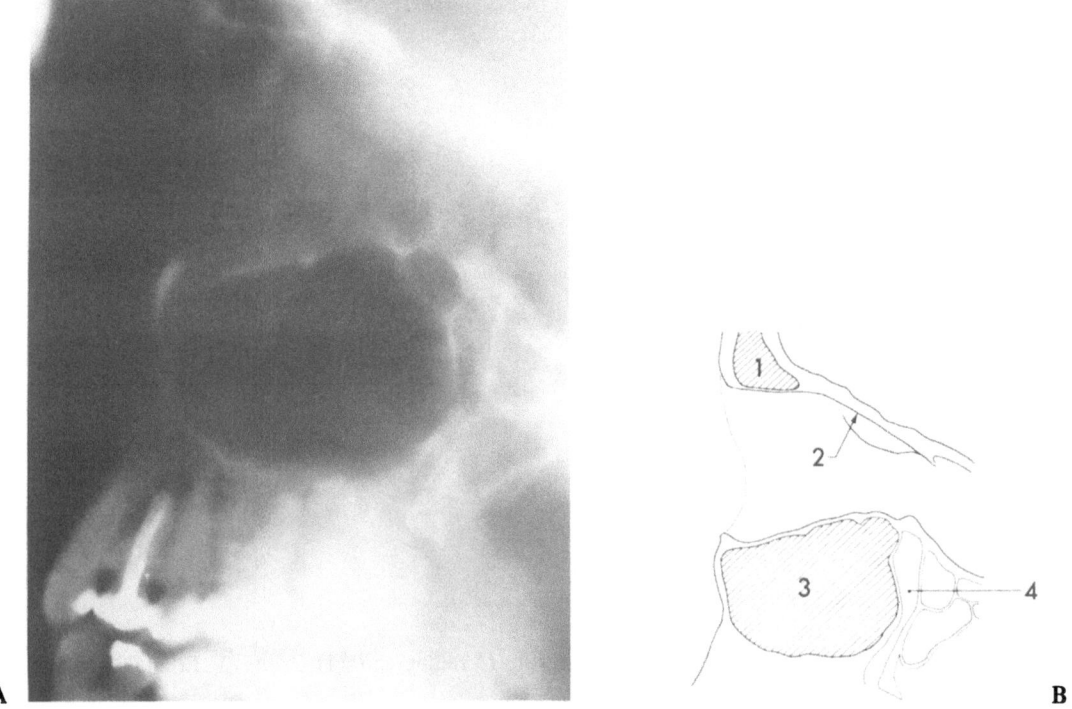

Figure 1.11 A. Lateral tomogram—section plane medial to Figure 1.10. **B.** Line drawing of radiograph. (1) Frontal sinus; (2) Orbital roof; (3) Maxillary sinus; (4) Pterygopalatine fossa.

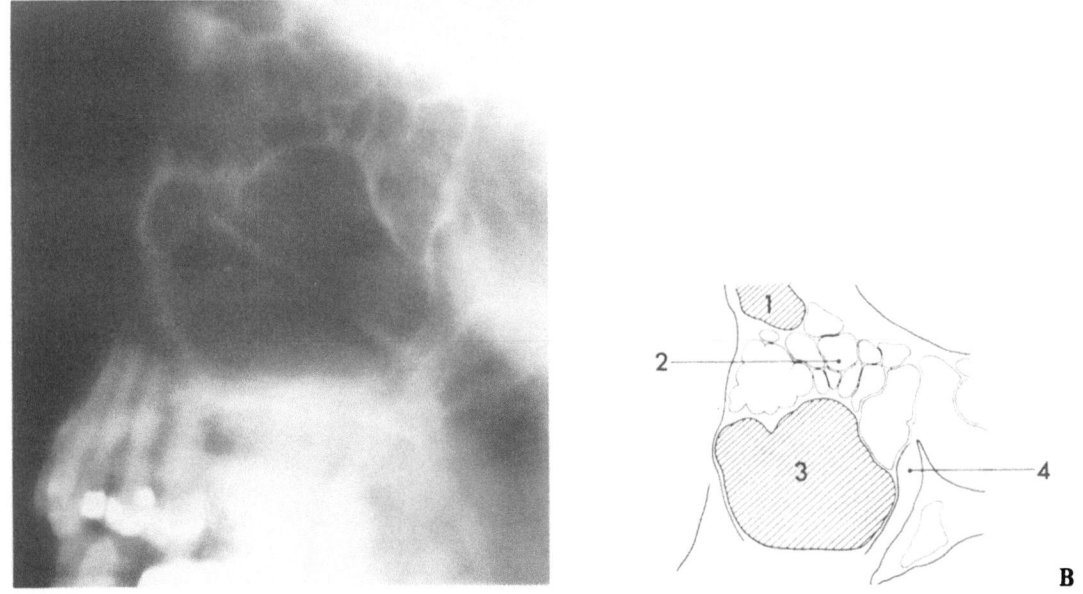

Figure 1.12 A. Lateral tomogram—section plane medial to Figure 1.11. **B.** Line drawing of radiograph. (1) Frontal sinus; (2) Ethmoid sinus; (3) Maxillary sinus; (4) Pterygopalatine fossa.

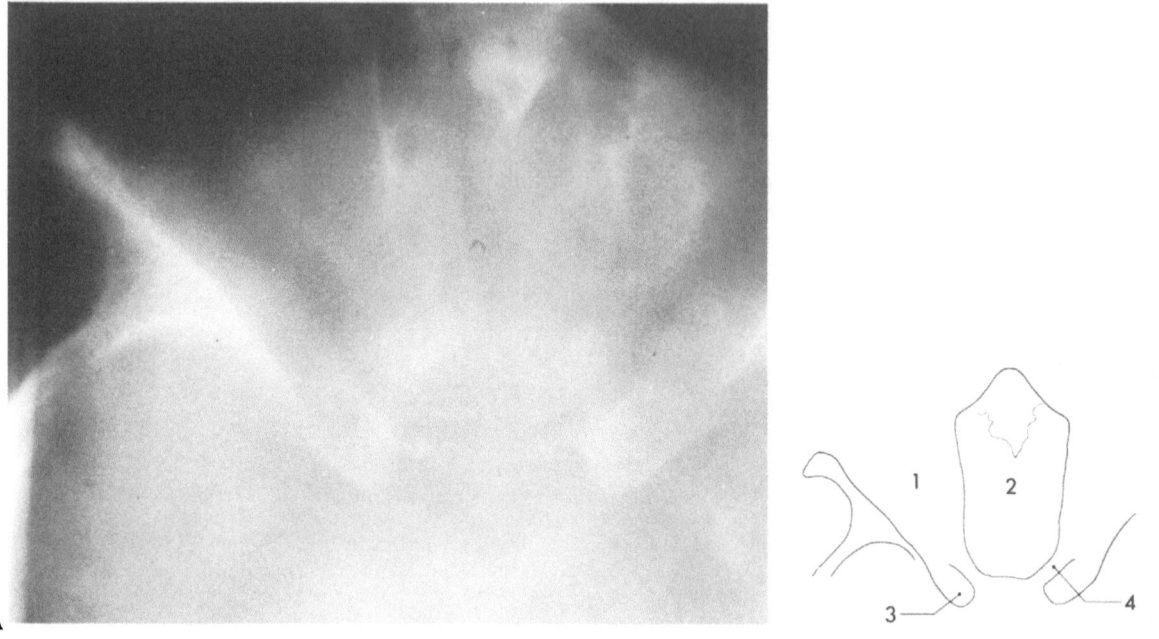

Figure 1.13 A. Tomogram in base projection. **B.** Line drawing of radiograph. (1) Orbit; (2) Ethmoid air cells; (3) Anterior clinoid; (4) Optic canal.

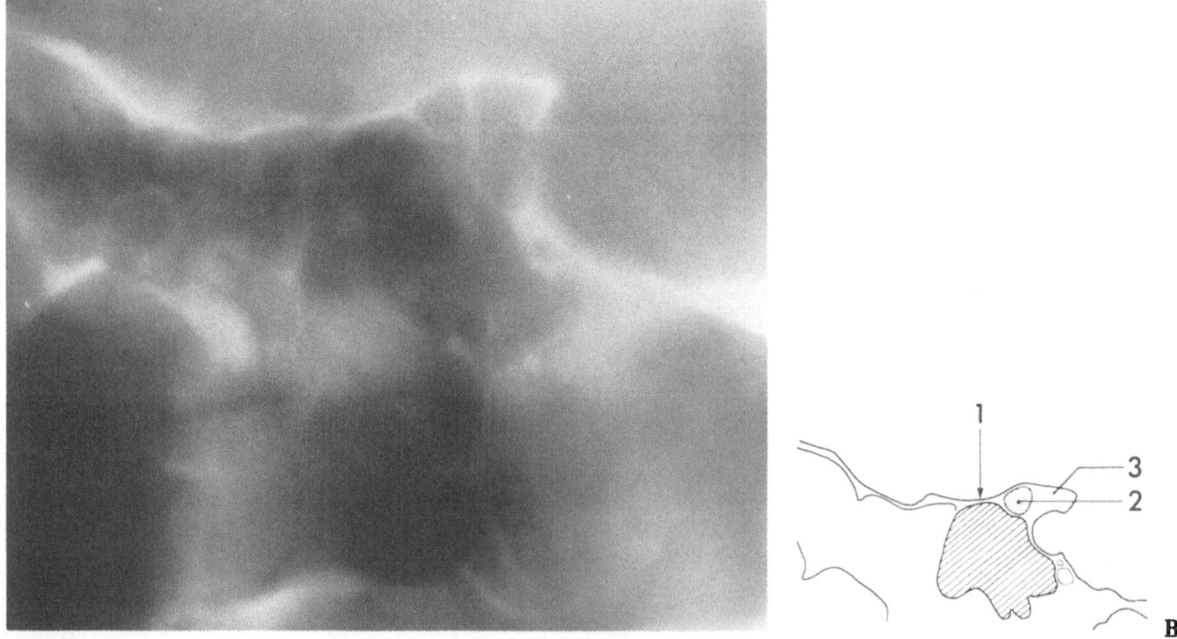

Figure 1.14 A. Tomograms in Rhese projection at cranial end. **B.** Line drawing of radiograph. (1) Planum sphenoidale; (2) Optic canal; (3) Anterior clinoid.

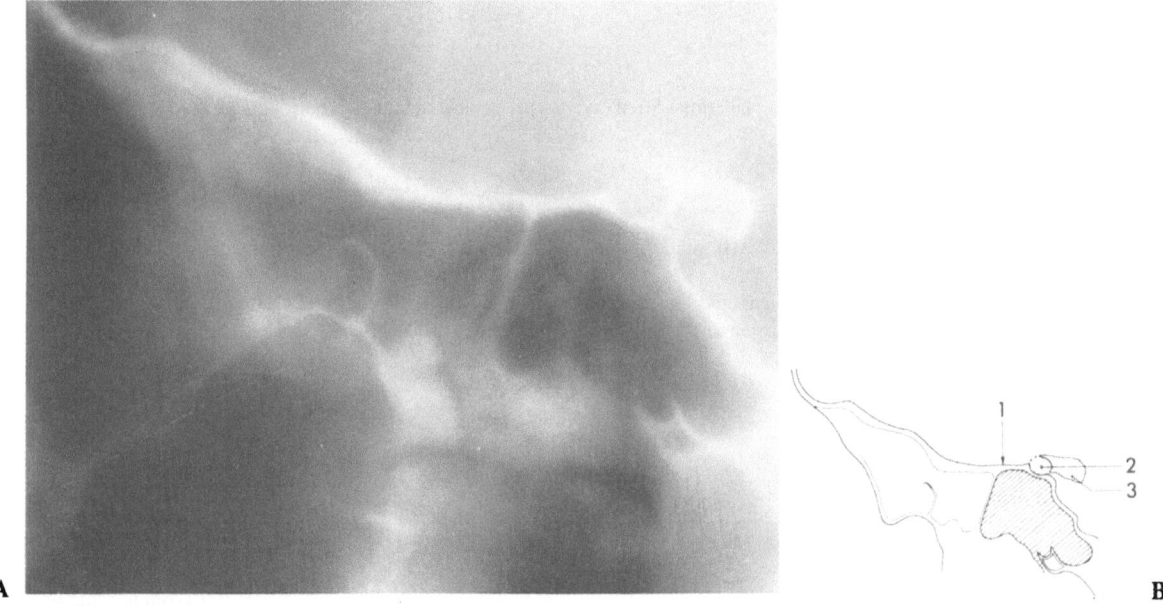

A   B

Figure 1.15 A. Tomograms in Rhese projection at midportion. **B.** Line drawing of radiograph. (1) Planum sphenoidale; (2) Optic canal; (3) Anterior clinoid.

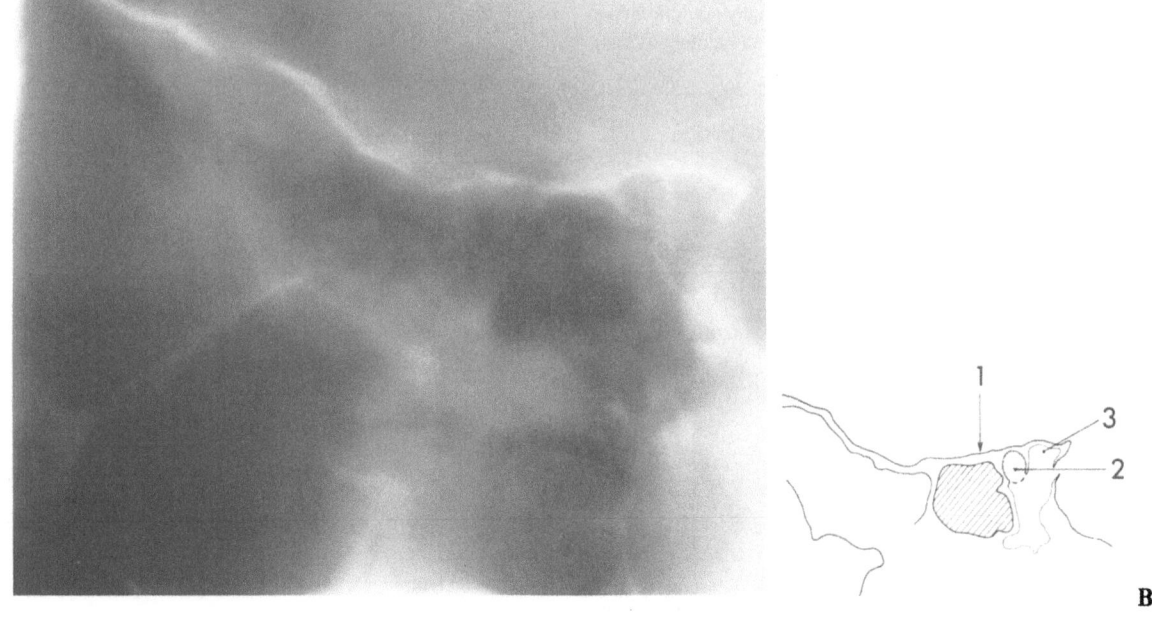

A   B

Figure 1.16 A. Tomograms in Rhese projection at orbital end. **B.** Line drawing of radiograph. (1) Planum sphenoidale; (2) Optic canal; (3) Anterior clinoid.

Table 1.1. Small orbit

Common

1. Enucleation in childhood
2. Radiation therapy

Uncommon

1. Anophthalmos, microphthalmos (e.g., Hallerman-Streiff syndrome, oculovertebral syndome—unilateral)
2. Cloverleaf skull
3. Craniostenosis of coronal suture
4. Crouzon's disease
5. Encroachment from adjacent mass (e.g., frontal sinus mucocele or neoplasm; antral neoplasm or cyst)
6. Increased bone density with encroachment on orbit (e.g., meningioma, fibrous dysplasia, Paget's disease, osteopetrosis, Pyle's disease, and thalassemia)
7. Marshall-Smith syndrome
8. Mucopolysaccharoidosis I-H
9. Neurofibromatosis
10. Osteitis (e.g., from sphenoid sinusitis)
11. Stanesco's dysplasia
12. Weill-Marchesani syndrome

Table 1.2. Large orbit

1. Congenital glaucoma (buphthalmos, hydrophthalmos)
2. Congenital serous cyst (often associated with anophthalmos or microphthalmos)
3. Exophthalmos (e.g., thyrotoxicosis)
4. Neurofibromatosis (orbital dysplasia)
5. Pseudotumor
6. Tumor within muscle cone (e.g., hemangioma, optic nerve glioma, neurofibroma, dermoid cyst, and retinoblastoma)
7. Varix of orbital vein

Table 1.3. Narrowed superior orbital (sphenoidal) fissure

Common

1. Fibrous dysplasia
2. Paget's disease
3. Normal variant; congenital asymmetry or narrowing

Uncommon

1. Bone tumor (e.g., osteoma, osteoblastic metastasis)
2. Meningioma with hyperostosis
3. Osteitis secondary to sinusitis
4. Osteopetrosis
5. Thalassemia, severe

Table 1.4. Enlarged superior orbital (sphenoidal) fissure (erosion and widening)

Common

1. Aneurysm of intracavernous portion of internal carotid artery
2. Normal asymmetry
3. Pituitary tumor (especially chromophobe adenoma)

Uncommon

1. Carotid-cavernous fistula
2. Chordoma
3. Chronic increased intracranial pressure
4. Craniopharyngioma
5. Extension from orbital or infraorbital mass (juvenile xanthogranuloma, lymphoma, Burkitt tumor, and neuroblastoma) or from paranasal sinus malignancy
6. Histiocytosis X
7. Meningioma
8. Metastatic carcinoma to sphenoid wing
9. Middle fossa mass (e.g., infratemporal chronic subdural hematoma or hygroma, arachnoid cyst with temporal lobe agenesis, and temporal lobe astrocytoma)
10. Mucocele of sphenoid sinus
11. Neurofibroma
12. Neurofibromatosis (orbital dysplasia)
13. Orbital varix
14. Posterior orbital encephalocele
15. Pseudotumor of orbit

Table 1.5. Intraorbital calcification

Common

1. Cataract
2. Foreign body
3. Phlebolith (e.g., orbital varices, hemangioma)
4. Phthisis bulbi (old trauma or infection of choroid or vitreous with shrunken globe)
5. Retinoblastoma

Uncommon

1. Aneurysm or atherosclerosis of internal carotid or ophthalmic artery; vascular calcification in sarcoidosis, syphilis, and diabetes
2. Collagen disease (e.g., band keratopathy of cornea in rheumatoid arthritis)
3. Hematoma; myositis ossificans of extraocular muscles
4. Hypercalcemia (metastatic calcification in conjunctiva and cornea; e.g., hypervitaminosis D, primary and secondary hyperparathyroidism, metastases, multiple myeloma, and milk-alkali syndrome)
5. Idiopathic
6. Intraocular infection (e.g., abscess, bacterial ophthalmitis tuberculosis, and syphilis)
7. Intraorbital neoplasm (e.g., meningioma, dermoid cyst, optic glioma, plexiform neurofibroma, lacrimal gland carcinoma, hemangioendothelioma, and metastasis)
8. Mucocele invading orbit
9. [Osteoma]
10. Parasitic disease (e.g., hydatid cyst, cysticercosis)
11. Retinal disease (e.g., detachment, retinitis, fibrosis, and retrolental fibroplasia)

Table 1.6. Unilateral exophthalmos (proptosis)

Bone Disease

Common

1. Fracture with retroorbital hematoma or orbital emphysema
2. Metastasis

Uncommon

1. Craniostenosis, severe
2. Histiocytosis X
3. Myeloma
4. Neurofibromatosis
5. Ossifying fibroma; fibrous dysplasia
6. Osteoma of a paranasal sinus
7. Osteomyelitis
8. Paget's disease
9. Primary benign or malignant bone neoplasm (e.g., osteosarcoma)

Paranasal Sinus or Nasopharyngeal Disease with Intraorbital Extension

Common

1. Carcinoma, lymphoepithelioma, or other neoplasm
2. Mucocele

Uncommon

1. Sinusitis

Primary Orbital Soft Tissue Disease (Including Extension from an Intracranial Lesion)

Common

1. Abscess or cellulitis (retrobulbar or periorbital)
2. Granuloma
3. Hemangioma
4. Lacrimal gland tumor
5. Meningioma (especially sphenoid ridge)

(continued on next page)

Table 1.6. *Continued*

Uncommon

1. Benign or malignant mesenchymal tumor (e.g., angioma, lipoma, myoma, fibroma [and their sarcomatous counterparts], and rhabdomyosarcoma)
2. Carotid artery aneurysm, carotid-cavernous fistula, cavernous sinus thrombosis, and arteriovenous malformation (congenital or traumatic)
3. Dermoid; teratoma
4. Epidermoid (cholesteatoma)
5. Foreign body
6. Hydatid cyst
7. Lymphoma
8. Neurofibroma
9. Optic glioma
10. Orbital meningocele or encephalocele (congenital or traumatic)
11. Orbital varices
12. Pseudotumor of orbit
13. Retinoblastoma, sympathicoblastoma, and neuroblastoma

Systemic Disease

1. Hyperthyroidism, thyrotoxicosis

Table 1.7. Syndrome with shallow orbital ridges

1. Acrocephalosyndactyly (Apert syndrome)
2. Aminopterin-induced syndrome
3. Cerebrohepatorenal syndrome (Zellweger syndrome)
4. Craniofacial dysostosis (Crouzon's disease)
5. Carpenter syndrome
6. Marshall-Smith syndrome
7. Osteogenesis imperfecta syndrome
8. Roberts syndrome
9. Stanesco dysplasia
10. Trisomy 13 syndrome
11. Trisomy 18 syndrome

Table 1.8. Sclerosis and thickening of the orbital roof or walls

Common

1. Fibrous dysplasia, leontiasis ossea
2. Healed fracture
3. Meningioma
4. Osteitis secondary to chronic sinusitis: mucocele or pyocele
5. Paget's disease

Uncommon

1. Dermoid
2. Histiocytosis X
3. Infantile cortical hyperostosis (Caffey's disease)
4. Lacrimal gland carcinoma
5. Lymphoma
6. Osteoblastic metastasis (e.g., breast, prostate)
7. Osteoma
8. Osteopetrosis
9. Osteosarcoma
10. Radiation therapy

Table 1.9. Optic canal enlargement (over 6.5 mm in diameter)

Common

1. Glioma of optic nerve
2. Neurofibromatosis with or without optic neurofibroma

Uncommon

1. Aneurysm of ophthalmic artery
2. Arteriovenous malformation
3. Hurler syndrome
4. Increased intracranial pressure
5. Inflammatory disease (e.g., tuberculous or sarcoid granuloma; chiasmatic arachnoiditis)
6. Meningioma of optic nerve sheath
7. Pituitary adenoma
8. Retinoblastoma with intracranial extension

Table 1.10. Localized bony defect or erosion about the optic canal

Common

1. Aneurysm of internal carotid artery
2. Malignant tumor arising in orbit, sphenoid sinus, or nasal cavity
3. Pituitary tumor
4. Tumor of orbital apex

Uncommon

1. Craniopharyngioma
2. Eosinophilic granuloma
3. Granuloma or other infection of sphenoid sinus
4. Metastasis
5. Mucocele or sphenoid sinus
6. Surgical defect
7. Tumor of anterior fossa (e.g., meningioma, astrocytoma, and glioma)

Table 1.11. Bony defect or radiolucent lesion of the orbit

Common

1. Extrinsic tumor invading orbit (e.g., meningioma, carcinoma or lymphoma of nasopharynx, nasal cavity, or paranasal sinus; carcinoma of skin or eyelid)
2. Metastasis (e.g., breast, lung, neuroblastoma, and Ewing's sarcoma)
3. Mucocele
4. Osteomyelitis secondary to sinusitis

Uncommon

1. Encephalocele; meningocele
2. Histiocytosis X
3. Juvenile xanthogranuloma
4. Lymphoma; Burkitt tumor
5. Myeloma
6. Neurofibromatosis (orbital dysplasia)
7. Primary bone tumor
8. Primary orbital tumor (e.g., hemangioma, hemangioblastoma, lacrimal gland tumor, dermoid, epidermoid, neurofibroma, melanoma, retinoblastoma, and rhabdomyosarcoma)

Bibliography

Arger PH: *Orbit Roentgenology.* New York, John Wiley & Sons, 1977.

Hanafee W: *Radiology of the Orbit,* in *Radiol Clin North Am.* Philadelphia, WB Saunders, 1972.

Korach A, Vignaud J: *Manual of Radiographic Techniques of the Skull.* New York, Masson Publishing, USA, Inc, 1981.

Lloyd GAS: *Radiology of the Orbit.* London, WB Saunders, Ltd, 1975.

Newton H, Potts G: *Radiology of the Skull and Brain. The Skull.* St Louis, CV Mosby, 1974.

Reeder MM, Felson B: *Gamuts in Radiology.* Cincinnati, Audiovisual Radiology of Cincinnati, Inc, 1975.

Taveras JM, Morello F: *Normal Neuroradiology.* Chicago, Year Book Medical Publications, Inc, 1979.

2
Computed Tomography of the Orbit

Robert G. Peyster

Computed tomography (CT) has attained a preeminent position for the evaluation of many orbital problems.

Technique for Orbital CT

A CT examination of the orbits most often consists of axial and coronal sectioning with 5-mm slices (Figs. 2.1, 2.2, and 2.3). This technique reliably detects the vast majority of intraorbital lesions. Occasionally, when finer detail is required, additional 1.5-mm slices are obtained.

Coronal sections are indispensable for lesions located at the inferior and superior areas of the orbit. Such lesions could be overlooked if the study were limited to the axial plane (Fig. 2.4). The optic nerves often are best evaluated in the coronal view, as are the superior and inferior recti and paranasal sinuses. The bony orbital floor and roof require coronal sections for evaluation. The coronal examination often is extended posteriorly to include the optic chiasm for patients suffering from visual loss and to evaluate for intracranial extension of orbital lesions. This procedure is essential for patients in whom orbital lesions represent a spread from an intracranial lesion, such as a meningioma of the sphenoid ridge.

Many CT scanners are now capable of performing computer reformation of data from axial scanning into coronal, sagittal, or oblique planes (Fig. 2.5). The facility of this process varies between scanners, but it is often time-consuming and produces images of lesser quality than those obtained from direct scanning. However, reconstruction is valuable in those cases where direct coronal scanning cannot be performed, as with young children,

patients with limited mobility of the neck, or those with excessive dental fillings. Occasionally, the sagittal- or oblique-reconstructed image may prove to be useful, as when it is desirable to follow the entire course of the optic nerve in a single section (Fig. 2.5C).

The need for intravenous (IV) contrast media administration for orbital CT is controversial. The intraorbital fat, due to its inherent low density, provides a natural contrast to all soft-tissue structures within the orbits, normal or abnormal. Muscles, vessels, and nerves clearly stand out against this background. Contrast material uniformly increases the density of all of the intraorbital soft-tissue structures, but it does not significantly enhance their visibility. Attempts to discriminate between lesions based on their density alteration after contrast media administration have been disappointing (4–6). However, contrast material is often necessary to evaluate intracranial extension of orbital lesions. For this reason, we usually employ IV contrast media except for cases where the process is known to be limited to the orbits, for trauma cases where hematoma is suspected, or when contraindicated because of an allergic history, renal failure, or other medical condition.

Normal CT Orbital Anatomy

Each orbit approximates the shape of a four-sided pyramid whose long central axis extends medially and superiorly from its anterior base to its posterior apex. Therefore, intraorbital structures such as the optic nerve, which are roughly aligned along the central orbital axis, lie in a plane at an angle

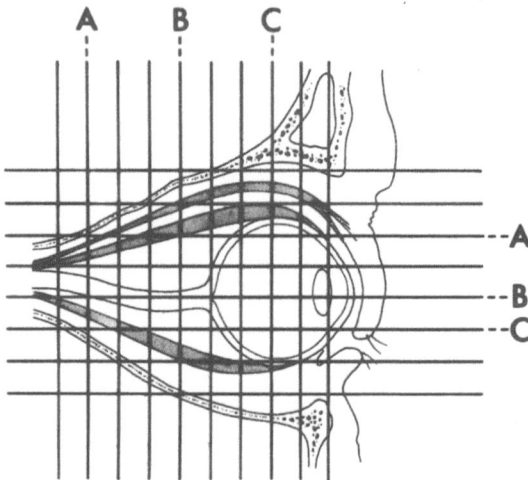

Figure 2.1. Line drawing of orbit showing reference planes for axial and coronal views.

from the plane through the orbitomeatal line. When the scan plane is parallel to the orbitomeatal line, fragmentation of these structures occurs, with different portions visualized on separate axial sections (Fig. 2.6). The orbits are bounded by the nasal cavity and ethmoid sinuses medially, the maxillary sinuses inferiorly, the frontal sinuses and anterior fossae superiorly, the middle fossae posteriorly and laterally, and the extracranial temporal fossae laterally.

The orbits may be divided into intraconal and extraconal portions (Fig. 2.7). The muscle cone is defined by the superior, medial, inferior, and lateral rectus muscles and the aponeurotic intermuscular membrane that connects them. This division of the orbits may be useful in the differential diagnosis of orbital lesions, as will be discussed below.

The globe is a roughly spherical-shaped structure that is situated in the anterior portion of the orbit (Fig. 2.8). Normally, approximately 40–50% of the globes lie behind the interzygomatic line, which is drawn by connecting the anterior margins of the zygomatic processes on a section including the lenses (Fig. 2.9). The percentage of the globes that lie behind this line may vary somewhat with the plane of section. A perpendicular drawn from the anterior margin of the globe to this line normally measures less than 21 mm, except when

proptosis is present. The outer margin of the globe is formed by its scleral investment, which is perforated by insertion of the optic nerve. The uvea, inside the sclera, and the retina form the innermost layer posteriorly. Together, they form a high-density boundary to the globe, which normally enhances with contrast material. The anterior margin of the globe is defined by the cornea centrally. The lens appears as a relatively dense structure in the anterior portion of the globe. The lens divides the globe into an anterior portion (filled with aqueous humor) and a posterior portion (filled with vitreous humor). The optic disc is located at the point of insertion of the optic nerve on the globe. The eyelids and conjunctiva may be seen anterior to the globe, where they will cause a thickening of the anterior globe margin. The orbital septum, which is a continuation of the periosteum, inserts on the tarsal plates of the eyelids and often can be seen on either side of the globe.

The optic nerve lies roughly along the central axis of the orbit. From its insertion on the posterior aspect of the globe, it passes posteriorly, superiorly, and medially to exit the orbit at the optic canal (Fig. 2.10). The optic nerve is contained within the optic nerve sheath, which is formed by all meningeal layers that are continuous with those of the intracranial cavity. On CT scan, therefore, it is the composite of the optic nerve and its meningeal investments that are seen and that may be referred to as the optic nerve/sheath. Enlargement of these structures may be due to processes enlarging the sheath without altering the actual size of the optic nerve itself. The subarachnoid space within the optic nerve sheath has been imaged during the course of metrizamide cisternography (3, 7). Enlargement of the subarachnoid space within the optic nerve sheath has been noted in patients with papilledema (1, 3, 7). The course of the optic nerve in the axial plane usually appears to be quite straight; occasionally, however, the nerve may ascribe a gentle curve. Changes in the position of the globe due to alterations in the direction of the gaze may affect the course of the nerve. On the coronal scan, the optic nerve/sheath may appear to be ellipsoidal, since the course of the nerve is also situated obliquely relative to the true coronal plane. The optic nerve/sheath measures between 3–5 mm in the axial plane and 4–6 mm in the coronal plane. On thin axial sections, the optic nerve often appears frag-

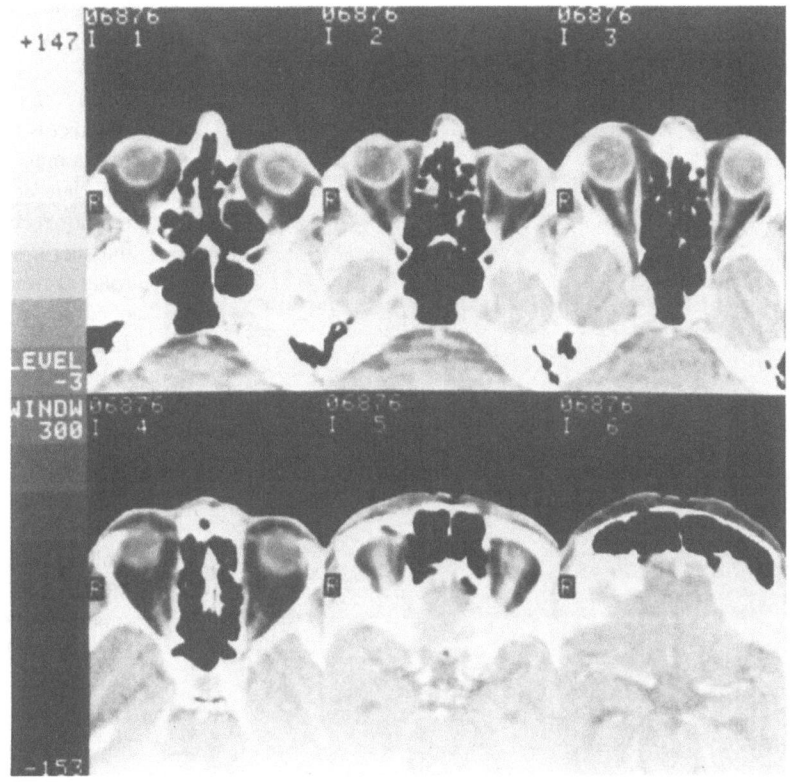

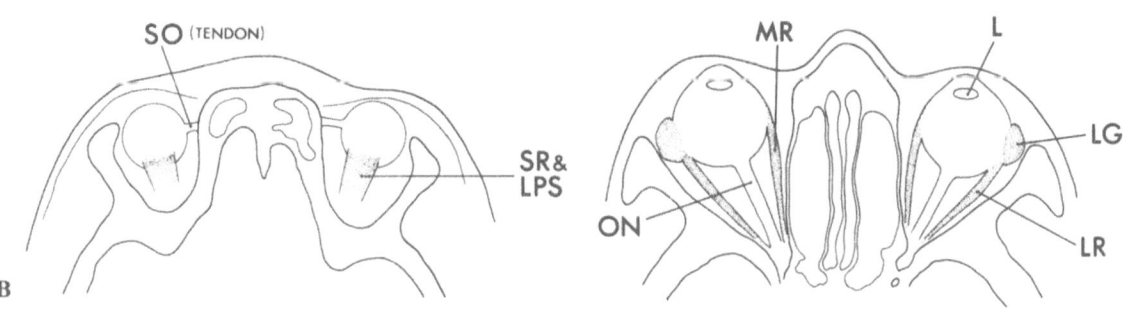

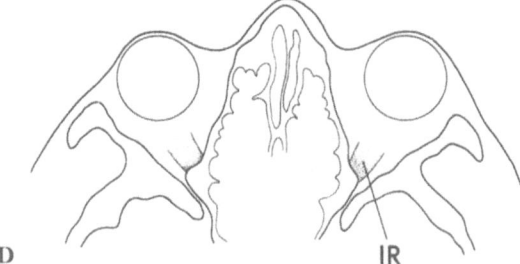

Figure 2.2 A. Normal axial CT scan of the orbit (5-mm slices). **B.** (I-5) Axial section taken at the level of axial plane A in Figure 2.1. *SO,* superior oblique (tendon); *SR,* superior rectus muscle; and *LPS,* levator palpebrae superioris. **C.** (I-3) Axial section taken at the level of axial plane B in Figure 2.1. *ON,* optic nerve; *MR,* medial rectus muscle; *L,* lens; *LG,* lacrimal gland; and *LR,* lateral rectus muscle. **D.** (I-1) Axial section taken at the level of axial plane C in Figure 2.1. *IR,* inferior rectus muscle.

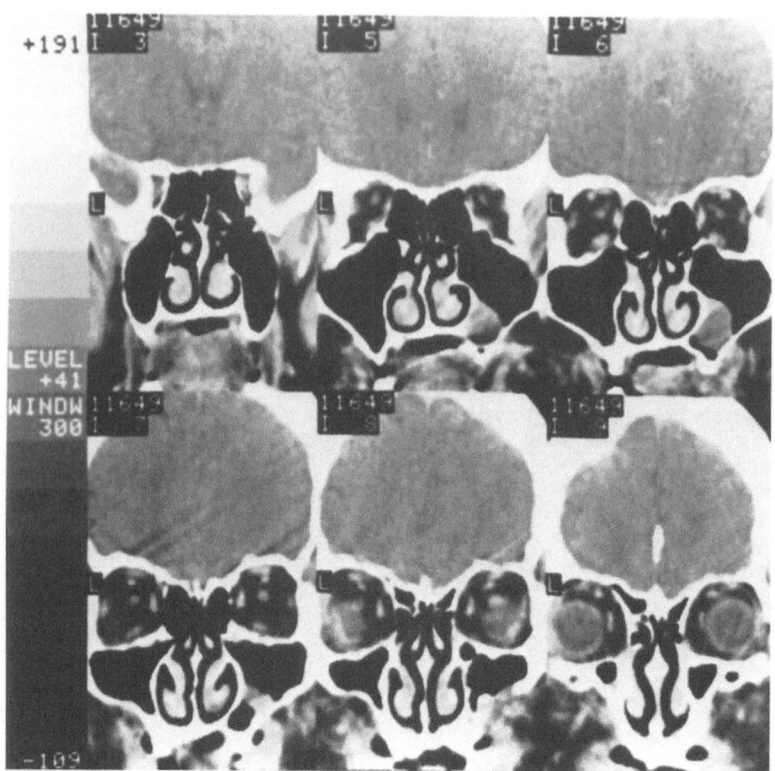

A

Figure 2.3 A. Normal coronal CT scan of the orbit (5-mm slices). **B.** (I-6) Coronal section taken at the level of coronal plane A in Figure 2.1. *SR*, superior rectus muscle; *MR*, medial rectus muscle; *ON*, optic nerve; *LR*, lateral rectus muscle; *IR*, inferior rectus muscle; and *MS*, maxillary sinus. **C.** (I-7) Coronal section taken at the level of coronal plane B in Figure 2.1. *LR*, lateral rectus muscle; *ON*, optic nerve; *SR*, superior rectus muscle; *MR*, medial rectus muscle; and *IR*, inferior rectus muscle. **D.** (I-9) Coronal section taken at the level of coronal plane C in Figure 2.1. *LG*, lacrimal gland; *SR*, superior rectus muscle; *LPS*, levator palpebrae superioris; *SO*, superior oblique muscle; *MR*, medial rectus muscle; *LR*, lateral rectus muscle; *IR*, inferior rectus muscle; and *IO*, inferior oblique muscle.

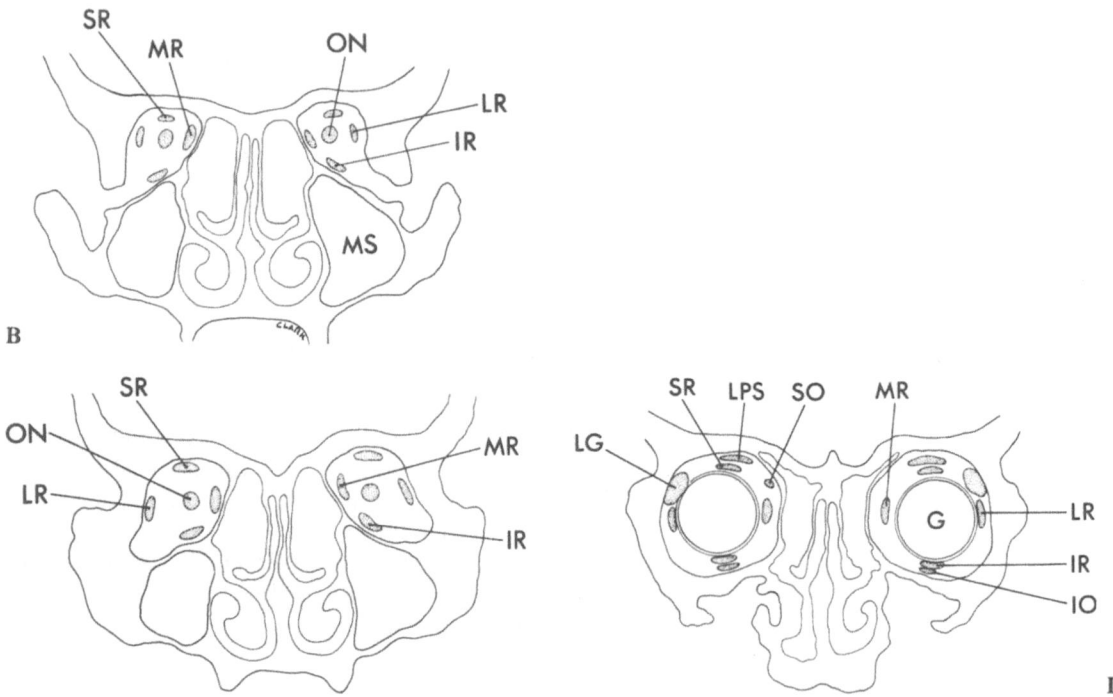

B

C

D

Figure 2.4. Hematoma of the right superior orbit. **A.** The right globe appears to be displaced forward. The superior margin of the right globe (lower left-hand slice) is obscured by tissue of higher density (arrow) than that seen in the opposite orbit.

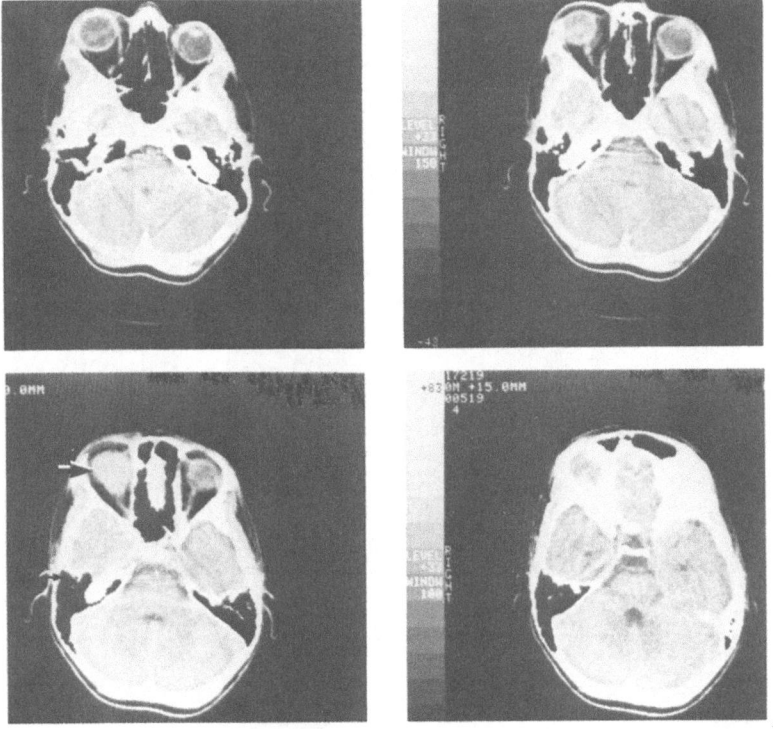

A

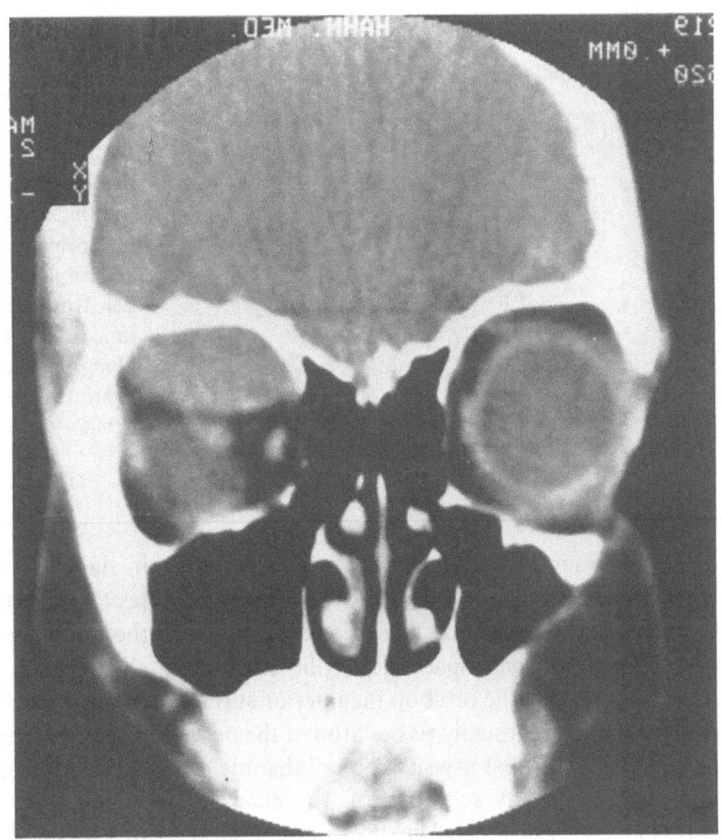

Figure 2.4 B. Coronal scan clearly delineates the hematoma in the superior aspect of the right orbit, and it is far superior to the axial examination in this case.

B

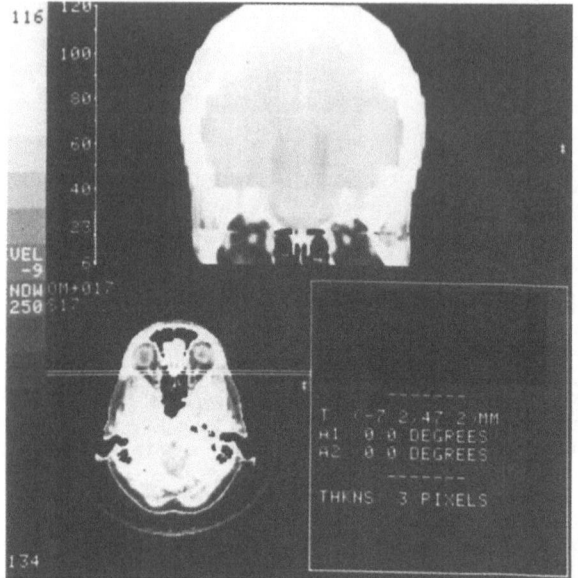

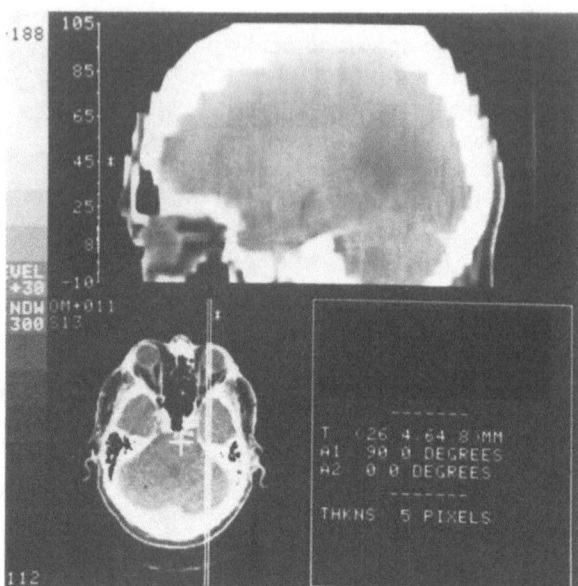

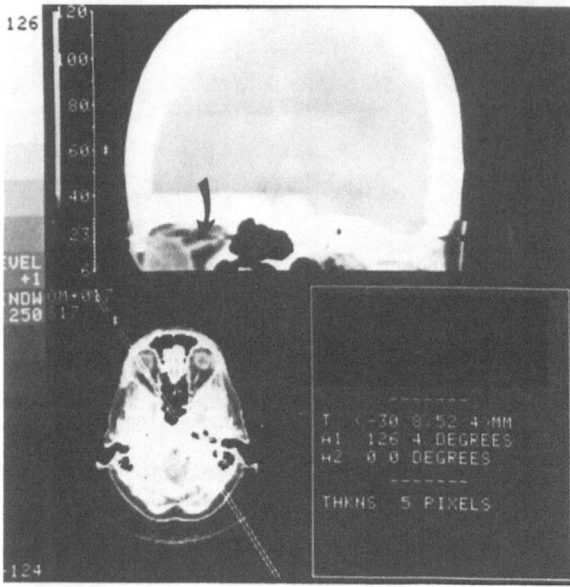

Figure 2.5. Computer-reconstructed views of the orbits from an axial orbital exam with 1.5-mm slices. **A.** Coronal reconstruction. The reconstructed view is seen in the superior half of the figure. The axial view appearing in the lower left-hand portion of the picture is employed to select the location of the reconstructed image. In this case, the two lines passing through the orbits demonstrate both the location of the coronal slice and the thickness of the slice. The delineation of soft-tissue intraorbital structures is quite good when 1.5-mm slices are employed for the axial examination. **B.** Sagittal-reconstructed image. **C.** Oblique paraaxial-reconstructed image. Note that the plane of reconstruction was chosen along the axis of the optic nerve (arrow), which is demonstrated essentially in its entire course through the orbit.

mented into several sections that are seen on different axial slices (Fig. 2.6).

Several small structures are frequently visualized in the intraconal space. The ophthalmic artery, which enters the orbit on the inferior surface of the optic nerve, usually passes around the nerve to its superior-medial aspect. The ophthalmic arteries are frequently seen both in the axial and coronal views (Fig. 2.11). The superior ophthalmic vein has a complex intraorbital course, originating in the extraconal space in the anterior-medial aspect of the orbit (Fig. 2.12). From here, it enters the intraconal space and travels medially to laterally beneath the superior rectus muscle to exit again from the intraconal space near the superior orbital fissure. It passes through this fissure to join the cavernous sinus. Therefore, on axial CT scan, it has a sigma-shaped course and may be seen just below the superior rectus muscle.

The extraocular muscles are well visualized on

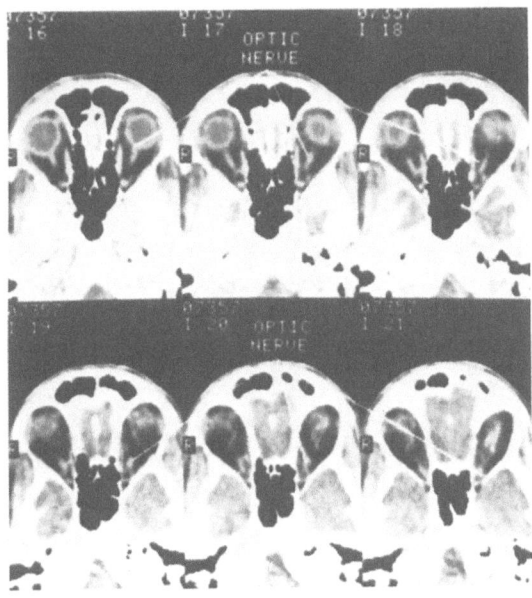

Figure 2.6. Axial orbital examination with 1.5-mm sections demonstrates fragmentation of the optic nerve with different portions visualized on each section.

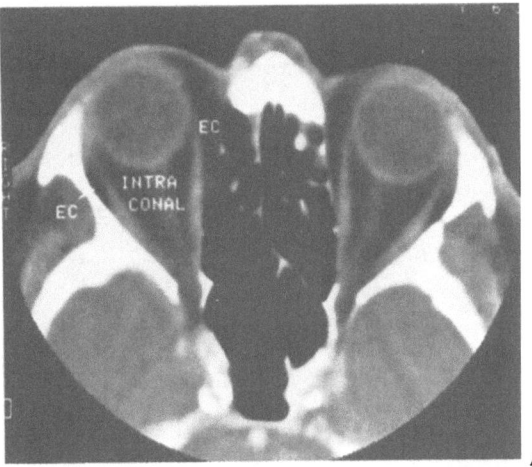

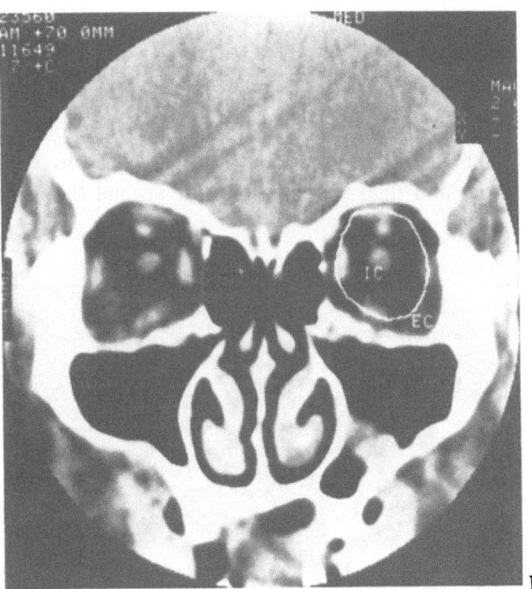

Figure 2.7. Demonstration of intraconal (*IC*) and extraconal (*EC*) spaces. **A.** Axial view. **B.** Coronal view. The circle through the rectus muscles approximates the position of the intermuscular membrane, which forms the boundary between the intraconal and extraconal spaces. The membrane itself is often seen on coronal slices.

orbital CT examination. They normally are enhanced uniformly with contrast material administration. There are six muscles that are normally seen on CT scan (Fig. 2.13). The four rectus muscles (superior, medial, inferior, and lateral) arise in the orbital apex from the fibrous annulus of Zinn, from which they extend forward to their separate insertions on their respective portions of the globe. As mentioned previously, these four muscles are joined by the intermuscular membrane. Posteriorly, the muscles lie along the bony orbital walls except for the superior rectus muscle, which is separated from the orbital roof by the levator palpebrae muscle. The levator palpebrae muscle inserts on the upper lid. The latter two muscles are so closely approximated that they often cannot be visually separated on CT scan and may be referred to collectively as the superior muscle group. The superior oblique muscle arises in the orbital apex and travels in the superior-medial corner of the orbit to the cartilaginous trochlea. It passes through the trochlea and extends posteriorly and laterally to insert itself on the superior lateral surface of the globe. The inferior oblique muscle, which is occasionally recognized on CT scan, arises from the floor of the anterior orbit beneath the globe and extends posteriorly and laterally beneath the inferior rectus muscle to insert itself on the inferior lateral surface of the globe. On coronal sections taken posterior to the globes, the inferior rectus will be seen along the floor of the orbit. However, on sections where the globe is present, the inferior oblique and inferior rectus muscles are difficult to separate visually. The me-

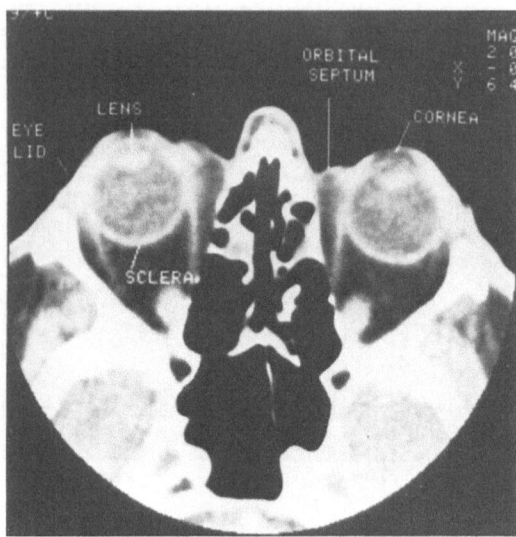

Figure 2.8. The globe. The various structures of the globe are indicated. The medial portion of the left orbital septum is identified as it passes between the globe and nasal bone. The structures of the eyelid cause increased density and thickening of the tissue around the globe, as noted.

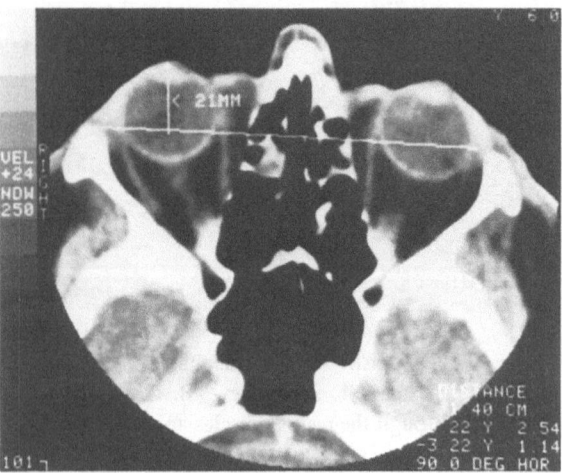

Figure 2.9. Computed tomographic guidelines for exophthalmos. Axial section at the level of the lenses. The horizontal line drawn between the zygomatic processes (the interzygomatic line) is illustrated. Normally, 40–50% of the globe should fall behind this line, but the percentage will vary with the slice angle, as in this example. On the right, a line from the anterior margin of the globe perpendicular to the interzygomatic line has been drawn. This distance should measure less than 21 mm. When this measurement exceeds 21 mm or when the globes lie entirely or nearly entirely in front of the interzygomatic line, proptosis is present.

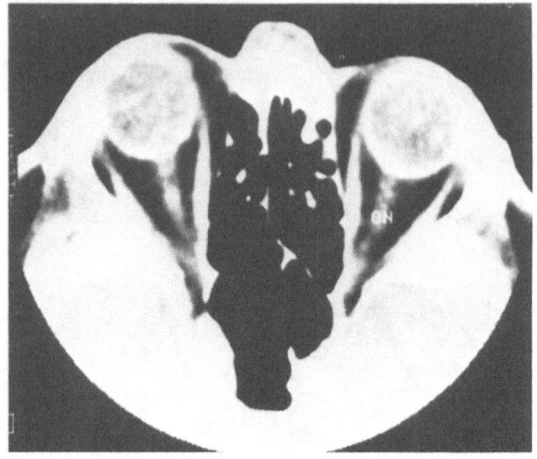

A

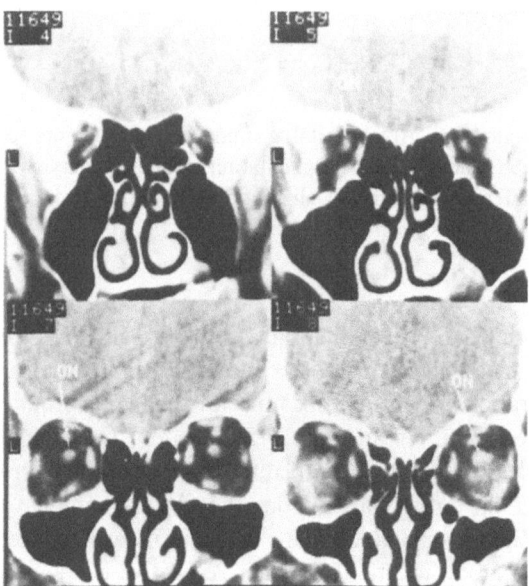

B

Figure 2.10 A. The optic nerve. Axial orbital section reveals the optic nerves (*ON*) crossing obliquely from the posterior margin of the globes toward the orbital apices. The optic canal entrance was just superior to this slice level. **B.** Four coronal slices demonstrate the relative position of the optic nerve within the orbit. On the most anterior section (lower right), where the nerve is about to insert on the globe, its position is relatively central within the orbit. On the most posterior section (upper left), the optic nerve lies in the superior-medial orbit near where it enters into the optic canal.

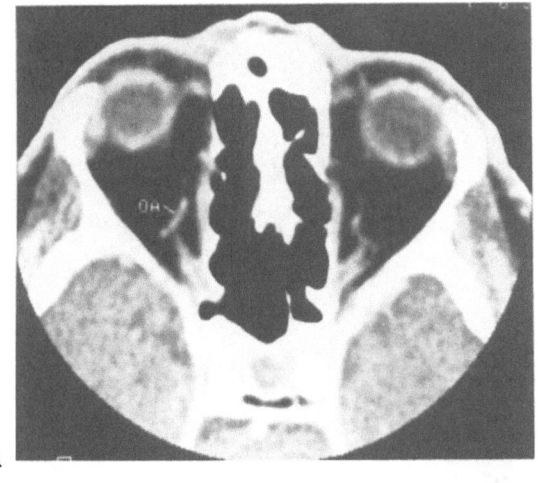

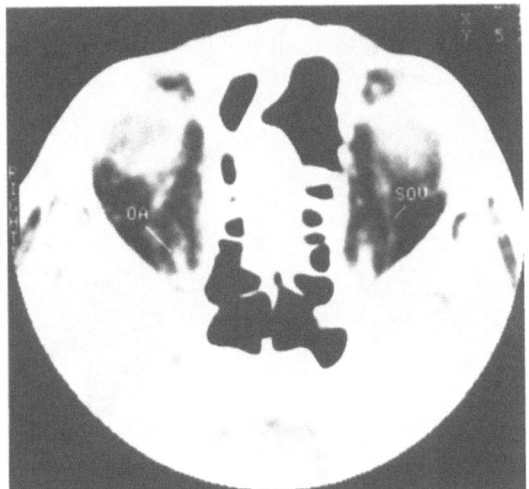

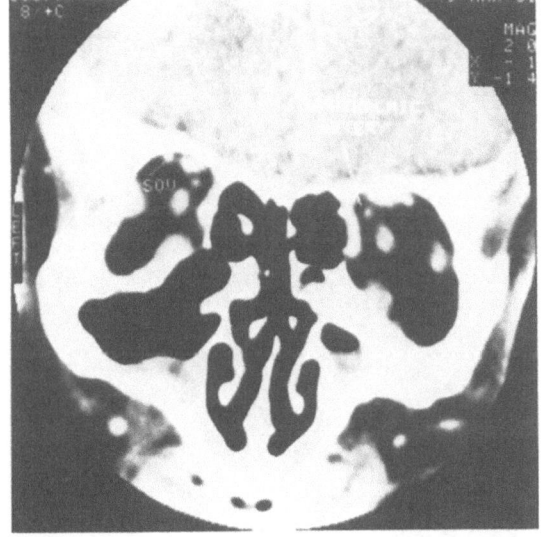

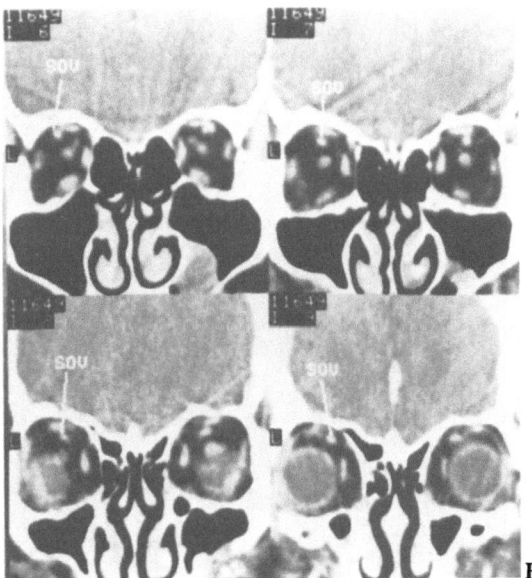

Figure 2.11. The ophthalmic artery. **A.** In the axial view, the ophthalmic artery (*OA*) is well shown as it passes anteromedially at a level just above the optic nerve. **B.** In the coronal view, the ophthalmic artery is also well shown (arrow). The superior ophthalmic vein (*SOV*) is labeled here to aid in its distinction.

Figure 2.12. The superior ophthalmic vein (*SOV*). **A.** High orbital axial section demonstrates the SOV traversing the orbit anteromedially to posterolaterally. The ophthalmic artery (*OA*) is faintly seen. **B.** Four coronal sections demonstrate the course of the SOV beneath the superior rectus muscle from its medial position anteriorly (lower right) to its lateral position more posteriorly (upper left).

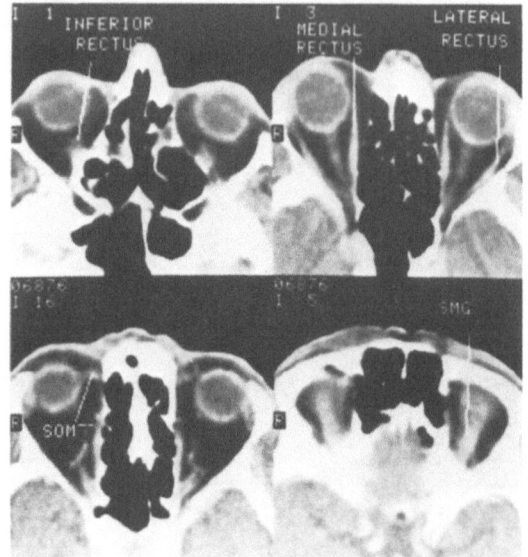

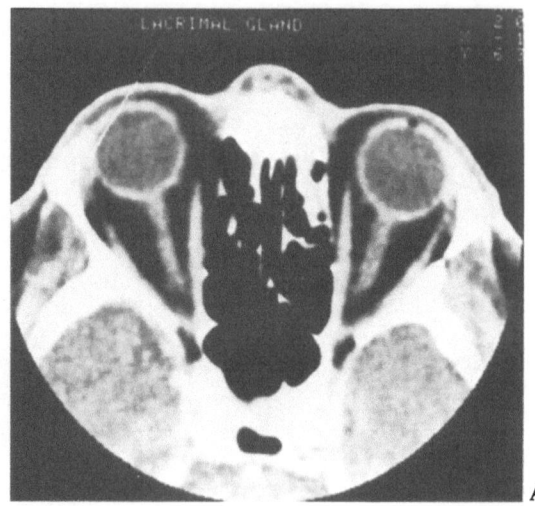

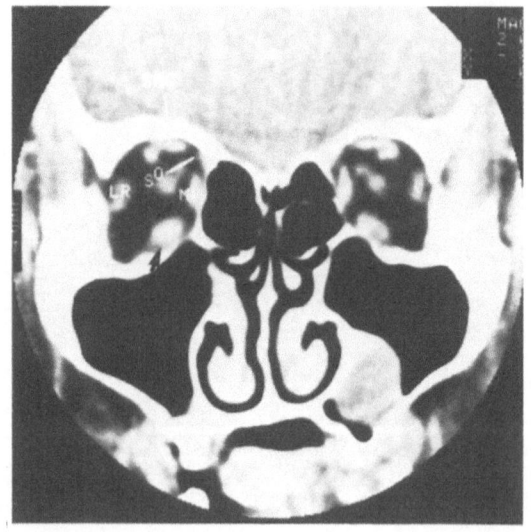

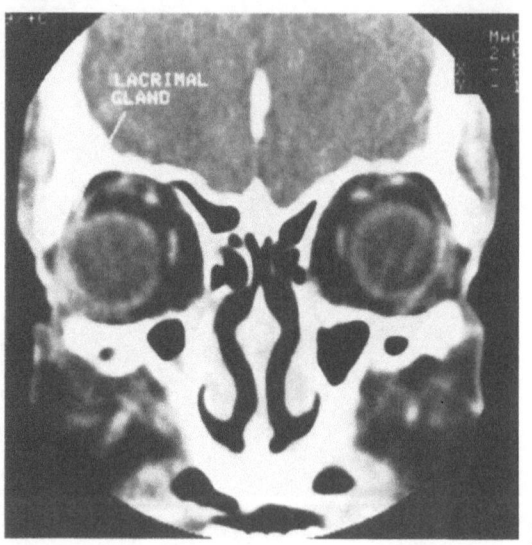

Figure 2.13. The extraocular muscles. **A.** Four axial sections extending from the inferior orbit (upper left) to the superior orbit (lower right). The superior oblique muscle (*SOM*) is seen both in its direct portion along the medial orbital wall and its reflected portion, extending from the trochlea to the medial surface of the globe. The superior muscle group (*SMG*) includes the superior rectus muscle and levator palpebrae muscles. **B.** Coronal view demonstrating the medial rectus (*MR*), lateral rectus (*LR*), inferior rectus (arrow), superior muscle group (*SMG*), and superior oblique muscle (*SOM*).

Figure 2.14. The lacrimal gland. **A.** In the axial view, the lacrimal gland has an almond-shaped configuration and lies between the zygomatic process and the lateral margin of the globe. **B.** The lacrimal gland is noted in the coronal view. Note that it lies lateral to the intermuscular membrane, which is seen passing between the superior muscle group and the lateral margin of the globe at the insertion of the lateral rectus muscle.

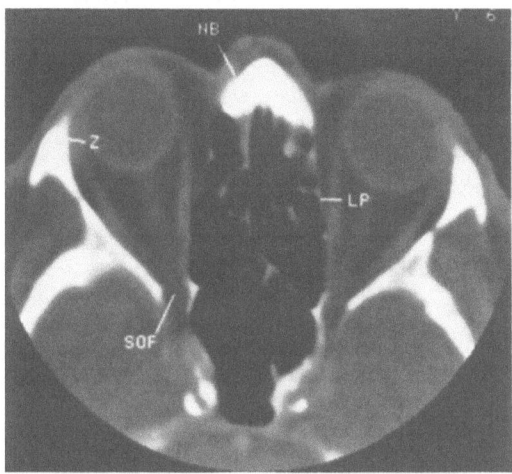

Figure 2.15. Axial orbital section photographed at a wide window setting to accentuate bone detail. The superior orbital fissure (*SOF*), the lamina papyracea (*LP*), nasal bone (*NB*), and zygomatic process (*Z*) are demonstrated.

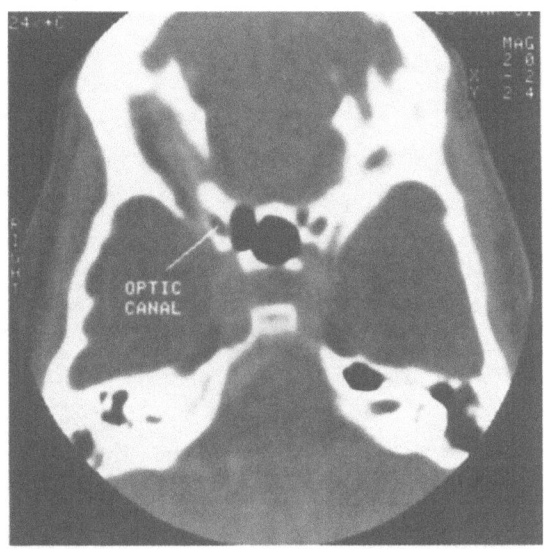

Figure 2.16. The optic canal is demonstrated in the axial view.

dial rectus is the thickest of the intraorbital muscles, and it usually measures close to 4 mm at its widest point.

The lacrimal glands (Fig. 2.14) are the only prominent structures located in the extraconal space with the exception of portions of the superior ophthalmic vein. The lacrimal glands are located within the lacrimal fossae on the medial surface of the zygomatic processes of the frontal bones in the anterior-superior-lateral aspect of the orbits. They are separated from the globe by the lateral rectus muscles. They are roughly almond-shaped and usually measure 4–5 mm in width.

Certain bony landmarks of the orbits deserve separate mention. The superior orbital fissures (Fig. 2.15) are formed at the orbital apices and permit passage of the superior ophthalmic vein and the third, fourth, and sixth cranial nerves and the first division of the fifth cranial nerve between the cavernous sinuses and the orbits. The lamina papyracea is a thin plate of bone forming most of the medial margin of the orbit and separating it from the adjacent ethmoid sinus. Since this bone is so thin, it often appears to be deficient on CT scan, erroneously suggesting bone destruction or fracture. The nasal bone forms the most anterior boundary of the medial orbit. The zygomatic process bounds the orbit anterolaterally. The optic canal often can be seen with aid of the bone win-

dow technique, especially when 1.5-mm thick sections are employed (Fig. 2.16). The optic canal is formed mostly by the anterior clinoid processes, with the thin optic strut forming a portion of the inferior wall of the canal.

Approach to Orbital CT Diagnosis

It is beyond the scope and intention of this chapter to illustrate the wide range of pathologies that may involve the orbit. A more comprehensive presentation of such lesions will be discussed in subsequent chapters.

While, in some cases, the diagnosis of an orbital lesion may be made confidently based on its CT appearance, more often the role of CT scanning is to outline the location and extent of the abnormality for guiding subsequent biopsy procedures. A patient presenting with proptosis may be found on CT scan to have a large lesion that principally involves the nasal cavity and paranasal sinuses with a smaller intraorbital component (Fig. 2.17). The most efficacious approach to a biopsy procedure for such a lesion is often via the nasal cavity or sinus, as a CT scan would suggest. While plain x-ray films or tomography should demonstrate nasal and sinus involvement, they are incapable of discriminating between a tumor and impacted mu-

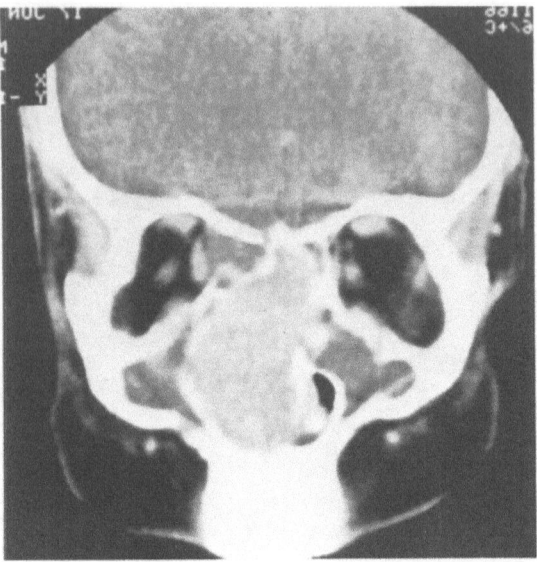

Figure 2.17. Carcinoma of the nasal cavity and adjacent paranasal sinuses, coronal section. The greatest bulk of the tumor mass is noted in the midline in the nasal cavity, with extension into the ethmoid and maxillary sinuses to some extent. Note that the central tissue, which represents the carcinoma, is of higher density than that occupying the majority of the sinuses. The latter represents impacted mucous, which results from drainage pathways blocked by the carcinoma. The tissue adjacent to the right medial rectus muscle has the density of impacted mucous in the ethmoid sinus. The ability to distinguish tissues by the density is helpful in planning biopsy specimens of lesions in this area.

Table 2.1. Location of more common orbital masses

I. Inside the eyeball
    Melanoma
    Retinoblastoma
    Metastatic tumor

II. Intraconal
    Optic nerve lesions
        Optic nerve glioma
        Optic nerve sheath meningioma
    Others
        Hemangioma
        Orbital pseudotumor
        Hemangiopericytoma
        Metastic lesion
        Lymphoma
        Hematoma
        Abscesses
        Orbital varices

III. Muscle masses
    Graves disease
    Orbital pseudotumor
    Metastatic tumor
    Lymphoma
    Arteriovenous malformation (carotid-cavernous fistula)

IV. Intraorbital extraconal masses
    Lacrimal gland tumor
    Dermoid-epidermoid tumors and teratoma
    Metastatic tumors
    Lymphoma
    Hemangioma-hemangiopericytoma
    Abscess
    Hematoma

V. Extraorbital masses
    Meningiomas
    Extension of primary malignant sinus tumors
    Metastatic tumor
    Mucocele from adjacent sinus
    Encephalocele
    Bone tumors of orbital walls

cous in these locations; they might lead to an inappropriate choice for the biopsy site.

The location of a lesion within the orbit may serve as a clue towards diagnosis. Certain lesions have predilections for involving either the intraconal or extraconal space (Table 2.1).

It is important to establish whether an orbital disease is unilateral or bilateral. Graves' orbitopathy, for example, was found to be bilateral in greater than 90% of the cases by Enzmann (2), and it would be the favored diagnosis in most cases of bilateral myopathies (Fig. 2.18). Of course, there are other CT features that might lead to an alternative diagnosis (e.g., orbital pseudotumor or metastases) with bilateral muscle enlargement. Bilateral or multicentric involvement of structures other than just the muscles would suggest metastases, orbital pseudotumor, or lymphoma (Fig. 2.19).

Specific lesion characteristics may be helpful in the differential diagnosis of orbital pathology. The character of the margin of the abnormality should be evaluated. Lesions with well-defined margins are often, but not always, found to be benign (Figs. 2.20 and 2.21). Vague, poorly defined margins suggest an infiltrative process such as orbital pseudotumor or lymphoma (Fig. 2.22).

The shape of the lesion is sometimes helpful in a diagnosis. This is particularly true in the case of vascular lesions—such as arteriovenous malformation or orbital varices, where the tubular shape of the components of the abnormality are characteristic (Fig. 2.23).

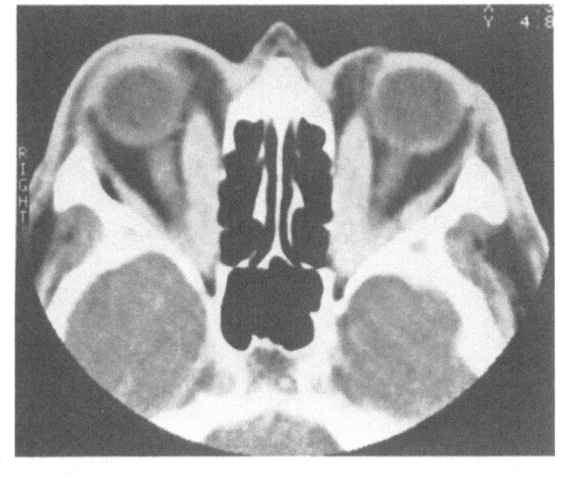

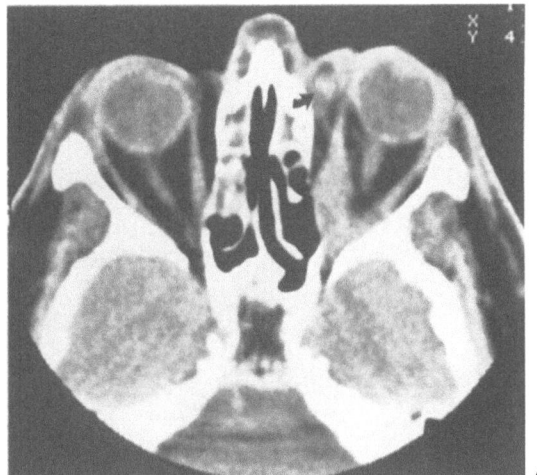

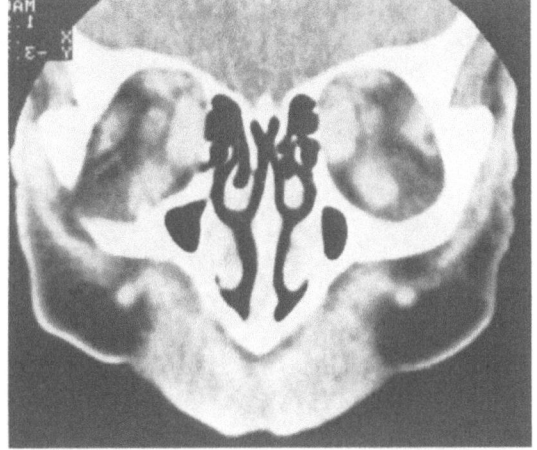

Figure 2.18. Bilateral Graves' orbitopathy. **A.** Axial view demonstrating massive enlargement of both medial recti and lesser enlargement of the lateral recti. Bilateral exophthalmos is present. **B.** Coronal scan reveals additional involvement of the inferior recti and, to a lesser extent, the superior muscle group bilaterally. Bilateral involvement is present in the vast majority of cases of Graves' orbitopathy.

Figure 2.19. Metastasis to the left orbit. **A.** Axial view. There is marked enlargement of the proximal portion of the left medial rectus muscle, with contiguous thickening of the proximal portion of the lateral rectus. The margins of the involved portions of the muscles are less well defined than was seen in a patient with Graves' disease in Figure 2.18. The sparing of the distal portions of the muscles is also not found in Graves' disease. Also note the abnormal soft tissue (arrow) located posterior to the left orbital septum, which represents a second metastatic deposit. **B.** The coronal view better demonstrates the anteromedially situated metastatic lesion in the left orbit.

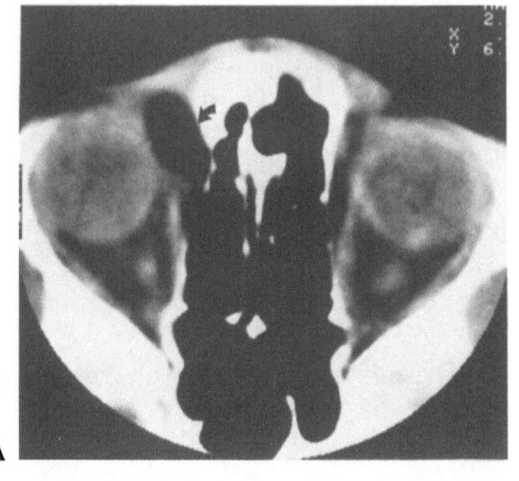

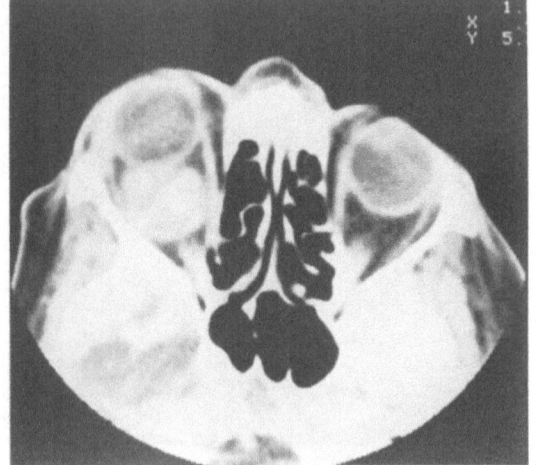

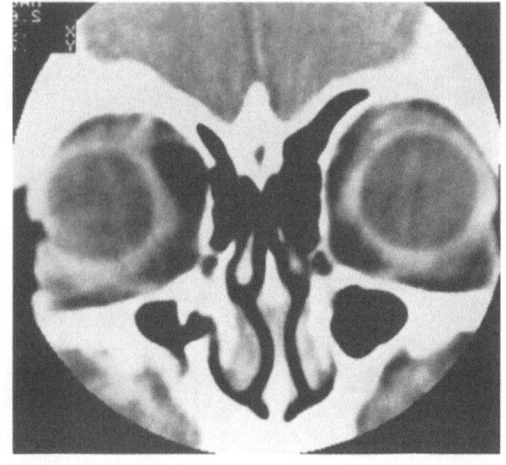

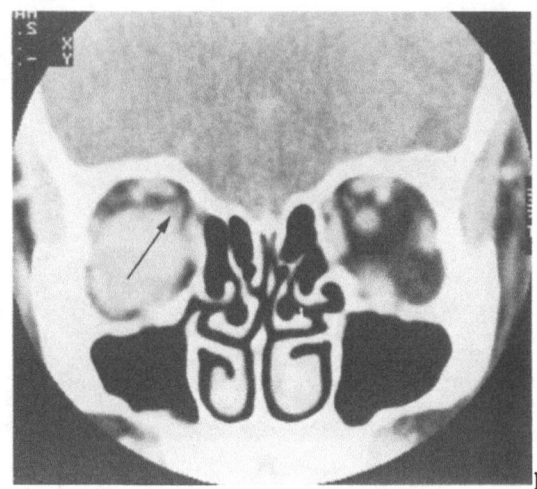

Figure 2.20. Dermoid cyst. **A.** Axial view reveals a low-density mass (arrow) in the anterior medial aspect of the right orbit between the nasal bone and the right globe. Density measurements of the mass placed it in the range of fatty tissue. The mass lies medial to the medial rectus muscle in an extraconal position. Note the erosion of the posterior aspect of the right nasal bone. **B.** The lesion is displacing the globe laterally. Erosion and molding of the adjacent bone around the lesion are noted.

Figure 2.21. Cavernous hemangioma of the right orbit. **A.** Axial view reveals a large high-density lesion centrally located posterior to the globe on the right. The lesion is confined within the intraconal space. On the axial view alone, this lesion potentially could be mistaken for an optic nerve tumor. In fact, the patient was scanned elsewhere, in which case a diagnosis of optic nerve meningioma was made. **B.** Coronal view reveals the large intraconal lesion on the right. The optic nerve (arrow) is displaced superomedially by the mass. Note that the displaced optic nerve distinguishes this lesion from a tumor arising from the optic nerve.

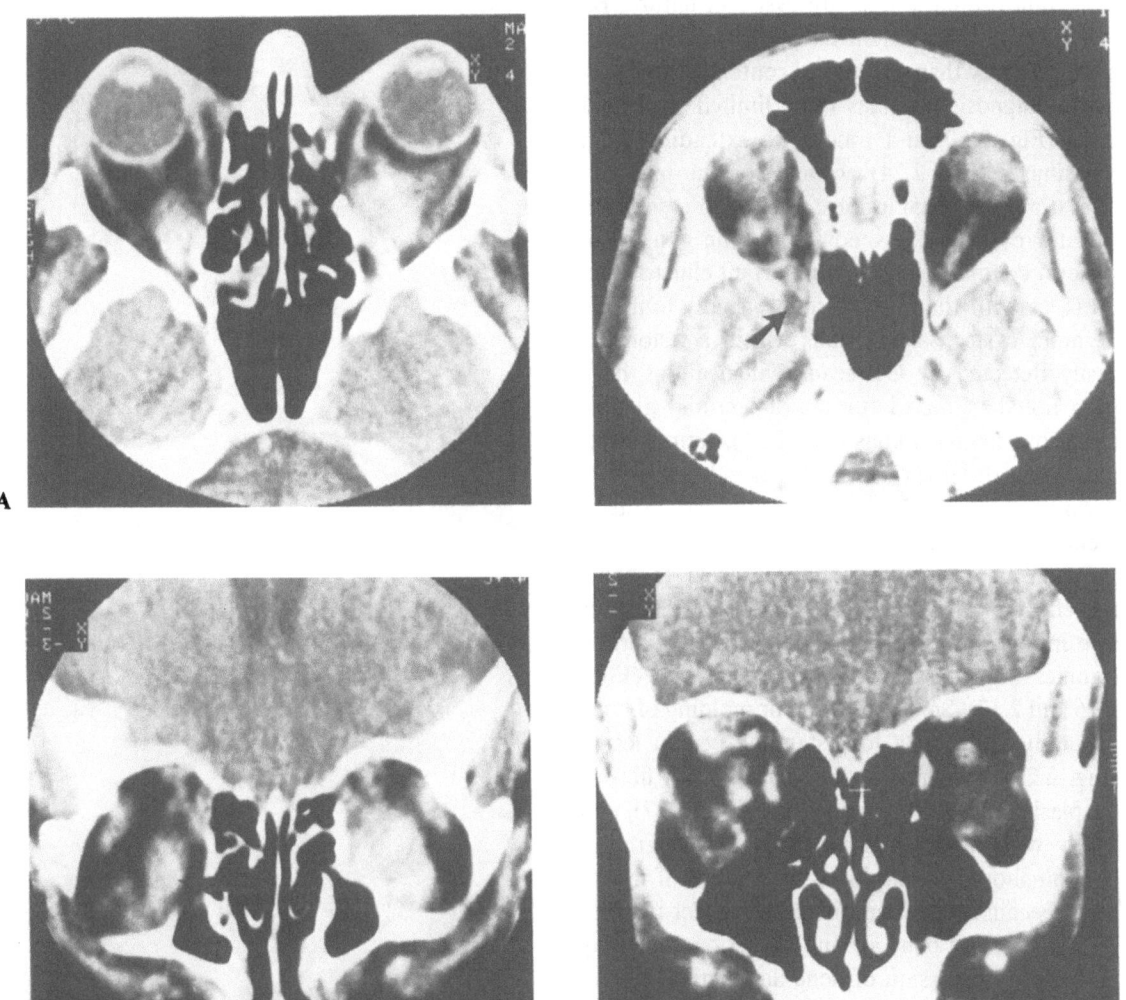

Figure 2.22. Bilateral orbital pseudotumor. **A.** Axial scan. Bilateral proptosis is noted. A large intraconal mass is noted on the left, obscuring the boundaries of the left inferior rectus muscle and presumably involving it. The boundaries of this lesion are ill defined, suggesting an infiltrative process. Similar, but less marked, involvement is noted in the right orbit. **B.** In the coronal view, the large left orbital mass clearly involves the inferior rectus muscle and, perhaps, infiltrates a portion of the medial rectus muscle as well. The smaller right orbital mass (arrow) appears to lie intraconally just above the inferior rectus muscle at this slice location.

Figure 2.23. Right orbital varices. **A.** Axial view reveals ill-defined soft-tissue density structures in the superior aspect of the right orbit. Note the widening of the right superior orbital fissure (arrow). **B.** Tubular-shaped soft-tissue abnormalities are noted in both the superior and inferior aspects of the right orbit, allowing the diagnosis of orbital varices. The superior and inferior ophthalmic veins appear to be enlarged in this case. The diagnosis was confirmed by orbital venography.

Certain orbital lesions are cystic in nature. By recognizing that a lesion has a capsule that is of higher density than the central contents, the differential diagnosis becomes quite limited. Dermoid cysts (Fig. 2.20) and mucoceles extending from the sinuses (Fig. 2.24) account for the majority of cystic intraorbital lesions. Orbital abscesses and hydatid cysts are less common. The density of the cyst contents can be an important clue to diagnosis, as with the fatty material usually found in dermoid cysts. Calcifications within a lesion are easily detected by CT scan. Calcifications have been noted in mixed tumors of lacrimal glands, cavernous hemangiomas (Fig. 2.25), retinoblastomas, and orbital varices, in the capsules of orbital dermoids, and occasionally in optic nerve sheath meningiomas and optic gliomas.

When an orbital lesion lies adjacent to bone, the effect of the lesion on the adjacent bone is also important. Frank bone destruction generally signifies an aggressive or malignant process (Figs. 2.16 and 2.17). Smooth erosion or molding of bone generally indicates a long-standing benign lesion (Fig. 2.20). Hyperostosis may occur with fibrous dysplasia (Fig. 2.26), meningioma (Fig. 2.27), and rarely with lacrimal gland tumors. A degree of caution should be employed in the case of mucoceles, because it is often difficult to detect the thin residual shell of bone around the lesion. One may get a false impression of bone destruction. Fortunately, the characteristic appearance of a mucocele, which is usually present, permits the proper diagnosis in most cases (Fig. 2.24).

CT scanning is extremely useful for identifying intraocular pathology. Neoplasms, such as uveal melanoma, retinoblastoma, and metastasis, when larger than 3 mm, are well shown (Fig. 11.22, 11.23). Retinal detachment can often be demonstrated, as can intraocular hemorrhage. Abnormalities of globe shape are readily categorized. Buphthalmos, enlargement of the globe usually secondary to congenital glaucoma, can be distinguished from axial myopia in which the globe is predominantly elongated (Figs. 2.28, 2.29, 2.30). An abnormally small globe can be seen with congenital microphthalmos and with phthisis which is due to prior trauma or infection. Defects in the globe margin may be noted with colaboma and staphyloma. Calcification of the globe not associated with neoplasia can be seen with drusen (Fig. 2.31), hypercalcemic states, retrolental fibroplasia, and phthisis.

Computed tomographic scanning is a valuable

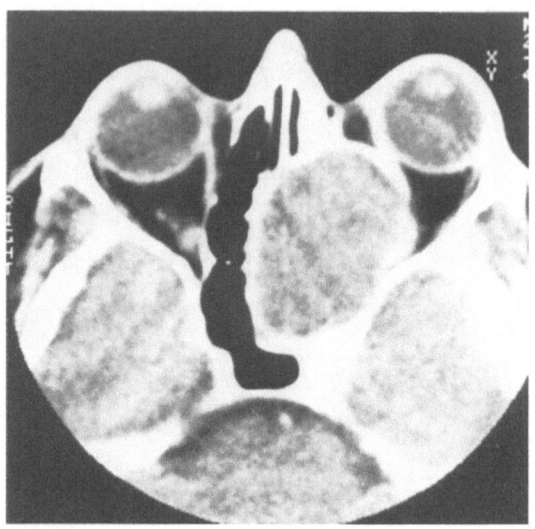

A

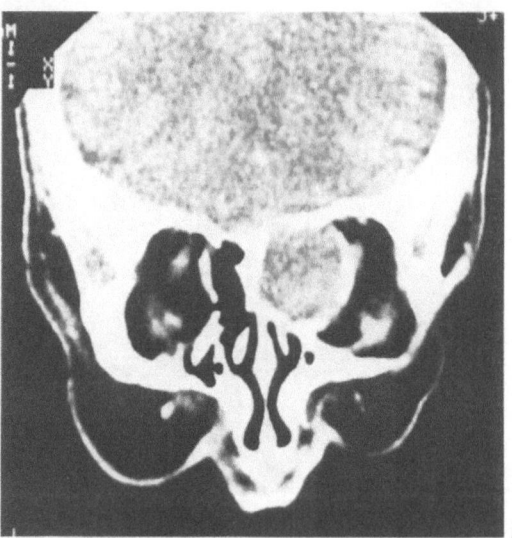

B

Figure 2.24. Left ethmoid sinus mucocele. **A.** Axial scan. A large mass is noted centered in the region of the left ethmoid sinus, which has been totally replaced by this abnormality. The lesion is extending toward the left orbit, producing proptosis. A reasonably well-defined bony shell remains around the mucocele in this case. However, in some cases, the bony rim is so thin that it cannot be distinguished from contrast-enhancing tissue; bone destruction is suggested. The contents of the mucocele are similar in density to brain tissue. **B.** Coronal view again reveals the lesion. There is a suggestion of early erosion of the cribriform plate.

tool for the diagnosis of orbital pathology when proper attention is paid to meticulous technique and careful observation of the general diagnostic features described above. Its role in evaluating the extent of lesions and in biopsy procedure planning is indispensable.

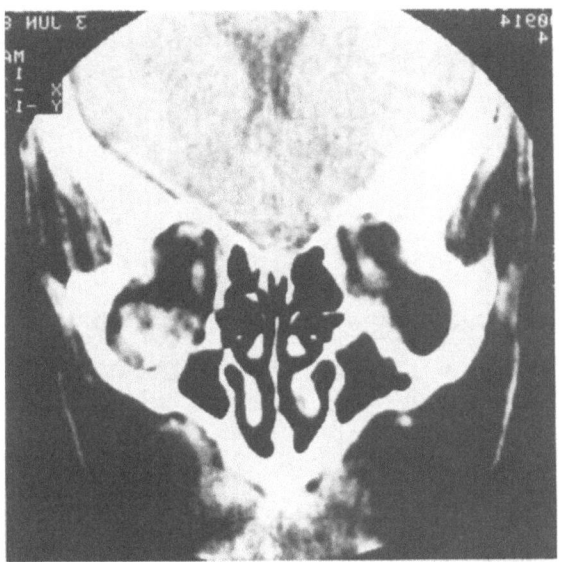

Figure 2.25. Partially calcified cavernous hemangioma in the inferior aspect of the right orbit, coronal view. Note the higher density areas, which represent calcification within the lesion.

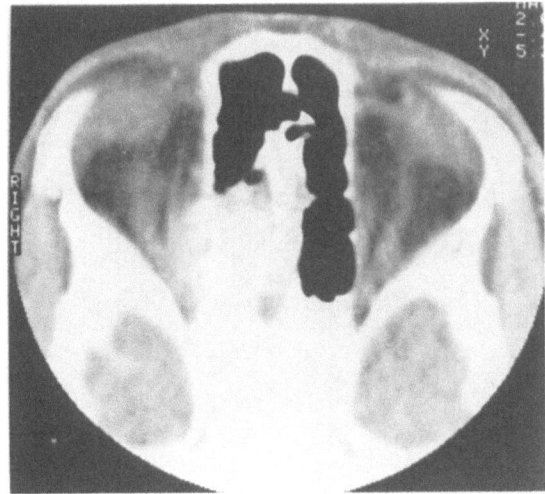

Figure 2.26. Fibrous dysplasia involving the right ethmoid sinus and orbit. An irregular high-density lesion, measuring in the range of bone values, occupies the posterior aspect of the right ethmoid sinus and extends into the right posterior orbit. The right medial rectus muscle is displaced laterally. This lesion was evaluated with a wide window setting of 500, which greatly improved the delineation of its architecture. At lower window settings usually employed for orbital soft tissues, this lesion appeared as a dense bony mass obscuring the characteristic irregular pattern of fibrous dysplasia.

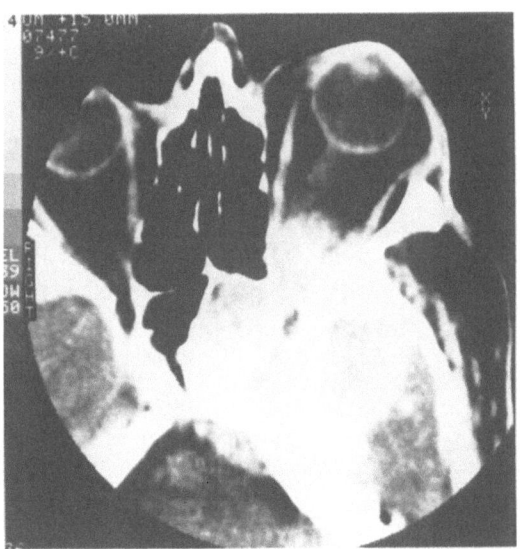

A

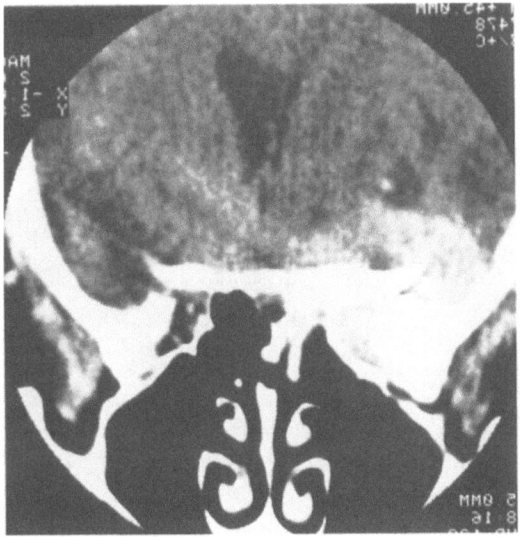

B

Figure 2.27. Sphenoid ridge meningioma. **A.** Axial scan reveals a large contrast-enhancing lesion arising from the sphenoid ridge, with extension into the left orbital apex, sphenoid sinus, pontine cistern, and middle fossa. Bony hyperostosis, which is typical of meningioma, is most marked along the medial aspect of the greater wing of the sphenoid. **B.** Coronal scan again reveals the large left meningioma. The left orbital apex appears to be filled with the contrast-enhancing lesion. Note the marked hyperostosis of the bony margin of the left orbit secondary to the lesion.

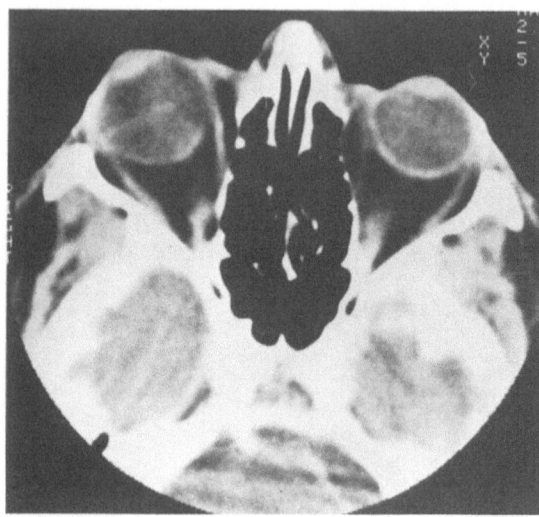

Figure 2.28. Buphthalmos secondary to congenital glaucoma. Axial view of the orbit shows the right side much larger than the left.

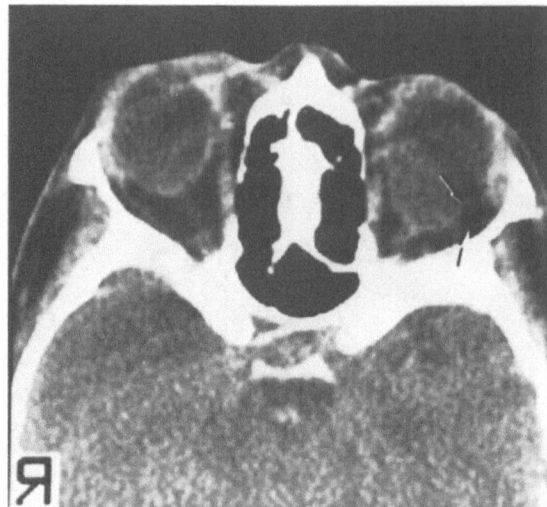

Figure 2.30. Axial myopia. Axial view reveals elongation of left globe in its anteroposterior diameter. A focal absence of scleral enhancement (black arrow) and a questionable bulge (white arrow) may represent a small staphyloma.

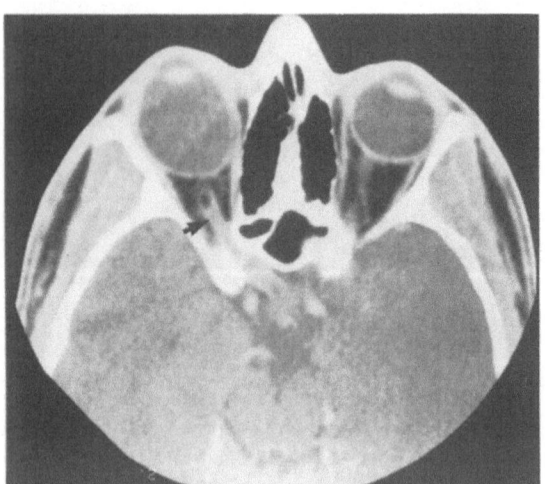

Figure 2.29. Buphthalmos in a patient with an optic nerve glioma. Axial CT view reveals enlargement of the right globe in a patient with neurofibromatosis. The enlargement of the optic nerve is consistent with an optic nerve glioma (arrow) extending into the optic canal and chiasmatic region.

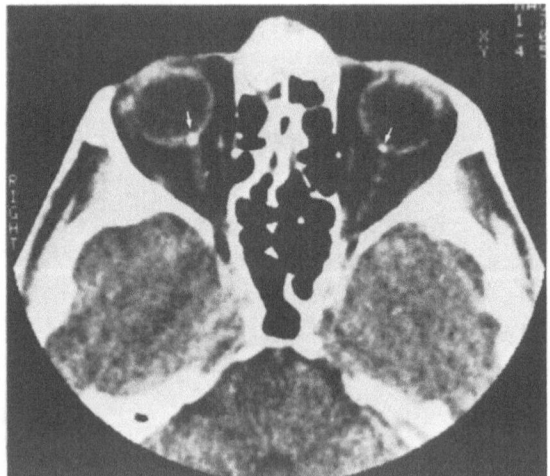

Figure 2.31. Optic nerve drusen. Axial CT shows bilateral calcifications at the insertion of the optic nerves on the globes (white arrows).

Acknowledgment. Figures 2.2A, 2.3A, 2.5–11, 2.12B, 2.13–15, 2.17–31 reproduced with permission from Peyster, R.G., and Hoover, E.D.: *Computerized Tomography in Orbital Disease and Neuro-ophthalmology.* Copyright © 1984 by Year Book Medical Publishers, Inc., Chicago.

References

1. Cabinis EA, Salvolini U, Radallec A, et al: Computed tomography of the optic nerve: Part 2. Size and shape modifications in papilledema. *J Comput Assist Tomogr* 2:150–155, 1978.
2. Enzmann DR, Donaldson SS, Kriss JP: Appearance of Graves' disease on orbital computed tomography. *J Comput Assist Tomogr* 3:815–819, 1979.
3. Fox AJ, Debrun G, Vinuela F, et al: Intrathecal metrizamide enhancement of the optic nerve sheath. *J Comput Assist Tomogr* 3:653–656, 1979.
4. Gyldensted C, Lester J, Fledelius H: Computed tomography of orbital lesions. A radiological study of 144 cases. *Neuroradiology* 13:141–150, 1977.
5. Hunsaker JN, Anderson RE, Van Dyke HKL, et al: A comparison of computed tomographic techniques in the diagnosis of Graves' ophthalmopathy. *Ophthal Surg* 10:34–40, 1979.
6. Lloyd GAS: CT scanning in the diagnosis of orbital disease. *Comput Tomogr* 3:227–239, 1979.
7. Manelfe C, Pasquini U, Bank WO: Metrizamide demonstration of the subarachnoid space surrounding the optic nerves. *J Comput Assist Tomogr* 2:545–547, 1978.

3
Computed Tomography Scanning in the Evaluation of Ocular Motility Disorders

Mahmood F. Mafee and Marilyn T. Miller

Computed tomography (CT) can aid in the diagnosis of a selected group of ocular motility disturbances. In some conditions, CT scanning can provide insight into the location of the pathologic process, allowing a specific treatment regimen to be applied.

Radiographic imaging of the extraocular muscles has been facilitated by the recent development of high-resolution CT scanners. For this examination, the patient's eyes are fixed in primary gaze and 1.5-mm axial sections are used. Then computer reconstruction of these sections can be made into coronal, sagittal, and oblique (para-axial or off-axis) planes. When additional information is needed to formulate a more accurate diagnosis or to treat the patient, other positions of gaze may be used or the standard technique may be modified.

Causes of Eye Motility Disturbances

Ocular muscle imbalances are fairly common; they occur in approximately 2–4% of the population. The onset usually is in infancy or early childhood, but acquired forms may occur at any age. Normally, the eyes are aligned so that the object being perceived falls on the macula of both eyes. If an ocular muscle imbalance exists, the object may fall on the macula of the fixing eye, but in a peripheral area of the retina of the other—or deviating—eye. This nonalignment is termed strabismus, squint, or heterotropia. 1) If the deviating eye points inward, the patient is said to have esotropia; 2) if the eye looks outward, exotropia exists; 3) if the deviating eye gazes up, hypertropia is pres-

ent; and 4) if the eye looks down, hypotropia is indicated. These deviations may be constant, variable, or intermittent.

Two major categories of strabismus have important diagnostic and therapeutic implications. Patients with nonparetic (concomitant) strabismus have no limitation of movement in any field of gaze; i.e., the degree of deviation is approximately the same when looking in any direction. The most frequent type of early childhood motility disturbance, nonparetic strabismus, may be present at birth or may start in the first few years of life. The etiology is not clearly known, but it may be due to a pathologic condition in higher brain centers that deal with the coordination of eye movement. Often, the family history of strabismus is present, but a more multifactorial pattern of transmission rather than a clear mendelian-type of inheritance may be present.

Patients with a nonconcomitant type of strabismus are seen less frequently. These cases are characterized by a limitation of movement in one or more fields of action. For example, a child with a sixth nerve palsy of the right eye will have restriction of abduction of that eye with no limitation in the other fields of gaze. This limitation produces an ocular deviation that varies in amount and, at times, type in the various fields of gaze (i.e., nonconcomitant strabismus). If the eyes are aligned in some fields of gaze, the patient may adapt an abnormal head position to achieve binocular vision and to avoid looking into the field of gaze of the paralyzed muscle, where an ocular deviation is present which may be associated with double vision. This nonconcomitant form of strabismus may be secondary to a central nervous system disease involving the nuclei or tracts of the cranial nerves supplying the extraocular muscles, or it may be due to congenital or acquired changes in the ocular muscles or orbital disease. Trauma or inflammatory processes involving the ocular muscles most commonly produce this type of strabismus.

Any pathologic process involving the nerve supply to the ocular muscles results in failure to move the eye in a predicted manner. For example, a right sixth nerve paresis causes the inability to abduct the right eye fully. Also, changes within the ocular muscles may restrict movement of the antagonistic muscle(s). Thyroid myopathy and blow-out fractures are common restrictive phenomena. In these conditions, damage or changes in the inferior rectus muscles often result in an inability to elevate the involved eye, although the superior rectus may be minimally involved or not at all. With the use of one or two forceps, passive rotation of the eye with the patient under local or general anesthesia will demonstrate this restrictive condition ("forced duction" examination). The CT scan may show changes in the size, structure, or location of involved ocular muscles that will explain these restrictive movements.

Anatomy of the Extraocular Muscles

Each eye has six extraocular muscles. The four rectus muscles arise from the annulus of Zinn, which is a funnel-shaped tendinous ring that encloses the optic foramen and the medial end of the superior orbital fissure (1, 2). The rectus muscles originate from the inner aspect of the annulus as two common tendons: the upper common tendon of Lockwood (superiorly) and the lower common tendon of Zinn (inferiorly). The inferior rectus originates from the common tendon of Zinn below the optic foramen. It inserts into the inferior sclera 6.5 mm from the limbus. The superior rectus (the longest of the four rectus muscles) originates from the common tendon of Lockwood above the optic foramen and from the sheath of the optic nerve. It passes below the levator aponeurosis and inserts into the upper sclera 7.7 mm from the limbus. The medial rectus (the thickest of these muscles) arises from the upper tendon of Lockwood, the lower tendon of Zinn, and the sheath of the

optic nerve (1, 2) and inserts 5.5 mm from the limbus. The lateral rectus originates from the lower common tendon of Zinn and the upper common tendon of Lockwood and inserts 6.9 mm from the limbus (1).

The superior oblique (longest and thinnest of the extraocular muscles) originates from the periosteum of sphenoid bone above and medial to the annulus of Zinn and the origin of the medial rectus (1–3). It passes anteriorly along the upper part of the medial orbital wall (1–3) as a slender tendon and enters the trochlea (a small fibrocartilaginous ring lined with a synovial-type sheath) (4). The tendon slides through the trochlea. It then turns sharply posterolaterally and downward beneath the superior rectus to insert in the lateral sclera, behind the equator of the eye. The inferior oblique muscle originates from the orbital plate of the maxilla just lateral to the orifice of the nasolacrimal duct. It passes under the lateral rectus and inserts to the posterior and lateral portion of the globe (3). The third cranial nerve (oculomotor) supplies the superior, inferior, and medial recti, the inferior oblique muscle, and the levator palpebrae. The lateral rectus is innervated by the sixth nerve (abducens), while the fourth nerve (trochlea) innervates the superior oblique muscle.

Use of CT Scan

The anatomy of the extraocular muscles is well visualized on a CT scan. However, some modification of routine views is needed to see certain muscles completely. For example, in a transverse axial CT scan of the orbit, only a portion of the inferior rectus muscle (which almost follows the floor of the orbit) can be seen on individual images. The entire muscle can be appreciated if the angulation of the cut is negative. Usually, it is best seen in an axial CT taken with −15° angulation. However, the best plane of section to evaluate vertical recti (inferior and superior rectus muscles) is a sagittal plane (Fig. 3.1). The horizontal recti are best seen in axial sections (Fig. 3.2).

The course of the superior oblique muscle, from its origin to the trochlea, can be best viewed in the axial plane (Fig. 3.3). The coronal plane only offers portions of the belly of this muscle on individual slices.

Figure 3.1. Direct sagittal CT scan of the orbit obtained with a Tomoscan 310. Note the inferior and superior rectus muscles in their entire course from the common tendon of Zinn (arrowheads) to their insertion at the globe. The inferior oblique muscle (large arrow) is below the inferior rectus muscle; the intermuscular fat and suspensory ligament of Lockwood (small arrow) are demonstrated. In oculoplastic surgery, the suspensory ligament of Lockwood plays an important role in preventing postsurgical differences in the width of the palpebral fissures of the eye (1) (CT scan courtesy of FW Zonneveld, MSC).

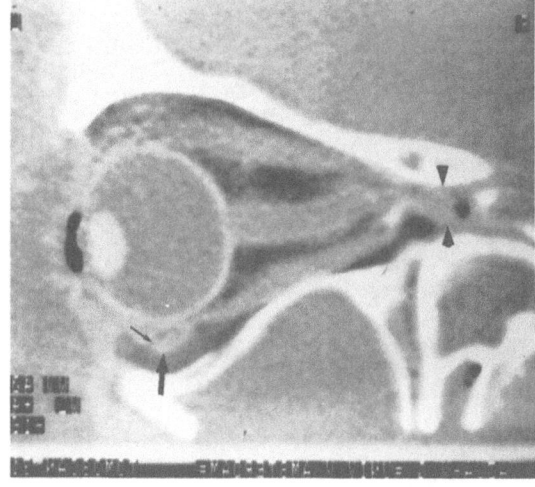

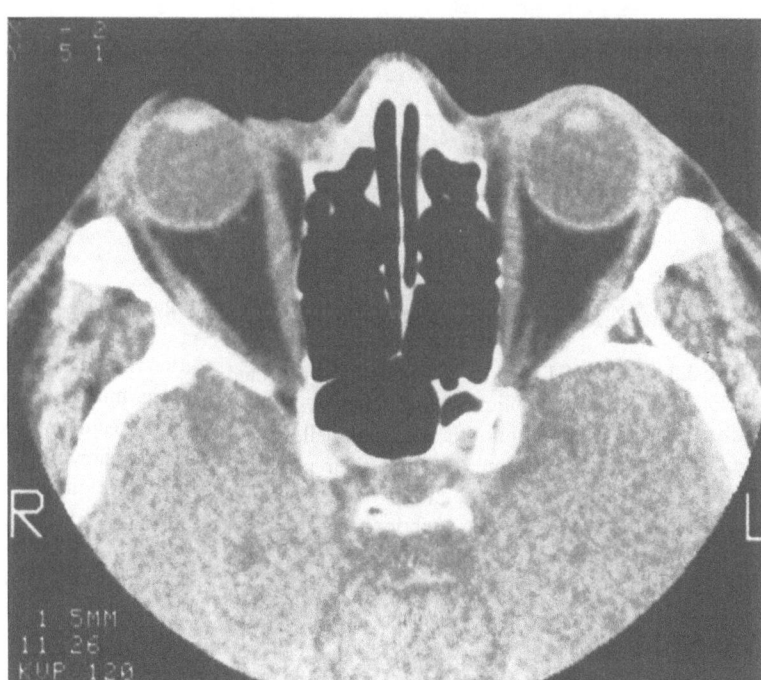

Figure 3.2. A CT scan showing the horizontal rectus muscles, from their origin (annulus of Zinn) to their insertions over the sclera.

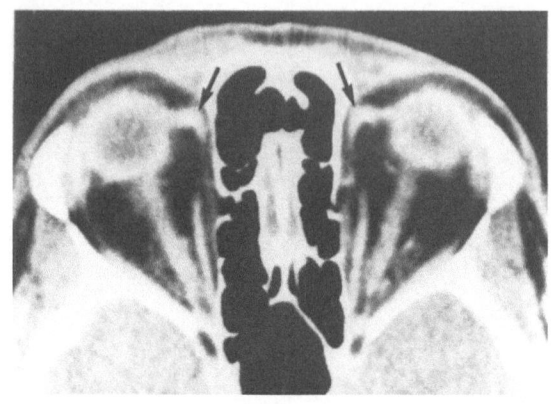

A

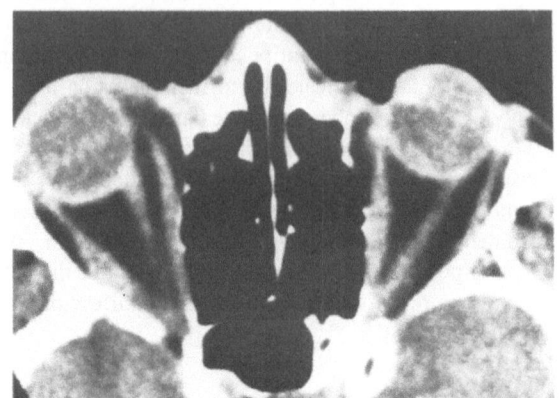

A

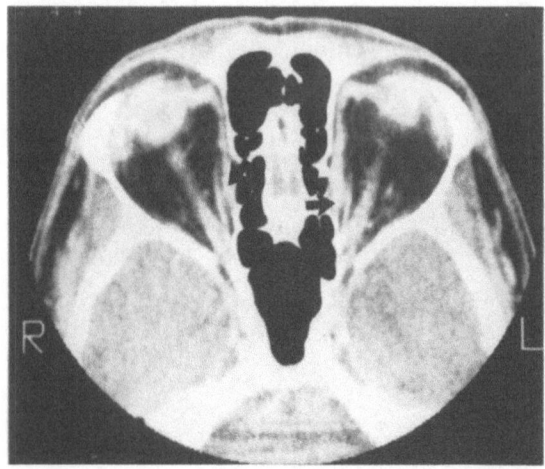

B

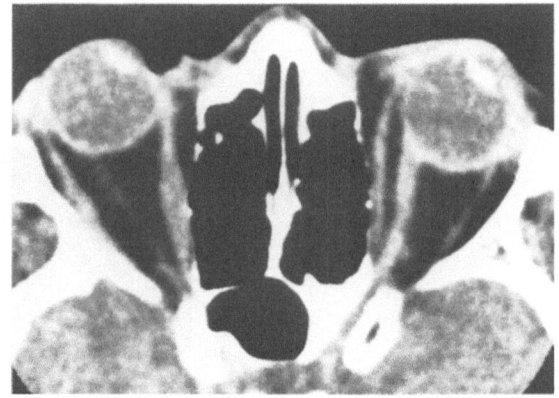

B

Figure 3.3 A. Axial CT scan demonstrating the reflected portion of the superior oblique muscles (arrows). Normally, the tendons are symmetric in size as well as density. The superior oblique muscles and their proximal tendons are just medial to the medial rectus muscles. **B.** This scan, obtained 1.5 mm superior to that shown in Figure 3.3A, demonstrates the entire course of both superior oblique muscles and their tendons (arrows). The partially volumed medial rectus is just lateral to the superior oblique muscles.

Figure 3.4 A. Axial CT scan obtained during right lateral gaze demonstrating Sherrington's law of reciprocal innervation. Note that the right lateral and left medial rectus muscles contract and the right medial and left lateral rectus muscles relax (lengthen). This is the same patient shown in Figure 3.2, with the eyes in primary gaze position. **B.** Axial CT scan obtained during left lateral gaze (same patient as in Figures 3.2 and 3.4A). The right medial and left lateral rectus muscles are contracted and the right lateral and left medial rectus muscles are relaxed (lengthened).

Sherrington Law of Reciprocal Innervation

The Sherrington law of reciprocal innervation states that when an agonist muscle contracts, an inhibitory impulse is sent to its antagonist, which relaxes and lengthens (1). These actions are essential for the normal full range of ocular movement. A CT scan of patients who are looking right and left will demonstrate this expected physiologic change function of the extraocular muscles (Fig. 3.4), with an increase in size of the contracting muscle and a decrease in size of the relaxed muscle.

Application of CT Scanning Imaging to Nonconcomitant Strabismus Conditions

Brown's Superior Oblique Tendon Sheath Syndrome

In 1950, Brown described a clinical syndrome (superior oblique tendon sheath or Brown's syndrome) characterized by an impaired ability to raise the eye in adduction (5). Typically, the patient may have straight eyes or a hypotropia (one eye lower in the primary position). Frequently, the palpebral fissure of the involved eye widens on adduction. Brown further classified this condition into true and simulated syndromes (6). True (congenital) Brown's syndrome includes only those patients with a congenitally short or taut superior oblique tendon sheath complex. Patients with simulated (acquired) Brown's syndrome acquire the clinical features of the syndrome, and may occur secondary to various etiologies (6–16). Most authors, including Brown (5, 6, 11, 16), have postulated that simulated Brown's syndrome is primarily a disease of the tendon sheath-trochlear complex of the superior oblique muscle secondary to an inflammatory process of the adjacent tissues.

Normal ocular movement requires a loose sheath and free movement of the tendon in the sheath (4, 11). When the eye is adducted, the primary action of the inferior oblique muscle is elevation (1). When the eye is elevated in the adducted position, the superior oblique muscle normally relaxes, causing its tendon to lengthen and slide freely through the trochlea. If the superior oblique muscle cannot relax or its tendon cannot lengthen, the eye cannot be elevated while adducted (Fig. 3.5A). This limitation of elevation in adduction simulates an inferior oblique palsy, although the pathologic process is postulated to be located primarily in the superior oblique complex. This restriction in the physiologic passage of the tendon through the trochlea may be permanent or occur on an intermittent basis in the acquired form (4, 6, 12). This restriction also is the most common cause of an isolated limitation of elevation in adduction (pseudopalsy of the inferior oblique muscle); it occurs in about 1 of 450 cases of strabismus (15).

In acquired Brown's syndrome, the symptom and findings often are intermittent. Affected patients usually complain of intermittent double vision (diplopia) on upward gaze; and sometimes a "clicking" sensation in the area of the trochlea when attempting to look up (11, 12). This clicking sensation often may be heard with a stethoscope, especially when the upward gaze is prolonged (11, 12).

In our experience, the CT appearance is characteristic of acquired Brown's syndrome. All of our patients demonstrated some degree of abnormality in the reflected portion of the superior oblique tendon. One patient (following head trauma many years before) had significant thickening of the reflected portion of the superior oblique tendon in

the involved eye (Figs. 3–5B and 3–5C), which was confirmed at the time of surgery. In the congenital form (true Brown's syndrome), a constant set of findings is noted in early infancy (Fig. 3.6A) (5, 6, 8, 11, 13, 15, 16). Full or near-full elevation is possible in adduction (Fig. 3.6A) (5, 6, 11), which distinguishes this ocular motility imbalance from that of a double elevator palsy (limitation of elevation in all upgaze positions). Many authors have described a widening of the palpebral fissure on adduction (5, 6, 11) in Brown's syndrome. Patients with straight eyes in downward gaze may assume a backward tilt of the head to achieve binocular vision (5, 6, 11). One of our patients who had a successfully treated right congenital Brown's syndrome (Fig. 3.6A and 3.6B) developed left Brown's syndrome after trauma (Fig. 3.6C). A CT scan showed an edematous reflected tendon of the superior oblique muscle in the involved eye (Fig. 3.6D). On the basis of history, motility examination, and CT findings, the patient was given a 2-week course of systemic steroid therapy followed by a locally injected steroid in the trochlear region of the left eye. Within 2 weeks, she had a complete remission of the left Brown's syndrome (Fig. 3.6E). Significant thickening of the reflected tendon of the left superior oblique muscle was demonstrated in another patient with rheumatoid arthritis associated with a left Brown's syndrome (Fig. 3.7). The association of acquired Brown's syndrome and rheumatoid arthritis has been well documented in the literature (6, 11, 16) and may spontaneously disappear.

The CT scan enables an evaluation of three features of the superior oblique muscle (8, 10, 12): 1) the angle that the reflected tendon makes with the medial wall of the orbit; 2) the thickness of the tendon; and 3) the density of the tendon compared with surrounding tissue. Under normal circumstances, these characteristics are nearly equal in both eyes (Fig. 3.3). The CT technique makes this comparison of both eyes possible in a manner that no other procedure allows (8, 10, 12). The angle of the reflected tendon may be altered by surgery. Also, CT scanning may be used to compare the angle of the reflected tendon with the clinical function of the superior oblique muscles and to determine damage to the trochlear region (Fig. 3.8). However, in true Brown's syndrome, relatively little abnormality of the superior oblique tendon has been demonstrated by CT scan. This factor may explain the frequent poor results generally attained by surgical stripping of the sheath

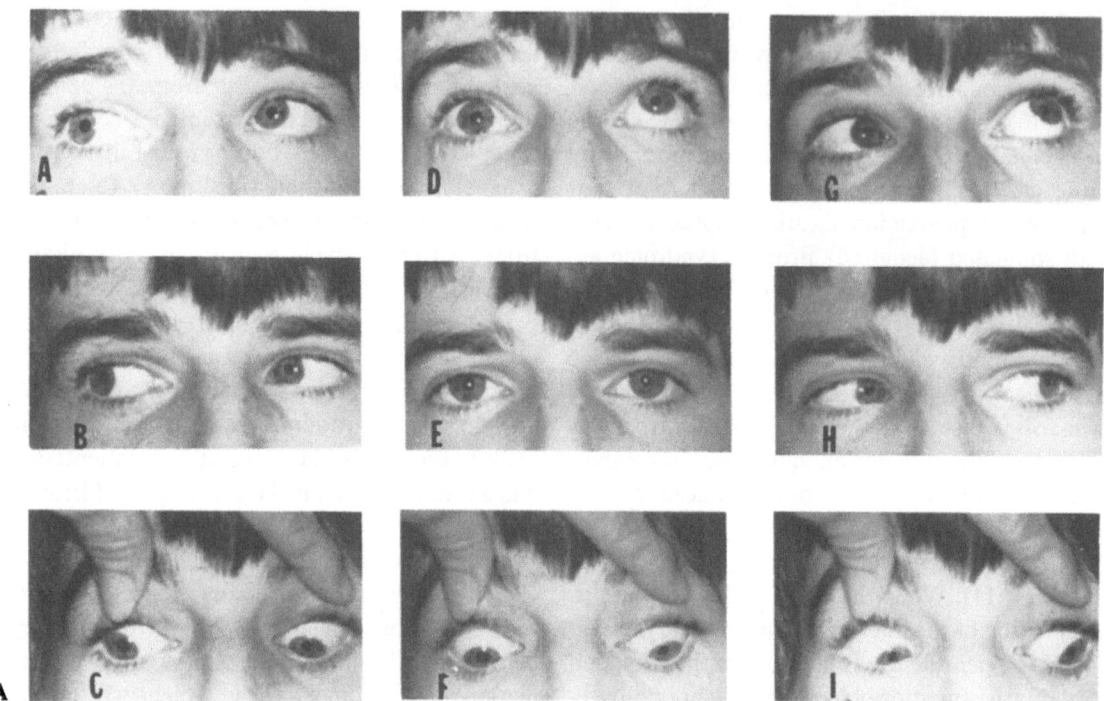

Figure 3.5 A. Acquired right superior oblique tendon sheath (Brown's) syndrome. Eyes are shown in various fields of gaze. The eyes are straight in the primary position (*E*); gaze right (*B*), gaze left (*H*), down and right (*C*), straight down (*F*), down and left (*I*). Notice failure of elevation of the right eye in upward midline (*D*) and up and left (adduction of right eye) positions of gaze (*G*). When the right eye is adducted nasally (*G*) from the primary position (*E*), the primary action of the right inferior oblique muscle in this position is elevation. Therefore, failure of elevation of the right eye in adduction (*G*) in this patient simulates paralysis of the right inferior oblique muscle (the hallmark of this syndrome). This is actually a pseudoparalysis that is not in the right inferior oblique muscle, but is due to the lack of appropriate relaxation of its antagonist; the right superior oblique muscle (Mafee, et al [12]).

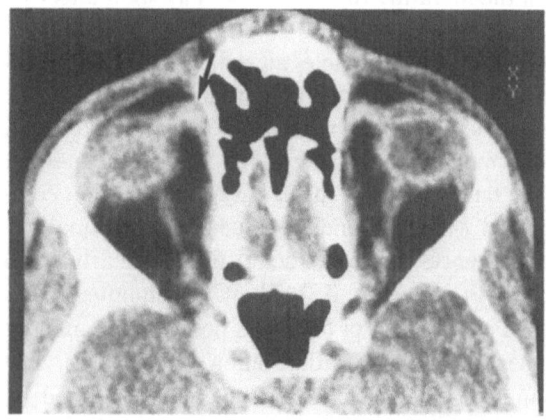

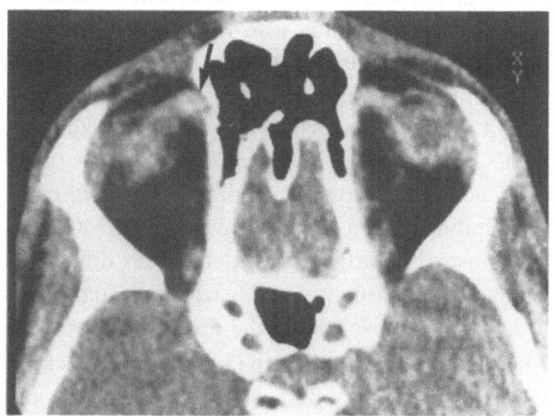

Figure 3.5 B. Acquired right superior oblique tendon sheath (Brown's) syndrome. Axial CT scan demonstrating thickening of the reflected portion of the right superior oblique tendon (arrow). The belly of the superior oblique muscle is seen on each side (Mafee, et al [12]).

Figure 3.5 C. Axial CT scan, obtained 1.5 mm superior to that shown in Figure 3.5B. Note marked thickening of the reflected portion of the right superior oblique tendon (arrow) (Mafee, et al [12]).

(12, 14). In contrast, patients with acquired Brown's superior oblique syndrome frequently show abnormalities of the superior oblique complex, which may assist the physician in the treatment of this condition.

Double Elevator Palsy

The major feature of double elevator palsy is a weakness of both elevators of the same eye (superior rectus and inferior oblique muscles). Double elevator palsy is almost always congenital (1), and elevation is limited through the entire upper field (Fig. 3.9A and 3.9B). Two patients with this syndrome demonstrated a small superior rectus muscle, although their inferior oblique muscle could not be definitely identified (Figs. 3.9C and 3.10) (17). Interestingly, one patient also had a large-sized inferior rectus (Fig. 3.9C and 3.9D). We do not know whether the size change is primary or secondary in nature (17). Congenital double elevator palsy must be differentiated from acquired conditions that cause a restriction in upward gaze, such as a blow-out fracture of the orbital floor, atypical Brown's syndrome, and endocrine myopathy with involvement of the inferior rectus (17). This differentiation is aided by forced duction testing and radiographic findings. Patients with double elevator palsy can be managed by transposing portions of the medial and lateral rectus muscles of the paretic eye to the superior rectus (Knapp procedure). One of our patients underwent a large recession of the inferior rectus, but a residual hypotrophia (Fig. 3.9E) still existed, requiring a secondary procedure.

Craniosynostosis Syndromes

Patients with craniosynostosis syndromes may have marked extraocular muscle anomalies, ranging from an apparent absence of ocular muscles noted at surgery (Fig. 3.11) to abnormally inserted or very small ocular muscles (Figs. 3.12 and 3.13) (18). One patient with Crouzon's syndrome had an unusual finding of absent superior oblique muscles on CT scan. In most of these patients, the inferior recti are displaced nasally and the superior recti are located more temporally (Figs. 3.12 and 3.13).

Endocrine Ocular Myopathy

Thyroid myopathy occurs most commonly in middle-aged women. It is ophthalmologically characterized by exophthalmos and in some patients by the gradual onset of diplopia, usually the vertical type. Initially, in the acute congestive phase, the retrobulbar orbital contents are markedly swollen and congested. Later, a more chronic, noncongestive phase follows, in which a restrictive type of limited eye movement often develops secondary to infiltration of the extraocular muscles and to subsequent loss of elasticity. The involvement can be unilateral or bilateral; when it is bilateral, it is often fairly asymmetric. The inferior rectus muscle is most commonly involved, leading to a limitation of elevation of the involved eye. The horizontal rectus muscles are also frequently involved, and the superior rectus and superior oblique muscles are less commonly affected. The forced duction test result is almost always abnormal.

Limitation of elevation is the most common disturbance of ocular motility in patients with Grave's disease (1). On attempted upgaze, intraocular tension may increase due to the restrictive process. The myopathy may occur at any time in the course of Grave's disease; laboratory evaluation may reveal hyperthyroidism, hypothyroidism, or euthyroidism. In fact, the disease occasionally is seen in patients who have been successfully treated for an overactive thyroid and who are euthyroid when first seen. Extraocular muscle enlargement in Grave's disease and associated compressive neuropathy, if any, can be visualized by CT scanning (Fig. 3.14) (18).

Unlike thyroid myositis, inflammatory myositis demonstrates an enlarged muscle cone and tendon, with conjunctival thickening over insertions of the muscles (19). The CT appearance of the extraocular muscles is very important in the differential diagnosis of orbital disease. Even slight changes of muscle size may be diagnostic in early stages of Grave's disease or ocular myositis (see also Chapter 10).

Traumatic Ocular Disorders

Computed tomography frequently is the diagnostic method of choice for radiologic evaluation of bones and soft-tissue disease of the craniofacial structures

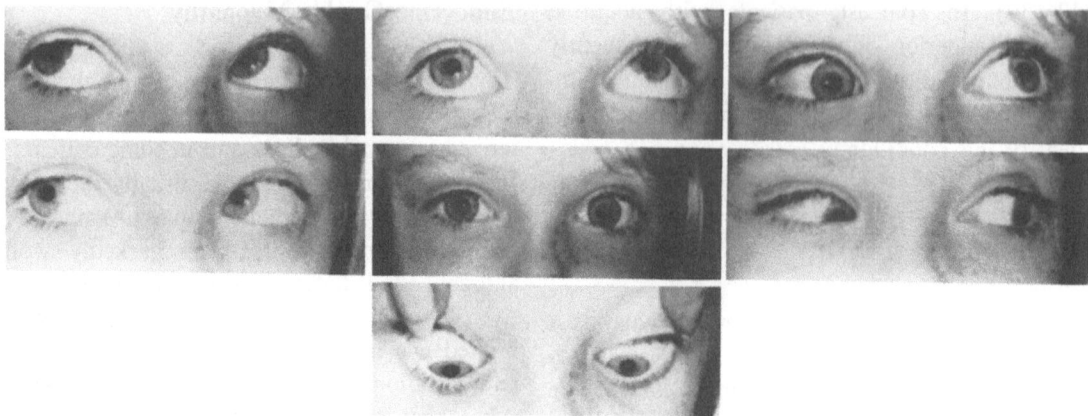

Figure 3.6 A. Congenital right superior oblique tendon sheath (Brown's) syndrome. Eyes are in various fields of gaze. Notice marked limitation of elevation of the right eye in upward midline (top middle) and, in particular, in adduction (top right) (Mafee, et al [12]).

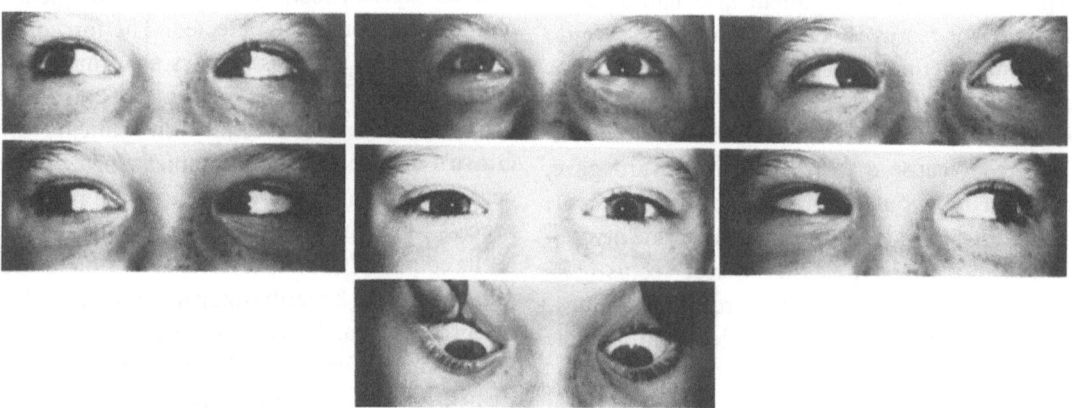

Figure 3.6 B. Same patient 11 months after tenotomy of the right superior oblique muscle. Note marked improvement in elevation of the patient's eyes both in adduction and abduction (Mafee, et al [12]).

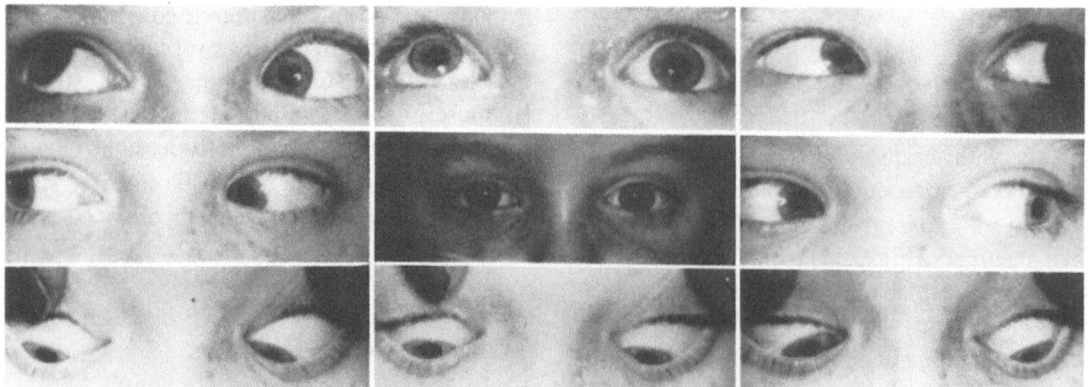

Figure 3.6 C. Same patient after acquired *left* superior oblique tendon sheath (Brown's) syndrome following trauma. Note limitation of elevation of the left eye in upward midline (top middle) and in adduction (top left) (Case courtesy of ER Folk, MD) (Mafee, et al [12]).

Figure 3.6 D. Axial CT scan demonstrates slight thickening of the reflected portion of the left superior oblique tendon (arrow). Note, however, a low-density image (hollow arrow) within the posterior aspect of the tendon that was considered to be due to edema or an old hematoma. The superior portion of the belly of the medial and lateral rectus muscles is visible (Mafee, et al [12]).

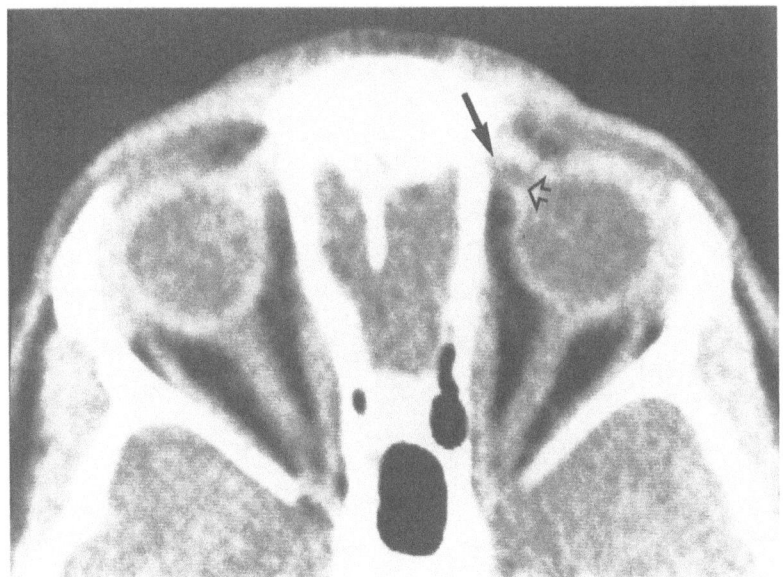

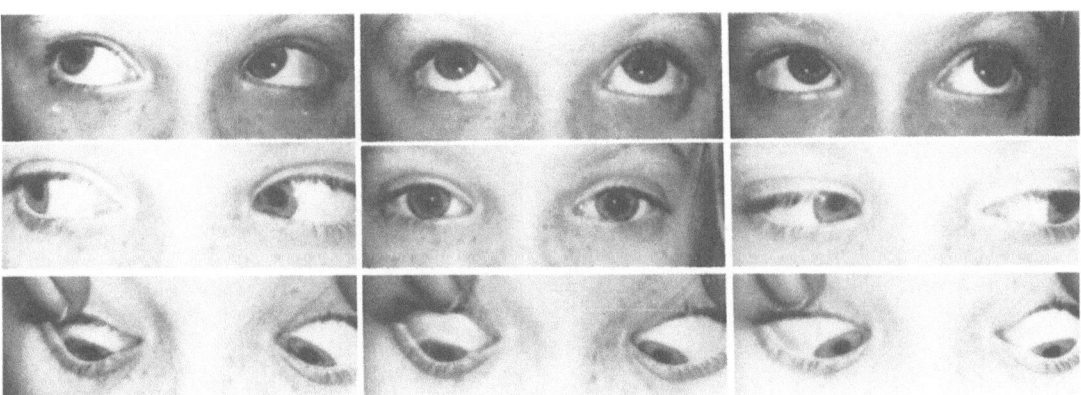

Figure 3.6 E. Two weeks after course of steroid therapy, there is marked improvement in the elevation of the patient's eyes both in adduction and abduction. (Mafee, et al [12]) (Case courtesy of ER Folk, MD).

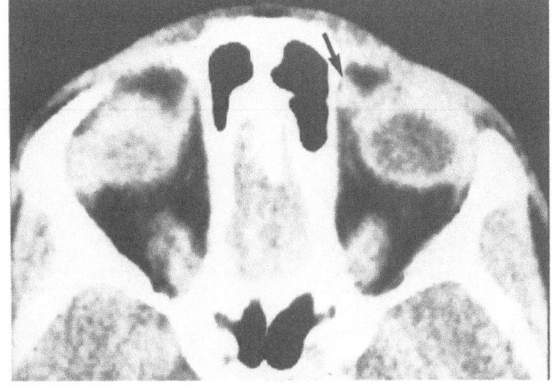

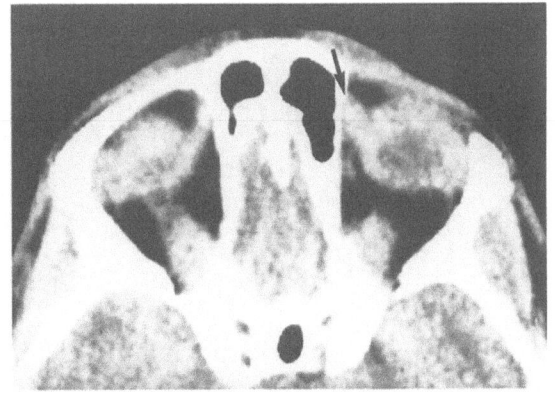

A   B

Figure 3.7 A. Acquired (rheumatoid arthritis) left superior oblique tendon sheath (Brown's) syndrome. Axial CT scan demonstrates thickening of the reflected portion of the left superior oblique tendon (arrow). **B.** Scan obtained 1.5 mm superior to that shown in Figure 3.3A demonstrates marked thickening of the reflected portion of the left superior oblique tendon (arrow) (Mafee, et al [12]) (Case courtesy of D Mittelman, MD).

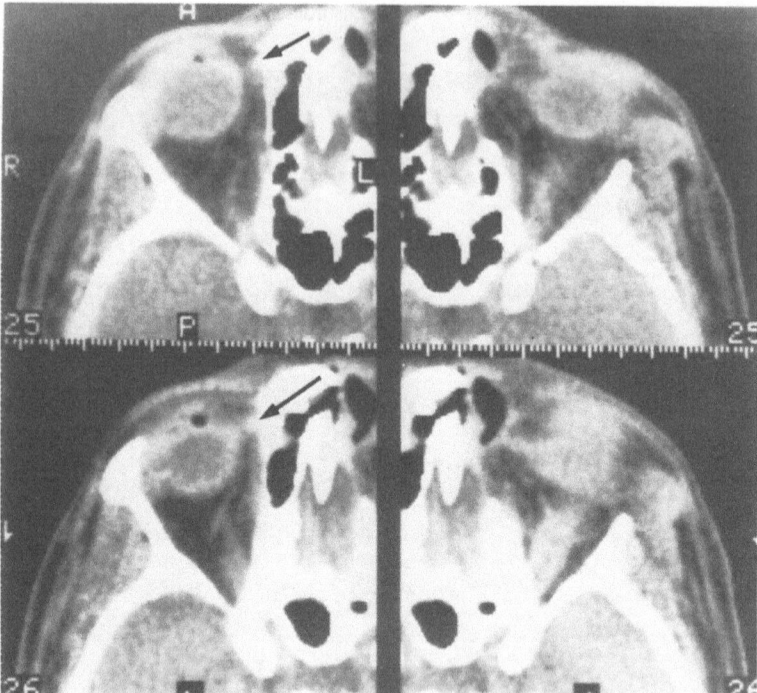

Figure 3.8. A 33-year-old woman developed left superior oblique muscle palsy after surgery for a frontal sinus osteoma. Note the normal reflected tendon of the right superior oblique muscle (arrows) and its absence on the left side. (Case courtesy of JZ Winkleman, MD) (Mafee, et al [12]).

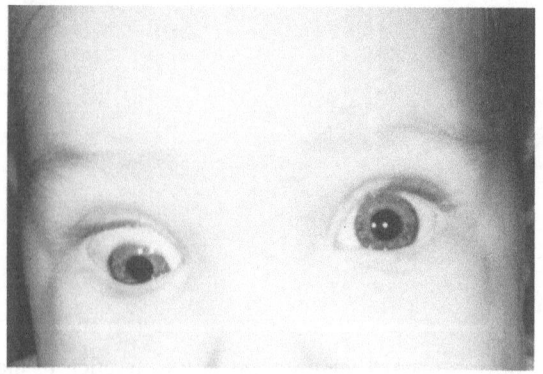

3.9A

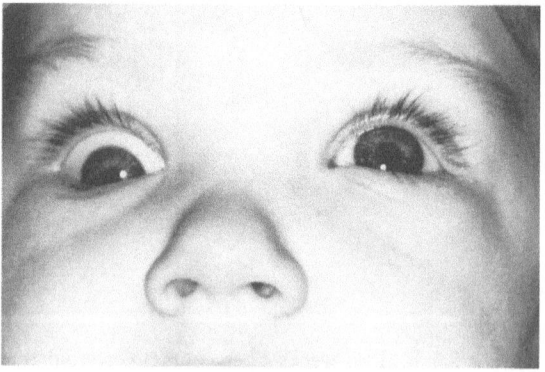

3.9B

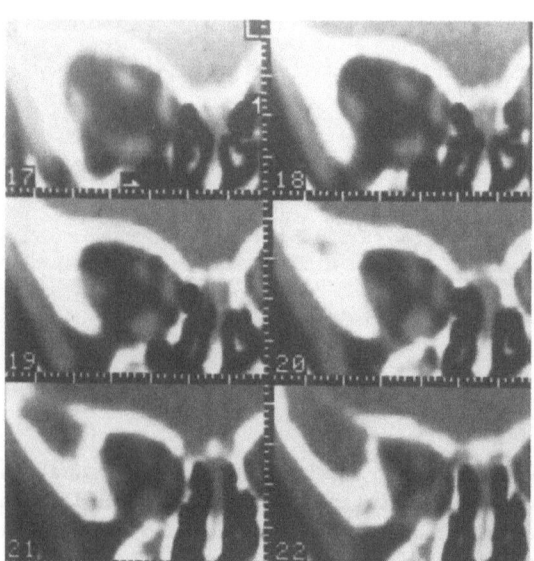

3.9C

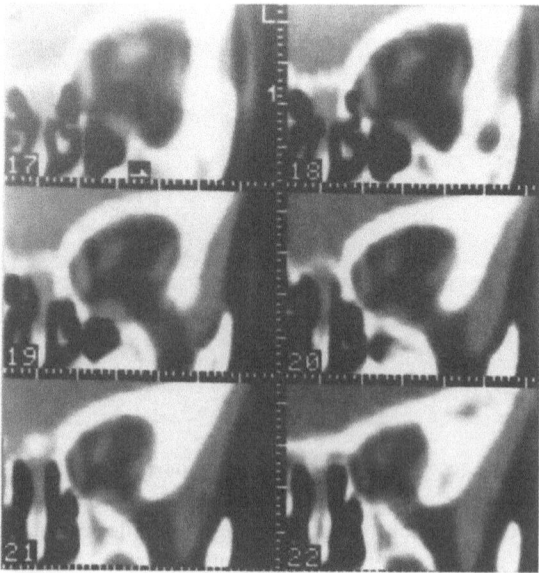

3.9D

(caption on facing page)

Figure 3.9 A. Double elevator palsy. Right hypotropia in the primary position in a patient with congenital double elevator palsy of the right eye (Courtesy of D. Mittelman, MD). **B.** Note limitation of elevation of the right eye (Courtesy of David Mittelman, MD). **C.** Double elevator palsy. Serial reformated coronal images showing enlarged right inferior rectus muscle. The superior rectus muscle is quite thin and hardly recognized as a distinct image. **D.** Serial reformated coronal images of the normal left eye of the same patient as in Figure 3.9C, for comparison. **E.** Note slight residual right hypotropia following recession of the right inferior rectus.

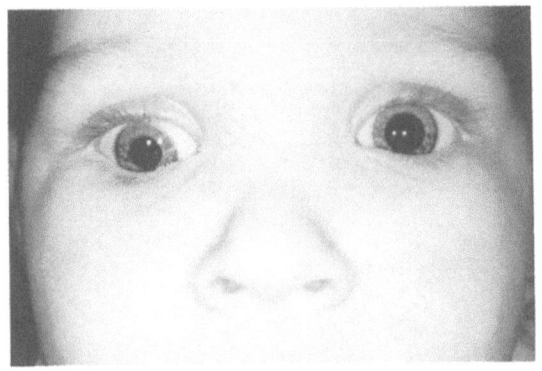

E

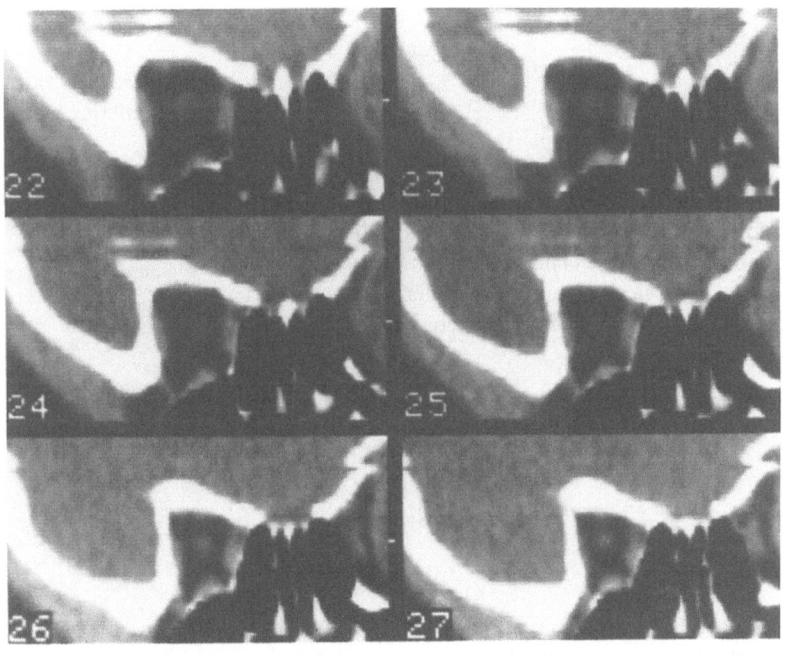

A

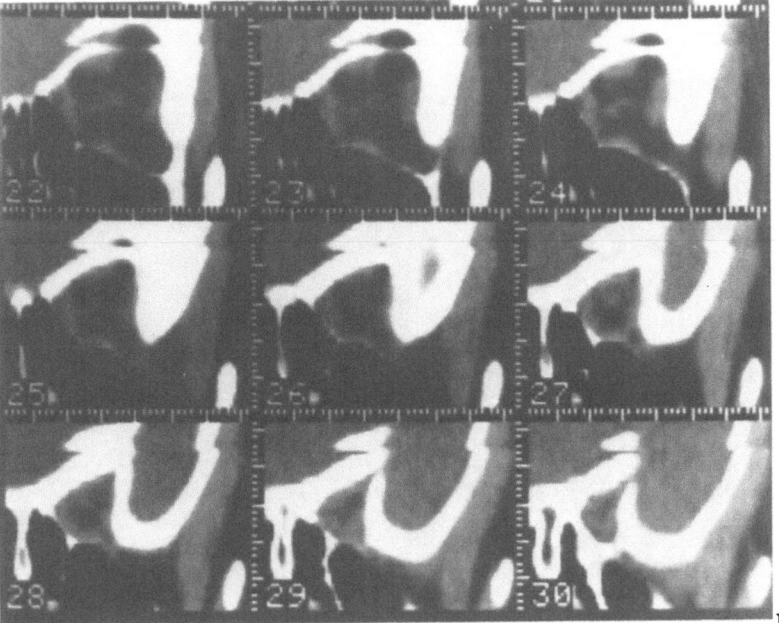

Figure 3.10 A. Double elevator palsy. Serial reformated coronal images showing flattening (thinning) of the superior rectus muscle. Unlike the patient in Figure 3.9C, the inferior rectus muscle in this patient is normal in appearance on CT scans. **B.** Serial reformated coronal images of the normal left eye of the same patient, for comparison. The superior rectus muscle is normal and is seen as a well-defined image.

B

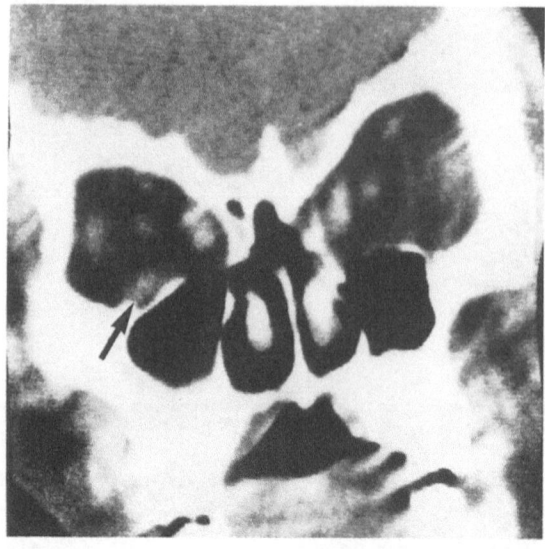

Figure 3.11. Coronal CT scan of the eyes of an 8-year-old boy with Crouzon's syndrome. The bony orbit is deformed and the left inferior rectus muscle is not visualized. On surgical exploration, no inferior rectus muscle was found. The right inferior rectus muscle is present (arrow).

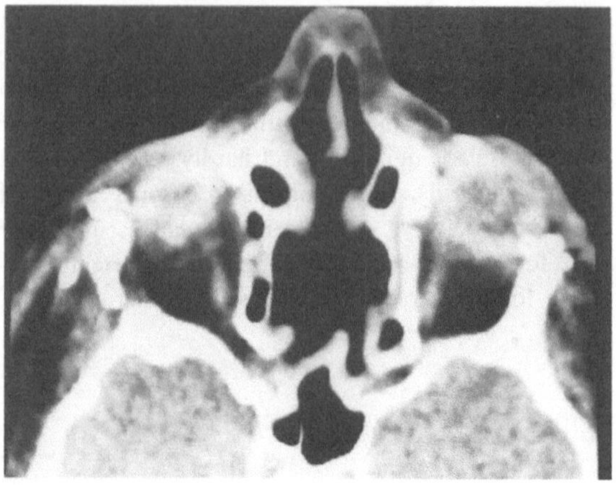

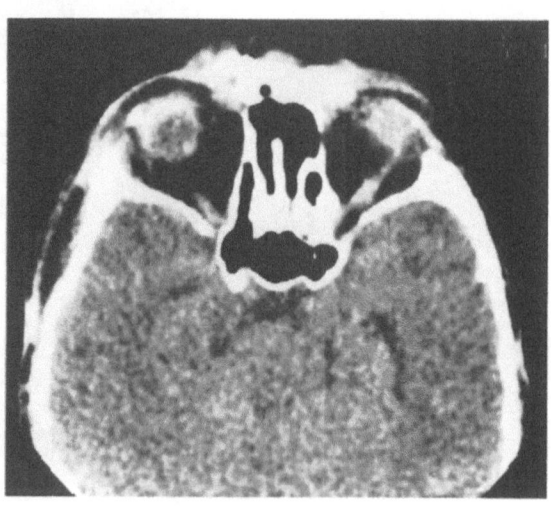

Figure 3.12. Crouzon's syndrome. Axial CT scan shows small inferior rectus muscles.

Figure 3.13. Crouzon's syndrome. Axial CT scan shows ▷ small superior rectus muscles, which are oriented more laterally than normal.

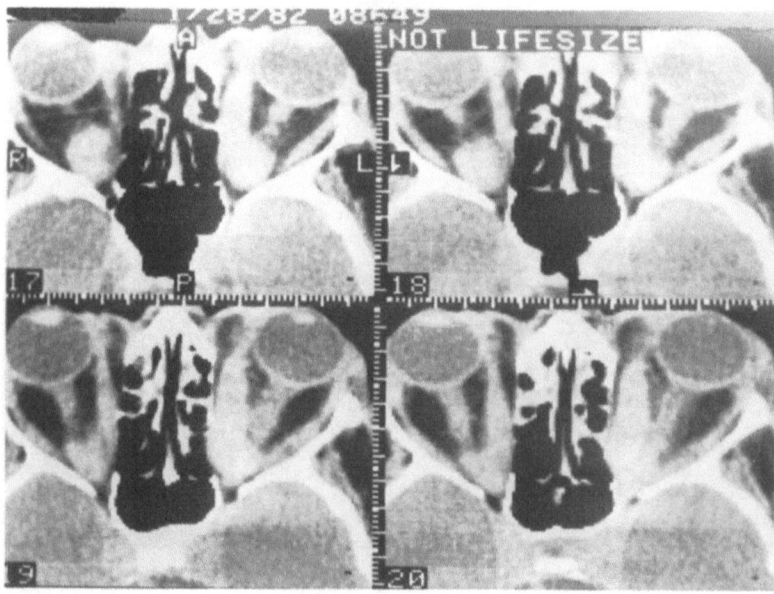

Figure 3.14. Thyroid myositis. A CT scan showing marked enlargement of the inferior rectus muscles. Notice enlarged left medial and lateral rectus muscles, resulting in strangulation of the left optic nerve.

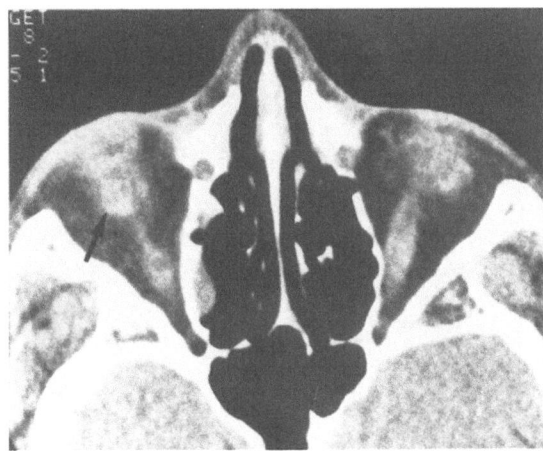

Fig. 3.15. Axial CT scan showing deformity of the right inferior rectus muscle (arrow) due to laceration of the muscle.

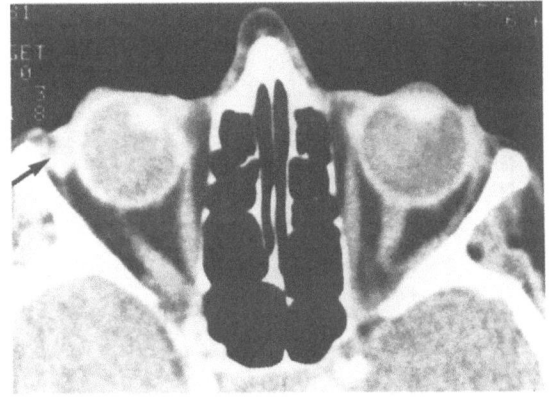

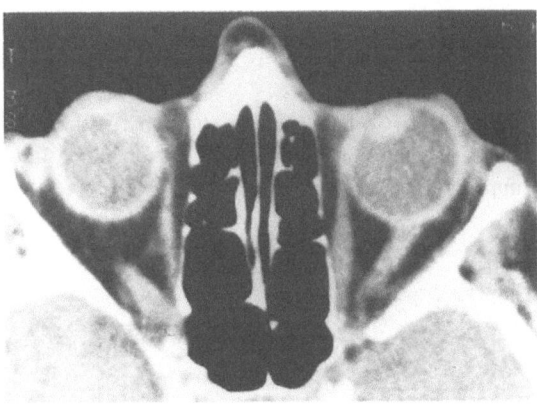

Figure 3.16. Atrophy of the right lateral rectus muscle. A CT scan in primary gaze shows nonvisualization of the right lateral rectus muscle. The right globe is turned to the left. Notice abnormal density (arrow) close to the insertion of the right lateral rectus, probably due to scar formation. This patient developed gradual loss of abduction of the right eye following a car accident. Nonvisualization of the inferior rectus was felt to be due to post-traumatic atrophy.

in injured patients. Figure 3.15 shows a posttraumatic CT scan of the right orbit some time after a knife stab wound in that area, after which the patient complained of vertical diplopia. Surgical exploration showed that the inferior rectus did not demonstrate any abnormality in the area of its insertion. Fibrous adhesions around the right inferior rectus and right inferior oblique muscles were lysed, but diplopia persisted. A CT scan of the eyes, with −15° tilt of the gantry, showed a laceration of the inferior rectus in the midportion of the belly (Fig. 3.15). Since the laceration was too far posteriorly to be approached surgically, a transplantation procedure in the form of a reverse Knapp procedure (i.e., the transposition of both the medial and lateral rectus muscles to the border of the inferior rectus muscle) was performed with excellent results.

The more serious complications of trauma or surgery on the extraocular muscles are torn or avulsed muscle and intramuscular hemorrhage. Therefore, the problem is a muscle that is not moving the eye in the desired direction. The CT scan is invaluable in providing information about the position of the muscle (Fig. 3.16).

Patients with blow-out fractures of the orbit may have significant ocular motility disorders. In such cases, the CT scan is a valuable way to evaluate the hard- and soft-tissue abnormality. Herniation of the orbital contents and extraocular muscles into the site of fracture (Figs. 3.17, 3.18, and 3.19) can be readily demonstrated by this technique. The CT scan also demonstrates any soft-tissue scarring

and the position of the prosthetic implant (Figs. 3.20 and 3.21) (20).

Conclusion

The investigation of abnormalities of ocular motility with imaging techniques is presently in an early stage. With CT, it is possible to demonstrate the anatomy and (to some extent) the physiology of the extraocular muscles as well as any intracranial neurologic cause. The magnetic resonance imaging technique has great promise for future use. It can show not only most of what is seen with CT, but also the brain stem and cranial nerves.

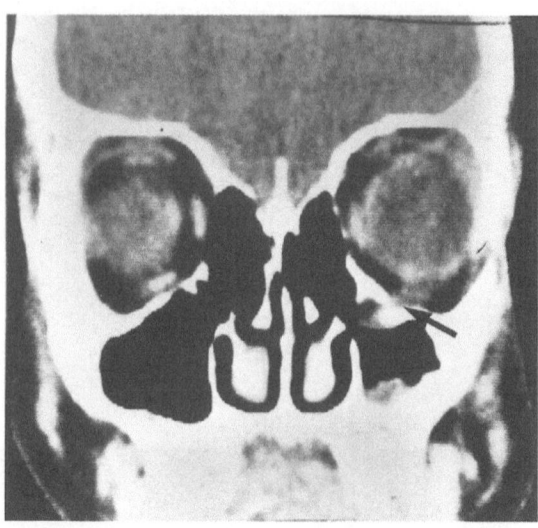

Figure 3.17. Coronal CT scan shows partial herniation of the left inferior rectus muscle (arrow). The muscle appears to be swollen.

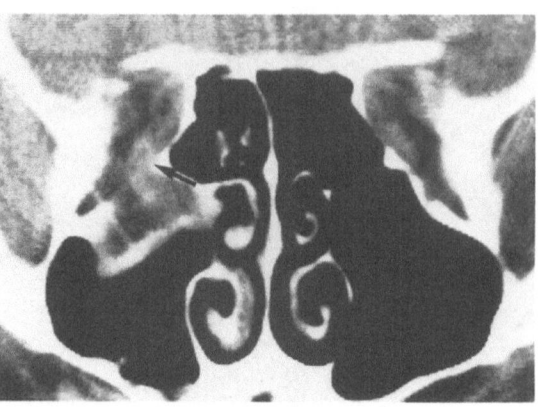

Figure 3.18. Coronal CT scan shows fracture of the floor of the right orbit and associated orbital fat herniation. Note the swollen right inferior rectus muscle (arrow), which is hooked over the site of fracture.

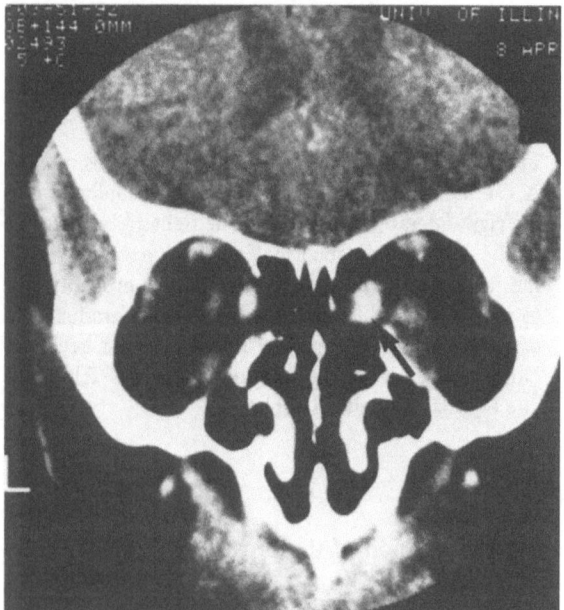

Figure 3.19. Coronal CT scan shows fracture of the medial wall of the left orbit. Note swollen, partially herniated left medial rectus (arrow) into the site of fracture.

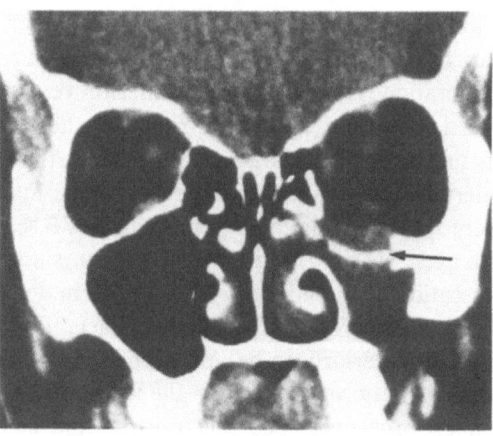

Figure 3.20. Coronal CT scan shows displaced silastic implant (arrow) and marked scar tissue along the left orbital floor.

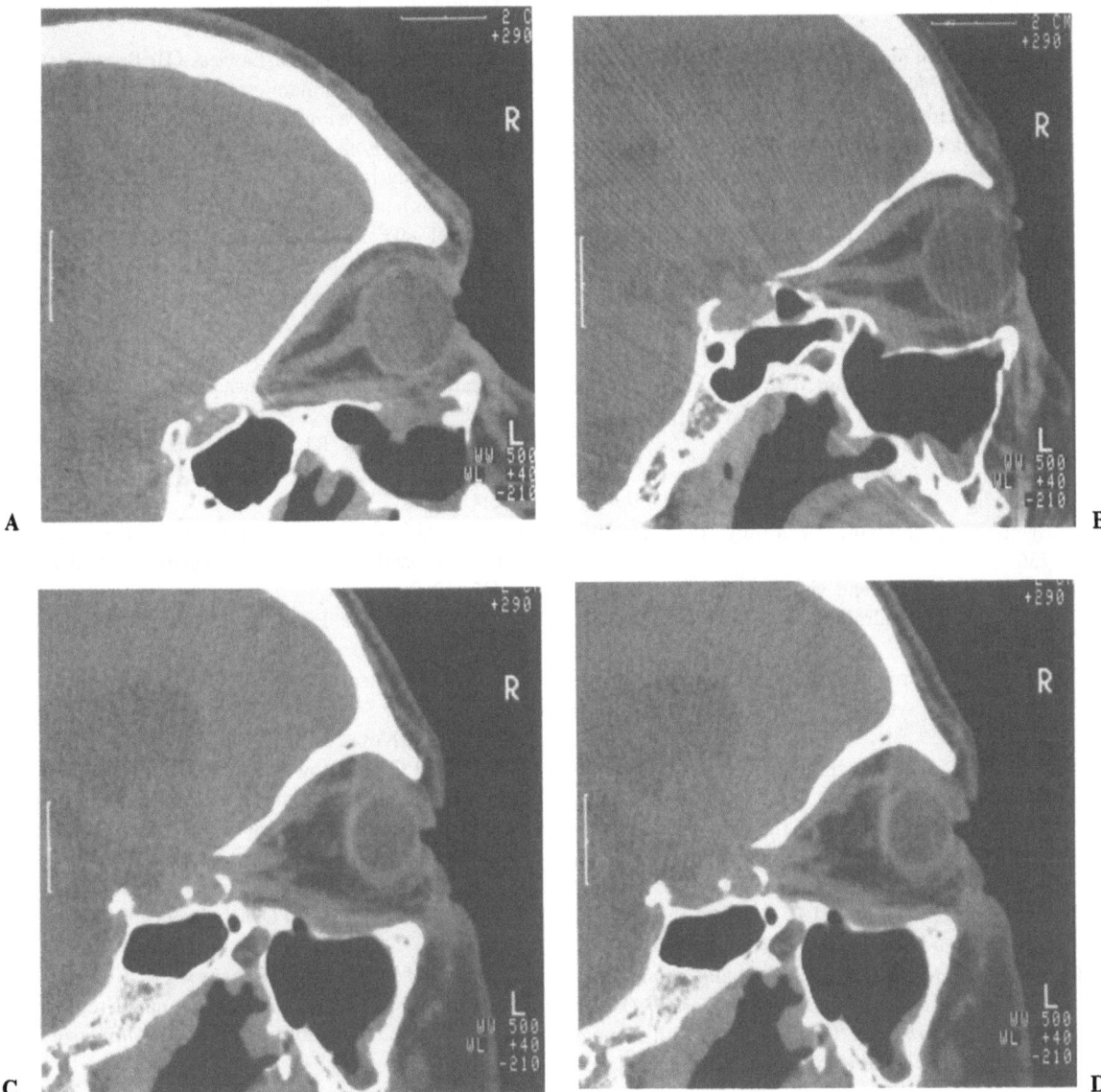

Figure 3.21 A. A 20-year-old boy, hit by a manhold lid of a Leopard tank, had a blow-out fracture, a motility impairment of inferior rectus without entrapment, and a prolapsed area filled with scar tissue. **B.** A 34-year-old man, punched in the eye during a fight, developed a blow-out fracture in the posterior part of the floor with scar tissue formation and a motility impairment of the inferior rectus muscle. Note fracture of the anterior wall of maxillary sinus. **C, D.** A 33-year-old man had motility impairment of the right inferior rectus muscle following reconstructive plastic surgery. Note scar tissue between inferior rectus and orbital floor (Case courtesy of L Koornneef, MD and FW Zonneveld, MSC).

References

1. Dale RT (ed): *Fundamentals of Ocular Motility and Strabismus.* New York, Grune & Stratton, 1982.

2. Sevel D, Hoyt C: *The Origin and Insertion of the Extraocular Muscles. Development, Histological Features, and Clinical Significance.* Presented at the 9th Annual Meeting of the American Association for Pediatric Ophthalmology and Strabismus. Vancouver, BC, Canada, August 3–6, 1983.

3. Fink WH: The anatomy of the extrinsic muscles of the eye, in Allen JH (ed): *Strabismus Ophthalmic Symposium.* St Louis, CV Mosby, 1950, pp 17–62.

4. Helveston EM, Merriam WW, Ellis FD, et al: The trochlea. A study of the anatomy and physiology. *Ophthalmology* 89:124–133, 1982.

5. Brown HW: Congenital structural muscle anomalies, in Allen JH (ed): *Strabismus Ophthalmic Symposium.* St Louis, CV Mosby, 1950, pp 205–236.

6. Brown HW: True and simulated superior oblique tendon sheath syndromes. *Doc Ophthalmol* 34:123–136, 1973.

7. Brown HW: True and simulated superior oblique tendon sheath syndromes. *Aust J Ophthalmol* 2:12–19, 1974.

8. Folk E, Miller MT, Mafee MF, et al: *Superior Oblique Tendon Sheath Syndromes.* Presented at the 9th Annual Meeting of the American Association for Pediatric Ophthalmology and Strabismus. Vancouver, BC, Canada, August 3–6, 1983.

9. Goldhammer Y, Smith LJ: Acquired intermittent Brown's syndrome. *Neurology* 24:666–668, 1984.

10. Mafee MF, Miller MT, Folk E, et al: *Computerized Axial Tomography as a Diagnostic Tool in Ocular Motility Disturbances.* Presented at the 9th Annual Meeting of the American Association for Pediatric Ophthalmology and Strabismus. Vancouver, BC, Canada, August 3–6, 1983.

11. Killian PJ, McClain B, Lawless OJ: Brown's syndrome, an unusual manifestation of rheumatoid arthritis. *Arthr Rheum* 20:1080–1084, 1977.

12. Mafee MF, Folk E, Langer BG, et al: Computed tomography in the evaluation of Brown's superior oblique tendon sheath syndrome. *Radiology* 154:691–695, 1985.

13. Mills PV, Coate MA: A case of acquired intermittent inferior oblique palsy. *Br Orthop J* 24:132–137, 1976.

14. Parks MM, Brown M: Superior oblique tendon sheath syndrome of Brown. *Am J Ophthalmol* 79:82–86, 1979.

15. Rayner J, Hiatt RL: Bilateral Brown's superior oblique tendon sheath syndrome. *Ann Ophthalmol* 5:412–417, 1969.

16. Sandford-Smith JH: Intermittent superior oblique tendon sheath syndrome. *Br J Ophthalmol* 53:412–417, 1969.

17. Mafee MF, Folk E, Miller MT, et al: CT in the assessment of ocular motility disorders. Presented at the 10th Scientific Assembly and annual meeting, Radiological Society of North America, Washington, D.C., Nov. 25–30, 1984.

18. Diamond GR, Katowitz JA, Whitaker LA, et al: Variations in extraocular muscles number and structure in craniofacial dysostosis. *Am J Ophthalmol* 90:410–418, 1980.

19. Trokel SL: Computed tomographic scanning of orbital inflammations. *Int Ophthalmol Clin* 22 (4):81–98, 1983.

20. Gilbard SM, Mafee MF, Lagouros PA, Langer BG: The diagnostic significance of computed tomography of orbital blow-out fracture. *Ophthalmology* (in press).

4
Ultrasonography of the Eye and Orbit

Richard L. Dallow

Ultrasonic techniques are essential for evaluation of the eye and orbital disorders. Ultrasound measures the eye accurately for calculating intraocular lens implants. More important diagnostic uses of ultrasound in the globe are to detect hidden hemorrhaging, retinal or choroidal detachment, vitreous organization, intraocular tumors, or foreign bodies. For orbital diagnosis, ultrasound identifies tumors with a high degree of tissue-typing and differentiates congestive and inflammatory orbital disorders.

Historically, ophthalmic applications of diagnostic ultrasound were first described in 1956 by Mundt and Hughes (11), using A-scan echo amplitude techniques. Two-dimensional ultrasonic imaging of the eye (B scan) was introduced in 1958 by Baum and Greenwood (1), and it was further developed separately by Purnell (14) and Coleman, et al (7). The water immersion system for ophthalmic ultrasonography devised by Coleman, Konig, and Katz (6) provided a practical means of combined A-scan and B-scan techniques that show both displays simultaneously and provide a maximum flexibility of electronic and mechanical adjustments. Bronson (4) reported a convenient motorized B-scan contact ultrasound system in 1972. A relief format showing A-scan amplitudes superimposed on the B scan image was reported by Coleman (7) to improve the appreciation of textures and contours. All of these techniques are currently in active clinical use, as summarized in publications of multiple authorship edited by Dallow (8), and by Chang, et al (5).

Technical Factors

Diagnostic ultrasonography is an imaging system that penetrates all soft tissues, and it is comparable in some respects to the radiographic technique of computed tomography (CT). When high-frequency sound is projected through soft tissues to be examined, the sound waves are partially reflected along the beam path at tissue interfaces that correspond to anatomic boundaries. These reflections are recorded on oscilloscopes either as echo spikes (A-scan format) or as dots (B-scan format). Although both displays are derived from the same original echoes, different information is gained from each of these presentations.

Ultrasound is defined as sound frequencies exceeding the audible range of 20,000 cycles per second (C/S), with the unit designation of (Hz). Medical diagnostic applications use a very high frequency in the millions of cycles per second: megahertz (MHz). The underlying physical basis for ultrasonography (meaning graphic presentation of sound echoes) is the piezo-electric effect of certain thin crystals and ceramic materials. This property is characterized by the emission of a specific sound wavelength through the deformation of the crystal when it is stimulated by an alternating electrical potential. Conversely, the crystal can receive echoes of the same wavelength and convert them into electrical potentials, which are then presented on an oscilloscope screen. This alternating emission-receiver arrangement is known as the pulse-echo system of ultrasound. The resonating crystal or ceramic, with its dampening, focusing, and electrical parts, is incorporated in a small instrument labeled the transducer.

Sound waves emitted by the transducer can be focused partially to produce a narrow beam of sound that is directed very precisely toward any object. Passage of the sound beam through soft tissues produces echoes at the interfaces between any two tissues of slightly differing densities (an acoustic impedance mismatch). The strength of the echo depends on the degree of contrast between these two adjacent tissues and the smoothness of the reflecting surface. Only a small portion of sound energy is reflected at most interfaces, with the remainder continuing through the tissues to be reflected at deeper interfaces. The power and exposure time are well below the levels that can produce burns in tissues when continuous-wave ultrasound is used therapeutically.

Oscilloscope displays of ultrasound echoes may present these echoes in several forms. A time-amplitude trace depicts the echoes as spikes with the vertical axis relating to the strength of reflectance properties, while the time scale on the horizontal axis indirectly relates a distance scale. Resolution between echoes anteroposteriorly in the tissue depends on the transducer frequency and the scanning technique used. The wavelength of the sound is the primary determinate of resolution, as it is inversely proportional to transducer frequency. A low frequency of 5 MHz resolves about 1 mm of tissue, while a 20-MHz transducer resolves 0.07 mm.

The ultrasound signals may be displayed as A-scan, B-scan, C-scan, D-scan (isometric), color-coded B-scan, M-scan, and Doppler. All displays are derived from the same tissue echoes, but different characteristics arise in each of these formats. The A-scan amplitude modulation is described above. The B-scan, or brightness modulation, presents echoes as dots rather than spikes, with the position of the echo being the same as on an A scan; but, with the intensity of the dot relating to the intensity of reflection. A complete B-scan image is composed of innumerable echo dots that are integrated from different beam locations as the transducer sweeps across the object in one plane. The resulting graphic two-dimensional image depicts outlines and internal tissue echoes of the object, resembling a thin histologic section. A C-Scan, or coronal section, is similar to a B-scan, except they are produced in the frontal or coronal plane. An isometric scan, or deflection modulation (D-scan), displays A-scan amplitudes superimposed on the two-dimensional B-scan image that has been tipped up on the Z axis of the oscilloscope. This produces an infinite gray scale of tissue densities. The resulting three-dimensional effect appears as a hilly terrain of echo amplitudes that enhances the examiner's appreciation of texture and internal echoes of lesions. One's perspective of this image is altered by rotating the tilted image through 360°, pivoted on a central axis at the transducer source. Another gray scale enhancement imaging technique is color-coding of the B-scan image. Color assignment is arbitrary, so the image colors can be manipulated at will. Resulting color images are quite vivid, but are rather coarse in amplitude differentiation. Motion characteristics of tissues are depicted ultrasonically with M scanning, which is a dot format with the transducer and the object stationary while the oscilloscope traces moves vertically. Thus, the relationship between two dots in time is depicted as wavy lines representing each reflectance interface. Motion of fluids, such as blood coursing through vessels, is detected with a Doppler ultrasound, which presents frequency alterations as fluids move towards or away from the transducer at variable speeds. Doppler signals are documented either by auditory changes in frequency or by a strip-graph charting.

Equipment and Techniques

Ultrasonography is a dynamic form of clinical examination. Echoes on the oscilloscope screen are constantly changing with alterations made by the examiner in probe position, transducer frequency, receiver sensitivity, and so on. Interpretation of findings is done during the course of this manipulative examination. Photographs are usually taken of the oscilloscope screen for documentation of findings, but these represent only a moment of the entire examination and are not truly representative of it. Unlike x-rays, interpretation of ultrasonography cannot be performed satisfactorily from still photographs in a retrospective fashion.

The three-dimensional character of the eye and orbit, and their abnormalities, can be appreciated by ultrasonography only through the entire manipulative process of examination from several different angles, with varying of electronic parameters and some educated guesswork. This process is similar to other clinical examination techniques (e.g., indirect ophthalmoscopy). In ultrasonography, the technical capabilities of the equipment are very refined, but the results of testing are no better than the individual examiner who performs the test. Thorough familiarity with ocular and orbital pathology is essential if the examiner is to obtain accurate diagnostic impressions from this technique. For these reasons, most ultrasonographers advocate that the test is performed by the ophthalmologist personally rather than by technicians.

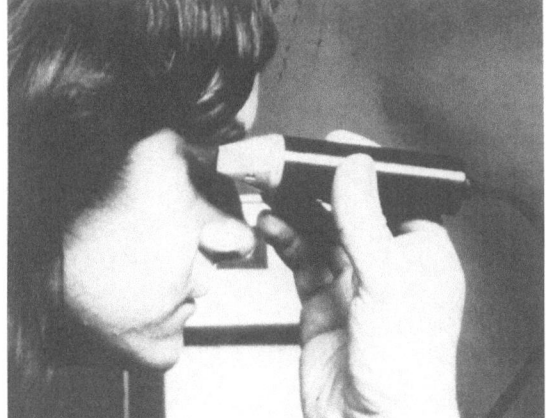

A

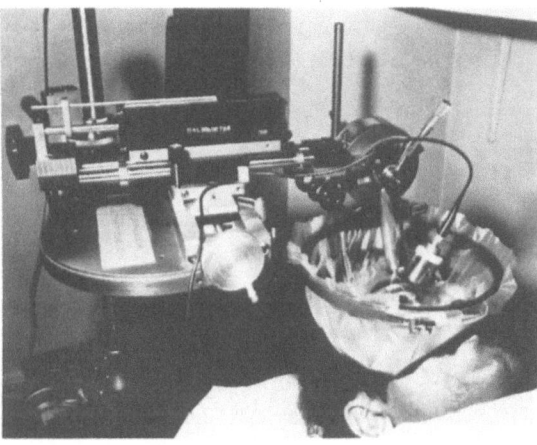

B

Figure 4.1. Techniques for ophthalmic ultrasound examination. **A.** Contact A-scan and two-dimensional B-scan probe with motorized-sector real-time capability. **B.** Immersion system for hand-operated real-time sector scan or storage static compound scan, with interchangeable transducers.

Both A-scan and B-scan ultrasonography can be performed by either a contact method or a water immersion method (Fig. 4.1). Some fluid coupling between the transducer and the object is necessary, because ultrasound does not travel adequately through air. For contact A-scan examination, the transducer probe is held directly against the eyelid or the globe, using a topical anesthetic drop and a viscous coupling agent. The probe may be directed from any angle, with the echo display from each position representing a narrow bore through the entire eye. Abnormal echoes are evaluated by modifying electronic variables on the instrument panel to characterize them in terms of location, density, thickness, shape, internal tissue echoes,

spontaneous movements, mobility, and other characteristics. A standardized A-scan instrument has been described by Ossoinig (13) for quantitative differentiation of tissues. Qualitative analysis of echo amplitudes can be performed with any instrument by relating abnormal echo amplitudes to the predictable echoes from any unvarying structure, such as the sclera. The two-dimensional morphology of tissue is not depicted with A-scan instruments, since this is a B-scan characteristic.

B-scan devices designed for contract use incorporate a small transducer within a fluid-filled compartment. The transducer is motorized to sweep continuously in a sector scan pattern. The smooth outside surface of the probe is placed against the eyelid with a viscous coupling agent similar to a contact A-scan examination. The B-scan image appears in real-time, continuously moving as the probe position or the eye internal structures move. The transducer must be moved manually to make it perpendicular to any abnormality, thus producing the maximal echoes from it. Contract methods of ultrasound examination are easily performed and have great flexibility. The equipment is portable, so that examination can be performed at the patient's bedside, in the operating room, or on uncooperative young children.

More sophisticated ultrasonography is possible with a more elaborate mechanical scanning device and electronics using a water bath placed over the eye. A practical water immersion technique incorporates a flexible plastic bag fixed around the orbital rim, with a large hole in it for the eye and lids to protrude through. The bag is suspended on a cantilevered hoop over the eye and filled with saline. The transducer is mounted on a hand-operated scanning apparatus in the water bath, but it is not in contact with the eye. Preparation for this method takes less than 3–5 minutes. While the technique is neither traumatic to the eye nor uncomfortable, the patient must lie still in the supine position. This immersion method is somewhat less convenient than contact methods, but improved scanning and electronics provide higher resolution and penetration for more accurate tissue differentiation. Transducer frequencies varying from 5–20 MHz are used with resolution of about 0.1 mm. The immersion system also permits more detailed examination of anterior portions of the eye because of the water stand-off. It enables better appreciation of the mobility of membranes within the eye as the patient looks from side to side with the transducer remaining stationary over it.

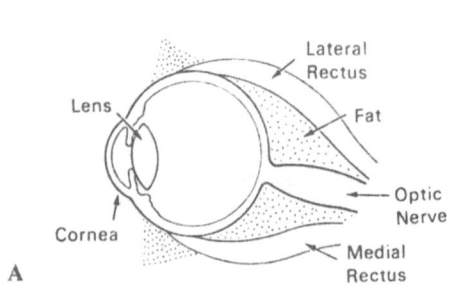

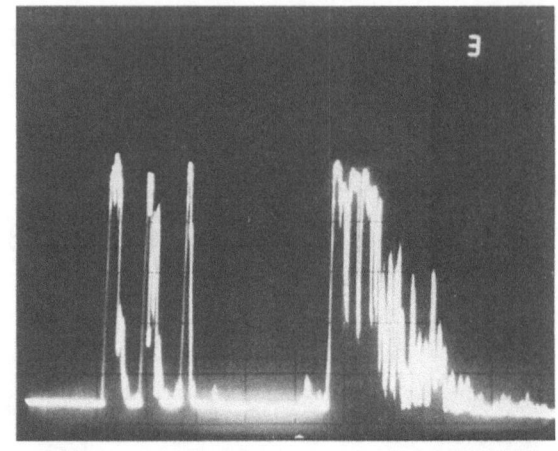

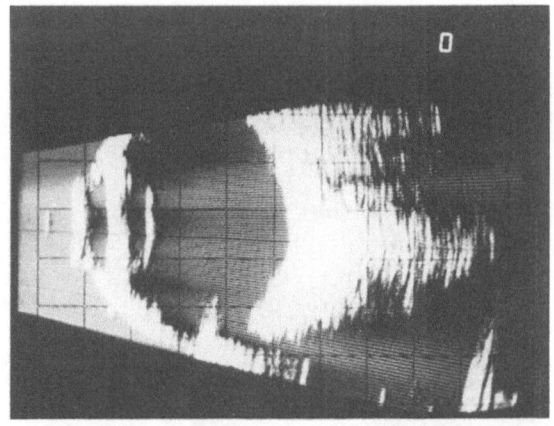

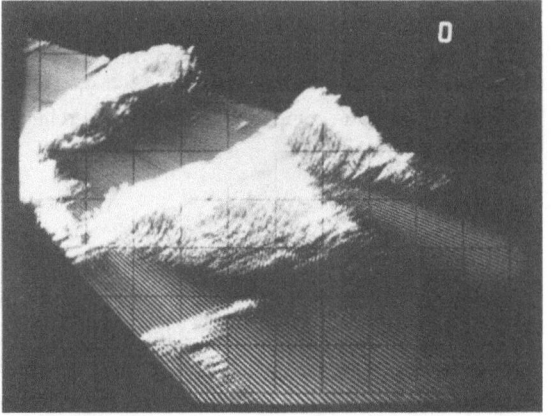

Figure 4.2. Normal eye. **A.** Diagram of major eye and orbit components, shown in horizontal (transverse) section. **B.** A-scan along the central axis. **C.** Contrast-enhanced (bistable) two-dimensional compound B-scan. **D.** Grey scale two-dimensional sector B-scan. **E.** Isometric D-scan demonstrating retinal surface; the bright vector line identifies the location of the displayed A-scan. **F.** Isometric D-scan with image rotated to allow the optic nerve to be viewed from behind the eye.

Ocular Diagnosis

A normal eye has a smooth, round contour with several internal reflecting surfaces: cornea, lens, iris, and the retina-choroid-sclera layers of the globe wall. Each of these structures produces high-amplitude, sharply defined echoes on A mode and smooth contours on B-scan images (Fig. 4.2). At its equator, the globe wall is incompletely depicted, because the ultrasound beam is oblique to this surface. Equatorial regions of the globe can be filled in by having the patient look from side to side or by reorienting the transducer laterally or medially so that the beam becomes perpendicular. Internally, the globe is filled with aqueous fluid (anteriorly) and a vitreous gel (posteriorly) through which sound is transmitted readily with no attenuation or internal echoes. The crystalline lens of the eye is composed of compactly organized tissue with no internal reflections unless a cataract is forming.

Retinal and Choroidal Detachment

Normally, the retina is appositioned with the choroid along the inner globe wall. Fluid or hemorrhage leaking beneath the retina causes it to detach and become elevated within the vitreous cavity. Even when fully detached, the retina retains its anatomic adhesion both at the optic nerve head posteriorly and to the ora serrata at the anterior periphery. Ultrasonically, a detached retina appears as a complete, smooth, and highly reflecting membrane within the vitreous cavity (Fig. 4.3). This membrane moves freely when visualized with real-time scanning as the patient turns his eye. There are many variations seen with retinal detachment. It may show only a localized area of elevation, instead of total detachment. Long-standing retinal detachment becomes organized and immobile, resulting in the late-stage appearance of a tight funnel configuration with connecting dense vitreous membranes and debris. A common retinal

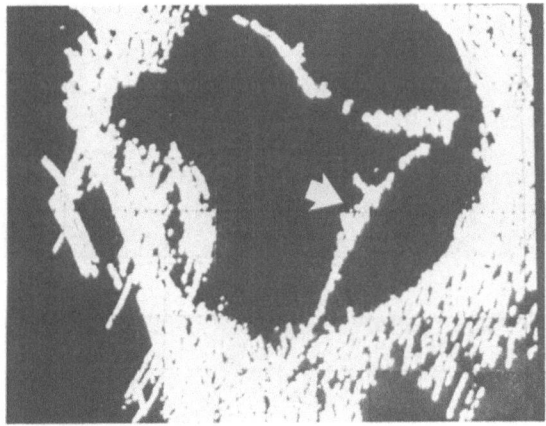

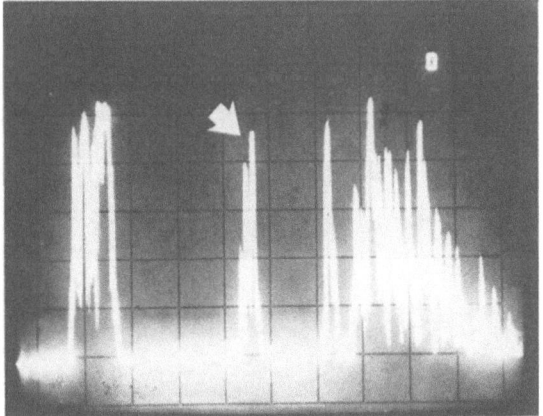

A   B

Figure 4.3. Retinal detachment. A. The two-dimensional B-scan shows a smooth membrane (arrow) emanating from the optic nerve and extending to the globe periphery. B. The A-scan shows a high-amplitude echo (arrow) in the midvitreous cavity. C. The isometric D-scan shows a sheet of uniform high-amplitude echoes (arrow).

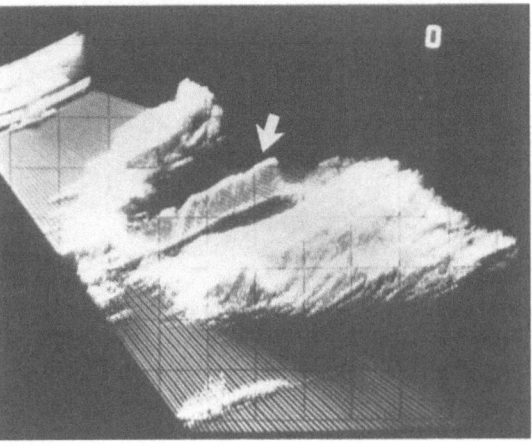

C

detachment pattern seen in diabetic, hypertensive, or trauma-related vitreous hemorrhage or fibro-proliferation is the appearance of a retina tented up in a peaked configuration with connecting vitreous membranes pulling it up.

Another major membrane configuration within the vitreous cavity is choroidal detachment, which appears as a smooth convex-elevated membrane located at the equatorial region of the eye, usually circumferentially. Because a choroidal detachment is thicker than the retina and inserts anteriorly near the lens equator and posteriorly near the globe equator, it is always distinguishable ultrasonically from a retinal detachment. The clinical implication of retinal and choroidal detachments are quite different.

Vitreous Opacities

Hemorrhage or inflammation occurring within the eye often spreads diffusely throughout the vitreous cavity, producing scattered low-amplitude echoes (Figs. 4.4 and 4.5). Denser debris of cellular aggregates may become confluent in some areas and layered along vitreous veils. Compared to a retinal detachment, vitreous veils appear somewhat incomplete, with irregular surfaces and only middensity echoes. These echoes tend to disappear on B-scan as the receiver sensitivity is lowered, whereas retinal detachment echoes persist at much lower sensitivity settings because they have more dense reflecting surfaces. The density, location, multiplicity, and configuration of the debris and mem-

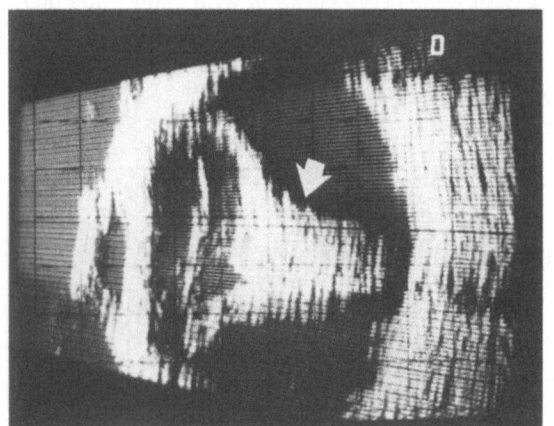

A

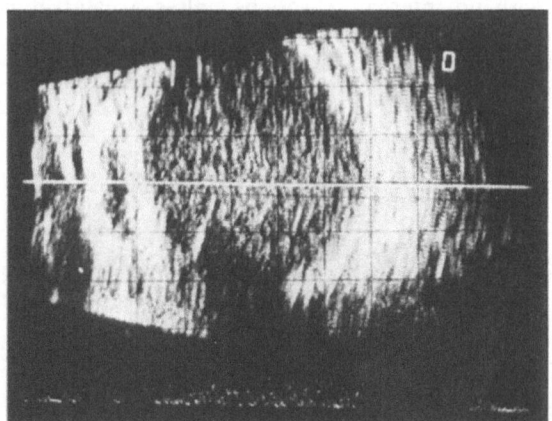

A

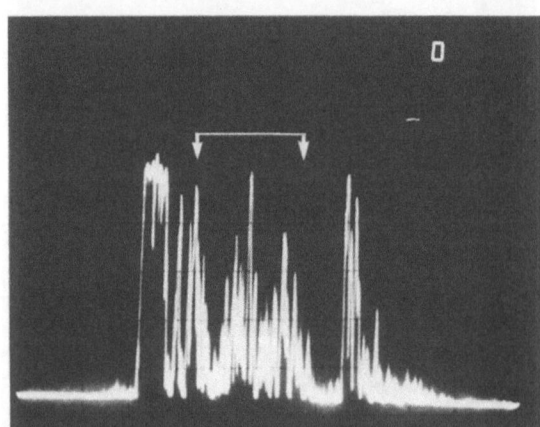

B

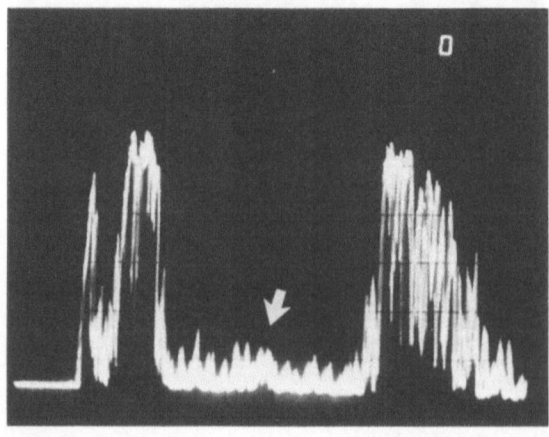

B

Figure 4.4. Vitreous cavity abnormalities. **A.** Total organized, inoperable retinal detachment seen on the two-dimensional B-scan as a funnel-like pattern (arrow) of moderate and (**B**) high-amplitude echoes from the disorganized fibrous tissue (arrows on A-scan).

Figure 4.5 A. Intraocular hemorrhage giving rise to diffuse low-amplitude echoes. **B.** Indicated by arrow on the A-scan.

branes is very important prognostically. Organizing membranes may detach the retina partially or totally by producing a progressively tightening traction within the eye. The vitreous gel is firmly attached to the globe wall at the same locations as the retina—the optic nerve head and the ora serrata region. Hence, dense vitreous membranes sometimes simulate the appearance of a retinal detachment, making their differential diagnosis impossible at times. Serial ultrasound examinations conducted over several weeks or months will show the evolving patterns of vitreo-retinal pathology and will serve as the primary guidelines for determining when vitrectomy and retinal surgery are appropriate.

Foreign Bodies

The eye is vulnerable to direct trauma from blunt as well as sharp objects. Blunt injury produces internal changes, such as retinal detachment or vitreous hemorrhage. Propelled, small foreign bodies (such as metal chips or glass fragments) may cause penetrating injury with the object retained within the eye, possibly with internal hemorrhage obscuring its location. Surgical removal of intraocular foreign bodies usually is advisable if they can be located precisely—ultrasound serves this purpose admirably. All foreign materials are detectable with ultrasound, but some significant limitations exist. Metal, glass, plastic, and stone are prominent reflectors, producing higher amplitude echoes than any normal structure except bone. Wood and vegetable matter reflect only intermediate amplitude echoes and thus may be quite difficult to distinguish. Ultrasound indicates not only the presence of foreign bodies, but also their relationship to the globe wall and the presence of associated disorders, such as retinal detachment (Fig. 4.6).

Foreign body detection is aided by the ultrasonic artifact of acoustic shadowing when the foreign body reflects sound totally. Lowering the receiver sensitivity on the oscilloscope demonstrates the persistence of a strong foreign body echo beyond that of all other echoes. The degree of foreign body response to a magnetic field can be graphically visualized by A scan or M scan. At the time of surgical removal of a foreign body, ultrasound can be of major importance for precision localization and extraction during the surgical procedure.

Foreign bodies do present several problems to

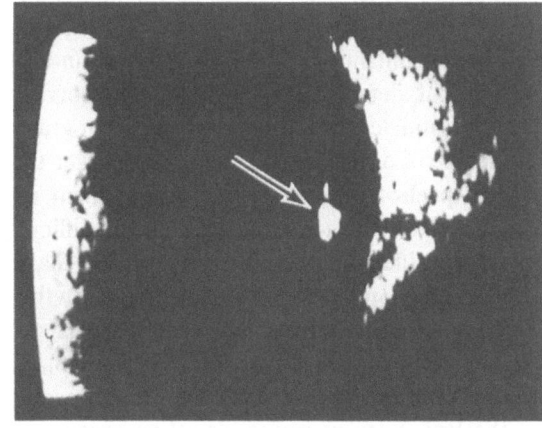

A

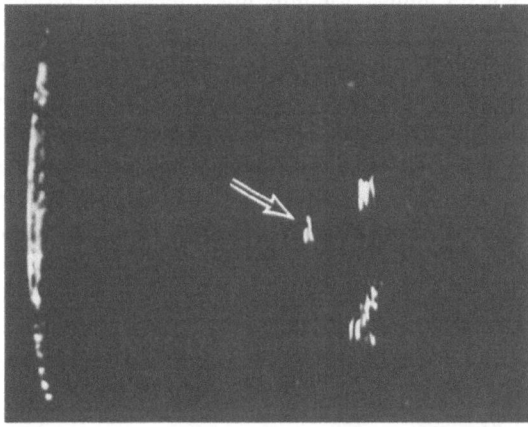

B

Figure 4.6. Foreign body within the eye. **A.** High-amplitude localized echo (arrow) with acoustic shadowing. **B.** The echo remains (arrow) with reduced receiver gain.

ultrasound diagnosis. They often are quite small and linear in shape. The ultrasound beam must be precisely perpendicular to the flat side of such foreign bodies to produce an echo. Thus, some foreign bodies may be missed on ultrasound scanning, because the orientation is not optimally perpendicular. It is sometimes easier to first identify the presence and general location of foreign material by plain x-ray films or CT; then ultrasound can be used for precise localization in reference to other ocular structures and for assessment of other soft-tissue abnormalities such as retinal detachment.

Intraocular Tumors

The most common intraocular tumors in adults are malignant melanoma, metastatic tumors, and hemangioma. In children, retinoblastoma is more significant. Other mass lesions may simulate a tumor clinically, such as subretinal hemorrhage, parasites, and inflammatory focci. A tumor underlying retinal detachment or vitreous hemorrhage may be undetectable clinically. Ultrasonography is capable of detecting all mass lesions larger than 1 mm in elevation and characterizing them into cystic, solid, or angiomatous types. Some difficulty exists in differentiating fibroproliferative masses from true neoplasms, but monitoring growth of a lesion on serial ultrasound examinations over time usually reveals the presence of a neoplasm. Ultrasound assumes a crucial role when opacities of the lens, vitreous cavity, or retina obscure the view for clinical examination of posterior portions of the eye.

The usual B-scan ultrasonic appearance of malignant melanoma is a mass along the inner globe contour, with a highly reflective, smooth convex contour. The internal tissue A-scan pattern is one of gradual decay (attenuation) of closely spaced echoes throughout the mass (Fig. 4.7). These ech-

oes derive from cellular aggregates, fibrous septae, and vessels within the mass; of course, this appearance can vary. Most melanomas consist of compact masses of similar cells; occasionally however, a necrotic center or a fungating growth pattern will alter the ultrasound findings. A polypoid or "button" appearance may be produced. Other types of tumors do not generally show this configuration. While melanomas expand primarily inward within the eye, they also frequently produce an apparent shallow "excavation" posteriorly by replacing the choroidal coat of the eye from which they originate. This appears as a concave indentation of the normal globe contour posterior to the tumor, and it is highly characteristic of malignant melanoma. An A scan can be critical in differentiating lesions, especially when the B scan image is equivocal. A localized vitreous hemorrhage may appear compact enough on a B scan to resemble a tumor mass. A-scan amplitudes show a high lead echo for tumors with a gradual decay of amplitudes; whereas, amplitudes from a hemorrhage are much

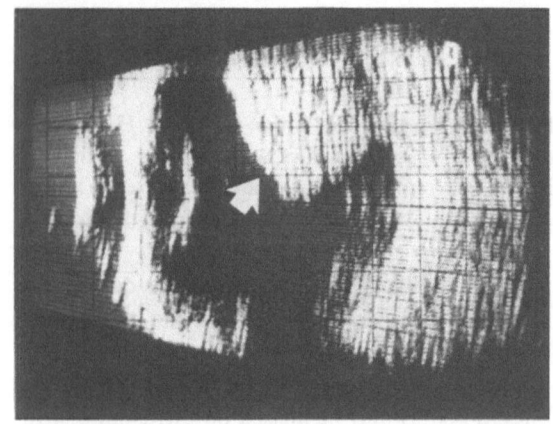

A

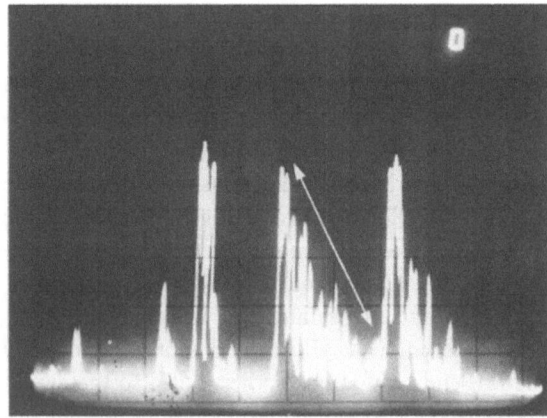

B

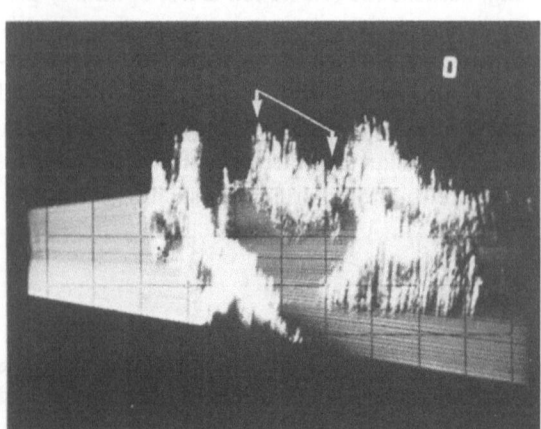

C

Figure 4.7. Intraocular tumor (malignant melanoma). **A.** The two-dimensional B-scan shows a well-defined, rounded mass of confluent echoes (arrow). **B.** The A-scan shows that the amplitudes of these echoes have a characteristic exponential decay (arrows). **C.** The isometric D-scan provides a better appreciation of the internal tumor texture of echoes.

lower, more closely arranged, and scintillating because of a slight motion of red blood cell aggregates producing the echoes. Tumors may be measured by ultrasound to document size and growth by using a high-resolution transducer (15 or 20 MHz) for accuracy greater than 0.1 mm in tumor height.

Metastatic tumors within the eye have the same locations as melanomas; i.e., within the uveal tract, and most frequently in the posterior pole of the eye. They may be due to any source, including tumors of the breast, gastrointestinal system, lung, prostate, and so on. In contrast to melanomas, metastatic tumors tend to have a flat configuration on B scanning, appearing as a low undulating mass elevated only to 1 mm, but having a broad base diameter. Metastatic tumors may be multiple, whereas melanoma is nearly always solitary. A-scan patterns differ little from melanoma patterns.

Hemangiomas also arise within the choroid component of the uveal tract. This benign and generally nonprogressive tumor has a very low elevation and a broad base dimension. The tumor composition of multiple small vascular channels and blood-filled spaces produces a characteristic A-scan appearance of sustained high-amplitude echoes throughout the mass, with a very regular spacing between them. If the lesion is large enough, it usually can be differentiated from solid tumors by ultrasonic criteria.

Retinoblastoma is the most common intraocular malignancy in children, but it is often masked by opacities such as cataract, hemorrhage, or vitreous membranes. It is often seen initially in a fairly advanced stage with a large fungating lesion having necrotic foci, calcium deposits, and associated vitreous debris and retinal detachment. The ultrasound pattern is quite variable because of these multiple elements. It always shows an irregular pattern of high-amplitude echoes and membranes. The detection of a multiple "foreign body" type of very high echoes reflected from the calcium deposits within the tumor is very suggestive of retinoblastoma. However, this sign is not always present.

Other nonneoplastic conditions may simulate the appearance of intraocular tumors, both clinically and ultrasonically. One particularly difficult lesion to differentiate is an organized subretinal hemorrhage (disciform maculopathy), which is a common abnormality found in elderly patients. It appears on B scan as a small elevated mass in the posterior pole of the eye, having the same size, shape, and configuration of a small melanoma. The A-scan pattern also may be indistinguishable from melanoma. Serial ultrasound examinations over time are necessary to demonstrate that a hemorrhage is static or regressing, rather than showing an increase in size that would imply a neoplasm. Many other lesions can resemble tumors on ultrasound examination, including vitreous hemorrhage, retinal and choroidal detachment, ciliary body cysts, brawny scleritis, lymphoid hyperplasia, melanocytoma, dislocated cataract, foreign bodies, parasites, and papilledema. Most of these disorders yield sufficient evidence on ultrasonography to be differentiated from neoplasms. The reliability of ultrasonic intraocular tumor differentiation has been documented by several investigators with a concensus of greater than 90% accuracy, regardless of the specific techniques and equipment employed.

Orbital Diagnosis

Soft tissues within the bony orbit have the potential for developing a large variety of tumors and inflammatory-congestive disorders. All of these may have similar clinical presentation of a protruding eye with no clinical evidence of the responsible disease. In fact, the most common causes of exophthalmos are inflammatory diseases, such as thyroid-related Graves' disease, pseudotumors, and cellulitis, rather than true neoplasms. The incidence of specific tumors varies in different series and for different age groups. A rough descending order of orbital tumor frequency is neurogenic tumors, cysts (mucocele or dermoid), hemangioma, lymphoma, metastatic tumor, lacrimal epithelial tumors, and secondary tumors invading from adjacent sinuses. Some arteriovenous anomalies can simulate orbital tumors, including varices and shunts. Radiography, CT, and ultrasound are essential tests for defining orbital abnormalities and for guiding surgical approaches to tumors.

Normal orbits produce a consistent picture on B-scan ultrasonography. The eye portion of the scan shows a clear delineation as a rounded structure. The retrobulbar pattern is derived primarily from the large fat pad, which has a triangular shape and is bounded both anteriorly by the globe concavity and on the sides by the extraocular muscles extending from the globe equator toward the apex of the orbit at the optic canal. The fat is quite heterogeneous, being composed of fat globules, fibrous septae, vessels, and nerves. High-amplitude echoes are produced throughout the fatty tissue complex, giving it a "filled-in" appearance on the B-scan image and a decaying high-amplitude pattern on A scan. The extraocular muscles and optic nerve are more compact, well-organized homogeneous tissue compared to the fat pad. These structures appear as relatively echo-free areas in contrast to adjacent fat. Hence, a B-scan section at the level of the optic nerve produces a W-shaped area of echoes posterior to the globe, with muscle and the optic nerve seen in negative contrast. The bony orbital wall is represented only by a few low-amplitude echoes, partly because the beam is not perpendicular to its surface and because the sound undergoes a shearing effect when it strikes bone. When the scan plane is directly above or below the optic nerve, a V-shaped fat pad is seen instead. Scanning may be performed in a horizontal, vertical, or oblique plane to visualize more peripheral structures. It is highly recommended that scans are performed in multiple meridians, as well as at multiple levels, so as not to overlook any pathology.

Several electronic and mechanical factors influence ultrasound imaging of the orbit. The transducer frequency that is necessary is somewhat lower than that used for intraocular diagnosis, because deeper penetration and more sensitivity are required; whereas, a high resolution is not as critical. Usually a 5- or 10-MHz transducer is best for orbital diagnosis. This will penetrate completely to the orbital apex and will bring out lower amplitude echoes. The scan pattern is another factor in imaging. A sector scan of the type produced by most contact B-scan instruments has the transducer pivot on a fulcrum, and it produces a pie-shaped sector image. Only about two thirds of the eye and orbit produce echoes in the sector scan, since many tissue interfaces are not perpendicular to the beam. A compound scan pattern produced only with the hand-operated transducer of the immersion system directs the beam from all angles, with the pivotal point being approximately in the center of the globe. Compound scan-

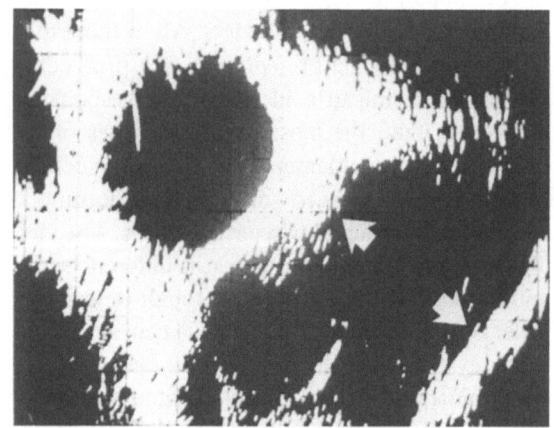

A

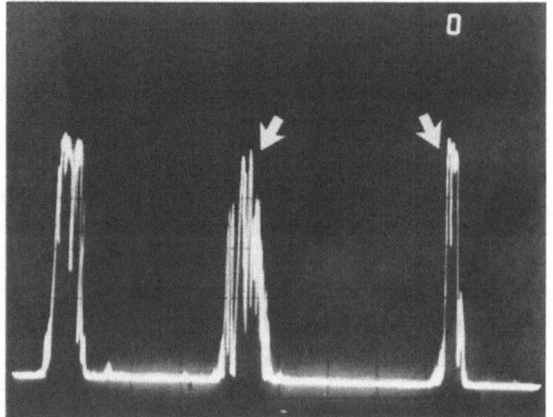

B

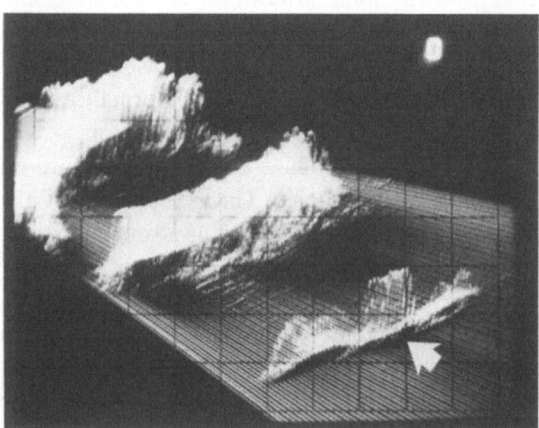

C

Figure 4.8. Large orbital cyst (mucocele). A. The two-dimensional B-scan shows a sharply demarcated ovoid mass with smooth walls (arrows). B. The A-scan shows strong interface echoes (arrows) with no internal tissue echoes. C. The isometric D-scan with image rotation displays the smooth posterior wall (arrow) of the cyst.

ning results in a more complete outlined image, deriving maximal echoes from all possible directions—but with some artifacts introduced and the gray scale sacrificed. A combination of these methods is best if appropriate equipment is available.

Orbital evaluation with ultrasound is a proven, reliable, and often unique detector of orbital pathology. With the convenience of examination and lack of morbidity of this test, ultrasonography often is the first procedure indicated when orbital pathology is suspected. Not only can it direct further studies, but it can properly direct the choice and route of any indicated surgery. Orbital abnormalities may be classified by ultrasonic criteria into four major categories: 1) mass lesions; 2) inflammatory congestive changes; 3) structural anomalies; and 4) foreign bodies. Each of these categories has several well-defined subdivisions of further ultrasonic classification.

Tumors of the Orbit

Orbital tumors, either malignant or benign, are classified by two-dimensional B-scan ultrasonography in terms of location, size, contour, and ability to transmit ultrasonic waves. A-scan criteria add additional information on the internal structures of tumors. Four general tumor types are easily identifiable: cystic, solid, angiomatous, and infiltrative.

Cystic tumors seen on a B-scan have a smoothly rounded contour that is sharply defined from adjacent structures and that often causes some distortion of normal tissues by compression. Cystic masses demonstrate good sound transmission with a clear definition of the posterior wall of the lesion and of tissues posterior to the tumor. Internally, cysts are generally devoid of echoes, because they have no significant tissue interfaces within the lesion. The exceptions to this are dermoid cysts, which may have considerable internal debris producing low-amplitude echoes throughout the mass. Cysts located anteriorly in the orbit generally represent dermoid or epithelial cysts, while those more posterior along the bony orbital walls frequently are mucoceles originating from the adjacent sinuses (Fig. 4.8.).

Solid tumors also demonstrate well-defined contours ultrasonically that contrast with adjacent tissues. The tumor contour may be smoothly rounded or somewhat irregular. In contrast to cysts, a solid tumor produces a significant sound

attenuation, so that penetration is poorer and so the posterior margin of the tumor may not be well defined ultrasonically with higher frequency transducers. Switching to a lower frequency transducer will usually permit better definition in these instances. Tissue interfaces within the tumor produce low-amplitude to midamplitude echoes within its substance, indicating a moderately heterogeneous tissue. A rounded outline with complete contour (encapsulated) and solid internal tissue characteristics may represent a glioma (Fig. 4.9) or meningioma if located within the retrobulbar fat; or, a lacrimal gland neoplasm if located along the temporal bony wall anteriorly. If the tumor has solid characteristics ultrasonically, but an irregular contour (nonencapsulated), this suggests an infiltrative neoplasm such as lymphoma (Fig.

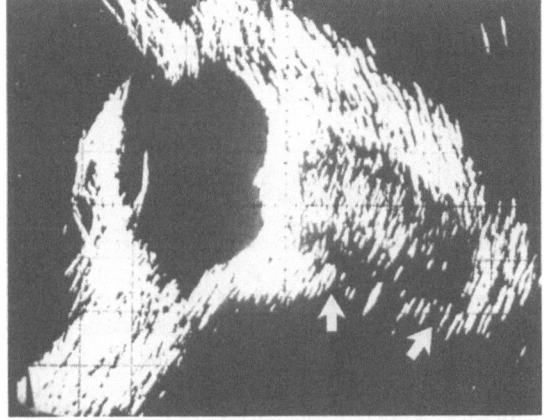

A

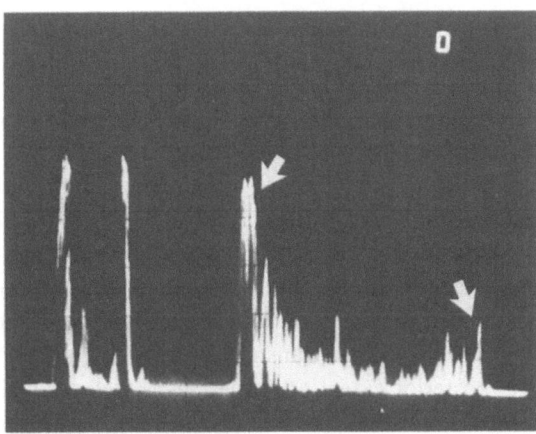

B

Figure 4.9 A. Solid circumscribed orbital tumor (optic nerve glioma). The two-dimensional B-scan shows a well-defined, rounded contour (arrows). **B.** The A-scan shows that these echoes are significantly attenuated with increasing depth (arrows).

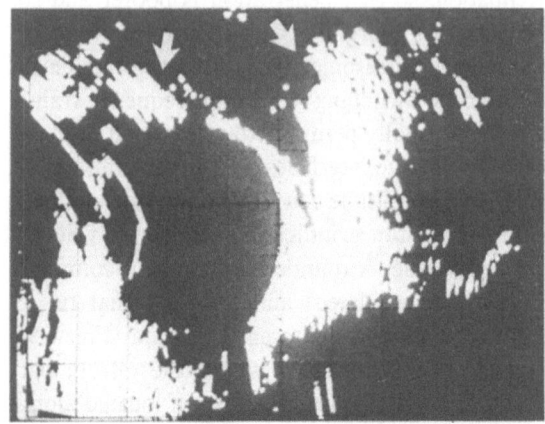

A

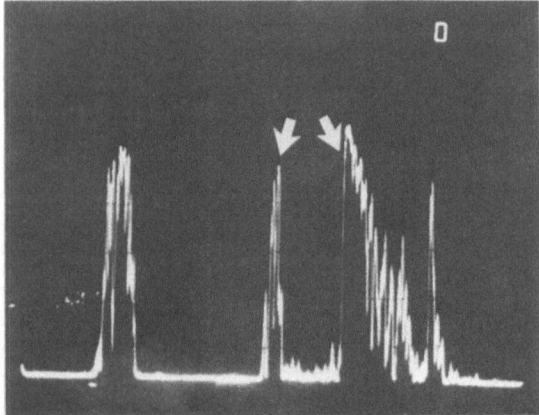

B

Figure 4.10. Infiltrative type of orbital tumor (lymphoma). **A.** The two-dimensional B-scan demonstrates irregular contour without complete boundaries (arrows). **B.** The A-scan shows low-amplitude internal echoes with good sound transmission (arrows); this characteristic is variable with tumor type and size.

4.10), sarcoma, or metastatic tumor. Tumors extending into the orbit from the intracranial space or from adjacent sinuses usually have a very flat configuration that follows the contour of the orbital walls.

Angiomatous tumors produce very high-amplitude echoes throughout the mass because of the fluid-filled character of these lesions with multiple vessel walls. Sound transmission is quite good and the posterior extent of the lesions is well defined. Anterior contours of hemangiomas sometimes are difficult to define, because the heterogeneous tissue pattern seems to merge with the retrobulbar fat pattern. Lowering receiver sensitivity permits one to differentiate between these two highly reflective masses. Lymphangiomas share some of these char-

acteristics, but the fluid spaces appear as multiple large cysts with prominent fibrous divisions; the general tumor outline is quite irregular instead of the circumscribed appearance of hemangiomas. Lymphangiomas do have excellent sound transmission, as one would expect from a fluid-filled lesion.

Some other irregular ultrasonic tumor patterns may be more difficult than the standard ones described thus far. Lymphomas and sclerosing pseudotumors show identifiable variations on these patterns. Lymphomas may have the circumscribed appearance of solid tumors with a very homogeneous internal tissue pattern because of the even, cellular composition of the mass. Other lymphomas of a more malignant and infiltrative type often demonstrate acutely angulated facets along the contour of a compact lesion, with some extensions along the posterior globe contour resembling infiltration of the sub-Tenon's space. Sclerosing pseudotumors, on the other hand, are so infiltrative and merged with fat and other structures that a single mass lesion is not identifiable. Instead, pseudotumors may produce an en-plaque type of lesion that extends along the orbital wall and may project into the retrobulbar fat. The more acute inflammatory pseudotumors are described below under "Inflammatory-Congestive Orbital Changes." Meningiomas arising in the optic nerve sheath cause generalized enlargement of the optic nerve, while those extending from the greater sphenoid wing produce en-plaque lesions similar to the sclerosing pseudotumor pattern. These represent the most difficult category of tumor for ultrasonic detection and classification. Primary orbital tumors are readily apparent with this test, while secondary tumors are more difficult to distinguish.

Inflammatory-Congestive Orbit Changes

In contrast to tumors that impose a new contour intruding on the normal orbital pattern, inflammatory and congestive diseases of the orbit involve structures normally present—sometimes causing only subtle changes in the normal ultrasonic pattern. Inflammatory ultrasound findings may be diffuse or localized to a particular area or tissue. A wide range of diseases produce orbital inflammation, including infections, lymphoid or granulomatous processes, or secondary passive congestion from arteriovenous anomalies. The etiology can only be inferred from ultrasonography, since the same findings may be present in several different pathologic disorders. Of major importance is the fact that inflammatory changes are clearly distinguished from the findings associated with true neoplasms.

Cellulitis and pseudotumor (idiopathic orbital inflammation) produce diffuse orbital ultrasound findings. The retrobulbar fat pad generally is the most involved tissue, with an abnormally diffuse mottled texture identified ultrasonically by widening the spaces between echoes. These changes probably result from interstitial edema abnormally separating fat globules and connective tissue. A granuloma or abscessed area may be identifiable ultrasonically as a focal mottled area, which is usually more evident after the area has become partially walled off from adjacent tissues. Edema in the posterior space enveloping the globe and around the optic nerve sheath is particularly characteristic of pseudotumor; it is referred to as sub-Tenon's edema.

Graves' disease, or dysthyroid exophthalmos, is the most common single cause of either bilateral or unilateral exophthalmos. The outstanding feature of this disease in the orbit is enlargement of extraocular muscles with accompanying clinical dysfunction. While the orbit becomes diffusely infiltrated with mast cells, lymphocytes, mucopolysaccharides, and accompanying edema, the extraocular muscles are the most affected tissues and increase greatly in volume. One of the most important uses of diagnostic ultrasonography in the orbit is demonstration of the fat and extraocular muscle changes accompanying active stages of Graves' disease (Fig. 4.11). The space between retrobulbar fat and the orbital wall shows a generalized widening; and, the usually echo-free area occupied by the muscles acquires internal tissue echoes from the histologic disorganization within them. Additionally, the muscle is compressed against the bony orbital wall, thus producing a better reflecting surface and a more defined outer margin of the muscle and orbital wall. It is noteworthy that lower frequency transducers may be necessary to bring out the muscle outlines fully; and, also that reduced sensitivity on the oscilloscope receiver may be necessary to avoid confusing the internal muscle echoes with the adjacent retrobulbar fat. The four rectus muscles may be visualized ultrasonically by scanning both the horizontal and vertical (sagittal) meridians. Superiorly, where the orbital roof slopes down toward the apex, one often can distinguish the levator muscle from the superior rectus muscle by the tissue plane separating them. The degree of muscle enlargement varies considerably from subtle to marked, depending on the amount of soft-tissue edema from the disease process. Bilateral changes are often evident ultrasonically, even when the exophthalmos appears to be unilateral clinically. Quantitative measurements of muscle enlargement are of questionable accuracy, depending on which portion of the muscle is measured and whether the beam is perpendicular or oblique. Both expansion of the retrobulbar fat volume and a slight enlargement of the optic nerve profile frequently accompany the enlarged muscles seen ultrasonically in Graves' disease.

Although these ultrasound signs are highly suggestive of Graves' disease, they are not pathogno-

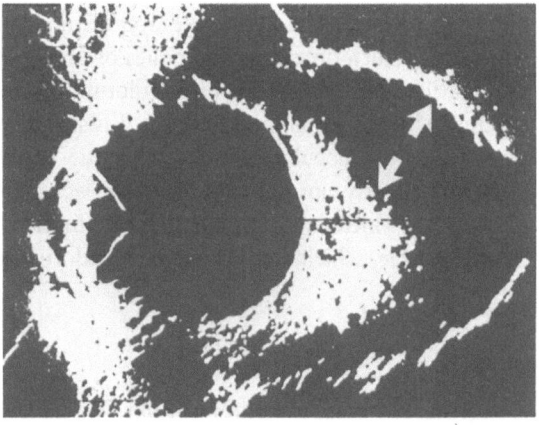

A

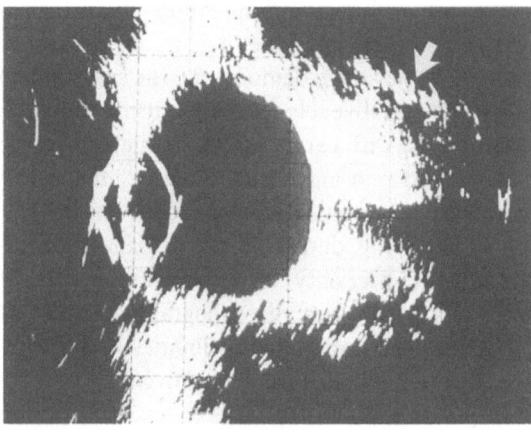

B

Figure 4.11 A. Enlarged extraocular rectus muscles extending from the globe equator to the orbital apex (arrows) indicate a congestive or inflammatory orbital disease process. B. The muscles of a normal orbit (arrow) contrast with the massive swelling that can occur.

monic for it—no more so than the enlarged muscles seen with CT. Passive congestion of the orbit secondary to arteriovenous anomalies or active inflammation, due to cellulitis or pseudotumor, may produce similar ultrasound findings. Enlargement of a single extraocular muscle, with the others appearing nearly normal in size, is characteristic of myositis—meaning an idiopathic inflammation of one muscle, which is a variant of pseudotumor.

Orbital Vascular Anomalies

Abnormal vascular communications, intracranially or intraorbitally, can cause exophthalmos with acute congestive or inflammatory clinical signs. These disorders produce no specific ultrasonic signs, but they often demonstrate the same inflammatory-congestive changes described above. In some cases, with careful study, a dilated superior ophthalmic vein may be detected in many orbits with arteriovenous malformations—particularly those involving dural shunts. Vascular contrast studies are necessary to document the vascular channels. The role of ultrasonography in these situations is to narrow the possibilities by failing to show gross tumor, or congestive-inflammatory changes.

Biometry

Precise measurement of eye dimensions to an accuracy of 0.01 mm is feasible with current ultrasound technology. Such accuracy requires a high-frequency transducer (15 or 20 MHz) with a weakly focused beam. Signal processing to truncate the returned echo enhances the apparent resolution. Electronic gating of the two echoes yields a much more accurate time measurement than is possible with visual analysis. Sound speed within each component of the eye tissues has been determined experimentally, and it must be applied to each segment of the time measurement of returned echoes when converting to a distance measurement. Besides these electronic factors, the ultrasonic beam must be optimally aligned toward the eye, with a maximum distance between the two echoes on the optical axis and perpendicular to their interfaces. Since there must be no compression of the cornea by a transducer, some type of water stand-

off is necessary. Measurements require only an A scan, whereas diagnostic applications of ultrasound require a combined A scan and B scan. The primary clinical importance of eye biometry is calculating diopter power for intraocular lens implants. A plastic prosthetic lens that is surgically placed into the eye at the time of cataract removal must have the proper focusing power for that individual eye. A wide range of lens powers are used, from +10 to +28 diopters. Clinical assessment of the appropriate lens implant for an individual eye is derived from three parameters. These are corneal curvature, axial eye length (by ultrasound), and the planned lens position in the eye. The lens power is then calculated by using a nomogram or formula derived from physiologic optics principles.

Summary

Ophthalmic ultrasonography has developed, since its introduction in 1956, into an essential diagnostic aid. Reproducible ultrasonic criteria are now well established for identification of vitreo-retinal disorders, foreign bodies, intraocular tumors, and orbital abnormalities (including tumors, inflammatory-congestive processes, and structural anomalies). An accuracy of 90–95% is obtainable by experienced examiners. Ultrasonic measurement of the eyes also aids in cataract surgery for lens implant power determination.

The thrust of current investigations in ophthalmic ultrasound is being directed toward improved techniques for acoustic characterization of tissues and the exploration of therapeutic applications in ocular disease. Conventional ultrasound systems fail to use all of the information contained in returned echoes. The simplified echo wave forms seen on oscilloscopes are designed to facilitate visual analysis. Computer spectral analysis of echoes has yielded far more detailed frequency components, thus making possible the identification of specific acoustic signatures for each type of ocular pathology. In relation to the therapeutic application of ultrasound, the destructive power of this energy is being used experimentally to produce filtering operations, to disperse vitreous hemorrhage, and to coagulate tumors of the eyes. The fruits of these research efforts will be evident in the future.

References

1. Baum G, Greenwood I: The application of ultrasonic locating techniques to ophthalmology: part 2. Ultrasonic visualization of soft tissues. *Arch Ophthalmol* 60:263–279, 1958.

2. Binkhorst RD: The optical design of intraocular lens implants. *Ophthalmol Surg* 6:17–31, 1975.

3. Bronson NR: Quantitative ultrasonography. Arch Ophthalmol 81:460–472, 1969.

4. Bronson NR, Fisher YL, Pickering NC, et al: *Ophthalmic Contact B-Scan Ultrasonography for the Clinician.* Baltimore, Williams & Wilkins, 1980.

5. Chang S, Coleman DJ, Dallow RL: Trends in ophthalmic ultrasonography, in Kurjak A (ed): *Progress in Medical Ultrasound.* Amsterdam, Excerpta Medica, 1980, vol 1, pp 279–312.

6. Coleman DJ, Koenig WF, Katz L: A hand operated ultrasound scan system for ophthalmic evaluation. *Am J Ophthalmol 68:256–263, 1969.*

7. Coleman DJ, Lizzi FL, Jack RL: *Ultrasonography of the Eye and Orbit.* Philadelphia, Lea & Febiger, 1977.

8. Dallow RL (ed): Ophthalmic ultrasonography: comparative techniques. *Int Ophthalmol Clin* 19(4):1–310, 1979.

9. Gernett H, Franceschetti A: Ultrasonic biometry of the eye, in Oksala A, Gernett H (eds): *Ultrasonics in Ophthalmology.* Basel, Karger, 1967, pp 175–200.

10. Jansson F: Measurements of intra-ocular distances by ultrasound. *Acta Ophthalmol* 74(suppl):1–51, 1963.

11. Mundt GH, Hughes WF: Ultrasonics in ocular diagnosis. *Am J Ophthalmol* 41:488–498, 1956.

12. Oksala A, Lehtinen A: Diagnostic value of ultrasonics in ophthalmology. *Ophthalmologica* 134:387–395, 1957.

13. Ossoinig KC: Clinical echo-ophthalmology, in Blodi F (ed): *Current Concepts in Ophthalmology.* St. Louis, CV Mosby, 1972, vol 3, pp 101–130.

14. Purnell EW: Ultrasound in ophthalmological diagnosis, in Grossman C, Homes JH, Joyner C, et al (eds): *Diagnostic Ultrasound.* New York, Plenum Press, 1966, pp 95–109.

5
Investigation of the Orbit by Contrast Techniques

Carlos F. Gonzalez

While carotid angiography and orbital venography were the procedures of choice in the investigation of intraorbital and paraorbital pathologies, the development of highly sophisticated computed tomographic (CT) and ultrasound techniques has decreased their use. Vascular studies are used only in the investigation of vascular malformations or vascular tumors within or around the orbit. Contrast injections into the orbital soft tissues (contrast orbitography or orbital pneumography) are dangerous techniques that are no longer used.

Carotid Angiography

The role of carotid angiography in the diagnosis of lesions within the orbit lies mainly in the investigation of paraorbital or intraorbital vascular abnormalities, such as ophthalmic artery aneurysms, arteriovenous malformation, and vascular intraorbital tumors (such as hemangiomas). Carotid angiography is also used to investigate the vascular supply of tumors around the orbit (such as sphenoid ridge meningiomas) and to demonstrate the intraorbital extension of intracranial, nasal, facial, or other periorbital vascular tumors.

Selective internal and external carotid injections are important to provide detailed knowledge of the internal and external supply of lesions—as well as the anastomosis between the vascular bed if embolization is to be used to treat vascular lesions.

Technique

Selective catheterization of the internal and external carotid arteries is accomplished via the femoral route using the Seldinger technique. Careful collimation, high magnification, and subtraction techniques are essential to demonstrate small vascular lesions. Serial views should be obtained in the lateral, caudal, and modified axial projections. The axial view is obtained by directing the central beam 75° cranially to the orbitomeatal line. Injections of 8 cc of contrast media (meglumine iothalamate USP 60%) into the internal carotid artery and 5 cc into the external carotid artery are usually performed. The complication rate is the same as in any catheterization of intracranial vessels. Complications found at the puncture site are vascular spasm, thrombosis, hematoma, and arteriovenous malformation. Intracranial complications caused by placing the catheter into the cerebral vessels are vascular spasm and intracerebral embolism.

Ophthalmic Artery

The ophthalmic artery is the first major branch of the internal carotid artery; it originates as the carotid artery perforates the dura matter close to the anterior clinoid process, after passing through the cavernous sinus. The ophthalmic artery also can originate from the middle meningeal artery, which is a branch of the external carotid artery. The course of the ophthalmic artery can be divided into three segments: intracranial, intracanalicular, and intraorbital (Fig. 5.1A and 5.1B). The intracanalicular segment of the ophthalmic artery lies beneath and slightly lateral to the optic nerve inside the optic canal. The orbital segment of the ophthalmic arteries first follows the optic nerve, then crosses over or under the optic nerve (Fig. 5.1C), and finally runs forward toward the medial

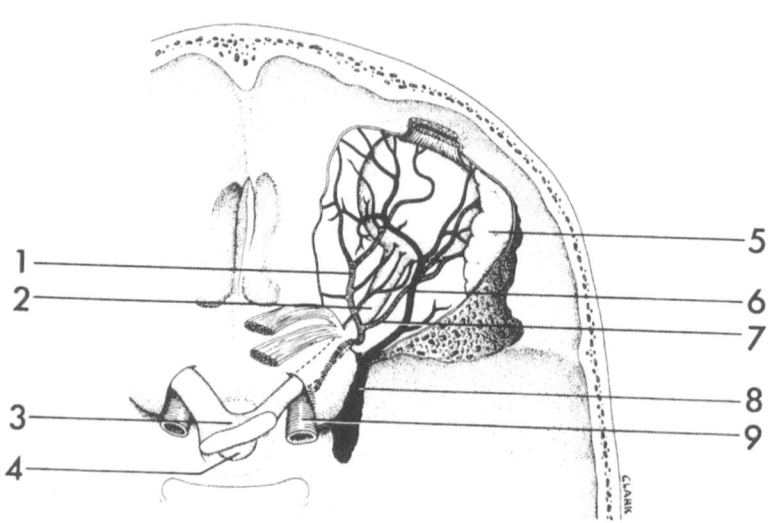

Figure 5.1. Vascular anatomy of the orbit: **A.** Axial diagrammatic representation of the orbit after removal of the orbital roof. (1) Ophthalmic artery; (2) Optic nerve; (3) Optic chiasm; (4) Pituitary gland; (5) Lacrimal gland; (6) Superior ophthalmic vein; (7) Lacrimal artery branch of the ophthalmic; (8) Cavernous sinus; (9) Carotid artery.

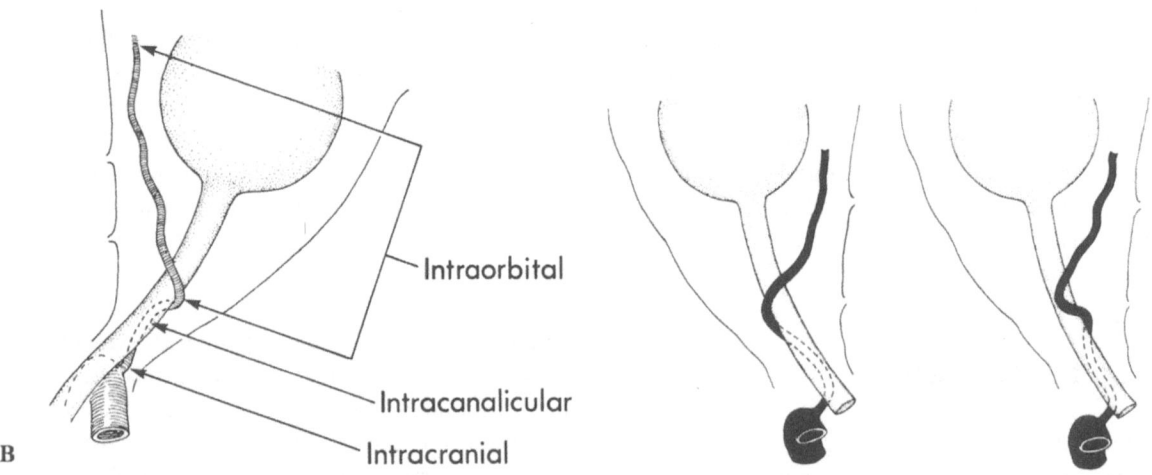

B. Ophthalmic artery segments. (1) Intracranial; (2) Intracanalicular; (3) Intraorbical. **C.** The artery crosses the optic nerve above the optic nerve (left); below the optic nerve (right).

wall of the orbit, terminating in the superior medial angle of the orbit. The radiographic appearance of the ophthalmic artery in the lateral view of the arteriogram is closely related to the artery's intraorbital segment. It may have a configuration suggesting a bayonet (4), or a broad L-shaped curve (Fig. 5.2A and 5.2B) (14), depending on whether the artery passes over or under the optic nerve. In the frontal projection, it is curved with a medial concavity. Later in its course, the artery has multiple branches—the most important of which is the central artery of the retina. Other branches are the posterior and anterior ciliary branches, the lacrimal artery, the supraorbital artery, and the ethmoidal arteries. Precise knowledge of the multiple anastomosis between the ophthalmic artery and middle meningeal artery is critical before embolization of the middle meningeal artery can be performed. At times, both occlusion of the ophthalmic artery and blindness have occurred after embolization of the middle meningeal artery due to blockage through anastomotic chains between the two systems (1). Occasionally, the ophthalmic artery may enter the orbit through the superior orbital fissure. Other anomalous origins of the artery are the intracavernous portion of the internal carotid artery and (very rarely) the middle cerebral artery.

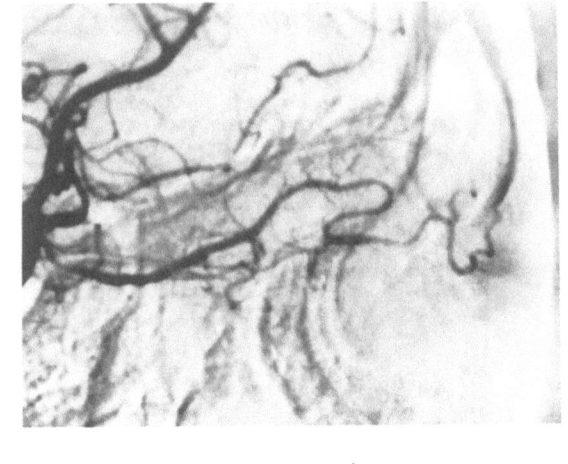

A

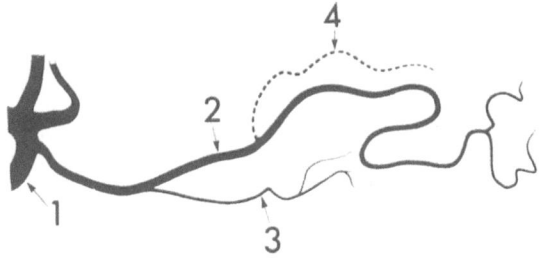

B

Figure 5.2. Ophthalmic arteriography. **A.** Lateral angiographic view. **B.** Diagrammatic representation of the radiograph. (1) Internal carotid artery; (2) Ophthalmic artery; (3) Long posterior ciliary arteries; (4) Lacrimal artery.

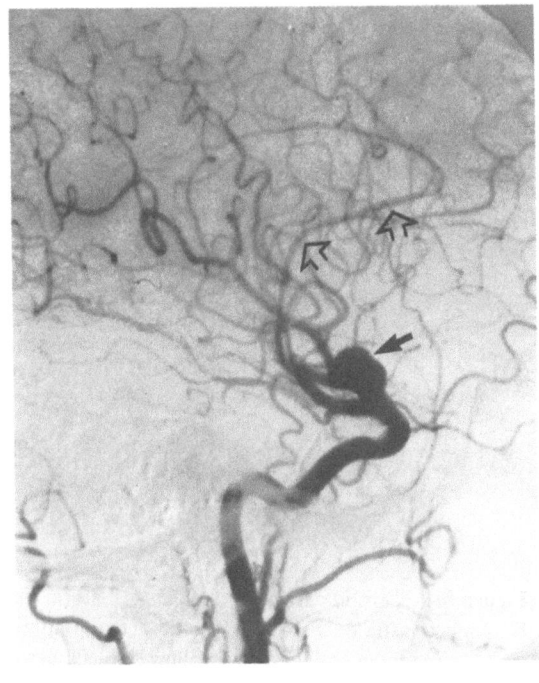

Figure 5.3. Giant carotid-ophthalmic artery aneurysm. A common carotid injection (oblique view) shows a large, partially filled aneurysm at the carotid-ophthalmic junction (arrow). Notice the significant displacement of the anterior cerebral artery (open arrows) due to a mass lesion produced by the clotted portion of the aneurysm.

Before the development of high-resolution CT scanning, displacement of the artery was used to indicate the location of vascular tumors within the orbit. At present, angiography is used mainly to demonstrate the pathologic circulation of vascular tumors. Indications for angiography include ophthalmic artery aneurysms (Fig. 5.3), carotid-cavernous fistulas (Fig. 5.4), and tumors with abnormal vasculature—such as hemangiopericytoma, capillary hemangioma (Fig. 5.5), cavernous hemangioma (Fig. 5.6), meningioma (Fig. 5.7), and malignant primary or metastatic tumors.

External Carotid Artery

Knowledge of the radiographic anatomy of the external carotid artery and its branches is important when orbital and periorbital tumors and vas-

cular malformations are to be treated by embolization of this artery's branches (Fig. 5.8) (8).

Orbital Venography

At one time, orbital venography was used to localize tumors within the orbit (2). Since the advent of CT—an easier method for showing these lesions—the use of orbital venography has decreased markedly. Currently, its use is limited to the demonstration of orbital venous malformations, and occasionally cavernous sinus thrombosis.

Technique

Several methods have been described historically. The most frequently used method is the percutane-

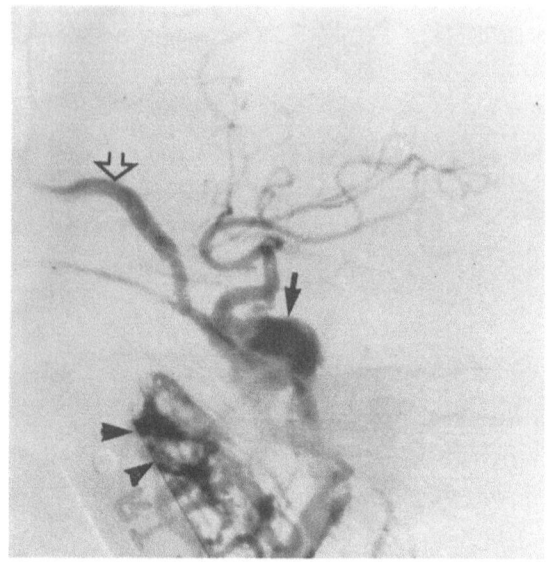
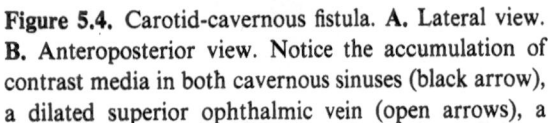

A

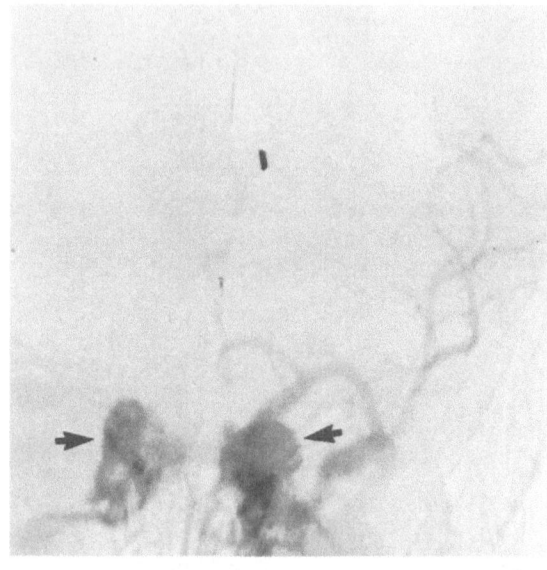

B

Figure 5.4. Carotid-cavernous fistula. **A.** Lateral view. **B.** Anteroposterior view. Notice the accumulation of contrast media in both cavernous sinuses (black arrow), a dilated superior ophthalmic vein (open arrows), a prominent pterygoid venous plexus (arrowheads), and poor filling of the internal carotid branches due to the fistula.

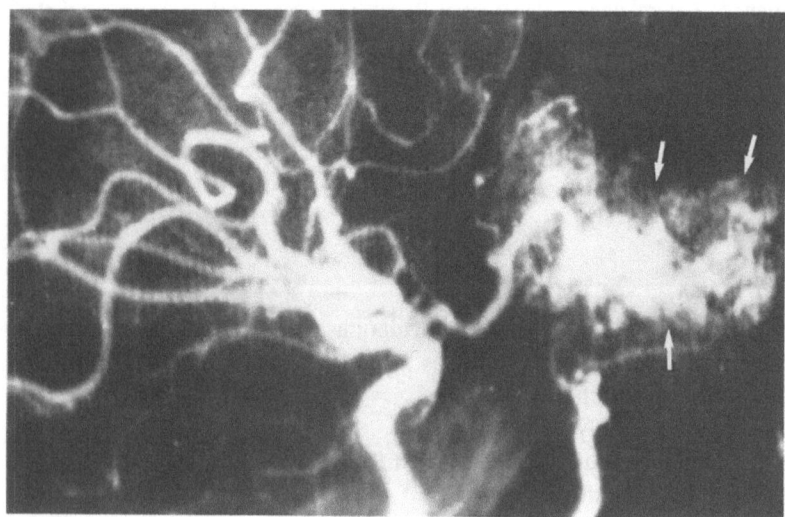

Figure 5.5. Capillary hemangioma. Carotid arteriogram showing the ophthalmic artery supplying a markedly vascular tumor in a young child (arrows). (Courtesy of Dilange D. Arteriography in angiomas of the orbit. *Radiology* 113: 355–361, 1974. Used with permission.)

ous puncture of the frontal vein, which was originally described by Vritsios (9, 11, 13). A 23–21-gauge scalp vein needle or presterilized 18-gauge catheter needle specially designed for this purpose (11)* is used to catheterize the vein. A total of 10 cc of water-soluble contrast media (meglumine iothalamate USP 60%) is delivered in 2 seconds. The films are taken in a sequence of one every half-second after the injection. Subtraction and magnification views are very helpful for visualizing the vascular detail. Three projections are usually obtained: routine anterior-posterior or under-tilted axial view (−20° from the orbitomeatal line) (Fig. 5.9), lateral view (Fig. 5.10), and basal view (Fig. 5.11). It is necessary to eliminate collateral venous

---

* Beckton-Dickinson and Co., Longdwell catheter needle, Rutherford, NJ.

Figure 5.6. Cavernous hemangioma. Selective internal carotid angiogram showing a small branch of the ophthalmic artery supplying an irregular collection of contrast media in the orbit corresponding to a cavernous hemangioma (arrow). Angiography does not always demonstrate this lesion. A CT scan is the procedure of choice (Courtesy of J Vignaud, Paris, France).

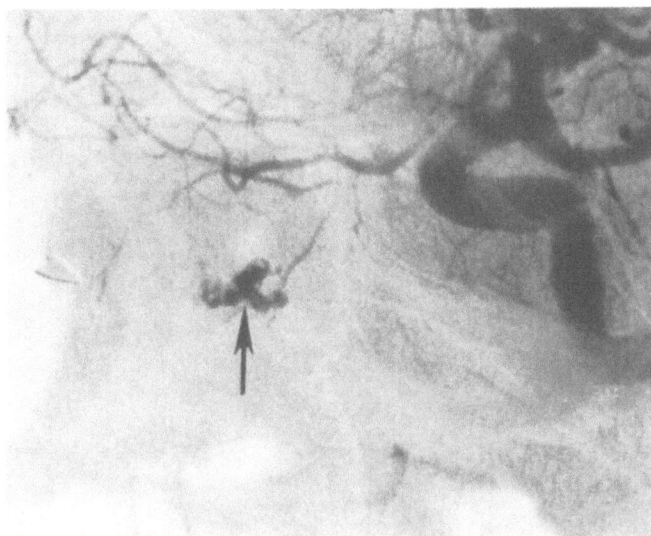

drainage. This is usually done with a rubber band placed around the forehead and digital compression at the inferior orbital rim, thus preventing the contrast agent from entering the facial veins. The rate of success with this technique is about 90% in most institutions (2).

Other techniques include injection into the angular vein (either by cut-down or percutaneous puncture), facial vein cut-down (9) and catheterization (3) and retrograde filling by injection into the inferior petrosal vein using catheter techniques (5).

Subcutaneous extravasation of the contrast media in the injection site is the most common complication of the injection technique in the frontal vein. Usually, the area clears without further problems. A few severe complications have been reported with the catheter techniques (6, 10, 12).

Anatomy

The superior ophthalmic vein originates near the roof of the nose from branches of the angular and

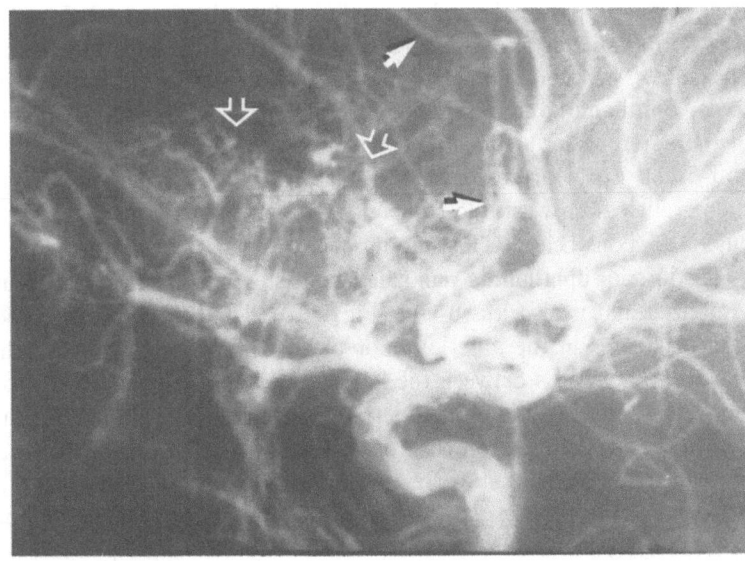

Figure 5.7. Subfrontal meningioma. There is significant superior and posterior displacement of the anterior cerebral artery due to the tumor (arrows). Multiple abnormal vessels are shown supplying the tumor coming from the ophthalmic artery (open arrows).

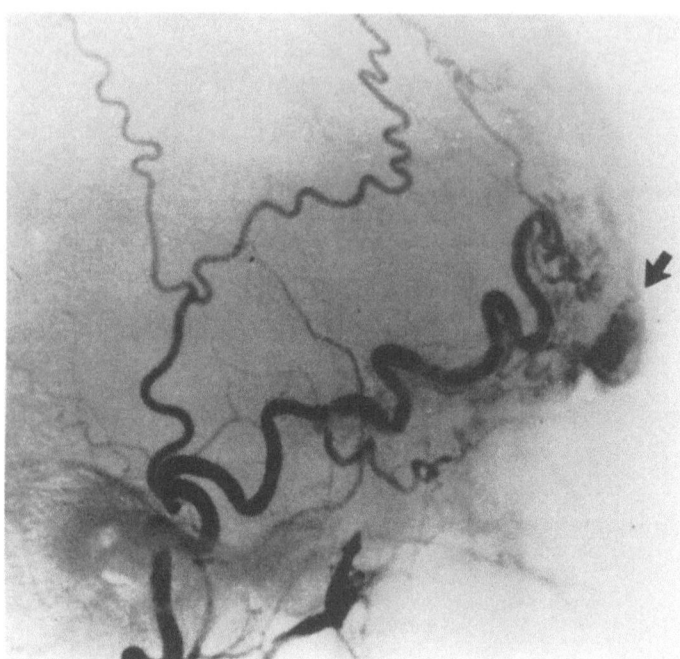

Figure 5.8. Superficial arteriovenous malformation of the eyelid. Selective external carotid injection is shown. Notice the enlarged superficial temporal artery supplying the malformation (arrow).

supraorbital veins. Three segments have been described (Figs. 5.1 and 5.9). The first extends from the origin of the vein in the inner wall of the orbit to the point of entrance into the muscle cone between the superior and medial rectus muscles. The second segment corresponds to the vein's posterior course laterally and above the globe, underneath the superior rectus muscle. The third segment begins when the vein changes its direction and runs backwards in the lateral part of the muscle cone; then, it finally passes through the inferior lateral part of the superior orbital fissure into the cavernous sinus. The radiographic appearance of the superior ophthalmic vein resembles a parallelogram in the anteroposterior and tilted views (Figs. 5.9 and 5.11). Local distortion and displacement of the parallelogram was used to diagnose space-occupying lesions before CT scanning.

The inferior ophthalmic vein is less consistently visualized and is also less useful (Fig. 5.10). The vein originates in the anterior floor of the orbit and runs backwards between the lateral and inferior rectus muscles to join the superior ophthalmic vein at the apex of the orbit. There also is a system of connecting veins that represents anastomosis between the superior and inferior ophthalmic veins.

Pathology

While nonopacification of the vein is usually the result of a faulty technique, it may represent a disease. The most common disorder associated with nonopacification of the vein is an arteriovenous fistula. Nonopacification of a single venous branch may be due to extrinsic compression by a tumor. This finding has also been described in inflammatory processes involving the orbit, including the Tolosa-Hunt syndrome (a nonspecific granulomatous inflammation that may involve the orbit, causing painful ophthalmoplegia) and other idiopathic inflammatory pseudotumors (7).

The current indication for orbital venography is demonstration of intraorbital venous varicosities. Congenital, traumatic, and secondary venous varices are easily identified. The radiographic manifestation is an unusual dilatation of the vein (Fig. 5.12). Large pools of contrast media (Fig. 5.12) are seen when the varices are associated with arteriovenous malformations. The malformation can be better demonstrated by direct puncture. The presence of a persistent stain that is seen on the delayed films often indicates the presence of arteriovenous malformation or hemangiomas.

At present, pituitary tumors and other lesions

Figure 5.9. Orbital venogram. **A.** Tilted anteroposterior view. **B.** Diagram of radiograph. The superior ophthalmic vein is well visualized in this view, and the radiographic appearance resembles a parallelogram. There is a good demonstration of the anatomic venous segments.

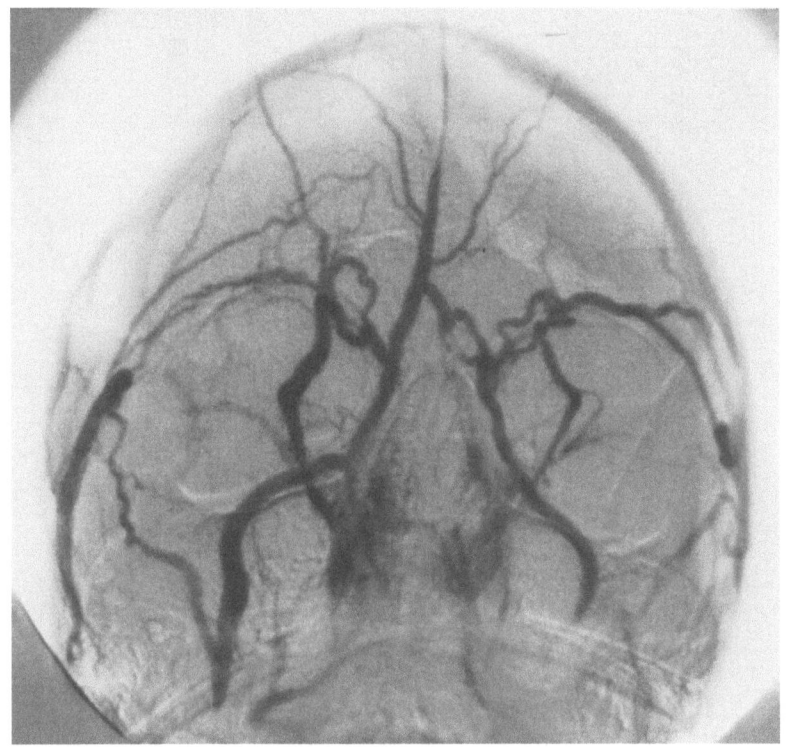

A

B

involving the sella turcica and the base of the skull are best studied by CT scanning, which almost totally eliminates the need for opacifying the cavernous sinus. Rarely, it may be necessary to inject the frontal vein in an attempt to diagnose cavernous sinus thrombosis or occlusion. In these cases, however, the preferred method of study usually is injection of contrast media into the inferior petrosal vein following selective-catheterisation of the vein. (5).

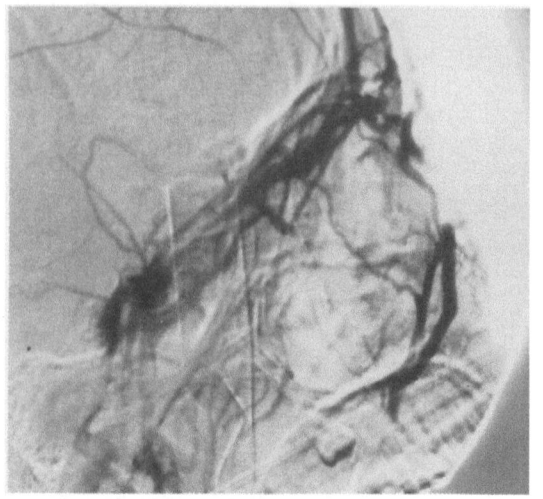

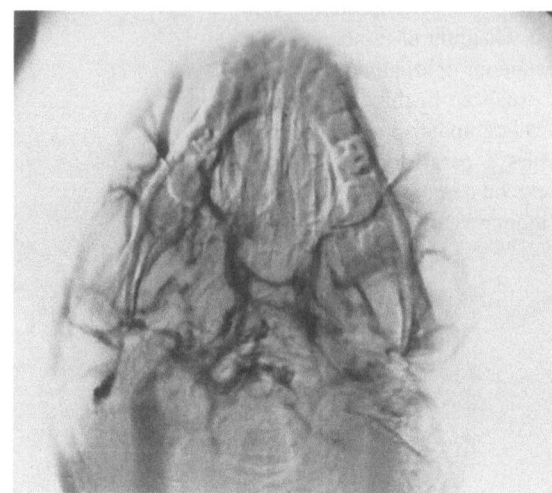

A

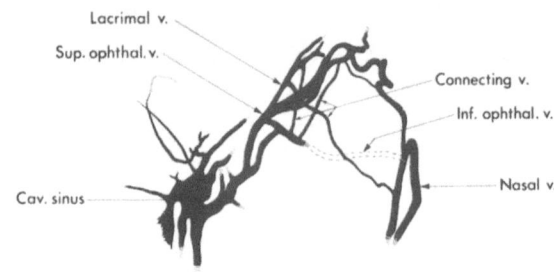

B

Figure 5.10. Orbital venogram. **A.** Lateral view. **B.** Diagram of radiograph. The superior ophthalmic vein is well visualized, as well as the inferior ophthalmic vein, when present.

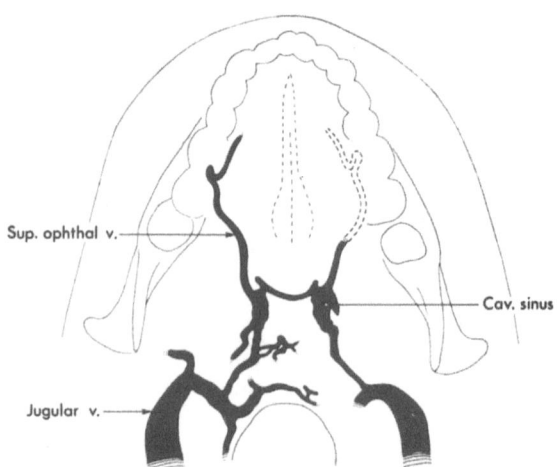

B

Figure 5.11. Orbital venogram. **A.** Base view. **B.** Diagram of radiograph showing excellent visualization of the superior ophthalmic vein. This is very useful when looking for pathology in the cavernous sinus and sellar or parasellar regions.

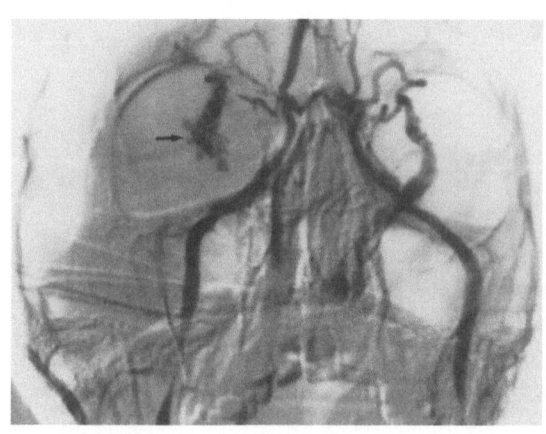

Figure 5.12. Orbital varix. Tilted anteroposterior view showing significant dilatation of the second and third segments of the right superior ophthalmic vein corresponding to an orbital varix (arrow).

References

1. Berenstein A, et al: Personal communication.

2. Bilaniuk LT, Vignaud J, Clay C: Orbital venography, in Arger P (ed): *Orbit Roentgenology.* New York, John Wiley & Sons, 1977, pp. 172–192.

3. Deodati F, Bec P, Espagno J, et al: Phlebographie orbitaire par catheterisme de la veine faciale. *Arch Ophthal Paris* 28:12, 1969.

4. Dilenge D, Fischgold H, David M: L'artere ophthalmique aspects angiographiques. *Neurochirurgie* 7:240–257, 1961.

5. Hanafee E, Rosen LM, Weidner W, et al: Venography of the cavernous sinus, orbital veins and basal venous plexus. *Radiology* 84:751–753, 1965.

6. Hanafee WN: Orbital venography. *Radiol Clin North Am* 10:63–81, 1972.

7. Klinel B: The Tolosa-Hunt syndrome. *Surv Ophthalmol* 27:79–95, 1982.

8. Lasjaunias P, Mont J, Vignaud J: External carotid supply to the orbit, in Arger P (ed): *Orbit Roentgenology.* New York, John Wiley & Sons, 1977.

9. Lombardi G, Casserini A: Venography of the orbit: technique and anatomy. *Br J Radiol* 41:282–286, 1968.

10. Shiu PC, Hanafee WN, Wilson GH, et al: Cavernous sinus venography. *Am J Roentgenol* 104:57–62, 1968.

11. Vignaud J: Technique de phlebographie orbitair epercutanee par la veine frontale. *Bull Soc Ophthal Fr* November, 1967, No 11.

12. Vignaud J, Clay C: Techniques d'opacification par voie veineuse du plexus caverneux. *Ann Radiol* 17(3):229–236, 1974.

13. Vritsios A: A new method for demonstrating ophthalmic veins, facial veins, and superficial venous system of head (in Greek). *Arch Soc Ophthal North Greece* 12:223–233, 1961.

14. Zimmerman RA, Vignaud J: Ophthalmic arteriography, in Arger P (ed): *Orbit Roentgenology.* New York, John Wiley & Sons, 1977, pp. 136–150.

6
The Lacrimal Drainage System

Melvin H. Becker

There are several conditions involving the lacrimal drainage system that may require imaging techniques for diagnosis and management. The most common of these is epiphora, which is the abnormal overflow of tears and usually is secondary to obstruction of the passages. Other conditions that require study are diverticula, fistulae, masses in the area of or within the lumen of the lacrimal passages, persistent drainage or obstruction after surgery on the passages, and persistent canaliculitis.

In evaluating a patient with excessive tearing, the physician should ask about painless overflow tearing, reading difficulties, the frequency of redness at the area of the inner canthus, history of entropion, absence of tears when crying, dry mouth, and the association between eating and tearing (23). The physical examination should evaluate the patient for abnormal orbicularis muscle action, eversion of the puncta, small puncta, tumor, large lacrimal lake, overflow tears, reflux of clear fluid, mucous, or pus when digital pressure is applied on the lacrimal sac, and signs of inflammation.

Anatomy

To evaluate the imaging studies of the lacrimal drainage system, one must be aware of its anatomy (Fig. 6.1) (12, 34, 58, 59). The drainage system for each eye usually has a superior and inferior canaliculus (47), a common canaliculus, a lacrimal sac, and a nasolacrimal duct. The tears enter the system through the superior and inferior puncta (about 0.3 mm openings) situated at the medial end of the upper and lower lid margins. Then the tears go into the inferior and superior canaliculi (lacrimal ducts). The canaliculi have vertical portions about 2 mm long and horizontal portions approximately 8 mm long. The vertical portion originates from the punctum, which is in the apex of the lacrimal papilla. As the vertical lumen joins the horizontal portion, it widens to about 2 mm to form the ampulla. The horizontal portions are about 0.5 mm in diameter and 2 mm in length, and they join to form the common canaliculus (lacrimal duct or sinus of Maier) in about 90% of all cases. The other 10% join the lacrimal sac, either independently or in some other variable fashion. Usually, the lacrimal duct opens into the lacrimal sac. The lacrimal sac is the widest portion of the drainage system, and it lies in the bony lacrimal fossa. The sac averages 10–12 mm in length and varies in diameter, depending on its state of dilation. Usually, it is not dilated. Its lumen is about 4–8 mm in anteroposterior diameter and 1–2 mm in lateral diameter. The nasolacrimal duct is the downward continuation of the lacrimal drainage system, extending from the neck of the lacrimal sac to the inferior meatus of the nose. The duct is 12–18 mm in length, with approximately 10 mm of its course passing through the osseous nasolacrimal canal. A short membranous portion of the nasolacrimal duct is situated between its junction with the neck of the lacrimal sac and the upper end of the bony nasolacrimal canal. Inferiorly, there is another small membranous portion, just before the duct exits into the nose. At the upper end of the nasolacrimal duct, there is a mucosal fold (the valve of Krause). Another narrowing mucosal fold (the valve of Taillefer) is located near the middle of the interosseous part of the duct. The meatal opening is usually about one-quarter of the way back from the anterior border of the lower turbinate. The valve of

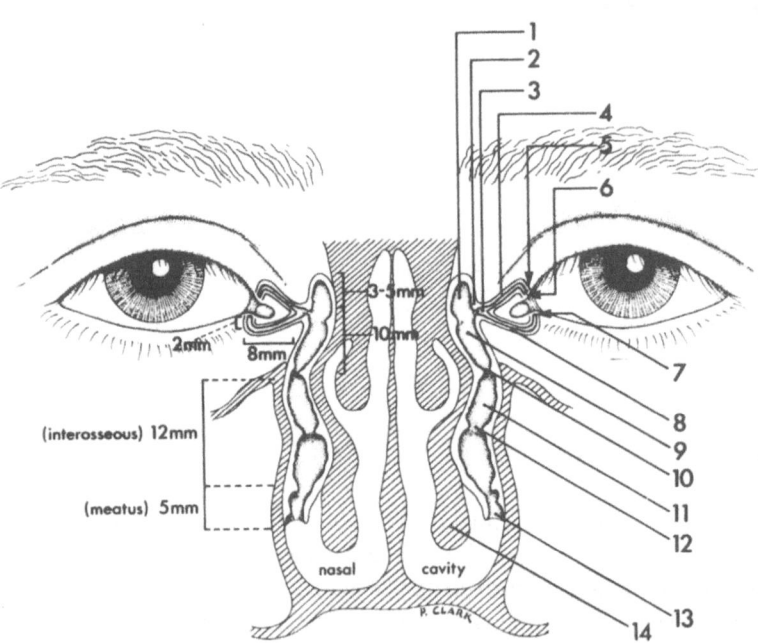

Figure 6.1. Normal anatomy of the nasolacrimal passages. (1) Fundus of lacrimal sac; (2) Valve of Rosenmüller; (3) Sinus of Maier; (4) Superior canaliculus; (5) Valve of Faltz; (6) Superior puncta (valve of Bochdalek); (7) Inferior puncta (valve of Bochdalek); (8) Inferior canaliculus; (9) Body of lacrimal sac; (10) Valve of Krause; (11) Nasolacrimal duct; (12) Valve of Taillefer; (13) Valve of Hasner (Horner, Bianchi, or Craveilhier) or plica lacrimalis; (14) Inferior turbinate.

Hasner is a mucosal fold that covers the ostium, through which the nasolacrimal duct opens into the nose.

Physiology

The elimination of tears from the conjunctival sac has been compared to the action of a pump (34). When the eyelids close during blinking, the superficial and deep heads of the pretarsal orbicularis oculi muscles close the ampulla and shorten the canaliculus. Also, with the lid closure, the punctum moves medially. Simultaneously, the deep heads of the preseptal orbicularis oculi muscles pull the orbital periosteum, to which the lateral wall of the tear sac is firmly attached laterally. This creates a negative pressure within the sac and, thus, draws fluid from the ampulla and the canaliculus into the sac. When the eye opens, these muscles relax; then the fibroelastic resilience of the orbital periosteum puts positive pressure on the tear sac, forcing tears into the nose. Also, the punctum moves laterally; fluid enters it, filling the ampulla and the lengthened canaliculus.

Evaluation Techniques

There are several studies to be employed in investigating the causes of overflow tearing in the absence of excessive lacrimation. In addition to the history and physical evaluation, these examinations include the Schirmer test (to evaluate the amount of tear formation), lacrimal irrigations, probing, the Jones dye tests, the saccharin test, isotope clearance studies, and dacryocystography (1, 11, 13, 23). Irrigation of the drainage system should be tried after checking that the eyelids are normal, the puncta are properly situated, and excessive lacrimation is not present via the Schirmer test. If the irrigation is successful, there should be either no obstruction or partial obstruction. If irrigation to the nose is impossible, there is complete obstruction, which may be investigated by probing the upper drainage system with a #0 Bowman probe. Normally, this probe will pass to a "hard stop" at the medial lacrimal sac, where the medial wall rests on bone. If a "soft stop" is encountered or the probe can be passed only a few millimeters, an obstruction is present. Reflux from the fellow punctum in the presence of a "soft stop" indicates normal upper and lower canals and a normal common canal.

Jones Tests

Several tests have been devised to determine if the tears are passing into the nose under physiologic conditions. A substance (fluorescein, saccharin, sodium pertechnetate, cyalume, and so on) is instilled into the conjunctival cul-de-sac, and examinations are done to check for the presence of the substance at various sites along the nasolacrimal system. The Jones tests are the most commonly used of these examinations (33, 35). In the Jones #1 test (a true test of normal physiology), a drop of 2% fluorescein dye is placed in the conjunctival cul-de-sac, and it should appear in the nose in about 5 minutes. The dye is detected on a cotton-tipped applicator placed under the inferior turbinate at the nasolacrimal duct opening. There are several variations of the method of detection of the dye in the nose. These include different positions of the head during the study, blowing the nose (23), and checking the nasal passage and oropharynx with ultraviolet light (19). If no dye appears in the nose, an obstruction is strongly suggested and the Jones #2 test is done. This is performed by irrigating the lacrimal drainage system with 1 cc of saline solution after the Jones #1 test. A cotton-tipped swab or tissue paper is placed in the nasal cavity under the inferior turbinate. A moderately stained yellow effluent detected on the probe proves that the dye reached the sac by the normal pumping mechanism, but could pass no further. The Jones #2 saline irrigation forces it to pass further. If colorless saline appears, the dye never entered the system. Therefore, the abnormality should be in the upper portion of the drainage system.

Taste Test

Another test of a physiologic nature is the saccharin test (24, 25, 31, 32). After a few drops of 2% saccharin are placed in the conjunctival sac, a healthy patient should taste the sweet substance within 5 minutes. This test is unreliable in nontasters. Some patients are so sensitive to the saccharin that even a symptomatic, partly obstructed drainage system may be erroneously considered normal. Only one eye may be reliably tested at a given time because of the persistence of the taste.

Isotope Studies

Radionuclide dacryocystography (lacrimal scintillography, nuclear lacrimal sac study, lacrimal scan, or radioactive imaging of the lacrimal apparatus) is the evaluation of the dynamics of tear drainage by using a radioactive tracer: technetium 99m sulphur colloid, or 99mTc pertechnetate (6, 7, 27, 28, 48, 49, 52, 53). The radioisotope with a viscosity approximate to that of tears is dropped into the conjunctival sac (a radioactive dose of 50–500 μCi); then the area of the drainage system

is scanned with the gamma camera with a pinhole collimator to follow the radioactive tracer into the canaliculi, the lacrimal sac, the nasolacrimal duct, and into the nose. Images usually are recorded for 30 minutes. During the first minutes, scan every 10 seconds after instillation; then scan once every 3 minutes for 10 minutes, and finally scan every 5 minutes until the 30-minute period has elapsed. This technique has been quantified (27, 28, 53) using a gamma camera interfaced with a computer, in which the transit time of the tracer can be compared with that of a normal subject. While this technique is helpful in exploring the excretory physiology of tears, it is not satisfactory for demonstrating pathologic anatomy. Some studies (8) have shown that the lacrimal scan is a sensitive test of canalicular function and of the adequacy of the lacrimal pumping mechanism. However, it is not a very sensitive test for the elimination of tears from the sac and nasolacrimal duct. Most investigators using the lacrimal scan consider it to be complementary to dacryocystography. In addition, this test is expensive and requires a technician who understands lacrimal anatomy. While some ophthalmologists feel that the isotope scan is a very useful study, others have had some reservations (Fig. 6.2).

The transit time from the conjunctival sac to

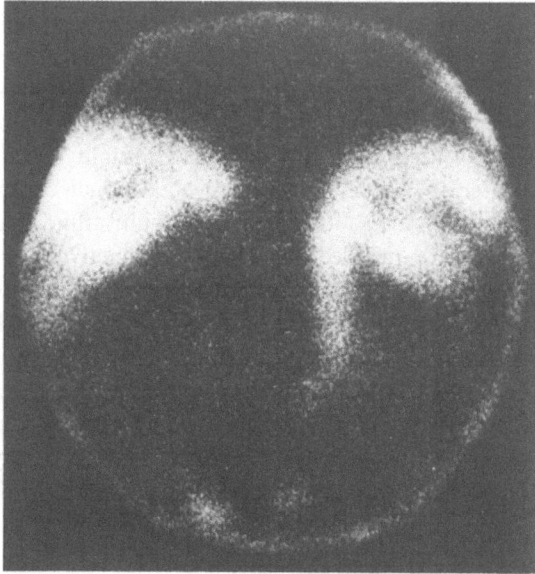

Figure 6.2. Radionuclide dacryocystogram showing a normal study (left) and a midlevel obstruction (right) (Case courtesy of A. Brackup, MD and M. Haller, MD, Queens, NY).

the nose has been determined by several different techniques (37). It is usually more rapid in the erect than in the supine position. Scintographic studies (6) using technetium pertechnetate revealed that the tracer substance reach the sac in 4–43 seconds, and the nose in 4–323 seconds (median, 43 seconds). With fluorescein staining of various solutions, it was found that aqueous solutions pass through in 60 seconds, 2.5% hydroxymethylcellulose in 90 seconds, and 2.5% methylcellulose in 255 seconds (37). Saccharin can be tasted in 3–17 minutes after conjunctival sac agent instillation (24, 38). Water-soluble contrast agents have a transit of 3–5 minutes (29). Iodized oil instilled into the sac usually leaves in 15 minutes (41) in normal eyes. The complete system should be empty within 30 minutes (40).

Experimental Studies

Currently, there is an examination being developed that uses a chemiluminescent material (cyalume) to demonstrate the structure and outflow patency of the lacrimal drainage system. The substance, which has been used only in monkeys and cadavers, is injected into the lower punctum. The chemical luminescence shows the canaliculi and lacrimal sac through the skin. In some cadavers, the common canaliculus and the upper portion of the nasolacrimal duct can also be seen. These structures are seen as areas of luminescence, but they are not sharply delineated (9, 46).

Several attempts have been made to use radiopaque substances for functional studies of the lacrimal drainage system (16, 29, 36, 42). The most recent trial involved the use of ultra-fluid lipiodol (29). With a cooperative patient, upright posteroanterior Waters views were obtained at 3, 15, and 30 minutes after two drops of ultra-fluid lipiodol were instilled into both conjunctival sacs without the use of anesthesia. After the 30-minute film, the patient was placed on the x-ray couch and an injection dacryocystography procedure was performed. Attempts to use currently available water-soluble contrast agents have not been very successful, probably due to their hypertonicity. It may be possible to do functional tear duct studies with the nonionic contrast media that are now in the process of development.

Radiologic Studies

Radiologic studies are necessary for a more definitive anatomic demonstration of abnormalities in the lacrimal drainage system. Routine x-ray films and/or computed tomograms of the orbits and paranasal sinuses can help in identifying diseases of the sinuses and nasal passages, which may be contributing factors in obstructions of the tear ducts (26). The osseous canal of the lacrimal apparatus can be shown on computed tomographic (CT) studies (Fig. 6.3). To demonstrate the bony lacrimal canal on routine radiographs, the patient bites on a large dental film; then the exposure is

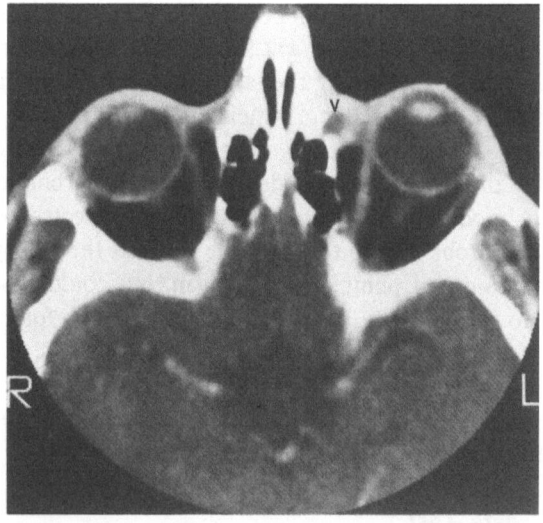

A

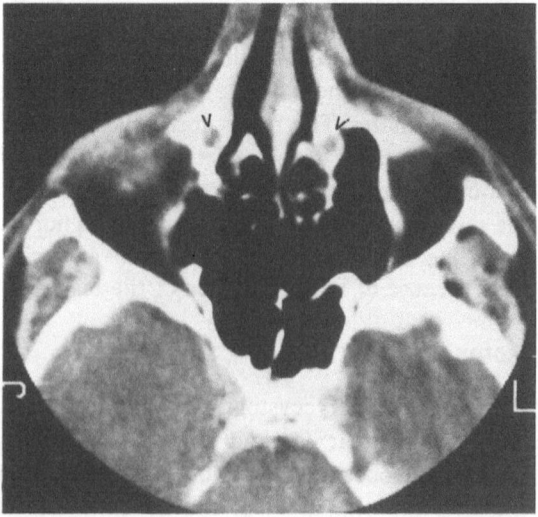

B

Figure 6.3 A. A 61-year-old man with purulent discharge from the upper punctum on the left with a soft mass present between the nose and the medial canthus. A CT scan performed with contrast shows a dilated tear sac on the left (*V*). **B.** A lower level CT view shows normal bony nasolacrimal ducts. (*V*).

made with the center of the x-ray beam perpendicular to the plane of the film. The beam traverses the frontal bone in the median line and exits at the level of the first molar tooth. Normally, the two orifices of the bony canal will appear as concentric, slightly oval shadows projected laterally to the median raphe (22). This view can be used to show stenosis of the lacrimal passages that are secondary to fractures of the bony canal.

The best method for visualizing the lacrimal drainage system at this time is the intubation dacryocystogram. This technique was first described in 1909 (17). Bismuth subnitrate was used as a contrast material and was injected into the inferior canaliculus via a metal cannula; then x-ray films were obtained. Since that time, many variations of the technique and various different contrast agents (water-soluble and oil-based) have been reported (4, 5, 14, 15, 21, 30, 32, 39, 43, 44, 50, 54). One technique used both a retrograde injection up the nasal ostium and a dental film intranasally as a substitute for the lateral and Waters positions (26). Another variation is distention dacryocystography—a method in which the radiographs are obtained during continuous injection of the contrast medium into the drainage system, via tubes placed in the canaliculi (30). In another technique—macrodacryocystography—the patient is placed at a greater distance from the x-ray cassette to provide greater magnification of the image on the film (4, 5, 39). X-ray subtraction techniques have been used to eliminate confusing bone shadows (Figs. 6.4 and 6.5) (39). Fluoroscopy and spot films of the lacrimal system during injection of contrast material is still another examination method (15). X-ray cinematography (16, 54, 56) may have some research value; but in our experience, it is generally not useful.

Our method of dacryocystogram begins with the patient in a supine position. After the physical examination, probing of the canaliculi and digital compression of the lacrimal sac to express any retained secretions (Fig. 6.4), the conjunctival sac is anesthetized with a few drops of a local anesthetic. A Rabinov (Cook, Inc., Bloomington, Indiana) sialography cannula or a similar-sized plastic tube (about 25 cm long) is attached to a 3 or 5 cc syringe containing either Ethiodol (Savage Laboratories, Missouri City, Texas), Salpix (Ortho Pharmaceutical Corp., Raritan, New Jersey), Sinografin (Squibb, Princeton, N.J.), or Renografin-76 (Squibb, Princeton, New Jersey). The contrast medium is flushed through the tubing to eliminate

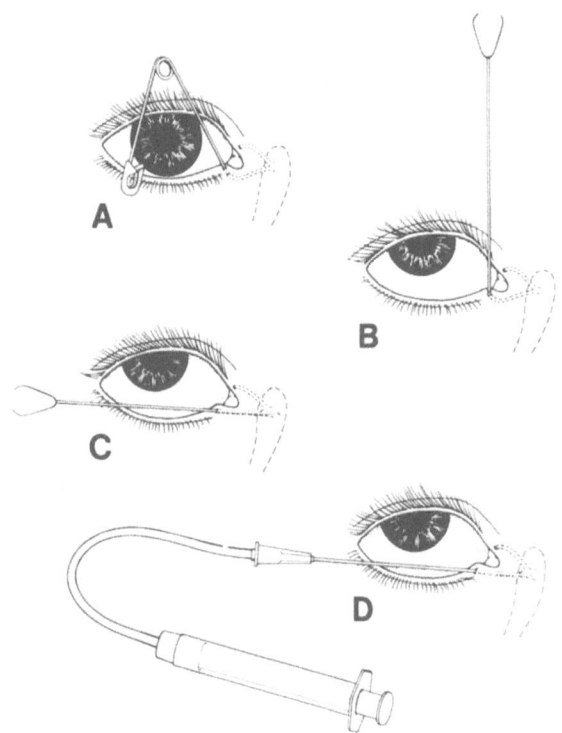

Figure 6.4. To cannulate the canaliculus for injection dacrocystography: **A.** Dilate the punctum. **B.** Then insert the Bowman dilator. **C.** Advance the dilator while stretching the lid. Remove the dilator and, in the same fashion, insert the cannula attached to the syringe of contrast media. **D.** Inject under fluoroscopic control, taking spot films before and after.

air bubbles; then the tip of the tube is inserted 3–5 mm through the punctum, usually into the inferior canaliculus. Under fluoroscopic control, the contrast agent is injected into the lacrimal drainage system. Appropriate spot films are obtained. If there is considerable reflux through the opposite canaliculus, it is occluded with a probe and the study is repeated. At present, we prefer to use Renografin 76 as the contrast agent, because it is an absorbable water-soluble agent, does not break up into globules as the oily agents may do, and is miscible with body fluids.

In a patient with an obstructed common canaliculus, the remainder of the distal lacrimal apparatus may be studied by using an injection technique (45). A 5/8-inch 25-gauge needle is inserted below the medial canthus and posterior to the anterior lacrimal crest until its tip meets the bony lacrimal fossa. Then 0.5 ml of a water-soluble contrast agent is injected. If there is no swelling of the

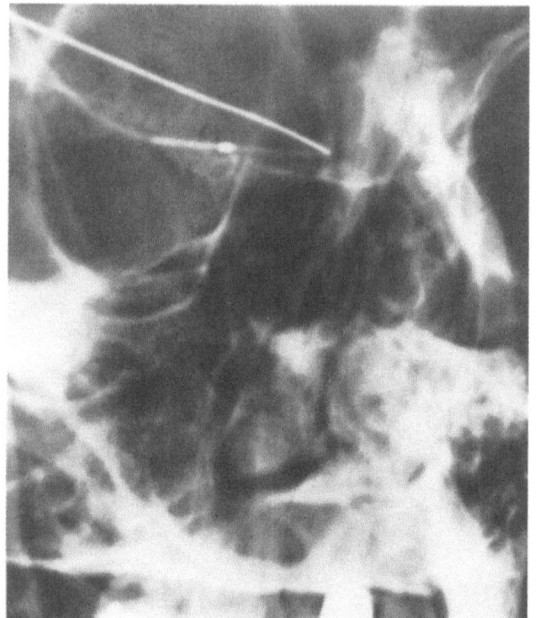

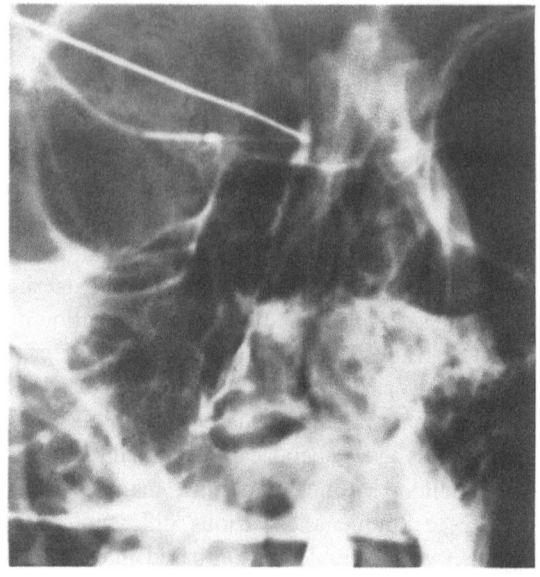

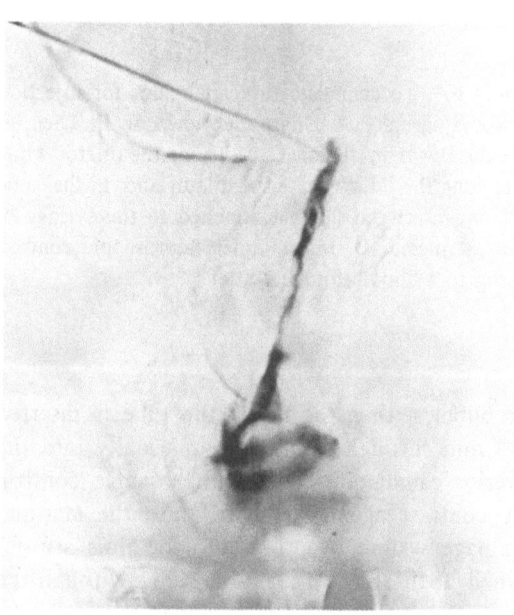

Figure 6.5. A. Scout film. **B.** Injection study made in the same position as the scout film, showing a normal drainage system. **C.** The subtraction study.

eyelids, an additional 1 ml is injected while a posteroanterior Caldwell view x-ray film is taken. Then the needle is withdrawn and a lateral view is obtained. These views are repeated in 30 minutes. If the lacrimal apparatus can be shown distal to the common canaliculus, this study can help to determine which patients can be treated by probing the common duct without performing a dacryocystorhinostomy procedure.

Clinical Aspects

The most common reason for patient referral for dacryocystography is the presence of epiphora. Other indications are masses in the area of the drainage system, trauma, and persistent overflow tearing after surgery. Obstructions of the lacrimal drainage system may be due to congenital causes, following facial bone fractures, tumors, foreign

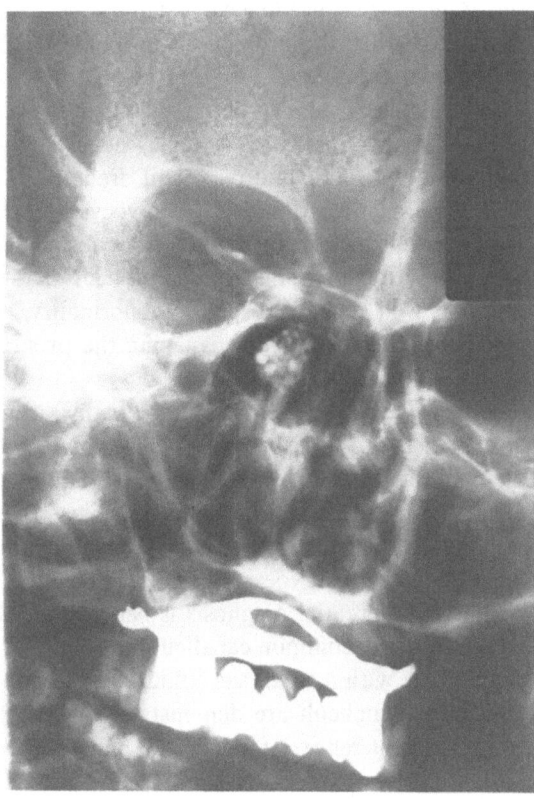

Figure 6.6. Contrast media (oily) in a cyst communicating with the tear sac, which had not been emptied prior to the injection.

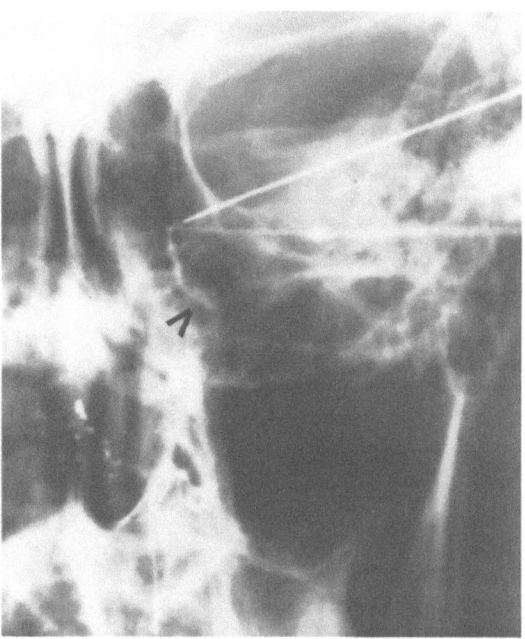

Figure 6.7. Deviation of the soft-tissue portion of the nasolacrimal duct by a sebaceous cyst. (V).

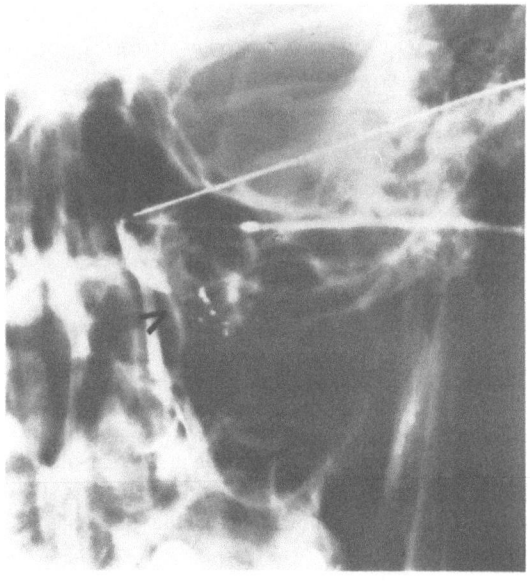

Figure 6.8. Demonstration of a posttraumatic fistula from the lower portion of the tear sac. (V).

bodies, casts, infections, scarring, ethmoiditis, and intranasal disease (Figs. 6.6, 6.7, 6.8, and 6.9).

Epiphora found in the young infant most often has a congenital etiology. An obstruction at the lower end of the nasolacrimal duct, presenting either as a persistent membrane or as a bony obstruction under the inferior turbinate, results from failure of complete canalization in the late embryologic period. There may be plugging of the lacrimal drainage pathway with inspissated meconium or debris (3, 44, 55). In 80–90% of infants with epiphora, the condition will spontaneously correct itself by the time the child is 4 months old (18). However, this condition may disappear as late as 21 months of age (55). Complications of this congenital obstruction include amniocele (amniotic fluid retained in the sac and a nonpatent nasolacrimal duct) and dacryocystitis (acute mucocele or pyocele). These conditions are treated by simple probing. At this age, other causes of masses in the area of the lacrimal sac are benign tumors

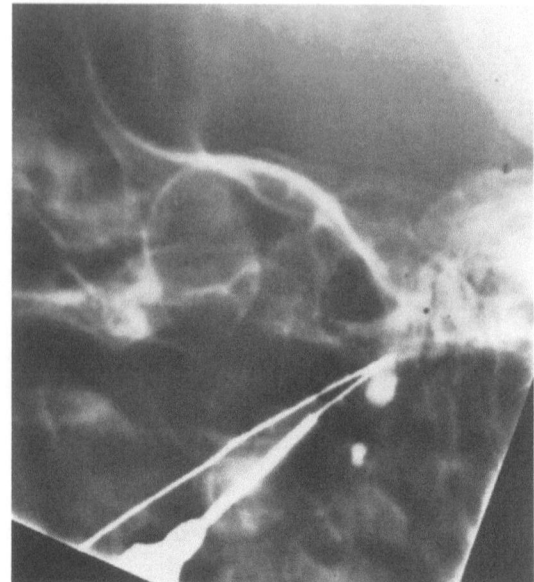

A

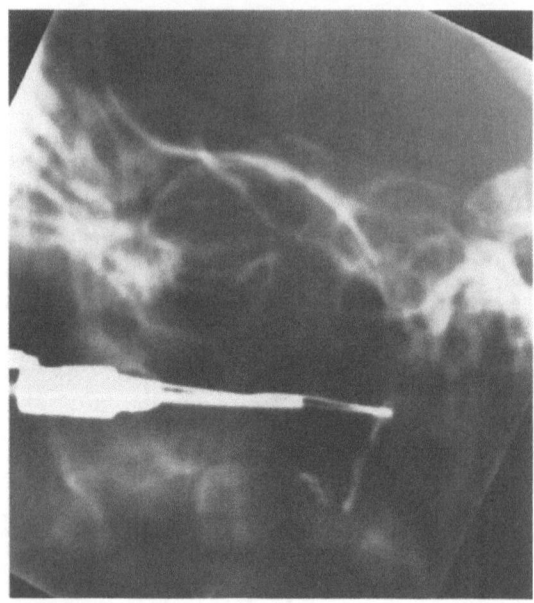

B

Figure 6.9 A. Midlevel obstruction in a 2-year-old child. **B.** Repeat study after probing, while patient is still on fluoroscopic table, showing that the duct has been opened.

(hemangioma, dermoid, and so on). Echography can help in the differential diagnosis by showing whether the mass is solid or fluid-filled (51). In infants 2 months of age or older, some investigators recommend probing for persistent epiphora (57). Dacryocystography may be considered in some of these patients (2, 20). The pressure from

the injections may, at times, be sufficient to open the drainage system. We have had one patient who was cured, with the probing being monitored by dacryocystography.

In adults, persistent epiphora, masses in the area of nasolacrimal pathway, trauma, persistent inflammation, tumors, and persistent drainage after surgery are indications for dacryocystography (44). Identification of the cause of the obstruction to tear flow and its localization on the dacryocystogram, as well as an unsuspected abnormality, are guides for the surgeon in managing the problem (41).

The obstructed site of the lacrimal pathway may be classified into three broad categories: high, middle, and low (44). The high-level obstructions are located in the canaliculi or sinus of Maier. These are usually diagnosed by physical examinations or probing. A dacryocystogram will be helpful when the differential diagnosis is between an obstruction of the common canaliculus or a midlevel obstruction with a small sac. Blocks in the upper and lower canaliculi are demonstrated when the contrast agent refluxes through the punctum that has been injected; on x-ray films, the injected canaliculus is outlined as far as the stenosis. A common canaliculus block is demonstrated by the regurgitation of the contrast agent through the nonintubated punctum and by outlining of both canaliculi on the x-ray film. There is no filling of the lacrimal sac if the obstruction is complete, and only partial filling of the sac if the obstruction is incomplete. Partial filling of the common canaliculus often indicates an obstruction of the medial end at the level of the lacrimal sac. Nonfilling of the lumen of the common canaliculus suggests a block involving its whole length.

The midlevel obstruction is the most common type studied by using dacryocystography. This is more common in adults. The obstruction includes the region of the neck of the sac to the lower third of the bony canal. The sac is dilated, and no contrast agent is seen in the lacrimal duct. These blocks may result in a mucocele.

The low-level obstruction is the one located at the lower end of the nasolacrimal duct. This usually is the congenital type, as discussed earlier. When a dacryocystogram is obtained on this type, no contrast agent will be seen in the nose.

Obstruction at the middle and lower levels in the lacrimal passageway results in the accumulation of secretions above the block and the gradual

Figure 6.10. A 20-month-old girl with persistent bilateral epiphora. **A.** Initial injection dacryocystogram showing midlevel obstruction on the left. **B.** After probing on the left, the nasolacrimal drainage system is opened, displaying a congenital diverticulum (arrow). **C.** Injection study after probing the right side, showing bilateral congenital diverticula (arrows) and open nasolacrimal ducts.

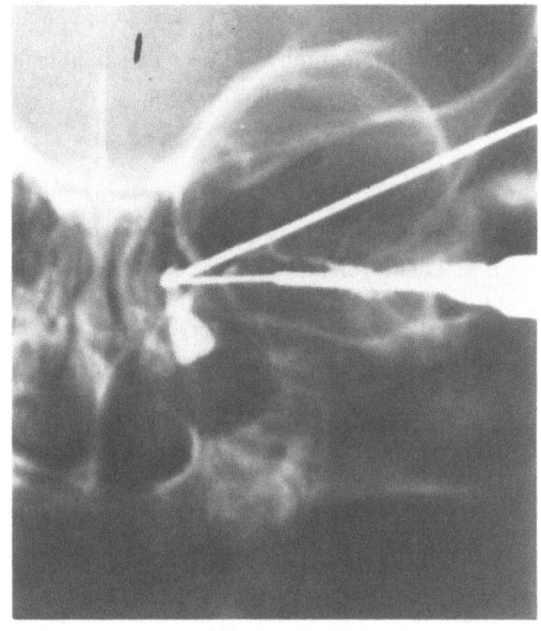

A

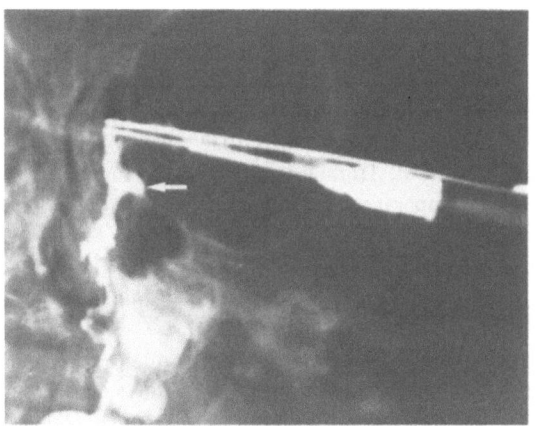

B

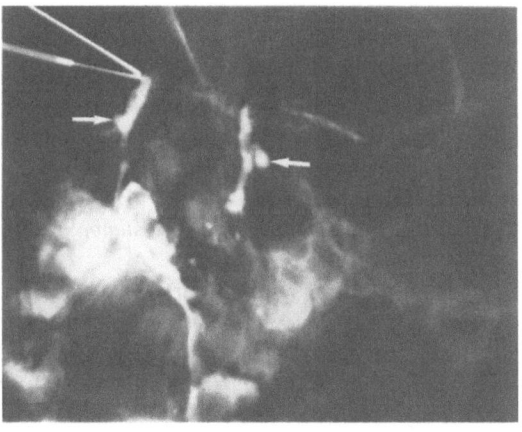

C

dilation of the duct or sac, where they are not confined by bone or restrictive fascial bands. This accumulation of stagnated secretions predisposes to infection and eventually to chronic dacryocystitis.

While dacryocystography may be useful in showing an intraluminal mass in the lacrimal drainage system, care must be taken in interpreting filling defects to exclude air bubbles, accumulations of mucous, and other debris. The intraluminal masses may be dacryoliths, tumors, or mycotic balls (often due to actinomyces).

Occasionally, an unsuspected diverticulum may be seen on the dacryocystogram. This often is congenital, and the knowledge of its presence is important to surgical planning. Also, congenital as well

as posttraumatic fistulae may be shown (Fig. 6.10) (10).

When a dacryocystorhinostomy is followed by persistent epiphora, a dacryocystogram is indicated to find the cause (42). The inadequate drainage may be due to an anastomosis, which is too high and/or too small. Sometimes, scarring or an inflammatory granuloma may be detected.

In patients with disorders of the lacrimal drainage pathway, the evaluation should include a history and ophthalmologic and nasal examinations. Then functional studies should be done, followed by routine x-ray films and an intubation dacryocystogram if an obstruction is suspected. Ultrasonic (echography) examination may be helpful if a mass is present. Dacryocystograms are valuable in therapeutic planning and in evaluating persistent epiphora after surgery.

Computed tomography is especially valuable for demonstrating the bony nasolacrimal duct.

References

1. Moses RA (ed): *Adler's Physiology of the Eye*, ed 7. St Louis, Toronto, London, CV Mosley, 1981, pp 16–37.
2. Agarwal ML, Geysta BP: Dacryocystography and lacrimal probing in cases of congenital obstruction of nasolacrimal duct. *Ind J Ophthal* 24:30–32, 1976.
3. Busse H, Muller KM, Kroll P: Radiological and histological findings of the lacrimal passages of newborns. *Arch Ophthalmol* 98:528–532, 1980.
4. Campbell W: Radiology of the lacrimal system: *Br J Radiol* 37:1–26, 1964.
5. Campbell W: Radiology of the lacrimal system. *Int Ophthal Clin* 4:399–441, 1964.
6. Carlton WH, Trueblook JH, Rossomondo RM: Clinical evaluation of microscintigraphy of the lacrimal drainage apparatus. *J Nucl Med* 14:89–92, 1973.
7. Chaudhuri TK, Saparoff GR, Dolan KD, et al: A comparative study of contrast dacryocystogram and nuclear dacryocystogram. *J Nucl Med* 16:605–608, 1974.
8. Chavis RM, Welham R, Maisey M: Quantitative lacrimal scintillography. *Arch Ophthalmol* 96:2066–2068, 1978.
9. Cohen SW, Sherman M, Schwartz GG, et al: Lacrimal outflow patency demonstrated by chemiluminescence. *Arch Ophthalmol* 98:126–127, 1980.
10. Dayton GO Jr, Hanafee W: Lacrimal sac fistulas. *Tr Am Ophth Soc* 78:301–310, 1980.
11. Demorest BH, Milder B: The pathologic lacrimal apparatus. *Arch Ophthalmol* 54:410–421, 1955.
12. Duke-Elder S, Wybar KC (eds): *System of Ophthalmology: The Anatomy of the Visual System*. St Louis, CV Mosley, 1961, vol II, pp 568–581.
13. Duke-Elder S, MacFaul PA (eds): *System of Ophthalmology: The Ocular Adnexa Part II*. St Louis, CV Mosley, 1974, vol XII, pp 675–773.
14. El Gammal T, Brooks BS: Amipaque dacryocystography. *Radiology* 141:541–542, 1981.
15. Eiferman RA: Fluoroscopy of the lacrimal system during intubation of contrast material. *Am J Ophth* 87:572–573, 1979.
16. Epstein E: Cine dacryocystography. *Trans Ophthal Soc UK* 81:284–287, 1961.
17. Ewing AE: Roentgen ray demonstration of the lacrimal abscess cavity. *Am J Ophthal* 26:1–4, 1909.
18. Ffooks OO: Dacryocystitis in infancy: *Br J Ophthalmol* 46:422–434, 1962.
19. Flack Q: The fluorescein appearance test for lacrimal obstruction. *Ophthalmology* 97:237–242, 1979.
20. Goldberg A, Hurwitz JJ: Congenital abnormalities of lacrimal drainage. Management of difficult cases. *Canad J Ophthal* 14:106–109, 1979.
21. Gullotta V von, Deuffer N von: Die dacryocystographie. *Forschr Roentgenstr* 124:466–471, 1976.
22. Hartmann E, Gilles E: *Roentgenologic Diagnosis in Ophthalmology*. Philadelphia, Montreal, JB Lippincott, 1959, pp 166–186.
23. Hecht SD: Evaluation of the lacrimal drainage system. *Ophthalmology* 85:1250–1258, 1978.
24. Hornblass Q: A simple taste test for lacrimal obstruction. *Arch Ophthalmol* 90:435–436, 1973.
25. Hornblass A, Ingis TM: Lacrimal function tests. *Arch Ophthalmol* 97:1654–1655, 1979.
26. Hourn GE: X-ray visualization of the nasolacrimal duct. *Ann Otol Rhinol Laryngol* 46:962–975, 1937.
27. Hurwitz JJ, Maisey MN, Welham RA: Quantitative lacrimal scintillography. I. Method and physiological application. *Br J Ophthal* 59:308–312, 1975.
28. Hurwitz JJ, Maisey MN, Welham RA: Quantitative lacrimal scintillography. II. Lacrimal pathology. *Br J Ophthal* 59:313–322, 1975.
29. Hurwitz JJ, Welham RA: Radiography in functional lacrimal testing. *Br J Ophthal* 59:323–331, 1975.
30. Iba GB, Hanafee WN: Distention dacryocystography. *Radiology* 90:1020–1022, 1968.
31. Ingis TM, Hornblass A: Lacrimal function tests: A comparative study. *Otolaryngol Ophthalmol Surg* 28:516–517, 1977.
32. Johansen JG, Udnaes I: Dacryocystography with amipaque (metrizamide). *Acta Ophthalmol* 55:683–687, 1977.
33. Jones LT: The cure of epiphora due to canalicular disorders, trauma and surgical failures on the lacrimal passages. *Trans Am Acad Ophthalmol Otolaryngol* 66:506–524, 1962.
34. Jones LT: Orbital anatomy, in Smith B, Converse JM (eds): *Plastic and Reconstructive Surgery of the Eye and Adnexa*. St Louis, CV Mosley, 1967, pp 30–45.
35. Jones LT, Linn ML: The diagnosis of causes of epiphora. *Am J Ophthalmol* 67:751–754, 1969.
36. Koszczynski Z, Nowicka L: Radiologiczne badanie morfologiczne oraz czynnosciowe, w Przypadkach niedroznosci drog Eowych. *Pol Przegl Radiol*, 32:701–703, 1968.
37. Linn ML, Jones LT: Rate of lacrimal excretion of ophthalmic vehicles. *Am J Ophthalmol* 65:76–80, 1968.
38. Lipsius E: Sodium saccharine for testing patency of the lacrimal passages. *Am J Ophthalmol* 41:320, 1956.
39. Lloyd GAS, Welham RAN: Subtraction macrodacryocystography. *Br J Radiol* 47:379–382, 1974.
40. Milder B, Demorest BH: Dacryocystography. I:

The normal lacrimal apparatus. *Arch Ophthalmol* 51:180–195, 1954.

41. Milder B: Dacryocystography in planning treatment of the lacrimal excretory system, in Veirs ER (ed): *The Lacrimal System. Proceedings of the First International Symposium.* St Louis, CV Mosley, 1971, pp 81–97.

42. Montanara A, Ciabattoni P, Rizzo P: Stenosis and functional disorders of the lacrimal drainage apparatus. Radiological examination. *Surv Ophthal* 23:249–258, 1979.

43. Montanara A, Catalino P, Gualdi M: Improved radiological technique for evaluating the lacrimal pathways with special emphasis on functional disorders. *Acta Ophthal* 57:547–563, 1979.

44. Pettit TH, Coin CC: Dacryocystography. *Radiol Clin North Am* 10:129–142, 1972.

45. Putterman AM: Dacryocystography with occluded common canaliculus. *Am J Ophthal* 76:1010–1012, 1973.

46. Raflo GT, Hurwitz JJ: Chemiluminescent evaluation of the human lacrimal outflow system. *Canad J Ophthalmol* 16:30–31, 1981.

47. Rodriguez HP, Kittleson AC: Distention dacryocystography. *Radiology* 109:317–321, 1973.

48. Rossomondo RM, Carlton WH, Trueblood JH, et al: A new method of evaluating lacrimal drainage. *Arch Ophthalmol* 88:523–525, 1972.

49. Saparoff GR, Chaudhuri T, Chandhuri T, et al: Nuclear lacrimal scan vs. dacryocystography. *Tr Am Acad Ophthalmol Otol* 81:566–579, 1976.

50. Sargent EN, Ebersole C: Dacryocystography: The use of Sinographin for visualization of the nasolacrimal passages. *Am J Roentgenol* 102:831–839, 1968.

51. Scott WE, Fabre JA, Ossining KC: Congenital mucocele of the lacrimal sac. *Arch Ophthalmol* 97:1656–1658, 1979.

52. Sorensen T, Taagehøj Jensen F: Methodological aspects of tear flow determination by means of a radioactive tracer. *Acta. Ophthal.* 55:726–737, 1977.

53. Sorensen T, Taagehøj Jensen F: Tear flow in normal human eyes, determination by means of radioisotope and gamma camera. *Acta. Ophthal.* 57:564–581, 1979.

54. Street DF, Howell MH: An alternative radiographic technique for macrodacryocystography. *Br J Radiol* 40:235–238, 1967.

55. Suckling RD: The natural history of congenital epiphora. *N Z Med J* 93:74–75, 1981.

56. Trokel SL, Potter GD: Kinetic dacryocystography. *Am J Ophthal* 70:1010–1011, 1970.

57. Veirs ER: Lacrimal disorders in infants and children, in Opt L (ed): *Diagnostic Procedures in Pediatric Ophthalmology.* Boston, Little Brown & Co, 1963, pp 213–221.

58. Whitnall SE: *The Anatomy of the Human Orbit and Accessory Organs of Vision.* ed 2. London, Edinburgh, Toronto, Oxford University Press, 1932, pp 208–252.

59. Wolff E: *Anatomy of the Eye and Orbit,* ed 7. Philadelphia, Toronto, WB Saunders, 1976, pp 226–237.

7
Foreign Body Localization

MELVIN H. BECKER

When an intraorbital foreign body is suspected, it is important for the management of the patient that the foreign body be identified and accurately localized. From the history of the patient's injury, the referring physician should have a good idea as to the nature of the suspected foreign body (wood, plastic, iron, or other metals). Since an examination of the eyeball may be interfered with by exudate or bleeding, the grave sequelae of a retained foreign body (infection, calcification, or siderosis) require imaging techniques (radiography, tomography, computed tomography [CT], ultrasound, or Berman locator) for a definitive diagnosis. These studies should determine if one or more foreign bodies are present, if the objects are radiopaque, and if they are inside or outside the globe. Also, the object's exact location and relationship to the wall of the eyeball should be established.

After the first recorded attempts at radiographic localization of an orbital foreign body in 1896 (2, 15), many techniques evolved. These techniques include those using only plain films, metallic markers, stereoscopic films, multisection tomography, CT, ultrasound, and electromagnetic devices (4, 5, 6, 8). In all of these techniques, a cooperative subject is necessary because a fixed gaze must be maintained.

When a foreign body is suspected, its presence or absence usually can be confirmed by a frontal and lateral radiograph of the orbit (Fig. 7.1). However, a radiolucent object cannot be excluded, because it cannot be differentiated from normal tissue. A radiolucent foreign body may be detected by ultrasonic techniques.

Radiographic Studies

If the foreign body is anteriorly situated, "bone-free" techniques are valuable (4, 7, 9, 13, 14). The bone-free examinations require the use of a topical anesthetic on the conjunctiva. A dental film is inserted between the eyeball and orbit; it is held in place either by the patient's hand or with a special film holder. One exposure is taken with the film held on the nasal side, (temporonasal view); the other is done with the film placed within the lower recess of the conjunctival sac (craniocaudal view) or preferably with the film inserted into the superior recess of the conjunctival sac (submento-vertex view) (Fig. 7.2). Each exposure should be made with the film positioned as deep as possible in the conjunctival sac, using a narrow cone with the central ray directed to expose as large a portion of the globe as possible to show tiny splinters of metal, glass, calcium compounds, or wood. These radiographic exposures should be made with low kilovoltage techniques (i.e., 40 kV, 20 mA, 0.4 seconds). It will be possible, at times, to demonstrate foreign bodies (such as glass and wood) that are not visible with higher kilovoltage studies.

Physiologic or dynamic methods may be employed to establish whether the foreign body is intraocular. In these techniques, the eyeball is rotated and movement is recorded on film (5, 7). The changes in position of the foreign body indicate whether the foreign matter is inside the eyeball and whether it is located anteriorly or posteriorly, superiorly or inferiorly, and temporally or nasally (Fig. 7.3). Although a specific axis of ocular rota-

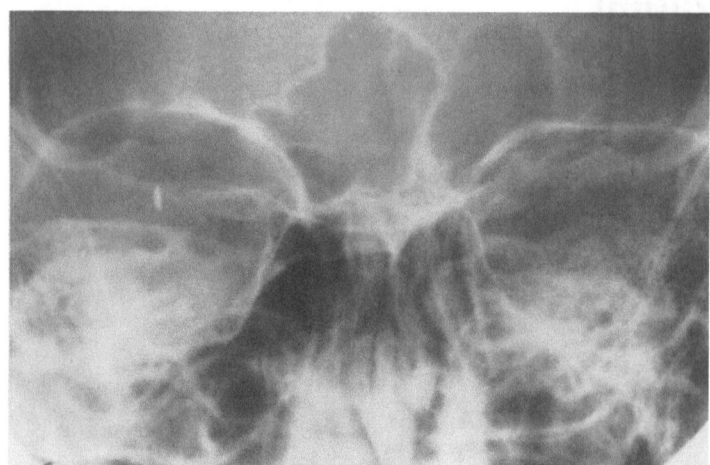

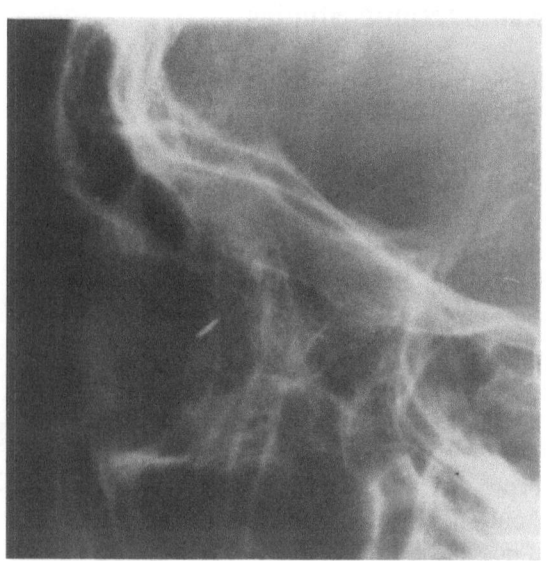

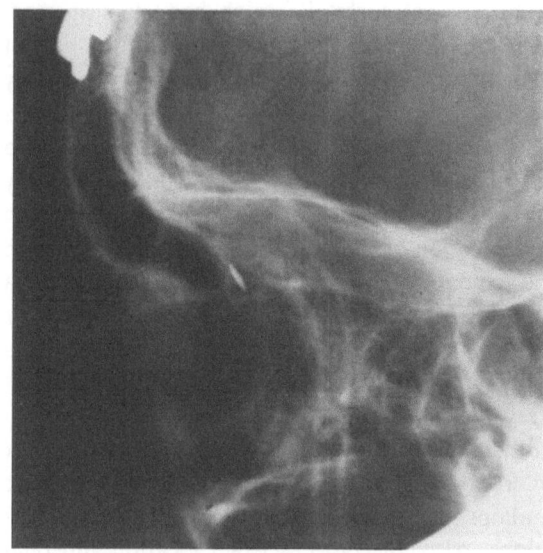

Figure 7.1 A. Posteroanterior view showing a metallic foreign body in the 12 o'clock position. **B.** Lateral view showing the foreign body located posteriorly. **C.** Lateral view with downward gaze showing the foreign body moving up, confirming that it is in the posterior area of the globe.

tion cannot be defined, a centrode of rotation lying 1.5 mm behind the equator of the globe may be used. If a foreign body is anterior to the centrode, films made after upward and downward gaze will show the fragment's movement in the direction of ocular motion. On the other hand, if the fragment is situated in the posterior portion of the globe, it will move in a direction opposite to the direction of gaze. Unfortunately, foreign bodies located in Tenon's capsule, ocular muscle, or orbital fat may move in relation to eye motion. Thus, a more specific means of localization is needed.

Metallic markers, in the form of a limbal ring embedded in a contact lens or placed extraocu-

larly, can be used to localize a foreign body precisely in three planes. The most commonly used of these techniques in the United States have been the limbal ring (10), the Sweet method, and the Comberg lens method (4, 5, 7, 10, 13). At present, this author has found only the Sweet method device to be available commercially. Since CT and ultrasonography are rapidly replacing these techniques, they will not be discussed. The details of how to use these methods may be found in texts written by Duke-Elder (4), Hartmann and Gilles (7), Lloyd (10), and Pendergrass, Shaeffer, and Hodes (3). The stereoscopic and multisection tomographic methods are also being replaced by CT and ultrasound techniques.

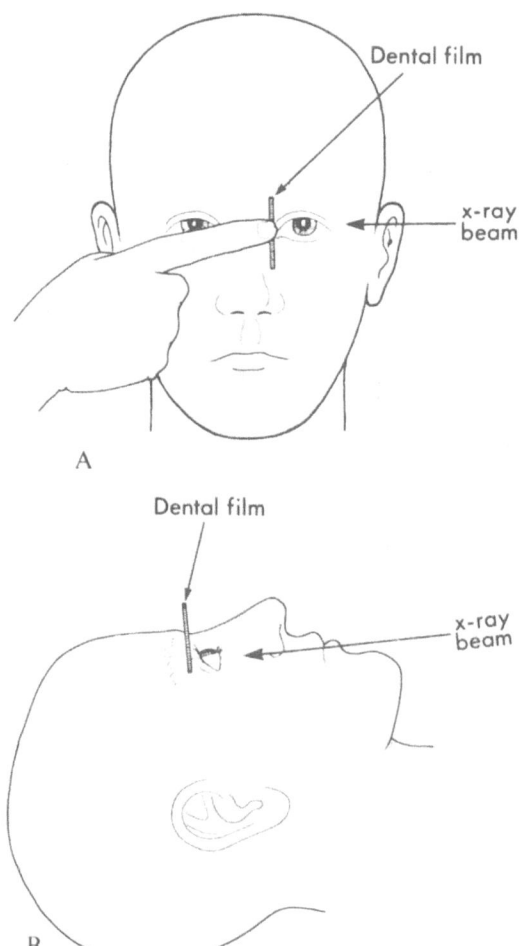

A

B

Figure 7.2. Positioning of dental film to obtain "bone-free" film of the globe. **A.** The submentovertical position with film deep in the upper fornix. **B.** The lateral or temporonasal view with film between the globe and the medial orbital wall.

Berman Locator

An instrument used for detecting metallic foreign bodies is the Berman locator (4). The principle of its use depends on the fact that if an alternating current is sent through a primary circuit, a current forms in a secondary coil by induction. If the voltages in the secondary coils are equalized, no current flows between them. However, if in this state the instrument approaches a metallic object, the balanced inductance is disturbed and a difference in potential is created in the secondary circuit, resulting in a flow of current which—when ampli-

fied—may be recorded by deflection of an ammeter needle for visual indication or by variations in the tone of a loudspeaker for an acoustic indication. The magnitude of this current varies with the magnetic properties of the particle, its size, and its distance from the instrument. While a magnetic foreign body profoundly affects the magnetic field created around the instrument, nonmagnetic metals also can be detected, but with lesser alterations in the magnetic field. The Berman locator can detect an iron or steel fragment at a distance of about 10 times the diameter of the particle. However, with a nonmagnetic metal, the effective range is 1 or 2 times the diameter of the particle. This method is not as accurate as radiography. However, it is valuable when accurate radiography is not available. Nonetheless, it is a useful adjunct to radiography. When covered with a sterile rubber shield, it can be used during surgery to confirm the position of the foreign body.

Ultrasound

Ultrasonic scanning units have been designed that are dedicated to studying the contents of the orbits. Transducers have been developed to allow both A-scan and B-scan evaluation of ocular structures. The A scan can determine the axial length of the eye by measuring the distance between signals reflected from the anterior and posterior orbital surfaces. This measurement allows for more precise localization of foreign bodies, since most other techniques have assumed this distance to be 24 mm. The B-scan ultrasonogram records a cross-sectional representation of the eye, and it can be used to determine accurate localization of a foreign body when a clear echo is received. (This is true for both radiopaque and radiolucent foreign bodies.) (see Fig. 4.6). The combination of ultrasound and radiographic studies increases the precision with which localization of a foreign body can be made (3). In addition, ultrasound studies are helpful in determining the presence of lens dislocation, retinal detachment, vitreous clots, and anatomic malformations.

Computed Tomography

Since the introduction of CT scanning in the early 1970s, the imaging of the orbit has been revolutionized. This is particularly true for foreign body lo-

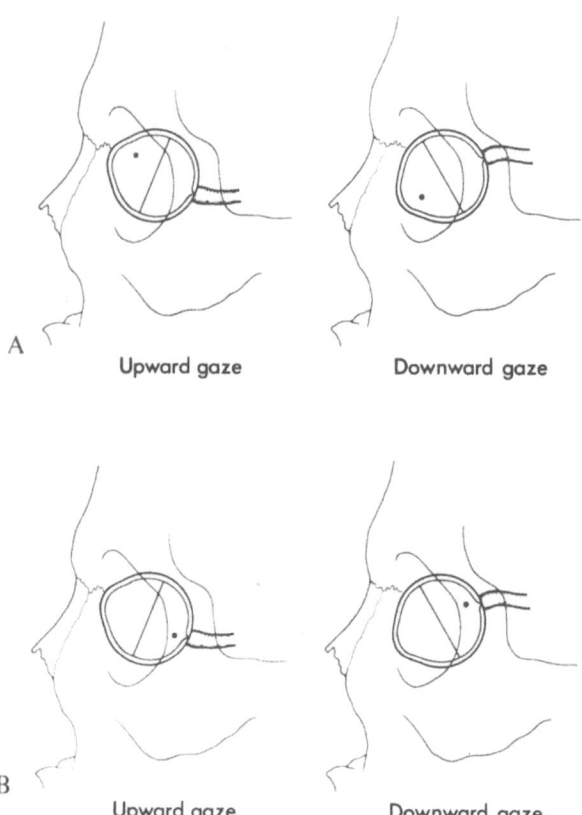

A

Upward gaze   Downward gaze

B

Upward gaze   Downward gaze

Figure 7.3. Drawings showing the change in location of a foreign body in the globe with different directions of gaze. **A.** An anterior foreign body moves in the direction of the gaze. **B.** A posterior foreign body moves opposite to the direction of the gaze.

calization (Fig. 7.4) (see also Figs. 15.22 and 15.23 and Fig. 16.19). With the newer generation of these units, the software has been programmed to reduce artifacts created by metal, and thereby has made it possible to very accurately localize foreign bodies. These foreign bodies, either metallic or nonmetallic, may be shown to be intraorbital or intraocular. The size and density of the object determines whether or not it will be seen (8). Metals may be visualized if they have a diameter of 1 mm or greater (6). Other materials (aluminum, glass, bone, and wood) must be somewhat larger to be detected (8). The absorption coefficient can help to define the material of the foreign body. In computed tomographic studies performed with the newer generation units, the studies can be done in both axial and coronal views. In these examina-

tions, the orbital anatomy is well outlined and precise localization of abnormalities is possible.

The two newest techniques of foreign body localization (i.e., ultrasound and CT) are complemental procedures. The ultrasound examination is particularly valuable in demonstrating radiolucent foreign bodies and in verifying the site of the foreign body. In addition, the ultrasound study yields considerable information about the abnormalities in the eyeball (e.g., retinal detachments, organized vitreous hemorrhage, or the differentiation of a choroidal prominence). However, the CT study will be helpful in the presence of unclear echogenic results in opaque media (1). A complementary CT scan is not needed in the study of foreign bodies involving the anterior third of the eyeball when a clear echogenic diagnosis is present. In problems of the middle third of the orbit, these two examinations complement each other. When the abnormalities are suspected in the orbital apex, the periorbital region, and the intracranial space, CT studies are more informative (1, 12). There is a case report (11) in which a wooden foreign body was abutting the optic nerve; this was demonstrated by a CT scan and not by ultrasonic study. In a severely traumatized patient, the CT study is easier to do.

Summary

When a foreign body is suspected in the orbit or eyeball that cannot be detected or localized by normal ophthalmologic examinations, imaging procedures should be performed using the simplest techniques first. Routine frontal and lateral films will identify radiopaque foreign bodies. If the foreign substance is anteriorly located, the "bone-free" radiographic study will be of further assistance. With a radiopaque foreign body, dynamic films can help to determine the object both in the eyeball and in which portion of it. If the foreign body is radiolucent, the ultrasonic study should be done. When detailed localization of the foreign body is desired, CT studies should be used, complementing the ultrasonic studies. If CT is not available, an older method is recommended, such as the limbal metal ring, the Comberg lens, the Sweet technique, or another method using metallic markers. When removing the foreign body, the ultrasonic method and/or the Berman locator can be helpful in the operating theater.

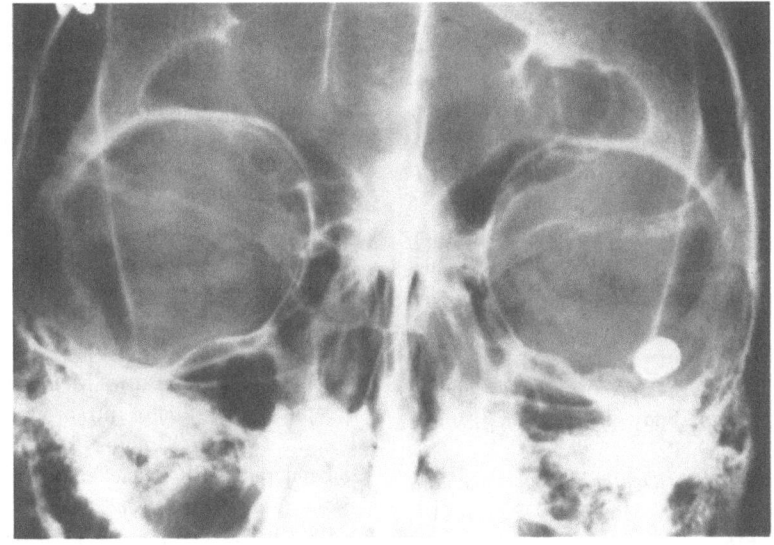

A

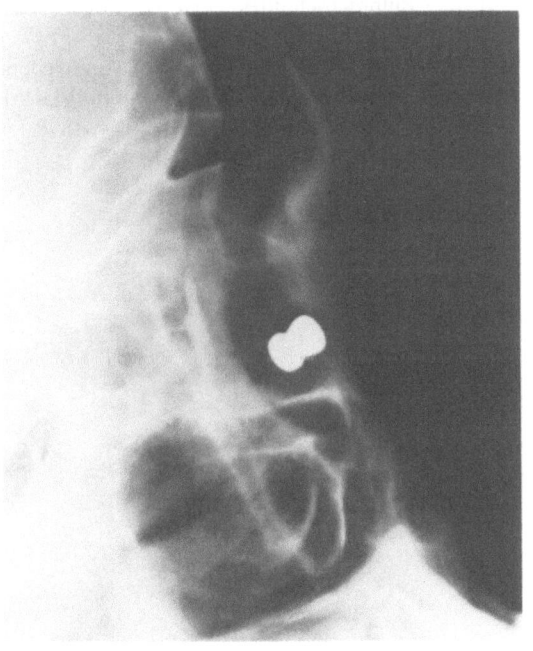

B

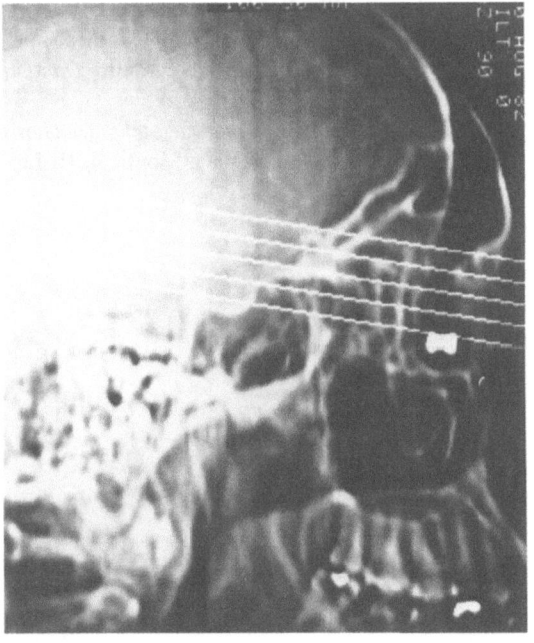

C

Figure 7.4 A. Anteroposterior view showing pellet from a gunshot in the lower lateral portion of the left orbit. **B.** Lateral view showing the pellet situated anteriorly. **C.** Lateral scout film used in CT localization. **D.** Axial CT view shows the pellet to be outside the globe. This was confirmed at surgery.

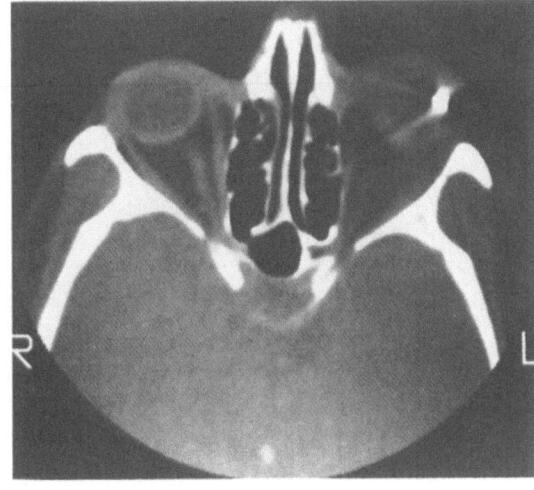

D

References

1. Bigar F, Spiess H, Gruber HU: Kombinierte Anwendung der Computer-Tomographie and Echographie in der Ophthalmologie. *Klin mbl Augenheilk* 174:806–815, 1979.
2. Clark CF: A question as to the presence and location of a minute fragment of steel in the eye determined by the roentgen rays—successful removal by the electromagnet. *Trans Am Ophthalmol Soc* 7:711–715, 1894–1896.
3. Coleman DJ, Trokel SL: A protocol for B-scan and radiographic foreign body localization. *Am J Ophthalmol* 71:84–89, 1971.
4. Duke-Elder S: *System of Ophthalmology: Mechanical Injuries.* St Louis, CV Mosley, 1972, vol XIV, part I, pp 565–616.
5. Erkonew W, Dolan KD: Ocular foreign body localization. *Radiol Clin North Am* 10:101–114, 1972.
6. Gaster RN, Duda EE: Localization of intraocular foreign bodies by computed tomography. *Ophthal Surg* 11:25–29, 1980.
7. Hartmann E, Gilles E: *Roentgenographic Diagnosis in Ophthalmology.* Philadelphia, Montreal, JB Lippincott, 1959, pp 128–165.
8. Kadir S, Arnow S, Davis KR: The use of computerized tomography in the detection of intraorbital foreign bodies. *Comput Tomogr* 1:151–156, 1977.
9. Lindblom H: Localisation des corps etrangers intraoculaires, par la radiographie sans squelette. *Acta Ophthalmol* 26:439–440, 1948.
10. Lloyd GA: *Radiology of the Orbit.* London, Philadelphia, Toronto, WB Saunders, 1975, pp 197–210.
11. Macrae JA: Diagnosis and management of a wooden orbital foreign body: case report. *Br J Ophthal* 63:848–851, 1979.
12. Mandelcorn MS, Brown M: Computed axial tomography localization of intraorbital foreign body. *Canad J Ophthal* 13:213–215, 1978.
13. Pendergrass EP, Schaeffer JP, Hodes PJ: *The Head and Neck in Roentgen Diagnosis,* ed 2. Springfield, Ill, Charles C Thomas, 1956, vol I, pp 811–863.
14. Vogt A: Skelettfreie: Rontgenanfnahme des vorderen Bulbusabschnittes. *Schweiz Med Wschr* 7:145–146, 1921.
15. Williams CH: A case of extraction of a bit of copper from the vitreous where x-rays helped to locate the metal. *Boston Med Surg J* 135:163–164, 1896.

8
Magnetic Resonance Imaging (MRI) of the Eye and Orbit

David F. Sobel, Ivan F. Moseley, and Michael Brant-Zawadzki

The contents of the orbit and its osseous margins have been particularly well imaged since the development of x-ray computed tomographic (CT) imaging. The greatly differing x-ray attenuation characteristics of the constituent tissues allow their separation and segregation into discrete compartments (11). Magnetic resonance imaging (MRI) is a newly emerging technique that may supplant or supplement CT for diagnostic imaging. MRI also has the potential to provide fine structural detail and tissue characterization in this region, while avoiding ionizing radiation to the globe and providing some unique information. The present discussion reflects our initial experience in examination of the eye, orbit, and structures therein by using this evolving imaging technology.

Basic Principles of MRI

Conventional radiographic techniques (including CT) rely on differences in atomic density between tissues to affect x-ray attenuation and, consequently, to produce contrast in the resulting images. Radiographic contrast media can be administered to enhance intrinsic contrast differences between tissues, based on the distribution of such agents in the capillary bed or their accumulation in the extracellular space. The magnetic resonance image is dependent on different tissue contrast parameters: hydrogen density, the state of motion of the hydrogen protons, and the relaxation times T1 and T2—which represent the behavior of hydrogen protons as influenced by the physicochemical properties of their host tissue when placed in a strong magnetic field (10). All of these play a major role in the formation of an image. Many

imaging techniques have been developed with MRI, the details of which are beyond the scope of this chapter. The very complexity of the physical processes involved affords new insights into tissue characterization and detection of disease. A somewhat simplistic explanation of the MRI process follows, but the interested reader is referred to a more comprehensive review (9).

Nuclei with an odd number of protons or neutrons act as small magnets when placed in a strong magnetic field. Hydrogen is the most ubiquitous of the body's elements having such a nucleus, and it is the focus of current MRI technology. An alignment of a small proportion of these hydrogen nuclei tends to occur in any given tissue, when it is placed in a static external magnetic field. A net magnetic vector or moment aligned with the magnetic field can then be described and quantified for the entire population of nuclei thus affected. Application of a radiofrequency (RF) pulse of a specific frequency (which is dependent on the strength of the magnetic field and the nuclei being imaged) introduces energy into the sample and displaces the net magnetic vector by an amount determined by the amplitude and duration of the RF pulse. After the pulse is removed, the protons tend to return to their original orientation (realign) while emitting the absorbed energy in the form of an RF signal, which is used to generate the magnetic resonance image. If a gradient is used to predictably alter the original magnetic field, the frequency signals emitted by the energized protons will be related to their position within that gradient. This is exploited by using Fourier analysis to obtain spatial information.

The nature of the surrounding tissue and the chemical state of the hydrogen atoms dictate the time required for protons to regain their original orientation or to relax within the magnetic field after the RF pulse. Two basic forms of relaxation can be studied that reflect a distinct physical characteristic of the tissue imaged. The realignment after an RF perturbation occurs exponentially with a "spin-lattice" time constant T1, which reflects thermal interactions of the hydrogen nucleus within its molecular environment. The more readily these nuclei can dissipate the energy bestowed on them by the RF excitation, the shorter the T1 value. During exposure to the RF pulse, not only is the proton vector or magnetization altered, but coherent resonance of the protons is induced (a rapid, repetitive alteration of their energy state). The RF signal detected from a sample of protons during relaxation is dependent on the magnitude of their collective vector at the time of excitation (a T1 function), while the decay of the signal is dictated by the loss of coherent resonance induced by local tissue nonhomogeneities in the magnetic field. This decay is characterized by the exponential "spin-spin" function (T2). Protons that rapidly traverse the plane being imaged, such as flowing blood, return relatively little signal during the acquisition sequence.

The characteristic tissue parameters (hydrogen density, motion of hydrogen protons, and T1 and T2 relaxation times of the tissue being imaged) contribute to the signal intensity detected by the imager and encoded in gray scale, but the manner in which information is gathered can be varied; thus, it can influence the relative contribution of each of these parameters to that signal intensity. For example, although the frequency of the pulse used to perturb the protons is characteristic of the magnet used, the amplitude and sequence of pulses can be varied as well as the time between the pulse applications and sampling of pulses for the excited nuclei. Since multiple tissue variables are expressed in a given image, a given choice of instrument parameters may produce a fortuitous similarity of signal intensities from disparate tissues. Since contrast on the magnetic resonance image is based on intensity differences emanating from distinct tissue types, such fortuitous similarity can cause lesions to be indistinguishable from their surrounding tissues. Therefore, the ability to vary the imaging sequence to highlight different combinations of T1 and T2 relaxation characteristics is crucial. For spin echo-type imaging, a long T1 relaxation time or short T2 relaxation time

will tend to decrease relative signal intensity; whereas a short T1 or long T2 relaxation time will tend to increase relative signal intensity. The pulse interval (TR) is the time between repetitive RF perturbations. The echo delay (TE) is the time elapsed between RF perturbation and the point in time when the signal (echo) emitted by the protons within the tissue is sampled. Both TR and TE are instrument parameters under computer control. Using a long TR diminishes the impact of differential T1 contributions from disparate tissues on image contrast, while enhancing the relative T2 contribution. Using a short TR helps to emphasize T1 differences between tissues. A short TR of 0.5 seconds and a long TR of 1.5 or 2.0 seconds are routinely employed at each plane of section in our imaging algorithm. We obtain two echo delay images at 28 and 56 msec (TE) for each pulse interval sequence (TR). This permits detection and quantification of signal decay (a T2 effect). Thus, four images are obtained at any given place. It should be noted that although absolute signal intensity increases with lengthening TR and decreases with lengthening TE, only relative image intensity (applied to a gray scale) is displayed on intensity images.

With our routine sequences, images obtained with a short TR and a short TE (TR, 0.5 seconds; TE, 28 msec) maximize the relative T1 contribution to signal intensity and tissue contrast; they are referred to as T1-weighted images. Similarly, images obtained with a long TR and long TE (TR, 1.5 or 2.0 seconds; TE, 56 msec) maximize the relative T2 contribution to signal intensity; they

---

Figure 8.1. Normal axial images. [In the legends of Figures 8-1 through 8-12: SE (spin echo), time in msec (TR)/time in msec (TE).] **A.** SE 500/28. **B.** SE 2,000/56. **C.** SE 500/28. **D.** SE 2,000/56. **E.** SE 500/28. **F.** SE 2,000/56. Sections (**A**) and (**B**) are at the level of the inferior rectus (arrows); (**C**) and (**D**) are at the level of the optic nerve; (**E**) and (**F**) are at the level of the superior rectus and trochlear tendon. The vitreous appear as low-signal intensities on the relatively T1-weighted SE 500/28 images (**A** and **C**) due to its long T1 relaxation time, but it appears as relatively high-signal intensity in the more T2-weighted SE 2,000/56 images (**B** and **D**) due to its long T2 relaxation time. The extraocular muscles yield an intermediate signal intensity. Note that the trochlear tendon (**E, F,** arrow) yields a weaker density of fibrous tissue. Note the inverse relationships of the relative intensity of the lens and vitreous on T1 and T2-weighted sequences.

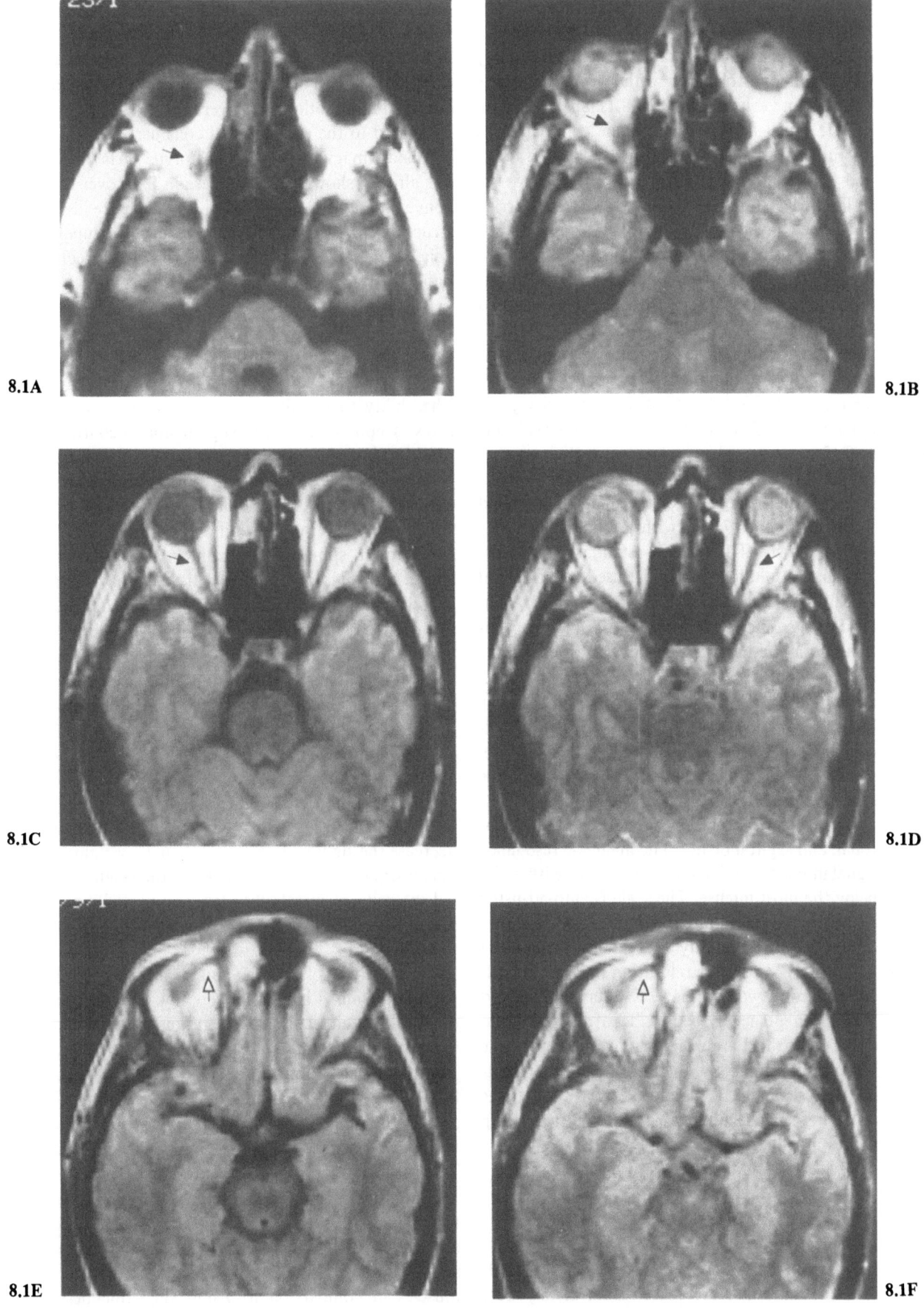

8.1A

8.1B

8.1C

8.1D

8.1E

8.1F

are referred to as T2-weighted images. The effect of varying instrument parameters is illustrated by a set of images obtained with a range of pulse intervals and echo delays (Fig. 8.1). Such variation of MR signal intensity (i.e., tissue contrast) with instrument parameters is an essential part of tissue and fluid characterization (3).

The MRI studies just illustrated were carried out at the University of California in San Francisco using apparatus for hydrogen imaging (2). The imager employs a superconducting magnet operating at 0.35 Tesla. The spin echo technique is used routinely with TR and TE intervals as described above. In addition, inversion recovery images (IR) occasionally are obtained with a pulse repetitive interval of (TR) 1.0 second and echo delays of (TE) 28 and 56 msec. The recovery interval (TI) is 0.42 seconds. This is another technique that emphasizes T1 differences between tissues.

The section thickness of the images illustrated in this chapter is 7 mm with a 2.6-mm interslice gap. A matrix of 128 × 128 (standard) or 256 × 256 (high resolution) Pixels was used with a spatial resolution in the X or Y axis of 1.7 mm for standard images and 0.8 mm for high resolution. Spatial resolution in the Z plane was equal to the slice thickness of 7 mm. The capability to obtain a 1.8-mm section thickness with our imager has been recently developed. Such images yield markedly improved spatial resolution in the Z plane, which results in improved delineation of structures such as the optic nerve.

Images can be routinely obtained in axial, coronal, and sagittal planes. The magnetic resonance signal intensity is related to a gray scale, with white being the most intense. The scale is auto-adjusted to render the most intense signal in any section as white and to modify the extent of the scale accordingly. Tissue T1 relaxation time can be calculated from two different TR intervals obtained at a given plane of section. Two different echo delay times (TE) are necessary to calculate tissue T2 relaxation time. Synthesized images representing these calculated T1 and T2 relaxation times on a gray scale (the longest relaxation time being white) in a Pixel matrix can be produced.

Surface Coil Imaging

Surface coil images are obtained by using specialized antennae that are placed immediately next to the bodily port of interest. The region sampled is limited; unlike the sample with the conventional antenna, which encircles the object. Such resulting images have been demonstrated as having a higher signal-to-noise ratio (S/N) over the limited volume compared to the conventional coils used for head and body imaging. A 10-cm prototype surface coil has already shown a 2.5 increase in S/N over the conventional head coil. The eye and orbit are ideal structures for surface coil imaging, because superficial structures are delineated best with this technique.

MRI of the Normal Eye and Orbit

The ability to visualize ocular and orbital structures is enhanced by the superb image contrast resulting from inherent signal intensity differences between vitreous, fat, muscle, and neural tissues (12, 13). These intensity differences are based on the tissues' disparate T1 and T2 relaxation times and proton spin density values. As discussed above, the spin echo intensity dictates that short T1 relaxation time or long T2 relaxation time tend to increase relative image signal intensity. Retrobulbar fat with a very short T1 relaxation time and intermediate T2 relaxation time yields the highest signal intensity of all normal orbital structures for all sequences of TR and TE that are clinically employed. The loss of the high-intensity or normal fat is useful in diagnosing infiltrative processes that tend to lengthen the relaxation time because of increased water content; therefore, they decrease the signal intensity of fat on T1-weighted image sequences. At the same time, the bright signal intensity of retrobulbar fat may partially obscure visualization of smaller structures due to spatial blurring.

The bony wall of the orbit and the air-containing paranasal sinuses have relatively low proton spin densities, which result in a generation of very weak signal intensities and a black appearance on MRI. The optic nerve and extraocular muscles (Figs. 8.2 and 8.3) produce an intermediate signal intensity (in the range of brain parenchyma) with little variation associated with alteration of TR and TE. The eyes are in the primary position during the 5–30-minute imaging time. Studies of muscle contraction and relaxation showed no associated changes in T1 or T2 relaxation time (15). The small diameter of the optic nerve and extraocular muscles in comparison to 7-mm slice thickness may result in their being obscured by the high-

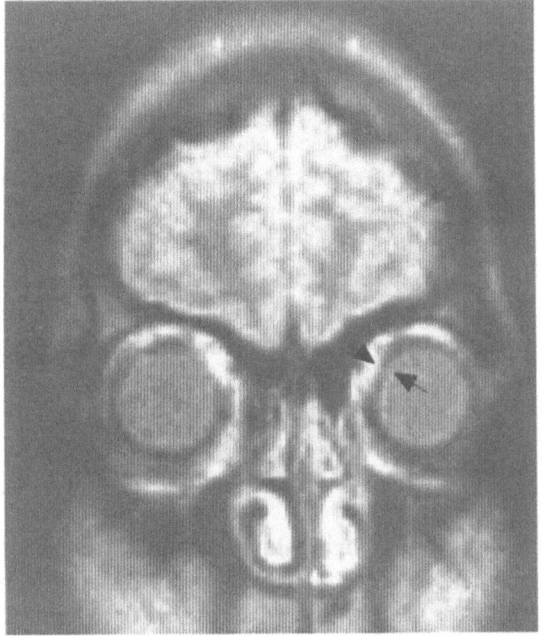

A

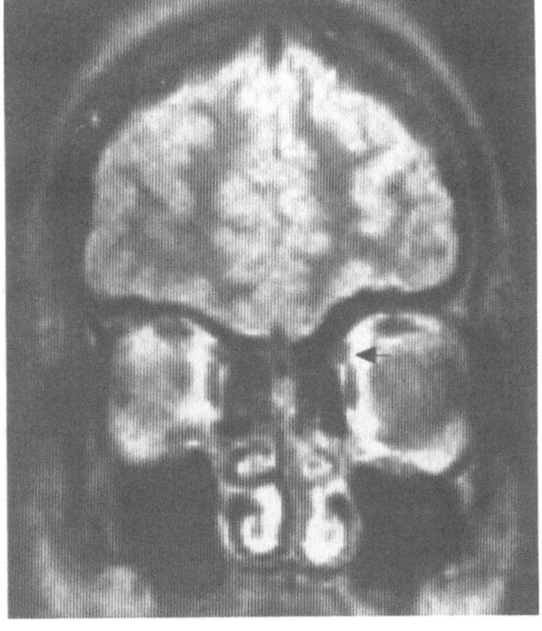

B

Figure 8.2. Normal coronal images (SE 2,000/56 sequence). The sclera, having a relatively low proton spin density, yields lower signal intensity than the adjacent vitreous (**A**). The extraocular muscles are well shown. The superior oblique muscle (arrows) is identified above the medial rectus (**B**).

signal intensity of surrounding fat. This problem is overcome with the use of thin sections of 1.8 mm.

The vitreous comprises two thirds of the volume of the globe. Its components are 99% water and 1% collagen and hyaluronic acid with traces of sodium chloride. The collagen and hyaluronic acid account for the gel-like characteristics of normal vitreous. A marked variation in signal intensity of the vitreous is observed when the imaging parameters are changed (Fig. 8.1). A weak signal relative to adjacent structures is obtained on a T1-weighted sequence; a relatively strong signal is obtained on a T2-weighted sequence, with a longer pulse interval and echo delay. This observation reflects the long T1 and long T2 relaxation times of water. Although the vitreous behaves in a manner similar to the cerebrospinal fluid, which

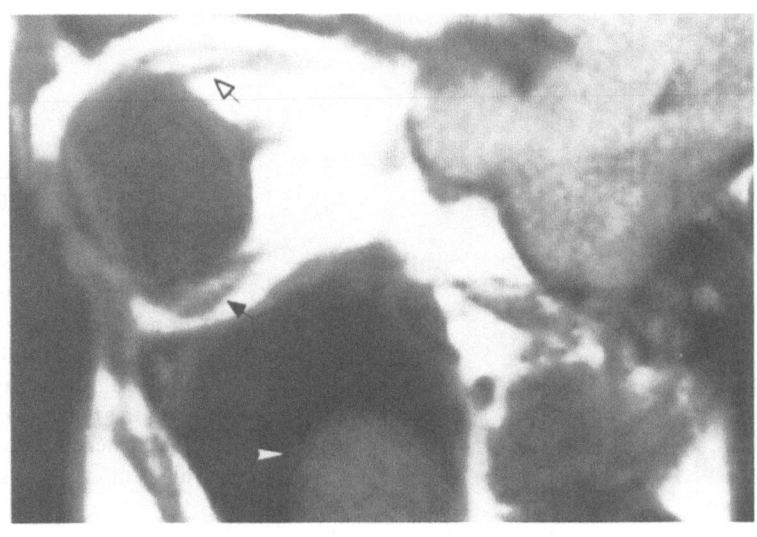

Figure 8.3. Normal sagittal image (SE 500/28). The inferior oblique muscle is seen (arrow) below the inferior rectus. The superior rectus muscle (open arrow) is seen inferior to the levator palpebrum. A retention cyst is incidentally noted in the maxillary antrum (white arrowhead).

is also greater than 99% water, subtle differences in signal intensity characteristics can be observed with long echo delay times. This can be explained by the slightly greater protein content of the vitreous, as compared to the cerebrospinal fluid. Increasing protein content within water tends to shorten the T1 and T2 relaxation times. Also, the gel-like state of vitreous compared to the liquid state of cerebrospinal fluid contributes to the subtle differences in their relaxation characteristics.

The lens is a dense structure made up of 65% water and 35% protein. It has an intermediate T1 relaxation time and short T2 relaxation time. On T1-weighted sequences, the lens appears bright in relation to the surrounding vitreous and aqueous. With longer TR and TE, there is greater image contrast dependence on T2 relaxation (i.e., disparate signal intensity is primarily based on T2 differences in tissue), which causes the relative signal intensity between the lens and vitreous to be re-versed. This is illustrated by the set of images in Figure 8.1.

Visualization of the sclera and cornea is best on long TR sequences, where they appear as foci of low-signal intensity bordering the vitreous (Fig. 8.2). The sclera consists of dense collagen and elastic fibers. In previous observations of such tissue, low-hydrogen proton spin densities and long T1 relaxation times have been noted, thus explaining the relatively low signal intensity. The cornea predominantly consists of multiple lamellar fibers with relatively low water content, which causes it to have similar intensity characteristics.

MRI of Ocular and Orbital Pathology

A discussion of ophthalmologic disease imaged by magnetic resonance, as with other imaging techniques, is best considered according to lesion loca-

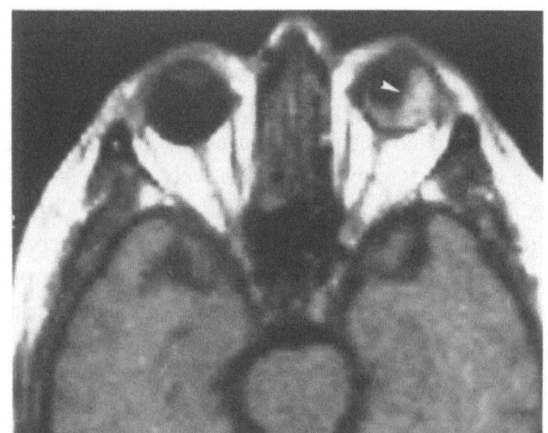

A

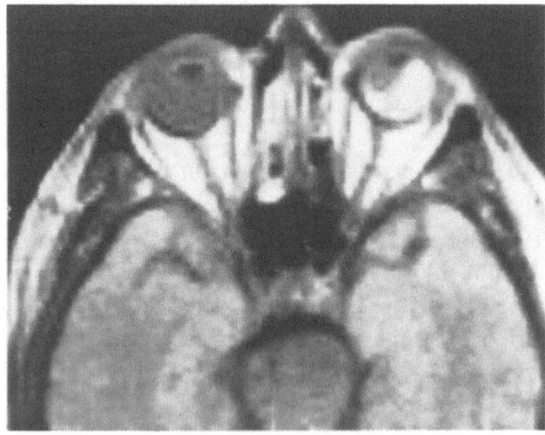

B

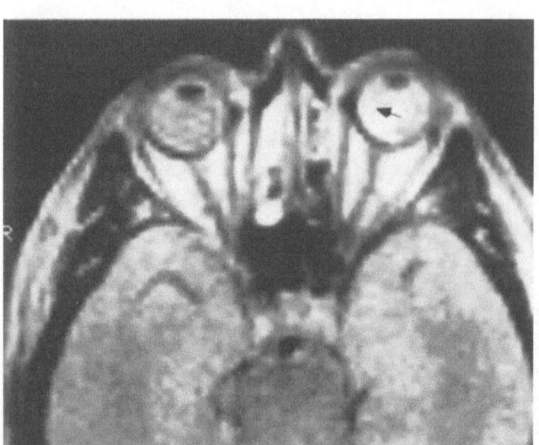

C

Figure 8.4. Choroidal melanoma. **A.** SE 500/28. **B.** SE 2,000/28. **C.** SE 2,000/56. The melanoma is most conspicuous on the T1-weighted image (**A**, white arrowhead). **B** and **C** have greater dependence of image contrast on T2 relaxation. As a result, the lesion increases in relative intensity, but so does the surrounding vitreous. Note that medial to the melanoma, there is a greater increase in intensity (arrow) than in the opposite eye. This was found to represent a subretinal fluid collection. Its greater-than-normal vitreous in **C** results from its different chemical state.

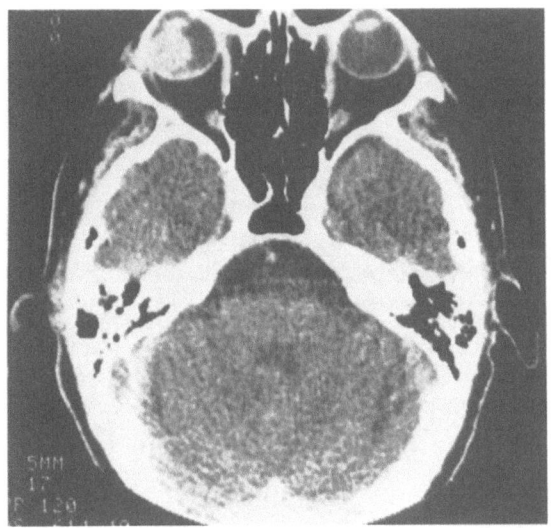

A

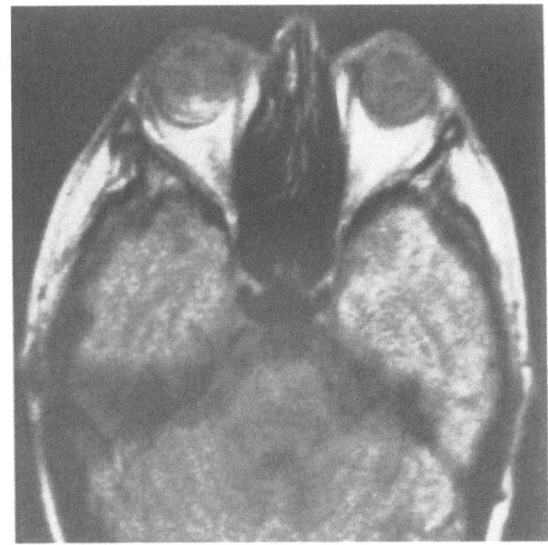

B

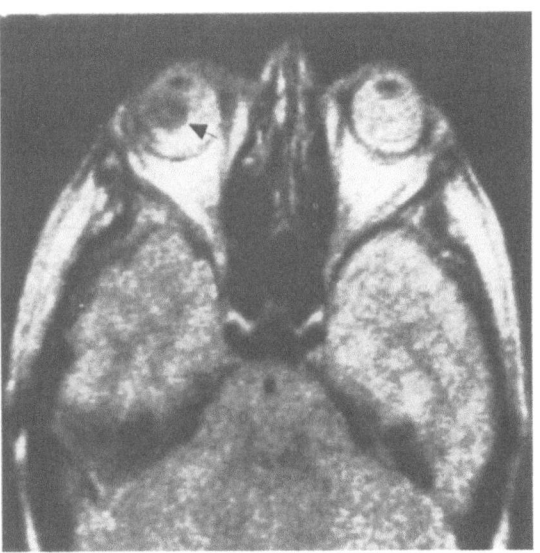

C

Figure 8.5. Choroidal melanoma. **A.** CT Scan. **B.** SE 2,000/28. **C.** SE 2,000/56. The CT scan shows a high-density lesion in the right globe. On MRI, the melanoma is best shown on the T2-weighted image (**C**, arrow), where it appears as a focus of low intensity. The melanoma in this patient is markedly more pigmented than in the prior patient (Figure 8-4). The low-intensity appearance (**C**) is explained by a greater effect on T2 shortening by the relatively high concentration of melanin (a paramagnetic substance), which results in decreased relative signal intensity on a T2-weighted image.

tion. Pathology is classified into ocular, extraconal, intraconal, optic nerve, and orbital apex.

Ocular Pathology

The vitreous renders pathologic processes of the eye ideally suited for MRI. The very long T1 relaxation time of the vitreous (2,800 msec) results in the appearance of relatively weak signal intensity on T1-weighted images. Neoplastic, hemorrhagic, and inflammatory processes have significantly shorter T1 relaxation times by comparison; therefore, they appear as foci of high-signal intensity in contrast to the vitreous on T1-weighted se-

quences. The relative behavior of these pathologic processes also can be compared to the behavior of the vitreous on T2-weighted sequences. Normally, the vitreous yields a strong signal intensity on images with long TR and TE due to the greater dependence on T2. Both primary and metastatic neoplasms of the globe are best visualized on the T1-weighted images, where they yield brighter signal intensity than the surrounding vitreous (14). In our experience, neoplastic lesions tend to increase in relative signal intensity on the T2-weighted images, which results in their being less conspicuous.

As previously reported (4), we found melanomas

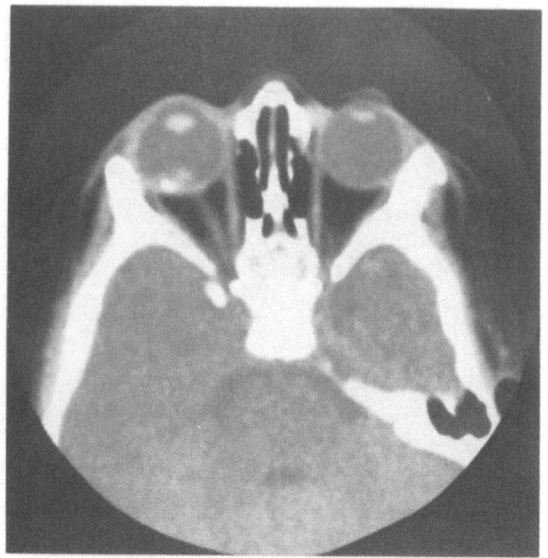

A

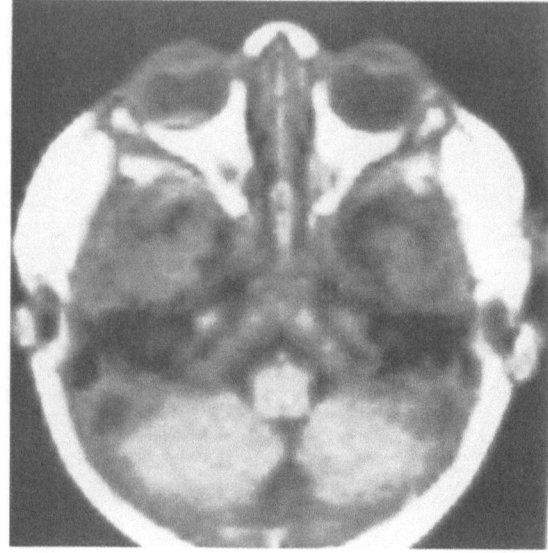

B

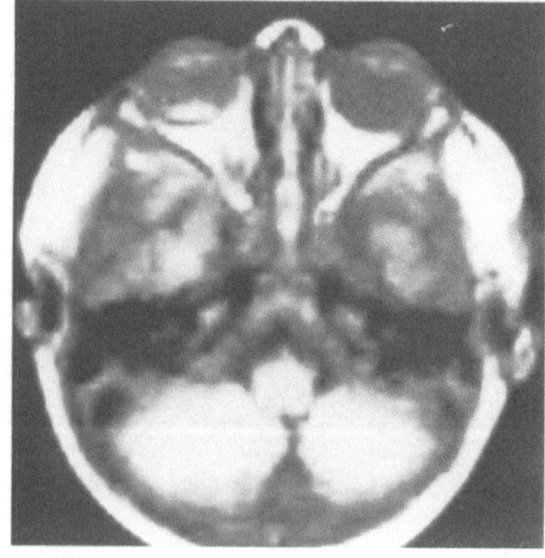

C

Figure 8.6. Retinoblastoma. **A.** CT. **B.** SE 500/28. **C.** SE 1,500/28. The CT scan shows a calcified mass in the right eye. The MRI shows the lesion as a high-intensity focus, but it fails to detect the punctate calcification. This is a significant shortcoming of MRI.

exhibiting a shorter T1 relaxation time (594 msec) and shorter T2 relaxation time (523 msec) than those generally observed in other nonhemorrhagic malignant neoplasms. This is partially explained by the unbound electron in melanin, which makes it a free radical. Free radicals are paramagnetic; i.e., they elicit "proton relaxation enhancement" by shortening the T1 and T2 relaxation times of protons. Despite the relatively shorter T1 and T2 relaxation times of the melanomas, they display intensity characteristics similar to other neoplasms of the eye (Fig. 8.4). An exception to this behavior was observed in the most densely pigmented melanoma that we have imaged, which yielded low-

signal intensity on the T2-weighted image (Fig. 8.5). This observation can be explained by reference to in vitro experiments that have shown low concentrations of paramagnetic substances having a predominant effect on shortening T1; whereas, higher concentrations have a greater relative effect on shortening T2, thereby resulting in decreased signal intensity with delayed echo sampling (1).

In our experience, retinoblastomas are well defined by MRI and CT. The intensity characteristics of retinoblastoma are similar to those observed for melanomas and other neoplastic lesions in the eye, despite the shorter T1 and T2 relaxation times of melanoma. This is due to the much longer T1

Figure 8.7. Dermoid **A.** CT scan. **B.** SE 500/28. The dermoid tumor is shown in the lacrimal fossa as a low-density mass on CT scan (arrow) and as a high-intensity mass on MRI (arrow). The MRI characteristics result from the short T1 of fat within the lesion. Note the erosion of the lateral orbital wall shown on MRI as a break in the black rim of cortical bone (open arrow).

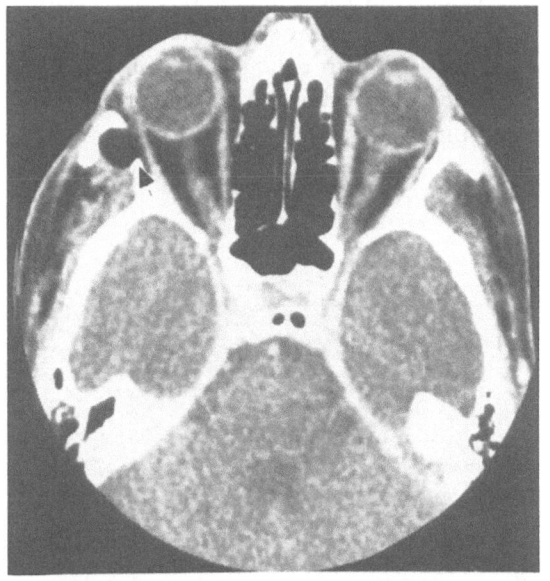

A

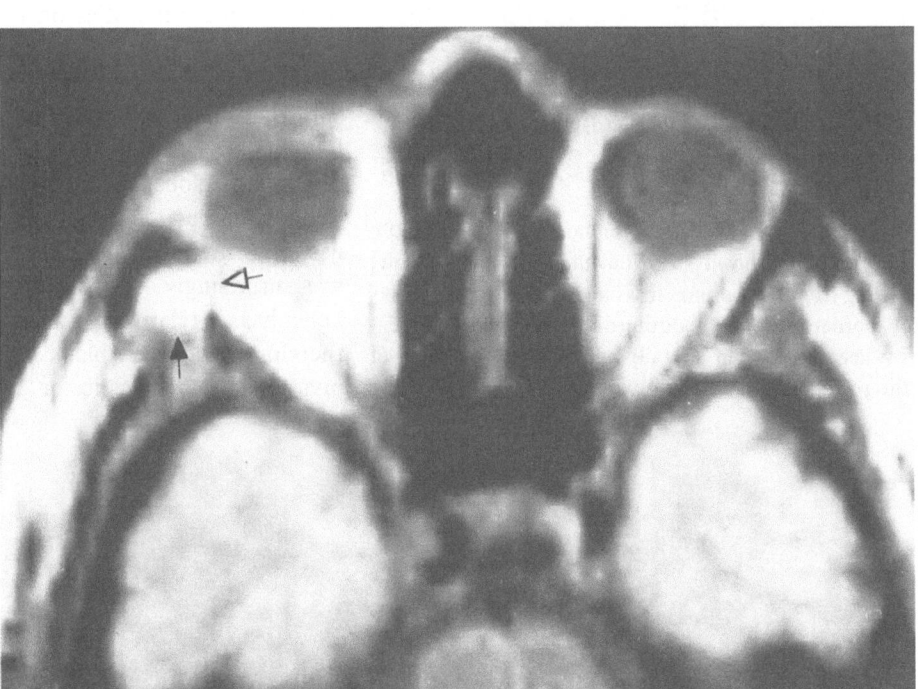

B

and T2 relaxation times of the vitreous compared to both retinoblastomas and melanomas. A significant shortcoming of MRI can be the failure to detect punctate calcification, as observed in Figure 8.6. This mitigates the utility of MRI in diagnosing retinoblastomas, because a small focus of calcification may be the only abnormality present (as has been observed with CT).

Magnetic resonance imaging may be unsuccess-ful in visualizing lesions less than 3 mm in size within the globe. This lack of detection occurs when thick sections are obtained with a gap between consecutive images. Thinner contiguous sections alleviate this shortcoming, as does the use of "surface coils."

Another potential application for MRI in ocular imaging is the demonstration of intraocular hemorrhage and vitreous liquefaction, which may occur in diabetes and collagen vascular disorders. Gonzalez, et al (6) have shown that vitreous transition from a gel to a liquid state in the bovine eye is demonstrated by the shortening of T1 relaxation time.

Orbit Pathology

Extraconal Pathology

Extraconal lesions tend to displace the extraocular muscles and the globe. These lesions are best shown by virtue of their disparate signal intensities with retrobulbar fat. Due to this reason, T1-weighted sequences are most useful in enhancing the intensity differences that result from the long T1 relaxational values of most neoplastic and inflammatory lesions, relative to the shorter T1 of fat. An exception is dermoid tumors, which yield the same signal intensity as retrobulbar fat due to their similar histology; however, these can be readily diagnosed by the presence of mass effect or bone destruction when present, as illustrated in Figure 8.7.

Epithelial and lymphocytic malignancies display similar signal intensities on MRI; in our experience, they cannot be differentiated from each other, nor can they be differentiated from benign epithelial or lymphocytic tumors. A lymphocytic lymphoma arising in the lacrimal fossa and displacing the globe is shown in Figure 8.8.

Bone destruction often is a helpful clue to suggesting the aggressive nature of a neoplasm; MRI was surprisingly sensitive in this regard. Cortical bone has a relatively low proton spin density; therefore, it appears black on MRI (7). Osseous invasion by neoplastic or infectious processes

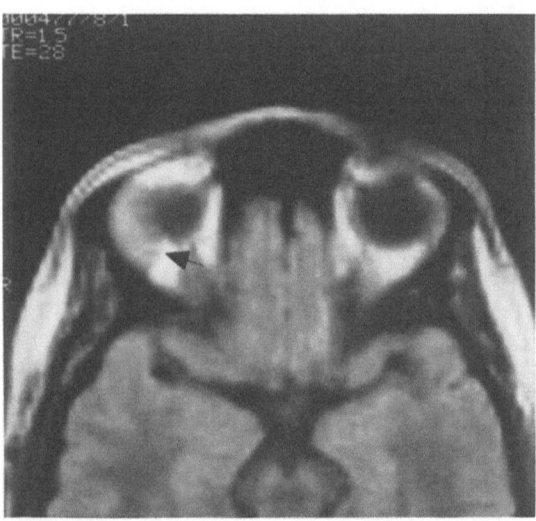

Figure 8.8. Lymphocytic lymphoma (SE 1,500/28). The lesion is shown as a low-intensity mass (arrow) arising from the lacrimal fossa and displacing the globe. Its borders are sharply outlined by the intact low-intensity osseous margin laterally and the high intensity of the retrobulbar fat medially.

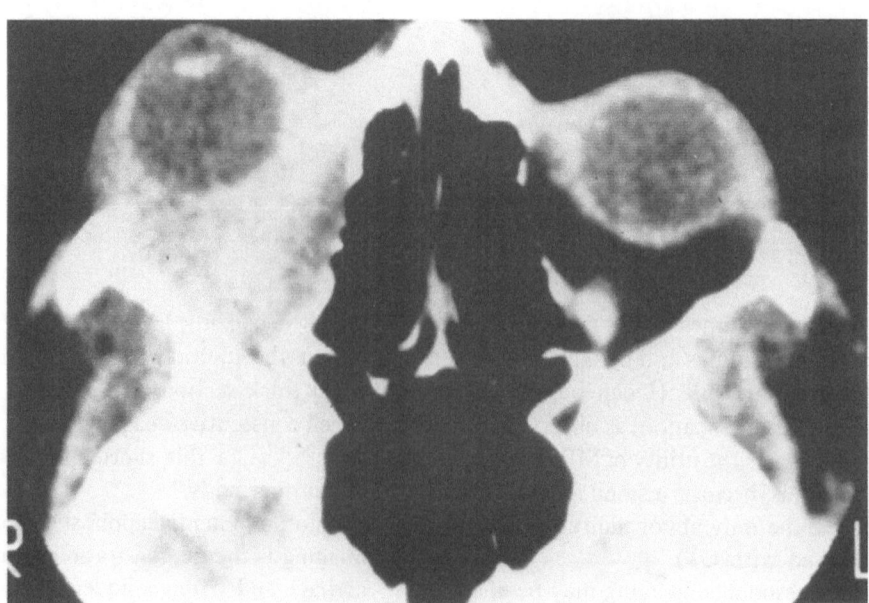

8.9A

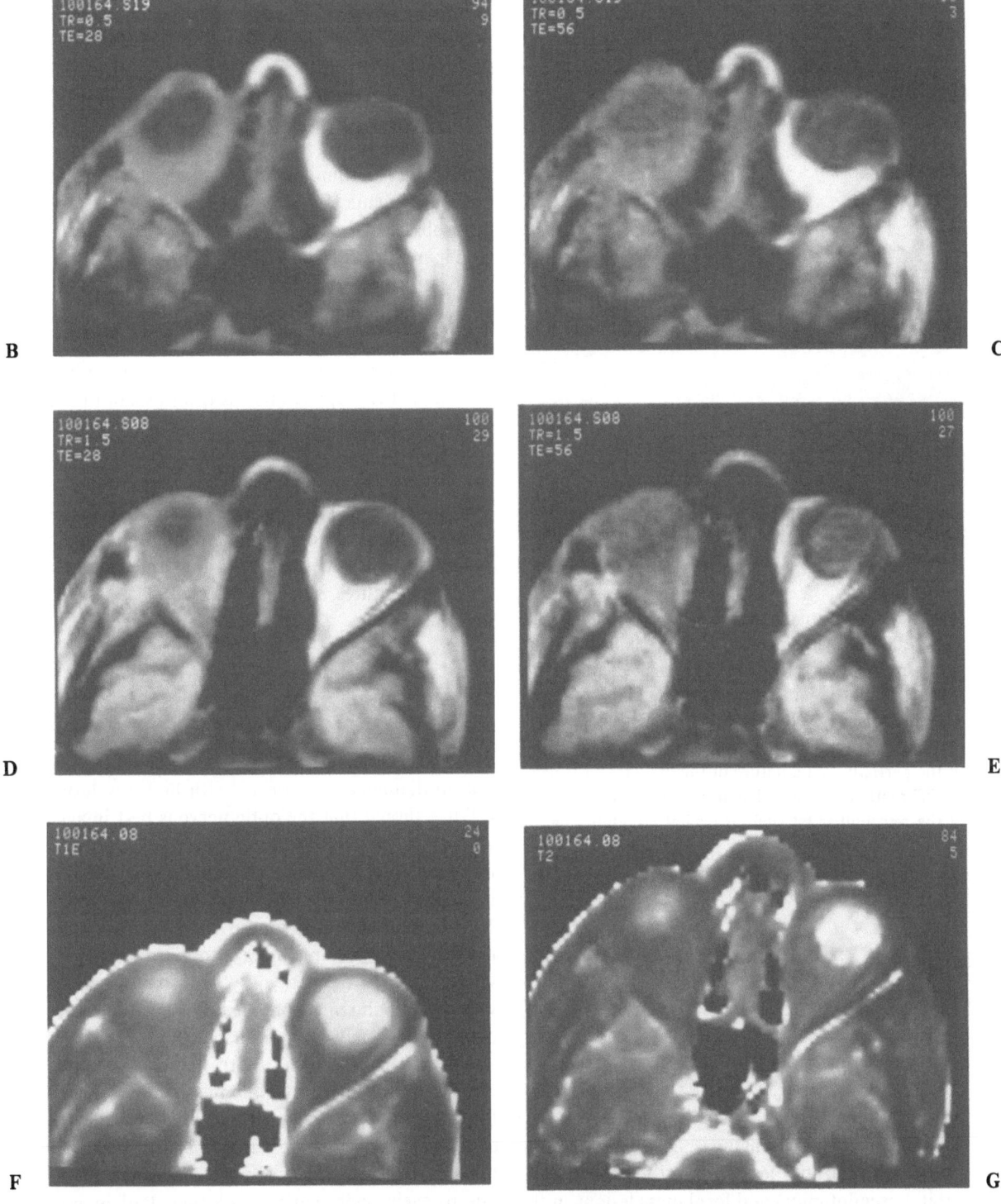

B

C

D

E

F

G

◁ **Figure 8.9.** Orbit pseudotumor. **A.** CT scan. **B.** SE 500/ 28. **C.** SE 500/56. **D.** SE 1,500/28. **E.** SE 1,500/56. **F.** T1-estimated calculated image. **G.** T2-calculated image. There is diffuse involvement of the retrobulbar fat in the right orbit. This appears as decreased relative signal intensity on T1- and T2-weighted sequences. On the calculated T1 and T2 images, relatively longer T1 and T2 values are arbitrarily assigned to appear brighter on the gray scale, respectively (i.e., a structure or lesion with a long T1 will appear relatively bright on the calculated T1 image; similarly, a structure with a long T2 will appear bright on the calculated T2 image). In this patient, the fat in the right orbit appears brighter than the opposite orbital fat on the calculated T1 image, reflecting the lengthened T1 due to edema or increased water content. Note that there is little disparity in appearance of the fat in the right and left orbit on the calculated T2 image.

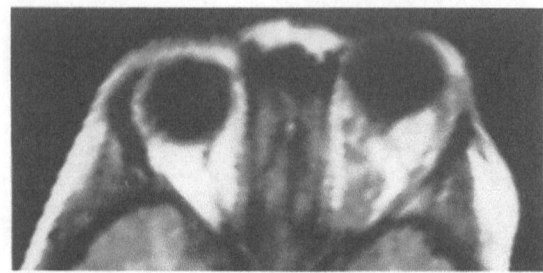

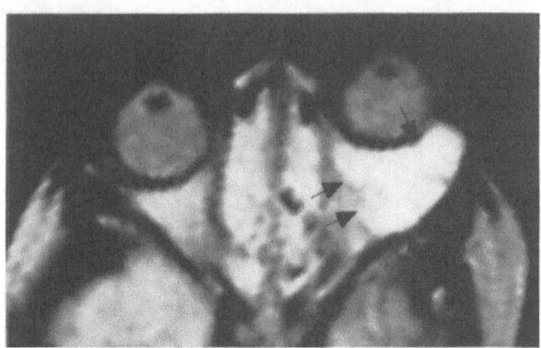

Figure 8.10. Cavernous lymphangioma. **A.** SE 500/28. **B.** SE 2,000/56. The lymphangioma has similar intensity as the retrobulbar fat on the T1-weighted image (**A**), but it actually becomes brighter than the fat on the T2-weighted image (**B,** arrows). The high-signal intensity on the T2-weighted intensity image probably is due to the partially cystic nature of this lesion, and it helps to differentiate it from edematous infiltrative processes of the retrobulbar fat such as orbital pseudotumor.

causes a relative increase in signal and a breeching of the black margin of cortical bone.

Intraconal Pathology

Magnetic resonance imaging is sensitive in defining both focal infiltrative lesions of retrobulbar fat (i.e., orbital pseudotumor) and focal mass lesions in the intraconal space. Infiltrative lesions are demonstrated by their alteration in signal intensity of the retrobulbar fat, which results from tissue edema (increased water content). Focal mass lesions demonstrate changes in signal intensity as well as in mass effect.

Orbital pseudotumor is an edematous inflammatory process associated with varying degrees of vasculitis, lymphocyte infiltration, and fibrosis. Pa-

tients with this diagnosis exhibit a relative decrease in signal intensity of the retrobulbar fat on both T1- and T2-weighted images (Fig. 8.9). Calculated T1 and T2 images can be obtained to confirm the lengthening of T1 relaxation time with minimal change in T2. Similar findings were observed in rat experiments (8), in which a direct correlation was observed between increasing water content and increasing T1 and T2 relaxation times for normal and abnormal tissue—except for the T2 of fat, which did not increase directly with an increase in water content. Thyroid ophthalmopathy is associated with similar tissue, therefore resulting in similar MRI appearance as orbit pseudotumor.

Focal mass lesions in the intraconal compartment generally exhibit an increase in relative signal intensity on T2-weighted images, which serve to differentiate them from orbital pseudotumor. Examples of a cavernous lymphangioma and malignant fibrous histiocytoma are illustrated, respectively, in Figures 8.10 and 8.11.

Optic Nerve

The intraorbital optic nerve is approximately 3 mm in diameter. Experience with high-resolution CT has shown that the optic nerve is best imaged with thin sections. We have found the use of 7-mm slice thickness to be unrewarding in visualizing optic nerve pathology. In contradistinction, 1.8-mm sections yield superb visualization of the nerve. It is important that appropriate scaling for visualization of the optic nerve is also used; otherwise, spatial blurring from the high-signal intensity of orbital fat may be a problem.

An example of a child with neurofibromatosis and bilateral optic nerve gliomas is illustrated in Figure 8.12. A CT scan showed bilateral enlargement of the optic nerves; MRI, 7-mm thick sections, failed to detect any abnormality of the nerves due to their poor spatial resolution. Patient motion, which also contributed to image degradation in this 3-year-old girl, usually is not a problem in children when they are properly sedated.

Daniels, et al (5) have been successful in visualizing a glioma and meningioma of the optic nerve with 5-mm MRI sections. However, the spatial resolution of these lesions with high-resolution CT was still superior to that of MRI. The optic nerve glioma showed similar intensity characteristics of

Figure 8.11. Malignant fibrous histiocytoma. **A.** SE 500/28. **B.** SE 2,000/56. In this patient, the lesion is most conspicuous on the T1-weighted image (**A**, arrow), and it becomes poorly defined on the T2-weighted image (**B**) due to a similar intensity as the surrounding fat.

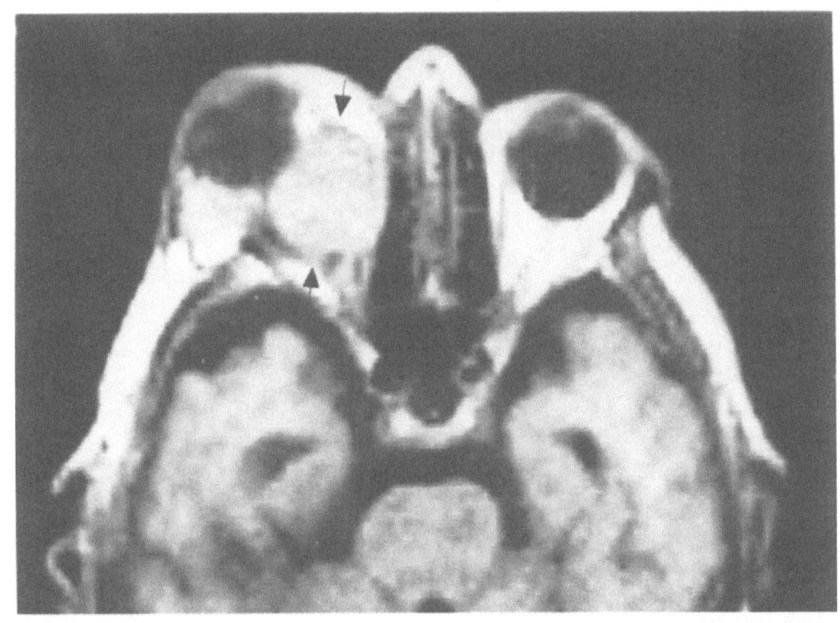

A

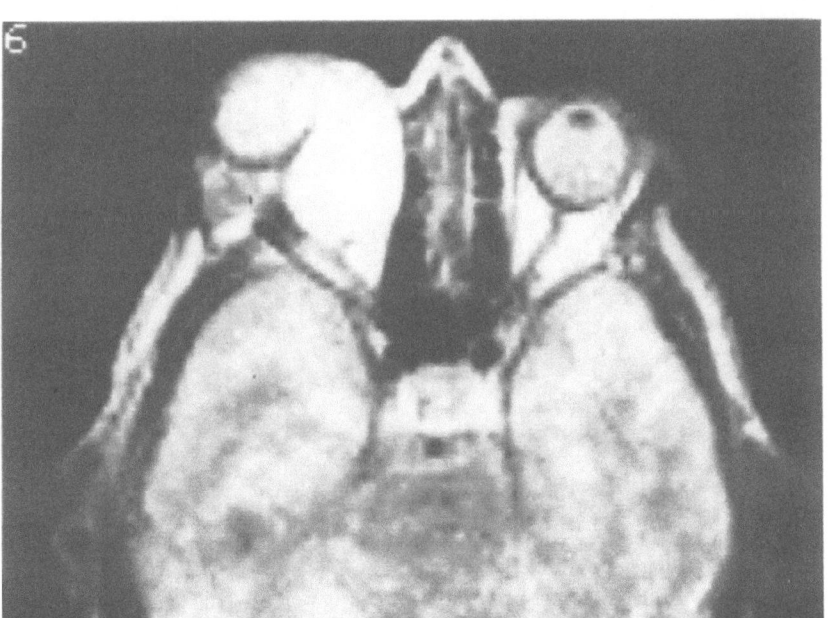

B

the opposite normal optic nerve, whereas the meningioma yielded a slightly stronger signal on both spin echo and saturation recovery images.

Early experience with surface coil images of the normal optic nerve demonstrated superb spatial resolution. This improved resolution allowed one to detect subtle alterations in tissue relaxation and signal intensity that could not be appreciated with greater section thickness. Surface coil technique combined with thin sections will allow MRI to

be equal—if not superior—to CT diagnosing of optic nerve pathology.

Orbital Apex

Lesions of the orbital apex are most commonly inflammatory, vascular, or neoplastic. In addition to being as sensitive as CT scanning in detecting these lesions, MRI also has been specific. In a

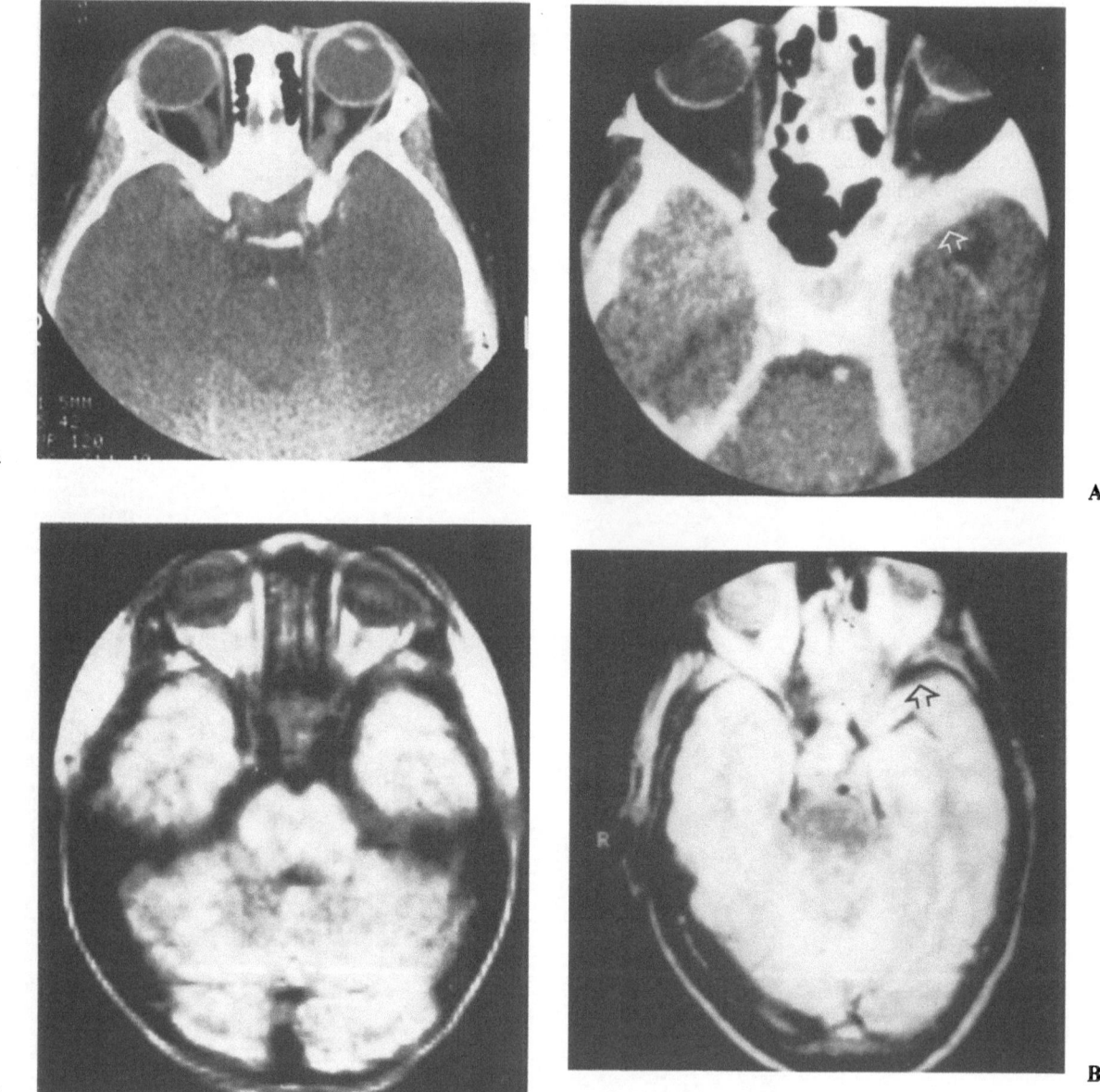

Figure 8.12. Bilateral optic nerve gliomas. **A.** CT scan. **B.** SE 500/28. Bilateral optic nerve enlargement is well shown on CT scan. On MRI, this cannot be appreciated due to the poor visualization of the optic nerves. Patient motion, present in this 3-year-old girl, is usually not a problem in children when they are properly sedated. Visualization of the optic nerves is markedly improved when 1.8-mm sections are obtained.

Figure 8.13. Tolosa-Hunt syndrome. **A.** CT scan. **B.** MRI **A** shows increased density (open arrow) applied to the left sphenoid wing and extending to the cavernous sinus. **B** shows the abnormal granulation tissue (open arrow) as decreased intensity applied to the sphenoid wing.

patient with biopsy-proven Tolosa-Hunt syndrome (painful ophthalmoplegia), MRIs show low-signal intensity on both T1- and T2-weighted sequences. This is consistent with the relatively low resonating proton density of granulation or fibrous tissue (Fig. 8.13).

Cavernous carotid aneurysms extending into the orbital apex are readily diagnosed on MRI due to the presence of blood flow within the aneurysm. Rapidly moving protons traverse the magnetic resonance plane of section without experiencing a full MRI cycle of alignment, excitation, and relaxation; therefore, they do not generate a detectable signal. In contradistinction, thrombus within the aneurysm is shown as a focus of higher signal intensity, and it can be readily detected.

Neoplastic lesions within the orbital apex are shown on T1- and T2-weighted sequences, as a result of their longer T1 and T2 relaxation times, than surrounding tissue. Again, bone destruction is a useful sign for suggesting their aggressive nature. Meningiomas tend to show only a slightly brighter signal than brain, whereas gliomas and other intraaxial neoplasms tend to show a markedly brighter signal on T2-weighted images.

Conclusion

In summary, our experience to date with MRI is very promising for ocular and orbital imaging. The diagnostic potential of any imaging modality is dependent on both tissue contrast and spatial resolution. In the case of the former, the tissue contrast in the eye and orbit with MRI is equal to that with CT. Unlike the brain, where the spatial resolution of MRI equals CT, this is not the case in the orbit—where the capacity to obtain thin sections is more crucial. As surface coils and thin section techniques are being developed, the limitations in spatial resolution are being resolved. The ability to characterize tissue according to T1 and T2 relaxation times and to determine relative flow are becoming more significant; they will allow MRI to surpass CT as the primary imaging modality for orbital and ocular disease.

References

1. Brasch RC, Wesbey GE, Gooding CA, et al: Magnetic resonance imaging of transfusional hemosiderosis complicating thalassemia major. *Radiology* 150:767–771, 1984.
2. Crooks LE, Arawaka M, Hoenninger J, et al: Nuclear magnetic resonance whole-body imager operating at 3.5 KGauss. *Radiology* 143:169–174, 1982.
3. Crooks LE, Mills CM, Davis PL, et al: Visualization of cerebral and vascular abnormalities by NMR imaging. The effects of imaging parameters on contrast. *Radiology* 144:843–852, 1982.
4. Damadian R, Zaner K, Hor D: Brain tumors by NMR. *Physiol Chem Physics* 5:381–402, 1973.
5. Daniels DL, Herfkens R, Cager WE: Magnetic resonance imaging of the optic nerves and chiasm. *Radiology* 152:79–83, 1984.
6. Gonzalez RG, Cheng HM, Barnett P, et al: Nuclear magnetic resonance imaging of the vitreous body. *Science* 223:399–400, 1984.
7. Han JS, Benson JE, Bonstelle CT, et al: Magnetic resonance imaging of the orbit: a preliminary experience. *Radiology* 150:755–759, 1984.
8. Herfkens R, Davis P, Crooks L, et al: Nuclear magnetic resonance imaging of the abnormal live rat and correlations with tissue characteristics. *Radiology* 141:211–218, 1981.
9. Kaufman L, Crooks LE, Margulis AR (eds.): *Nuclear Magnetic Resonance Imaging in Medicine.* Tokyo, Igaku-Shoin, 1981.
10. Ling CR, Foster MA, Hutchison JMS: Comparison of NMR water proton T1 relaxation times of rabbit tissues at 24 MHz and 2.5 MHz. *Phys Med Biol* 25:748–751, 1980.
11. Moseley IF, Sanders MD: *Computerized Tomography in Neuro-ophthalmology.* London, Chapman and Hall, 1982.
12. Moseley I, Brant-Zawadzki M, Mills C: Nuclear magnetic resonance imaging of the orbit. *Br J Ophthalmol* 67(6):333–342, 1983.
13. Sobel DF, Mills C, Char D, et al: NMR of the normal and pathologic eye and orbit. *American Journal of Neuroradiology* 5:345–350, 1984.
14. Sobel DF, Kelly W, Kjos BO, et al: Magnetic resonance imaging of orbital and ocular disease. *American Journal of Neuroradiology* 6:259–264, 1985.
15. Taylor DA, Bore CF: A review of the magnetic resonance response of biological tissue and its applicability to the diagnosis of cancer by NMR radiology. *J Comput Tomogr* 5:122–134, 1981.

9
Congenital Abnormalities

MELVIN H. BECKER and JOSEPH G. MCCARTHY

There are many congenital disorders that involve the orbit, globe, and adjacent soft tissues (e.g., muscles, nerves, lacrimal apparatus, and skin) (90). The conditions that involve the bony structures are the ones in which imaging techniques—such as routine radiographs, tomograms, and computed tomography (CT)—are of most value. A knowledge of both the embryologic development and anatomic measurements of the orbits is helpful in understanding the disorders that affect the orbit.

Embryology and Development

In the embryo, the earliest developmental changes that can be recognized as the face and eyes appear at approximately the 23rd day. At this time, the head region of the developing embryo still contains a neural groove—or unclosed brain. The eyes begin as shallow depressions or grooves (the optic sulci) on the lateral aspects of the forebrain. The grooves become the optic placodes, which subsequently evaginate to form the optic vesicles. These can be seen projecting through the overlying ectoderm in the 28-day-old embryo. On the 13th day, the optic vesicles swell and become attached to the brain by the optic stalks. Approximately 1 day later, the lens placodes appear as areas of thickened ectoderm overlying the optic vesicles. The distal wall of the optic vesicles indent by rapid marginal growth, bringing about the formation of double-layered optic cups, which are incomplete inferiorly as the choroidal fissures. The cups are then attached to the diencephalic region of the brain by thickened optic stalks. The optic cups eventually become the retinae, and the optic stalks become

the tissue through which optic nerve fibers grow back from the retinal regions to the brain. By the 32nd day, the lens placodes have moved inward to form lens vesicles, occupying the concavities of the optic cups. Toward the end of the fifth week, the lens placodes and their vesicles have completely separated from the surface ectoderm to form the lens.

Initially, the axes of the primitive eye regions are located at an angle of about 180° to each other. The divergence of the primitive eyes is reduced during the subsequent months of embryonic and fetal development. During the fourth month, the angle is reduced to about 65° by the broadening of the shape of the head, both adjacent and posterior to the orbits. At the time of birth, this angle has been reduced sufficiently to make binocular vision possible (Fig. 9.1).

During the sixth week, the embryonic development of the face has progressed, with the forward extension of the maxillary process beneath the corresponding optic vesicles. This results in the fusion of the paired maxillary processes with the lateral borders of the lateral nasal processes (Figs. 9.2 and 9.3). Pigment appears in the optic vesicles. The incomplete inferior portion of the optic cups (the choroidal fissures) becomes continuous, with grooves on the inferior sides of the optic stalks near the attachment to the optic cups. Along these grooves, blood vessels pass into the optic cups and through the choroidal fissure to supply the thickened inner layer of the cups. The inner layers are destined to become a portion of the retina, the lens vesicles, and the intervening mesenchyme. Normally, the choroidal fissures are fused and completely obliterated. If only partial fusion or

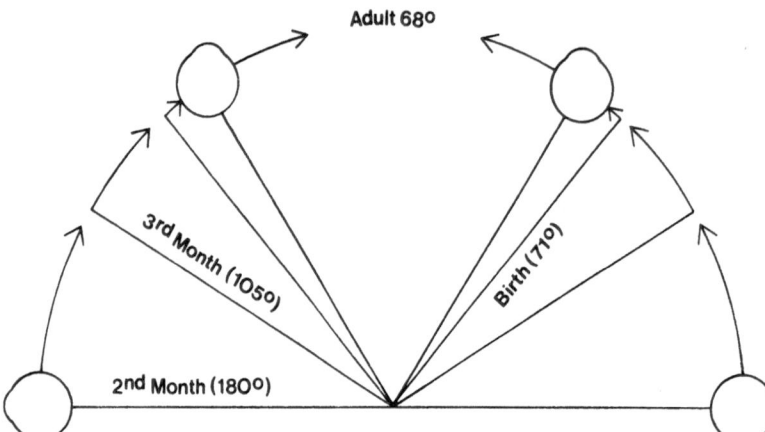

Figure 9.1. The orbital axis swings forward from 180° (in the second-month embryo) to 71° (at birth) to 68° (in the adult) (From Mann [187]).

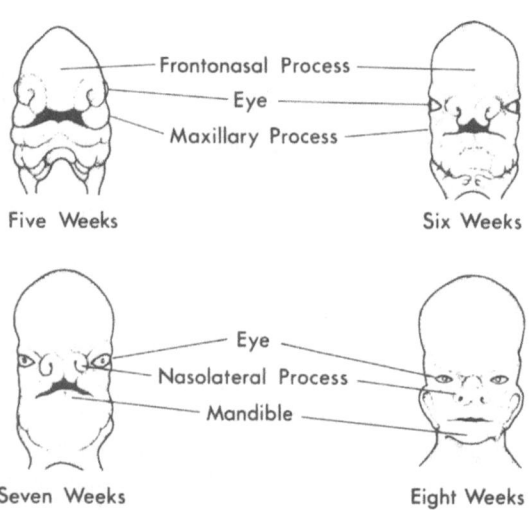

Figure 9.2. Development of the human face (From Patten [210]).

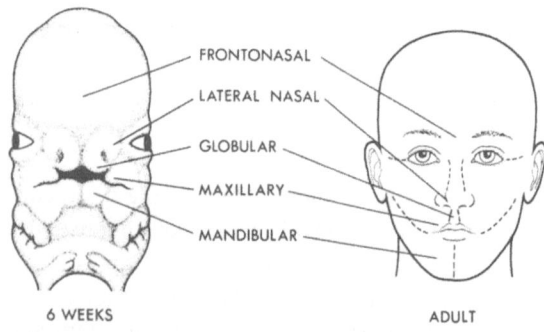

Figure 9.3. Contribution to the adult face from embryonic processes (From Kawamoto [155]).

nonfusion occurs, the resulting deformity is known as coloboma of the iris or coloboma of the iris and choroid.

During the seventh week, there is obvious development of the nose, lips, and chin. Facial clefts are almost completely closed. The eyes continue their forward and medial movement and become more prominent. The eyelids begin to form as upper and lower arch-like folds, lying superficially above and below the developing lens and optic cups. The free edges of the eyelid folds grow rapidly, with their margins coming into contact with each other about the middle of the ninth week. Then, they unite by an epithelial fusion that cuts off a space—the conjunctival sac—from the exterior of the fetus. The eyelids remain fused until the seventh fetal month. The eyelashes, glands, and other accessory eyelid structures form in a manner similar to other parts of the integumentary system. By the eighth week, the last week of true embryonic development, the face has assumed features that make it recognizable as human (13, 88, 90, 129, 168, 185, 208).

Development and Pathology

Faulty development of the embryo and fetus will result in congenital abnormalities. During the late embryogenic period (about the 17th day), the anterior portion of the neural tube contains the cells that will form the optic anlage. Disturbance of the prosencephalic organizing center (prechordal mesoblast) can cause cyclopia, synophthalmia, or arhinencephaly. During the early organogenetic period (about the 19th day), failure of the neuroectoderm of the optic pit to develop from the anterior portion of the neural plate will cause primary an-ophthalmia. An abnormality in the development of the blastemic stage of skull bone formation at approximately the 28th day can result in cranio-stenosis. At about the 42nd day, abnormal fusion of the maxillary and lateral nasal processes (meso-derm) will result in facial clefts. Mandibulofacial dysostosis and otocephaly probably are due to inhi-bition of mesodermal differentiation of the facial structures derived from the first visceral arch on approximately the 44th day. On approximately the 50th day, anencephaly can be the result of failure of the cephalad closure of the neural tube due to a break in the continuity of the roof plate.

The orbit is formed from a combination of mem-branous and cartilaginous anlage, while the base of the skull, the cranial bone, and the ethmoid and sphenoid bones (which contribute to the orbit) arise from the cartilage of the more primitive chon-drocranium. The superior portions of the orbit and calvarium develop from a membranous anlage.

In the postnatal period, considerable changes take place in the orbit. At birth, the margins are sharp and almost circular in outline, closely fitting around the globe. Their horizontal diameter is slightly greater than their vertical diameter. From age 3 months to 5 years, the orbital height in-creases and the vertical diameter approaches that of the horizontal diameter (89, 195). At 7 years of age, the orbital margin is less sharp, and the coronal section has the shape of a quadrilateral with rounded corners (Table 9.1) (271).

The shape and size of the orbit is determined by a combination of factors; one being the presence of the globe. In the absence of the eyeball, the orbit tends to be deformed and small, depending on the amount of tissue present in the orbit. The superior and lateral portions of the orbit are deter-mined, to some extent, by brain growth and the presence or absence of premature synostosis of the cranial sutures. Patients born with microphthal-mia or anophthalmia tend to have smaller and differently shaped orbits than normal. Growth ar-rest in fetal life may result in orbits being too far apart (such as in the fetal face syndrome). There are some developmental arrest situations in which facial clefts may result in asymmetric formation of the orbit. Enucleation of the globe in infancy or very early childhood, if untreated with a prosthesis, leads to arrested development with a small orbit. The earlier in life that the eye is removed, the more evident is the disparity in size of the two orbits (156, 243).

The changes in the orbit during the growth pe-riod depend, in part, on the development of the cranium and facial skeleton, between which the orbit is situated. The growth of the neighboring paranasal sinuses is another factor (88, 269, 271).

At birth, the globe has attained 75% of its adult size, and the development of orbital size and shape is almost complete. The interorbital distance changes with growth (69, 88, 116, 130). Adult configurations usually have been achieved at 12 years of age.

The newborn orbits are pointed more laterally than in the adult. Their orbital axes (lines drawn from the middle of the orbital opening to the optic foramen) make an angle of 115°; if projected poste-riorly, they meet in the middle of the nasal septum. In the adult, the orbital axes make an angle of 40–50° with each other; if projected backward, they meet at the upper part of the clivus of the sphenoid. These axes lie in the horizontal plane in the infant; but in the adult, they slope down-wards from 15–20° (271).

In the young child, the orbital fissures are rela-tively large due to the narrowness of the orbital surface of the greater wing of the sphenoid.

The optic canal, having no length at birth, be-comes 4 mm long by 1 year of age and up to 9 mm in adults (269).

The orbital walls, with advancing age, become much thinner due to bone resorption. Occasion-ally, they are so thin as to suggest holes in the orbital roof (271). The orbital fissures tend to widen.

After puberty, the skull and orbit develop differ-ently for males and females. In the female, the orbital walls tend to be delicate, and the orbital opening is circular. In the male, the orbital margins are more strongly developed and a prominent su-praorbital ridge develops (269).

Table 9.1. Growth changes of the orbital opening

Age	Form	Height (mm)	Width (mm)	Index
Fetus (8 mo)	Oval	14	18	77.7
Newborn (6 mo)	Rounded	27	27	100
Child (7 yr)	Quadrilateral	28	33	84.8
Adult	Quadrilateral	35	39	89.7

From (271).

Anatomy

The orbits are bony cavities located on either side of the root of the nose, and they have a general shape resembling a pear. The ethmoid, frontal, lacrimal, nasal, palatine, sphenoid, zygomatic, and maxillary bones contribute to the four walls of the orbit that contains the globe, associated muscles, vessels, and nerves. The central axis of the orbit is directed posteromedially, and it is approximately 25° from the sagittal plane. The axes of both orbits, when extended posteriorly, would cross each other at an angle of about 40–45°. The roof of the orbit is composed of the orbital plate of the frontal bone and the orbital surface of the lesser wing of the sphenoid. The lateral wall of the orbit is formed by the greater wing of the sphenoid, the orbital process of the frontal bone, and the orbital process of the zygoma. If the lateral walls are projected posteriorly, they form an angle of approximately 90°. The lateral wall forms an angle of about 45° with the medial wall (Fig. 9.4). The medial wall of the orbit is formed from the body of the sphenoid, the lamina papyracea of the ethmoid bone, the lacrimal bone, and the frontal process of the maxilla. The floor of the orbit is composed of the orbital plate of the maxilla and the orbital surface of the zygoma. The infraorbital fissure separates the greater wing of the sphenoid and the maxilla. The superior orbital fissure, which separates the greater and lesser wings of the sphenoid, and the optic nerve canal are at the apex of the orbit (88, 269, 271).

Orbital measurements are valuable in the evaluation of congenital malformations and in planning surgical treatment. These may be in the form of cephalometric studies, which are measurements obtained directly from skull x-ray films taken with the subject 6 feet from the radiographic tube (103, 273). The measurements may be obtained in other ways, such as from regular films, tomograms, and CT scans if the distortion factors are taken into consideration. The size of the globe may be measured by CT or echography. The globe lies slightly nearer the upper and lateral sides, but it does not normally come in contact with the orbital bones. The average distances in adults are 4.5 mm from the lateral and superior wall, 6.5 mm from the medial wall, and 6.2 mm from the inferior wall. The apex of the cornea usually is equidistant from the superior and inferior orbital margins. The lateral orbital margin is recessed, leaving about half of the globe unprotected. The average distances between the equator of the globe and the orbital walls are 4 mm from the roof, 4.5 mm from the lateral wall, 6.8 mm from the floor, and 6.5 mm from the medial wall (269).

Many measurements have been obtained from anatomic specimens, patients, and radiographic studies. The sagittal diameter of the globe is about 17 mm at birth, and it increases rapidly until 3 years of age, when it is about 22.5 mm. Growth is slow thereafter, so that the adult sagittal diameter is about 24 mm (89). There are changes in the orbital opening with advancing age. The height ranges from 14 mm (fetal) to 39 mm (adult) (271) (Table 9.1). The relationship between the orbital height and width can be expressed as the "orbital index": orbital height × 100 divided by orbital width. Using this index, three types of orbits are recognized: 1) orbital index exceeding 89 is designated as the round orbit (megaseme) and is characteristic of the yellow race, except the Eskimos; 2) an orbital index of 84–89 (mesoseme) is characteristic of whites; and 3) an orbital index less than 84 is designated as the rectangular orbit (microseme) and is characteristic of blacks (88, 269).

Different investigators have given variable measurements for some orbital dimensions. In adults,

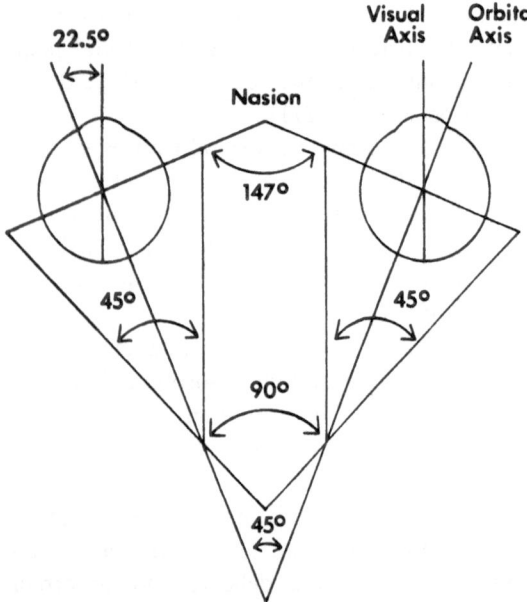

Figure 9.4. Diagram (horizontal section) to show the angles formed by the orbital walls (From Whitnall [271]).

a useful average is 40 mm for the depth of the orbit, 35 mm for the height of the orbital opening, 40 mm for the width of the orbital opening, 25–29 mm for the interorbital distance, 30 cc for the orbital volume, and the ratio of volume of the orbit to volume of the globe as 4.5:1 (271).

The measurement of the interorbital distance is of considerable use in the evaluation of congenital abnormalities. The soft-tissue distance (i.e., the space between the inner canthi, the pupils, and the outer canthi) is of limited value. The distance (skeletal) between the medial orbital walls must be differentiated from the distance between the inner or medial canthi. Several investigators have compiled these measurements for various ages (5, 62, 69, 116, 130, 241). Table 9.2 is taken from a recent study of the distance between the medial bony orbital walls (130). In general, the measurements approximate those of previous studies. The interorbital distances were measured as the narrowest distance between the medial orbital walls, as seen on paranasal sinus x-ray films. A focal-film distance of 30 inches was used. However, at times, it may be difficult to identify the landmarks

for this measurement. Tables 9.3A and 9.3B are taken from a recent study in live whites (76) and are similar to other studies. The intercanthal distance (the space between the apices of the medial canthi) does not have a consistent relationship with the interorbital and interpupillary distances, and thus cannot be used to determine orbital or ocular spacing (Fig. 9.5) (19, 51, 82, 99). The interpupillary distance is not easy to measure, especially in infants, uncooperative patients, and those with disturbances of fixation or nystagmus. The interpupillary measurement is invalid in cases of strabismus (99, 166, 221).

The lateral orbital distance is measured with calipers whose points are held at the external canthi against the inner bony surface, where the zygomatic bone forms a palpable notch at the site of the suture. The medial intercanthal distance is taken with the caliper points held at the internal canthus, where the upper and lower lids meet. The interpupillary distance is measured with the caliper points held at the middle of each pupil, while the subject's eyes are directed straight ahead to a point beyond 2 meters.

Table 9.2. Interorbital distance[a]

Age (yr)	10th Male	10th Female	25th Male	25th Female	50th Male	50th Female	75th Male	75th Female	90th Male	90th Female
0.5[b]					1.69	1.68				
1.0[b]					1.75	1.75				
1.5	1.524	1.514	1.651	1.632	1.773	1.733	1.920	1.854	2.063	1.988
2	1.578	1.567	1.700	1.682	1.822	1.784	1.971	1.905	2.114	2.039
3	1.680	1.657	1.795	1.764	1.909	1.859	2.056	1.992	2.201	2.130
4	1.760	1.729	1.877	1.837	1.994	1.929	2.143	2.070	2.292	2.215
5	1.830	1.790	1.952	1.906	2.073	2.007	2.229	2.146	2.382	2.288
6	1.896	1.842	2.022	1.964	2.143	2.078	2.308	2.218	2.466	2.362
7	1.957	1.896	2.076	2.021	2.199	2.144	2.371	2.288	2.537	2.431
8	2.025	1.949	2.132	2.087	2.256	2.207	2.429	2.352	2.607	2.487
9	2.069	1.989	2.187	2.140	2.310	2.270	2.480	2.409	2.656	2.542
10	2.114	2.044	2.236	2.180	2.357	2.313	2.534	2.458	2.716	2.596
11	2.164	2.102	2.288	2.234	2.412	2.359	2.592	2.510	2.780	2.649
12	2.220	2.148	2.344	2.284	2.468	2.419	2.643	2.573	2.834	2.710
13	2.278	2.196	2.405	2.328	2.529	2.466	2.704	2.623	2.904	2.766
14	2.328	2.228	2.460	2.363	2.590	2.498	2.760	2.646	2.964	2.786
15	2.374	2.243	2.515	2.385	2.650	2.524	2.817	2.668	3.024	2.803
16	2.407	2.275	2.553	2.416	2.697	2.547	2.868	2.693	3.084	2.833
17	2.438	2.306	2.586	2.442	2.723	2.563	2.894	2.704	3.101	2.849
18	2.454	2.309	2.608	2.453	2.741	2.581	2.915	2.724	3.119	2.865
19	2.456	2.314	2.616	2.459	2.759	2.588	2.937	2.738	3.148	2.882
20	2.469	2.318	2.629	2.460	2.778	2.585	2.971	2.743	3.196	2.890

[a] In centimeters.
[b] Average of minimum and maximum.
Modified from (130).

Table 9.3A. Intercanthal and interpupillary distances in males*

Age	Lateral orbital distance		Medial intercanthal distance		Inter-pupillary distance	
	Mean	SD	Mean	SD	Mean	SD
7 days	6.1	1.05	2.1	0.20	3.8	0.32
6 mo	6.6	0.32	2.5	0.30	4.0	0.33
1 yr	7.1	0.39	2.7	0.32	4.4	0.32
2 yr	7.2	0.39	2.7	0.20	4.4	0.32
3 yr	7.3	0.36	2.7	0.20	4.7	0.33
4 yr	7.6	0.32	2.7	0.24	4.9	0.28
5 yr	7.7	0.36	2.7	0.22	4.9	0.30
6 yr	8.0	0.47	2.8	0.17	5.3	0.26
7–8 yr	8.2	0.37	2.9	0.22	5.5	0.30
9–10 yr	8.4	0.42	2.9	0.17	5.5	0.32
11–12 yr	8.6	0.39	3.0	0.28	5.7	0.28
13–14 yr	8.8	0.40	3.1	0.14	5.9	0.28
15–16 yr	9.0	0.45	3.2	0.24	6.1	0.32
17–18 yr	9.2	0.36	3.2	0.30	6.3	0.35
19–20 yr	9.4	0.41	3.2	0.26	6.3	0.32

* In centimeters. Modified from (76).

Table 9.3B. Intercanthal and interpupillary distances in females*

Age	Lateral orbital distance		Medial intercanthal distance		Inter-pupillary distance	
	Mean	SD	Mean	SD	Mean	SD
7 days	6.0	0.22	2.1	0.44	3.7	0.24
6 mo	6.6	0.44	2.4	0.22	4.0	0.28
1 yr	6.8	0.39	2.5	0.24	4.2	0.28
2 yr	7.0	0.39	2.5	0.30	4.4	0.28
3 yr	7.3	0.47	2.6	0.29	4.5	0.28
4 yr	7.5	0.40	2.6	0.22	4.7	0.36
5 yr	7.7	0.24	2.7	0.26	4.9	0.33
6 yr	7.7	1.17	2.8	0.17	5.2	0.39
7–8 yr	7.9	0.39	2.9	0.22	5.4	0.30
9–10 yr	8.1	0.41	3.0	0.24	5.6	0.59
11–12 yr	8.4	0.37	3.0	0.24	5.8	0.30
13–14 yr	8.9	0.33	3.0	0.20	5.8	0.33
15–16 yr	8.9	0.30	3.0	0.17	5.8	0.20
17–18 yr	8.9	0.44	3.1	0.26	6.1	0.20
19–20 yr	9.3	0.37	3.2	0.28	6.1	0.30

* In centimeters. Modified from (76).

• • • medial orbital wall
-—- pupil distance from midline
medial canthal distance from midline

(Conticanthus: bony interorbital distance is greater than expected from the intermedial canthus distance.)

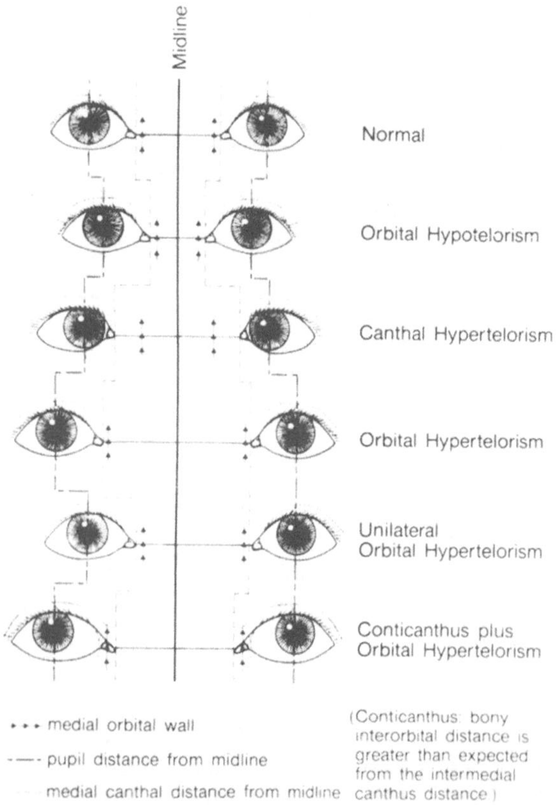

Figure 9.5. Diagram to show relative distance between medial orbital wall, inner canthi, and pupils in the normal and abnormal conditions.

Diagnostic Imaging Techniques

Imaging techniques are not usually used to diagnose congenital syndromes, but they are helpful in defining the anatomic defects. A complete genetic evaluation (including family history), physical examination, and (at times) laboratory studies are necessary to define a given condition.

Most of the congenital abnormalities seen by the ophthalmologist—including those involving the eyelids, the cornea, the uveal tract, the lens, and the retina—can be diagnosed on physical examination. Diagnostic imaging is of value in the examination of those conditions that involve the orbit and the globes. The echogram or ultrasonogram can show the size and shape of the eyeball, as well as some abnormalities of the lens and the vitreous. Routine x-ray films and tomograms reveal the size, shape, and position of the orbits and its various components. In some patients, the anatomy of the base of the skull may be shown.

The cephalometric radiographic study is obtained with the patient's head positioned in a cephalostat. The x-ray tube is in a fixed relationship to the cephalostat, with a known object-film distance. In general, measurements obtained from x-ray films in one institution can be compared with those from another institution, provided that identical methods are employed. Tracings made from serial x-ray films on the same subject are used to study the growth pattern or the effect of surgical reconstruction. Normal cephalometric measurements are available on whites (43, 62, 84, 228, 248, 273), blacks (7, 85), Mexican-Americans (112), Chinese (191), and Japanese (192).

The multidirectional tomographic study (frontal, lateral, and basal views) shows the relationship of the craniofacial bones and provides a record upon which measurements can be made. The basal view, which is especially helpful in evaluating asymmetric deformities, is of value in demonstrating horizontal widening of the ethmoid sinuses, the axis of the orbits, and the shape and position of the orbital walls.

The CT study adds additional information to that obtainable by other imaging techniques. The basal view of the orbits is easier to obtain than by any other method; in addition, it shows details of the globe and orbital contents. Intracranial disorders—such as hydrocephalus, cerebral ventricular anomalies, and encephaloceles that may be associated with congenital malformations—can be demonstrated (25). Demonstration of bone and adjacent soft-tissue anatomy in the axial and coronal planes can be very helpful in planning surgical treatment. Currently, at several institutions, three-dimensional reconstructions are being done. We find that they are very useful in treatment planning.

Congenital Abnormalities

There are many abnormalities that involve the orbits. Some are hereditary and some are sporadic. It is impossible to list all of the congenital malformations or syndromes, because much confusion and controversy exists in the literature. The study of these conditions is complicated by the variety of names for the same concept or syndrome. Also, there are overlapping criteria for the diagnosis of a syndrome. The ambiguity of the anatomic measurements and the frequency with which new syndromes are being reported are additional complicating factors. There are several excellent books that have attempted to compile descriptions of these disorders (33, 123, 138, 198, 244, 254).

Developmental abnormalities of the orbits occur with some frequency. Most are minor, and they

are considered to be anatomic variations. The orbits may be deformed in association with widespread dysostoses of the skull and/or skeleton. Since the globe and the orbit develop somewhat independently in disorders such as clinical anophthalmos, the orbit may be well formed but small; and, the muscles and lacrimal apparatus may be relatively unaffected. Anomalies of ossification may result in accessory sutures and supernumerary ossicles in the orbital walls. Rarely, there may be congenital absence of bone in the frontal, maxillary, and orbital areas with resulting displacement of the eye. Pulsating exophthalmos may result from an absence of bone in the roof or posterior wall of the orbit (216).

Unilateral enlargement of the orbit may be symmetric or asymmetric. A tumor located posteriorly in the muscle cone is likely to cause symmetric enlargement of the orbit due to the uniform pressure that results from its presence. Asymmetric enlargement of one orbit may be due to eccentrically located lesions, such as hemangioma, dermoid, or neurofibroma. These lesions may cause local thinning of the orbital wall. Hemangioma usually occurs in the superior quadrant of the orbit, dermoids in the superior temporal area, and neurofibromas in the posterior part—where they may be associated with bony defects (159).

A small orbit may be seen with clinical anophthalmia, microphthalmia, fibrous dysplasia, and expansile infective or neoplastic disease in adjacent structures such as the paranasal sinuses (198, 274). Enucleation of the globe in infancy, if not followed with prompt prosthetic treatment, may cause a small orbit (156, 255).

Lacrimal Drainage System

Most of the congenital abnormalities that involve the lacrimal drainage system can be identified by physical examination. Others are demonstrated via dacryocystograms. Occasionally, supernumerary and displaced puncta can be seen opening into a normal canaliculus or into a separate duct that empties into the tear sac. Supernumerary puncta have been seen on a familial basis (215). The size and position of the puncta and canaliculi may vary. Medial or lateral displacement of the puncta that is associated with displacement of the canthi has been noted (207, 224). Atresia and total absence of the puncta may be hereditary (8, 169, 215, 223).

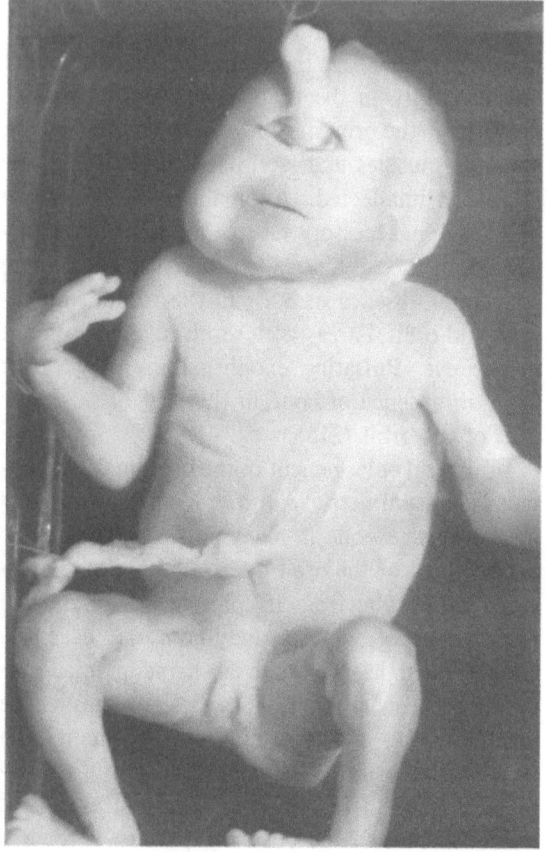

A

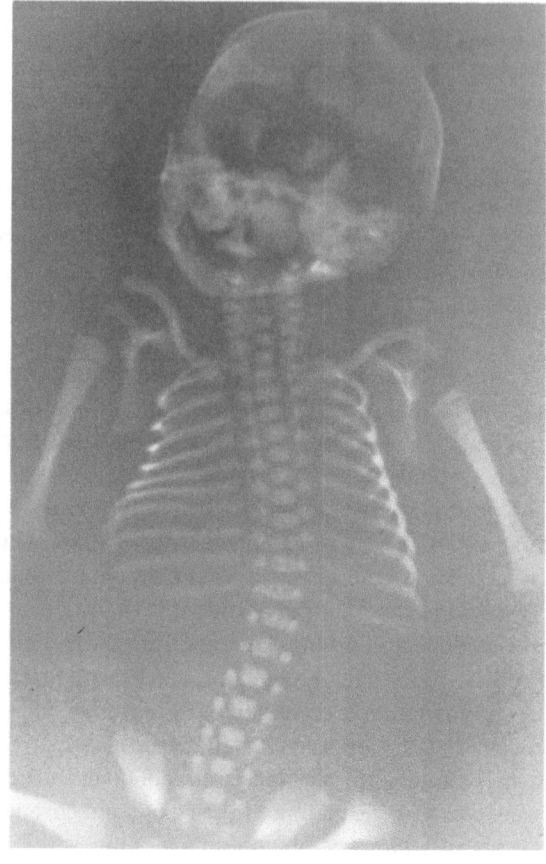

B

Figure 9.6. A. Photograph of preserved specimen with cyclopia. **B.** Radiograph of the specimen obtained with the fetus in the specimen bottle. Note the single large orbit. (Courtesy of The New York City Medical Examiner's Office and E Gross, MD, Chief Medical Examiner).

There may be congenital absence of both the punctum and canaliculus (158). Rarely, fistulas occur either secondary to congenital obstruction of the drainage system or from persistence of facial fissures, or from actual aberrant outpouching of the nasolacrimal sac (40, 89). Congenital abnormalities of the nasolacrimal apparatus often occur in conjunction with cleft lip and cleft palate (89, 215).

While abnormalities of the nasolacrimal apparatus in major facial anomalies are not common, they have been reported in Treacher-Collins syndrome (59, 232), lateral nasal proboscis (181), blepharonasofacial syndrome (207, 224), median facial cleft (162), Waardenburg syndrome (20, 117), and with epicanthus, telecanthus (196), and ectodermal dysplasia syndrome (27, 38, 42).

Abnormalities of the Globe

The eyeball or globe develops from ectodermal elements and the orbit develops from mesodermal elements. Defects in the development of the globe may result in a small orbit, but the major orbital changes are found in association with deformities of the skull and skeleton (165, 183).

Cyclopia, synophthalmia, clinical anophthalmos, microphthalmos, and buphthalmos are developmental abnormalities of the globe that are rarely seen. The first four abnormalities may be seen in association with problems in forebrain differentiation (holoprosencephaly) (Figs. 9.6 and 9.7).

Holoprosencephaly is often seen in association with facial dysmorphia. These facial disorders (i.e.,

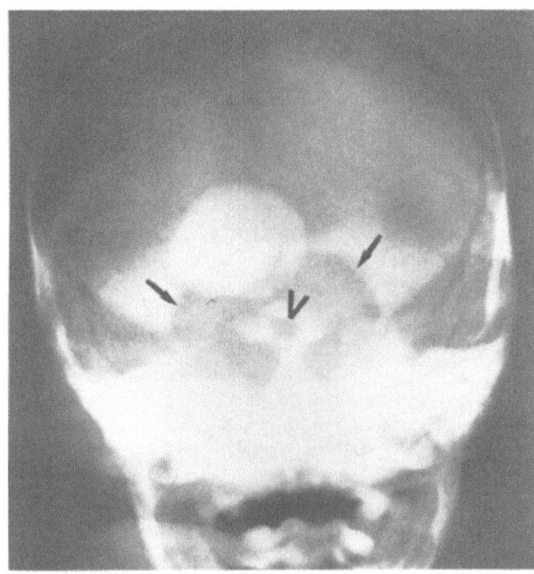

Figure 9.7. Radiograph of a fetal head with cyclopia. The rounded density above the single orbit is the probosis. The foramen magnum can be seen through the orbit. Orbit (arrows); foramen magnum (*V*).

cyclopia, ethmocephaly, cebocephaly, premaxillary agenesis, and less severe facial dysmorphia) probably represent a developmental spectrum (78); and they are sometimes called holoprosencephalies. Since prosencephalic and median face development are related, severe brain malformation may be predicted on the basis of the midline face configuration (81). In the severe form of holoprosencephaly (alobar), the prosencephalon remains as a holosphere with a single ventricular cavity. This cavity is covered by cerebral cortex. The frontal poles of the frontal lobes do not develop. A dorsal sac that contains fluid, posterior to the prosencephalon, represents the invaginated roof of a monoventricle. The unseparated thalami are contained in the cerebrum, which has been arrested in development. A spectrum of less severe malformations may be encountered if the cerebral development is arrested at a later stage. Although this brain malformation was originally called arhinencephaly, the term holoprosencephaly is preferred because it means an arrest in cleavage of the prosencephalon of the cerebral hemispheres; this stresses the holistic, primitive nature of the undivided prosencephalon (199).

The most severely deformed of the holoprosencephalic facies is *cyclopia or synophthalmia.* These are regional congenital anomalies of the upper midface. In cyclopia, only a solitary median eye is present. In synophthalmia, the ocular rudiment is comprised of mirror-image parts of two incomplete eyes jointed in the midline. In either disorder, the ocular structure is in a solitary median cavity or pseudoorbit. The ocular structure usually has associated abnormalities, such as cystic formations, colobomas, retinal dysplasia, and aplasia of the optic nerve. Alobar holoprosencephaly, absent corpus callosum, and septum pellucidum are the abnormalities found in the brain. The bones of the face and skull are abnormal. There may be hypoplasia or absence of the frontal, ethmoid, nasal, vomer, turbinate, and palatine bone. The crista galli is absent. The maxillary processes fuse with each other to form a large maxilla without a nasal structure between them. The absence of the nasal septum and ethmoids leaves a solitary cavity to function as the orbit or pseudoorbit. There may be total absence of a nose; or a proboscis-like structure may be present above the median eye. In both conditions, death usually occurs in utero or shortly after birth. Since cyclopia and synophthalmia are lethal disorders, imaging studies are rarely done. If done, routine x-ray films should show an absent crista galli, the solitary pseudoorbit, and the bone abnormalities described above. The CT scan should show the brain abnormality.

Ethmocephaly, which is associated with alobar holoprosencephaly, is a disorder in which two orbits are present with definite orbital hypotelorism. The nose may be absent or replaced by a proboscis. The forehead is small and the frontal suture is obliterated. There is an absence of the nasal bones, premaxilla, ethmoid, and turbinates. The lacrimal and palatine bones are fused. The olfactory nerves and lobes are either absent or underdeveloped. The optic nerves may bifurcate at the dura after a single origin (69, 123, 254).

Cebocephaly, which is usually associated with alobar holoprosencephaly, is a condition in which the face somewhat resembles that of a monkey. The skull and face are small. A flat rudimentary nose with a single nostril is in its normal position. The anterior cranial fossa is narrow and the sphenoid and ethmoid are hypoplastic. There are two orbits, which are close to each other. The maxillae are fused. Additional abnormalities that may be seen are microphthalmia, clinical anophthalmia, malformations of the pinna, congenital heart dis-

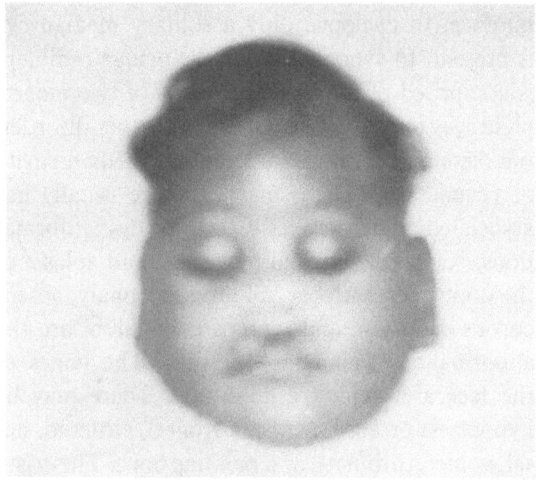

A

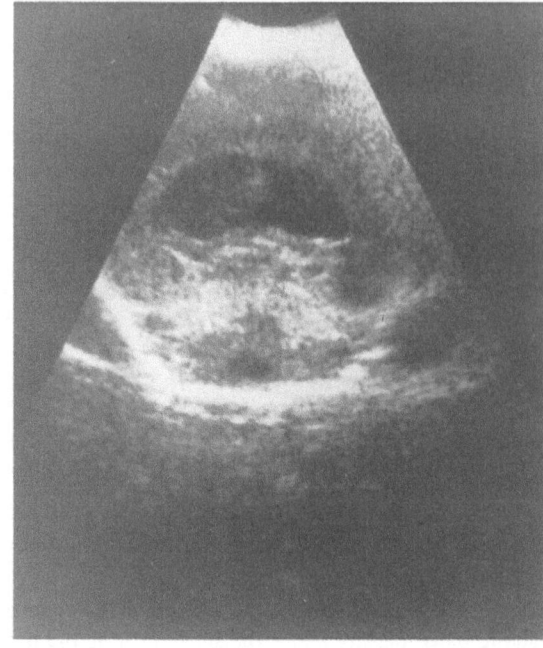

C

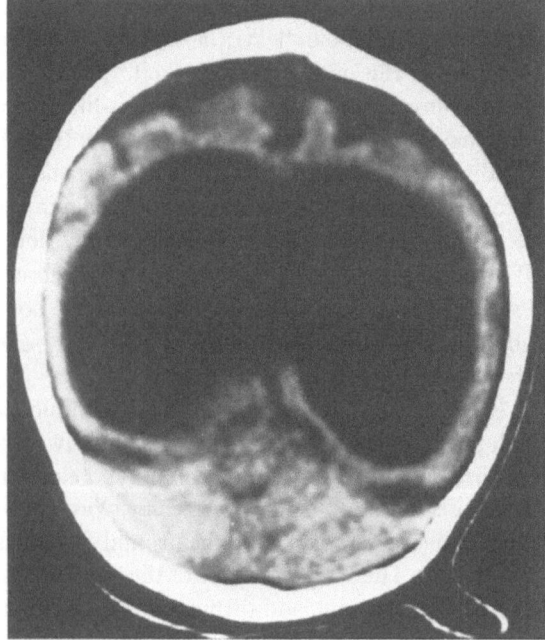

B

Figure 9.8. A. Patient with premaxillary agenesis with cleft palate and the narrow space between the eyes. **B.** Computed Tomogram of the brain showing a large single ventricle (holoprosencephaly) (Courtesy of I Fish, MD, New York, NY). **C.** Midcoronal ultrasound scan of skull demonstrating a single, large midline ventricle (lobar holoprosencephaly) (Courtesy IA Engle, MD, New York Hospital-Cornell Medical Center, New York, NY)

ease, micrognathia, and bicornuate uterus. Transition forms to cyclopia have been described (69, 123).

Premaxillary agenesis with cleft palate usually is associated with alobar holoprosencephaly. It is the most common form of holoprosencephaly to be seen in living subjects. There is a wide-open median cleft corresponding to the missing philtrum. It is confluent with the single nasal opening. The nose is flat, and orbital hypotelorism is present. The premaxilla, nasal septum, horizontal plate of the ethmoid, and crista galli are absent. The single nasal cavity is narrow, and choanal atresia may be present. The optic foramina are fused.

There are variable degrees of severity of this disorder. Other associated abnormalities may be present, such as polydactyly, congenital heart disease, microphthalmia, ear malformations, and spina bifida (Fig. 9.8) (69, 123).

Less severe facial dysmorphia is associated with semilobar or lobar holoprosencephaly. It has variable features, including orbital or ocular hypotelorism or hypertelorism, a flat nose, unilateral or bilateral cleft lip, iris colomba, and (at times) other anomalies. There is minimal facial dysmorphia in some cases (123).

In many cases, the etiology of holoprosencephaly is unknown. Many different factors have been found to be associated. The distinct chromosome syndromes, which may be associated with holoprosencephaly and facial dysmorphia, include trisomy 13, 18 p-syndrome, 13 q-syndrome, trisomy 18, triploidy, plus a number of other unusual karyotypes (90, 123, 131, 157). Normal karyotypes have been reported as well. Most cases are sporadic (123). Occasionally, holoprosencephaly with facial dysmorphia has been reported to be autosomal-recessive. Teratogenic agents such as lithium, magnesium, Veratrum alkaloids, the Vica alkaloid vinblastine, vitamin A, and others have been reported as causal factors (157, 201).

A rare syndrome that sometimes includes cyclopia is *Otocephalia* (microstomia, agnathia, and synotia). In this disorder, there is failure in the formation of the mandibular arch, often with fusion of the external ears in the midline area, which is usually occupied by the mandible. The mouth is small (123).

Holoprosencephaly and facial dysmorphia have been observed in some cases of Meckel syndrome (123).

Anophthalmos, strictly defined, means a complete absence of the eye. However, this is rarely the case, since histologic studies usually reveal a rudimentary eye. The terms clinical anophthalmos or extreme microphthalmos are more appropriate. The condition often is bilateral. When it is unilateral, the existing eye is frequently abnormal and microphthalmic. Clinical anophthalmos may be classified into three types. Primary clinical anophthalmos, which is the most usual type, is due to failure in the development of the optic primordium that is unassociated with gross abnormalities of the medullary tube. It tends to appear sporadically in an otherwise well-formed child, and it is bilateral. The secondary clinical anophthalmos forms as part of a widespread maldevelopment of the anterior end of the neural tube. The resulting fetus is a nonvariable monster with multiple abnormalities. The third type, consecutive anophthalmos, occurs when the optic vesicle has formed and has subsequently undergone degeneration. This type may be unilateral and should be called extreme microphthalmos (90). The radiographic findings are a small, shallow, and conical orbit with underdeveloped bony walls. In the older patient, the stunted orbit will show encroachment from the paranasal sinuses. The optic canals will be small or absent. The sphenoid bone may be poorly formed (Figs. 9.9 and 9.10).

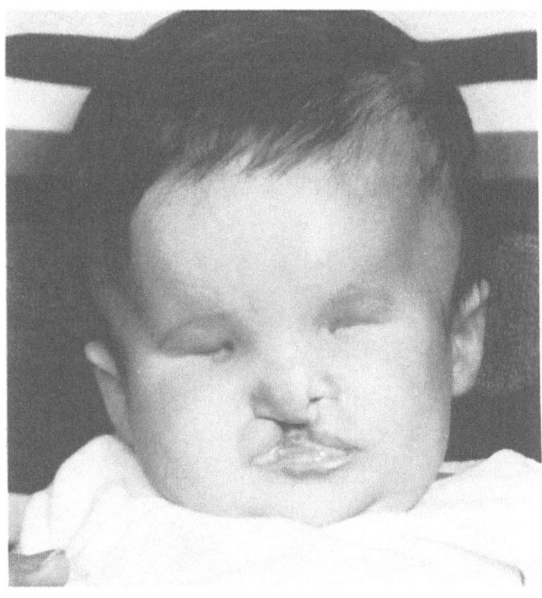

A

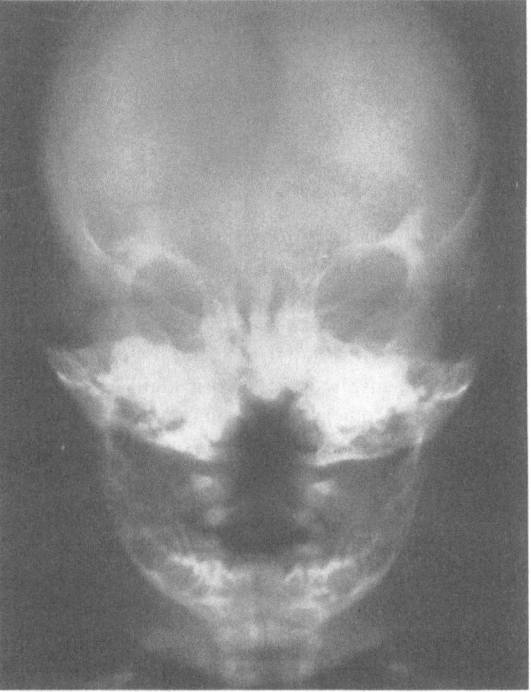

B

Figure 9.9. A. Patient with bilateral clinical anophthalmia and a cleft lip and palate. **B.** Frontal radiograph showing small orbits, some degree of orbital hypertelorism, and the cleft palate.

Clinical anophthalmos may be found as a sporadic bilateral disorder (primary anophthalmos); or it may be found in other conditions, such as trisomy 13, focal dermal hypoplasia (Goltz syndrome), Goldenhar syndrome, Lenz syn-

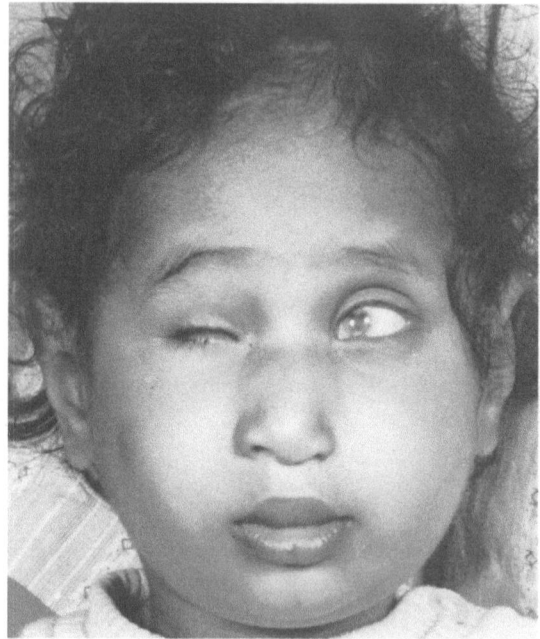

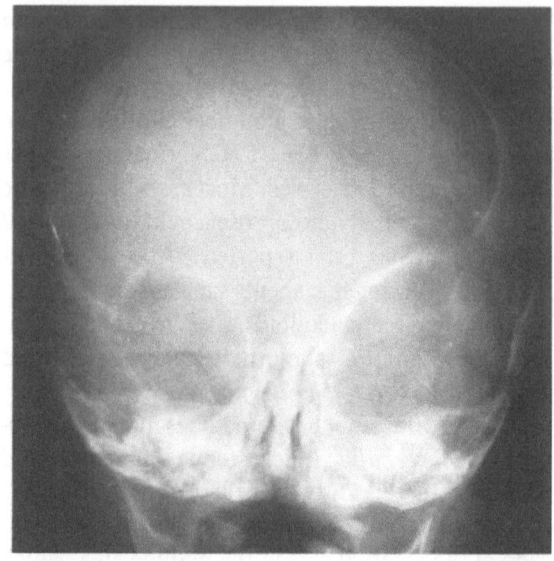

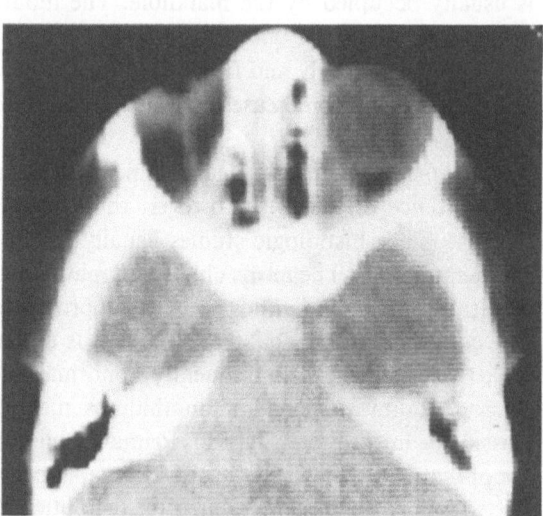

Figure 9.10. A. Two-year-old boy with unilateral clinical anophthalmos. **B.** Frontal radiograph showing a small orbit on the involved side and a high arched palate. **C.** Computed tomogram showing an amorphous mass and cyst where the eye should be on the involved side.

drome, Meckel syndrome, microphthalmia with digital anomalies, thalidomide embryopathy, and X-linked anophthalmia (138, 254).

Cryptophthalmos syndrome is a rare autosomal disease with an absence of the palpebral fissure, either unilateral or bilateral. There are no eyelids nor eyelashes on the involved side. The lacrimal ducts may be deformed or absent. Small eyeballs are often palpable under the skin-covering. The involved globe has abnormalities of the anterior portion, but the posterior portion usually is functional. Some of the reported cases have had orbito-palpebral cysts, which give the appearance of a protrusion in the region of the globe (92). When unilateral cryptophthalmos is present, the opposite side (with the palpebral fissure) usually will have

ocular abnormalities such as symblepharon, upper lid coloboma, microphthalmia, and others. In addition to the ocular anomalies, there may be total or partial soft-tissue syndactyly, coloboma of the alae nasi, an unusual hairline, and various urogenital abnormalities. In about 20% of the reported cases, malformed temporal and parietal bones have been noted. Calcification has been reported in the falx cerebri; and the foramen magnum has been found to be heart-shaped, with incomplete closure of the exoccipital portion of the occipital bone. Approximately 10% of the patients have a meningoencephalocele. Computed tomographic studies of the orbits are helpful in evaluating the globes (123, 138).

Microphthalmos is a term used to include a

great variety of abnormalities of the globe when it is smaller than normal, even though the literal definition would be "small eyeball." Pure microphthalmos or nanophthalmos is a small but otherwise normal eye. Microphthalmos may be divided into three major types: nanophthalmos, colobomatous microphthalmos, and complicated microphthalmos (90).

Nanophthalmos (pure microphthalmos) is an uncommon condition in which there is an arrested development of the globe in all dimensions after the embryonic fissure has closed. The eye is reduced in volume (usually about one-third) without other gross abnormalities. The palpebral fissure is narrow, and the globe is set deep in a small orbit. In unilateral cases, the side of the face and, possibly, the entire side of the body on the involved side may be underdeveloped. Bilateral cases usually are seen as part of a generalized dwarfing syndrome. While nanophthalmos may be hereditary, sporadic cases are more common. Nanophthalmos may be seen in association with other syndromes (90).

Colobomatous microphthalmos is a small globe associated with a failure of closure of the embryonic cleft. It is seen with other ocular abnormalities, and it sometimes is seen with a colobomatous cyst. If the colobomatous microphthalmos is unilateral, the other eye may be microphthalmic and deformed. This condition may be hereditary, sporadic, or associated with other syndromes (90).

Complicated microphthalmos is a small eye with many anomalies. The globe may be very small, or it may be represented by a small ectodermal nodule in the orbit (clinical anophthalmos). Clinical anophthalmos may occur on one side, while the other side may have microphthalmia. With complicated microphthalmia, many diverse abnormalities may be present, such as corneal opacities or staphylomata, cataract, aniridia, corectopia, persistence of the pupillary membrane, thickening or ossification of the choroid, and various abnormalities of the retina. This condition may be hereditary, sporadic, or associated with other syndromes (90) (Figs. 9.11 and 9.12).

Table 9.4 is a listing of many syndromes and conditions that have been reported to have microphthalmia. However, the association is not always seen in all cases, and the type of microphthalmos is often not recorded. It is hoped that with the advent of CT scanning and its ability to show the globe and orbit, better descriptions of the anatomy will be made and the syndromes will be better defined (110).

Aicardi syndrome is a dominant X chromosome disease characterized by infantile spasm and convulsions, subnormal intelligence, lacunar chorioretinopathy, microphthalmos, colobomas, iris synechia, optic atrophy, facial asymmetry, and plagiocephaly. Imaging studies may show agenesis of the corpus callosum, heterotopic gray matter, hydrocephalus, Arnold-Chiari malformation, Dandy-Walker syndrome, block vertebrae, hemivertebrae, butterfly vertebrae, spina bifida, abnormal costovertebral articulation, and scoliosis (254).

The *cerebro-oculo-facio-skeletal syndrome* is an autosomal-recessive disease characterized by prenatal growth retardation, craniofacial dysmorphia, microcephaly, a sloping forehead, a high nasal

Table 9.4. Conditions with reported microphthalmos

1. Aicardi syndrome
2. Cerebro-oculo-facio-skeletal syndrome (COFS syndrome)
3. Chromosome 6 r-syndrome
4. Chromosome 10 q + syndrome
5. Chromosome trisomy 13 syndrome (Trisomy D1)
6. Chromosome 13 q-syndrome
7. Chromosome 13 r-syndrome
8. Chromosome trisomy 18
9. Congenital cytomegalovirus infection
10. Congenital Rubella syndrome
11. Congenital toxoplasmosis syndrome
12. Cryptophthalmos syndrome
13. de Lange syndrome
14. Fetal alcohol syndrome
15. Fetal Herpes simplex infection
16. Focal dermal hypoplasia (Goltz syndrome)
17. Gingival fibromatosis, microphthalmia, mental retardation, athetosis, and hypopigmentation (Cross syndrome)
18. Goldenhar syndrome (oculoauriculovertebral dysplasia)
19. Hallerman-Streiff syndrome (oculomandibulodyscephaly)
20. Holoprosencephaly (holoprosencephaly and facial dysmorphias)
21. Lenz microphthalmos syndrome (microphthalmia and digital anomalies)
22. Meckel syndrome (dyscephalia, splanchocystica, and Gruber syndrome)
23. Microphthalmia, corneal opacity, mental retardation, and spasticity syndrome
24. Microcephaly, microphthalmia, falciform retinal folds, and blindness
25. Norrie disease
26. Oculodentodigital syndrome (oculodentoosseous dysplasia)
27. Thalidomide embryopathy
28. Treacher-Collins syndrome (mandibulofacial dysostosis)
29. Warfarin embryopathy

From (33, 123, 138, 150, 254).

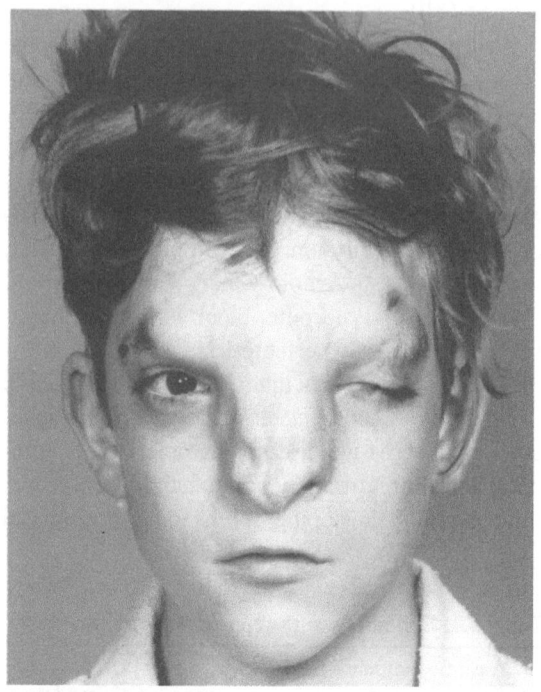

A

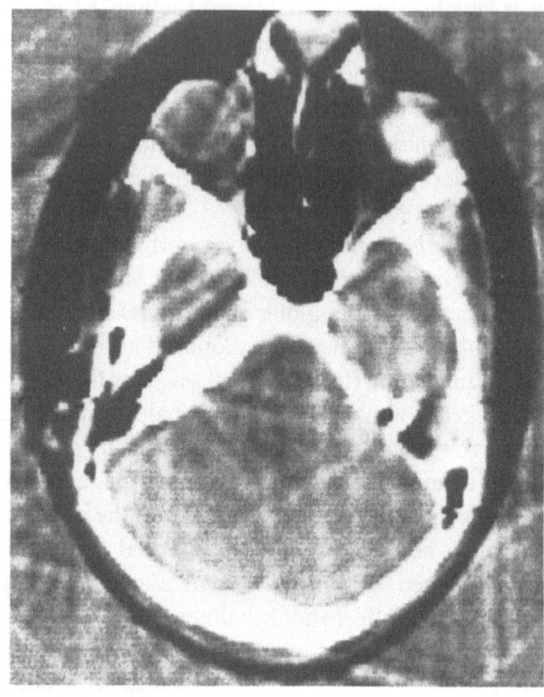

C

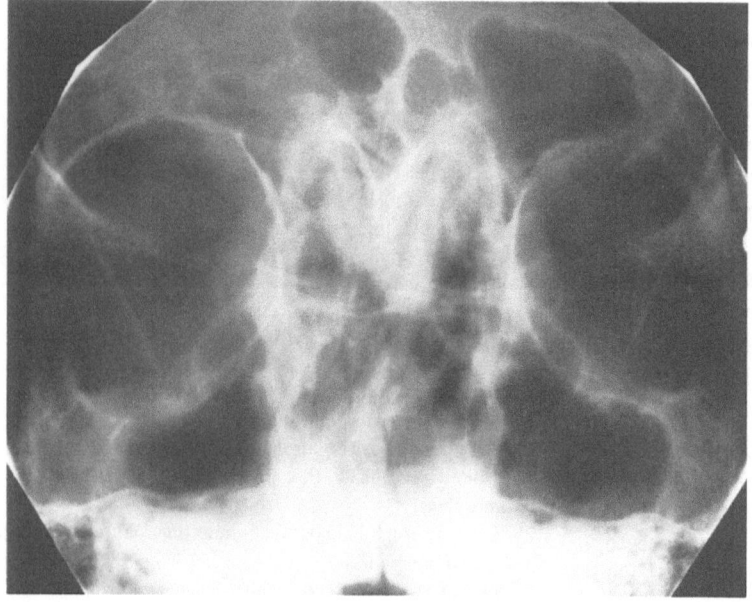

B

Figure 9.11. A. Eleven-year-old
boy with unilateral complicated
microphthalmos—a broad bifid
nose. **B.** Waters view radiograph showing that the orbit on
the involved side is smaller than
normal. A frontonasal cleft is
present as well as orbital hypertelorism. **C.** Computed tomogram shows a round, dense tissue mass instead of a normal eye
on the involved side.

bridge, overhanging upper lip, micrognathia, narrow palpebral fissures, microphthalmia, cataract,
short neck, kyphosis, scoliosis, camptodactyly, and
foot deformities (254).

Focal dermal hypoplasia or Goltz syndrome is
a disease consisting of atrophy and linear hyperpig-
mentation of the skin, localized deposits of superficial fat, multiple papillomas of the mucous membranes, limb abnormalities, and anomalies of the

nails. Other reported abnormalities include absent
uvula, split soft palate, facial asymmetry, and deafness. About 50% of reported cases have eye anomalies (microphthalmia, coloboma, and strabismus)
(123, 138, 254).

Hallermann-Streiff syndrome or oculomandibulodyscephaly is a syndrome consisting of proportionate dwarfism, congenital cataracts, microphthalmos, dyscephaly with a hypoplastic

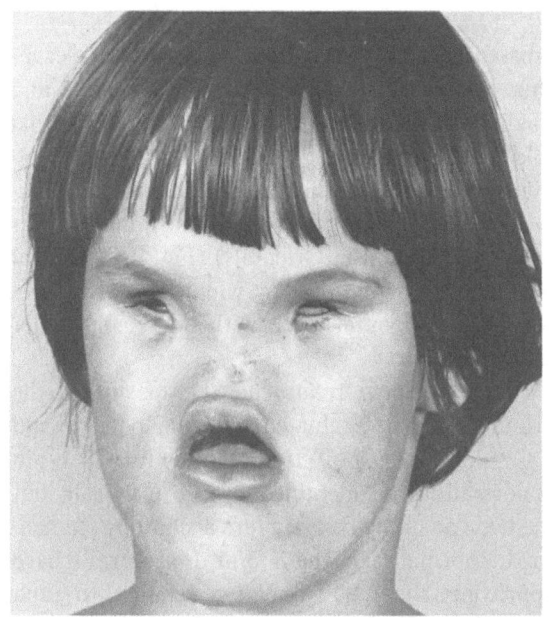

A

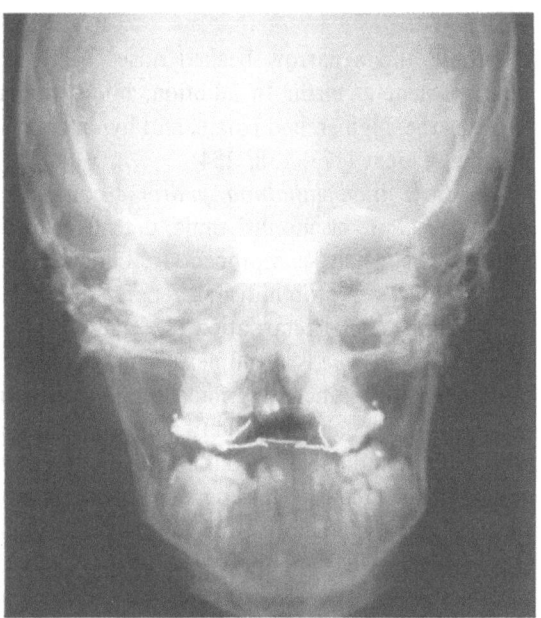

B

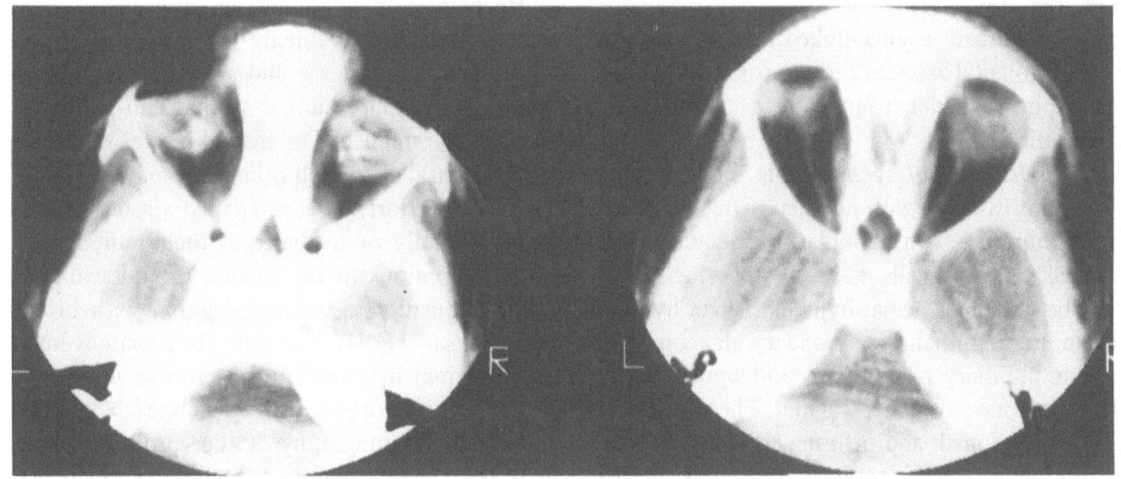

C

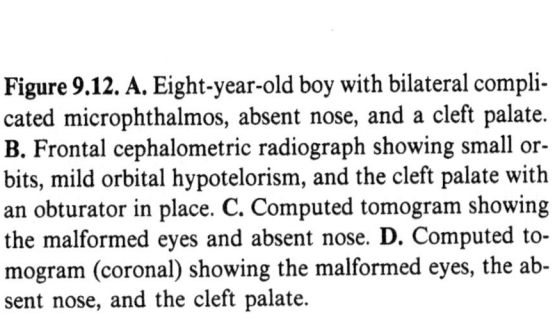

Figure 9.12. A. Eight-year-old boy with bilateral complicated microphthalmos, absent nose, and a cleft palate.
B. Frontal cephalometric radiograph showing small orbits, mild orbital hypotelorism, and the cleft palate with
an obturator in place. **C.** Computed tomogram showing
the malformed eyes and absent nose. **D.** Computed tomogram (coronal) showing the malformed eyes, the absent nose, and the cleft palate.

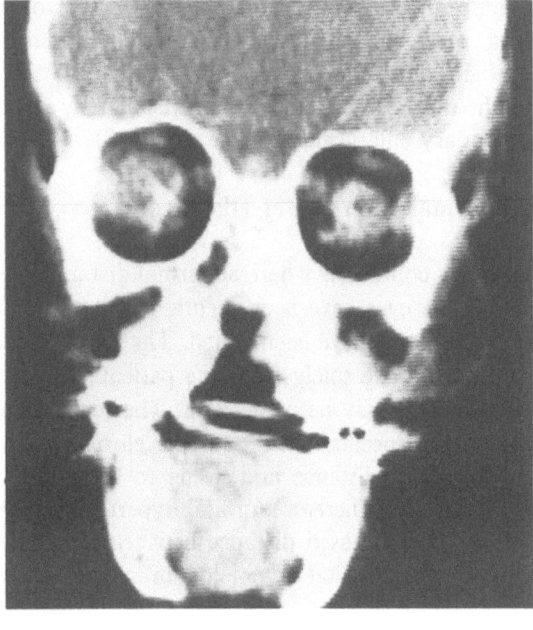

D

mandible and a narrow beaked nose. Teeth are often present at birth. In addition, microstomia, blue sclerae, high arched palate, and hypotrichosis may be evident (123, 138, 254).

The *Lenz microphthalmia syndrome* consists of microphthalmia or anophthalmia, defective dentition, microcephaly, camptodactyly, clinodactyly, hypospadias, cryptorchidism, renal anomalies, growth and mental retardation (123, 254).

Meckel syndrome is a complex group of congenital abnormalities, including microcephaly with an occipital encephalocele, cleft palate, postaxial polydactyly, and polycystic kidney, liver, and pancreas. Other frequent findings are microphthalmos, orbital hypothelorism or hypertelorism, absent olfactory tracts, congenital heart disease, and genital abnormalities. In one case, a chromosomal abnormality, 46,xx,3 p+, has been reported (33, 123, 138, 144, 254).

Norrie disease is an x-linked recessive disorder with retrolental vascular masses, iris atrophy, cataracts, phthisis bulbi at birth, deafness, and mental retardation (138).

Oculodentodigital syndrome is an autosomal-dominant disorder with characteristic facies, having a thin nose with hypoplastic alae and narrow nostrils. The eyeballs have microcornea. There may be associated ocular hypotelorism or hypertelorism, microphthalmos, secondary glaucoma, persistent pupillary membranes, and optic atrophy. The teeth have defective enamel. There is syndactyly of the fourth and fifth fingers (33, 123, 254).

Buphthalmos or congenital glaucoma is a hereditary disorder of the drainage system of the anterior chamber of the eye that causes the eyeball to enlarge as the increased tension acts on an immature eyeball. When this occurs prior to or shortly after birth, the enlargement of the eyeball may cause secondary enlargement of the orbit (90).

Abnormal Interorbital Distance

In many conditions where abnormal distances between the eyes have been mentioned, no specific measurements have been stated. The descriptions often are made solely from the patient's appearance, which may be misleading. The terms used may not be specific. The term hypertelorism means an increased distance and needs to be modified to be specific. Therefore, orbital hypertelorism refers to the increased distance between the orbits (Table 9.2). Orbital hypotelorism means a de-

creased space between these structures. Telecanthus is a lateral displacement of the puncta and medial canthus relative to the iris. An epicanthal fold (plica palpebronasalis) is a fold of skin extending from the root of the nose to the inner termination of the eyebrow, overlapping the inner canthus (a normal finding in Orientals) (Fig. 9.5). Orbital dystopia is a condition in which the orbits are not on a horizontal level, with one being higher than the other.

When planning treatment, the spacing of the orbits should be evaluated by cephalometric and CT studies (25, 186, 194). Not only will brain abnormalities be identified by the CT scan, but the bone anatomy can be more accurately studied. In the normal face, the lateral orbital walls have approximately a 90° angle in relation to each other. In orbital hypertelorism, the angle becomes more obtuse; in hypotelorism, it is more acute. Exact angle measurements are not possible, because both the lateral and medial orbital walls tend to be slightly curved so that end-points are difficult to establish. The medial orbital walls usually are parallel to each other, but may be wedge-shaped anteriorly, wedge-shaped posteriorly, or bulge laterally or medially at their midportions. These variations in the medial orbital walls are most frequently seen in association with orbital hypertelorism (194). The cribriform plate is lower than normal in orbital hypertelorism in relation to the superior orbital walls which are best evaluated on polytomography or the coronal CT scan (63, 186). Alterations in the angle of divergence of the optic nerve with globe movement, as shown with dynamic ocular CT scanning, have demonstrated that the optic axis is not a reliable method for evaluating ocular hypertelorism (186).

Orbital hypertelorism may seem to be present in a given patient when a normal or smaller than normal distance between the eyes is found by measurement. Conditions that can cause an illusion of orbital hypertelorism are blepharophimosis, dystrophia canthorum, epicanthal folds, external strabismus, flat nasal bridge, internal ankyloblepharon, microcephaly, microphthalmos, clinical anophthalmos, small face with normally spaced eyes, small nose, symblepharon, and widely spaced eyebrows (82). Two good examples of this illusion are Down syndrome (chromosome 21 trisomy syndrome or mongoloidism) (4), and trisomy 13 (Patau syndrome) (149). Both syndromes have been described as having hypertelorism as a manifestation. When subsequent studies were done with measurements, orbital hypotelorism was present (31, 79, 81, 82, 176).

The degree of orbital hypertelorism varies from patient to patient. In some patients, the distance from the medial orbital wall to the facial midline may be normal on one side, while the distance may be greater or less than normal on the other side. The severity of increased orbital spacing in adults has been classified into three groups (259): 1) first-degree orbital spacing has an interorbital distance of 30–34 mm; 2) second degree has an interorbital distance of greater than 34 mm, with a normal shape and orientation of the orbits; and 3) third degree has an interorbital distance greater than 40 mm, with a prolapse of the cribriform plate and a decreased distance between the outer canthus and the external auditory canal.

Orbital Hypotelorism

Orbital hypotelorism, which is a narrowed space between the orbits, is usually seen in conjunction with hypoplasia of the ethmoids. It has been reported to occur in several syndromes (Table 9.5).

Binder syndrome (maxillonasal dysplasia) is not as rare as the scarcity of reports would suggest. This is probably due to the fact that the features of this syndrome are not very striking. This disorder is characterized by a flat vertical nose with flattened alae and nasal tip. Radiographic study will show an absence or hypoplasia of the anterior nasal spine, thinness of the labial plate of alveolar bone over the upper incisors, and the frontal sinuses being hypoplastic. Mild orbital hypotelorism may be noted (Figure 9.13) (34).

Craniotelencephalic dysplasia is characterized by protrusion of the frontal bone, craniosynostosis (brachycephaly), and orbital hypotelorism. Encephaloceles, hemangiomas, and mental retardation are also seen (138).

Orbital Hypertelorism

Orbital hypertelorism (telorbitism) should be considered a physical finding that is common to many disorders—and not a separate entity. It has been reported in a multitude of conditions, many of which are listed in Table 9.6. The original reports may have described the syndrome as being associated with wide-spaced eyes, or hypertelorism. Only in a few cases have measurements been made to

Table 9.5. Orbital hypotelorism syndromes

1. Baller-Gerold syndrome (craniosynostosis-radial aplasia syndrome)
2. Binder syndrome (maxillonasal dysplasia)
3. Chromosome 13 trisomy syndrome (Patau syndrome)
4. Chromosome 18 p-syndrome
5. Chromosome 21 trisomy syndrome (Down syndrome, or mongolism)
6. Craniotelencephalic syndrome
7. de Lange syndrome
8. Elfin facies syndrome
9. Holoprosencephalia and facial dysmorphia spectrum of disorders
10. Meckel syndrome
11. Median cleft lip and orbital hypotelorism without holoprosencephalia
12. Microcephaly (often proportionate hypotelorism)
13. Oculodentodigital syndrome
14. Trigonocephaly
15. Williams syndrome (Idiopathic hypercalcemia-supravalvular stenosis syndrome)
16. Other rare miscellaneous disorders

From (22, 32, 33, 61, 82, 138, 244, 254).

verify that orbital hypertelorism is actually present. The reports of some of the conditions indicate that either hypotelorism or hypertelorism may be present.

The Greig syndrome was among the first syndromes to be reported that involved orbital hypertelorism (125). It was originally described as ocular hypertelorism or as a great breadth between the eyes without other associated abnormalities (Fig. 9.14). Since then, some investigators have included it as part of the median cleft face syndrome (or the frontonasal dysplasia malformations complex) (77, 237). Other investigators have noted the association of orbital hypertelorism with a variety of other anomalies (178, 210). One of these is the Sprengel deformity (154).

A syndrome related to the Greig syndrome is the *frontodigital syndrome* (*Greig cephalopolysyndactyly syndrome*). This is an autosomal-dominant disorder with frontal bossing, scaphocephaly, or brachycephaly, hypertelorism, and ear anomaly. The hand and foot abnormalities may be postaxial or preaxial polydactyly, broad first digit, and syndactyly (254).

The frontonasal dysplasia malformation complex (*median cleft face syndrome*) is a disorder consisting of orbital hypertelorism, broad nasal root, anterior cranium bifidum occultum, median facial clefting involving the nose or both the nose and

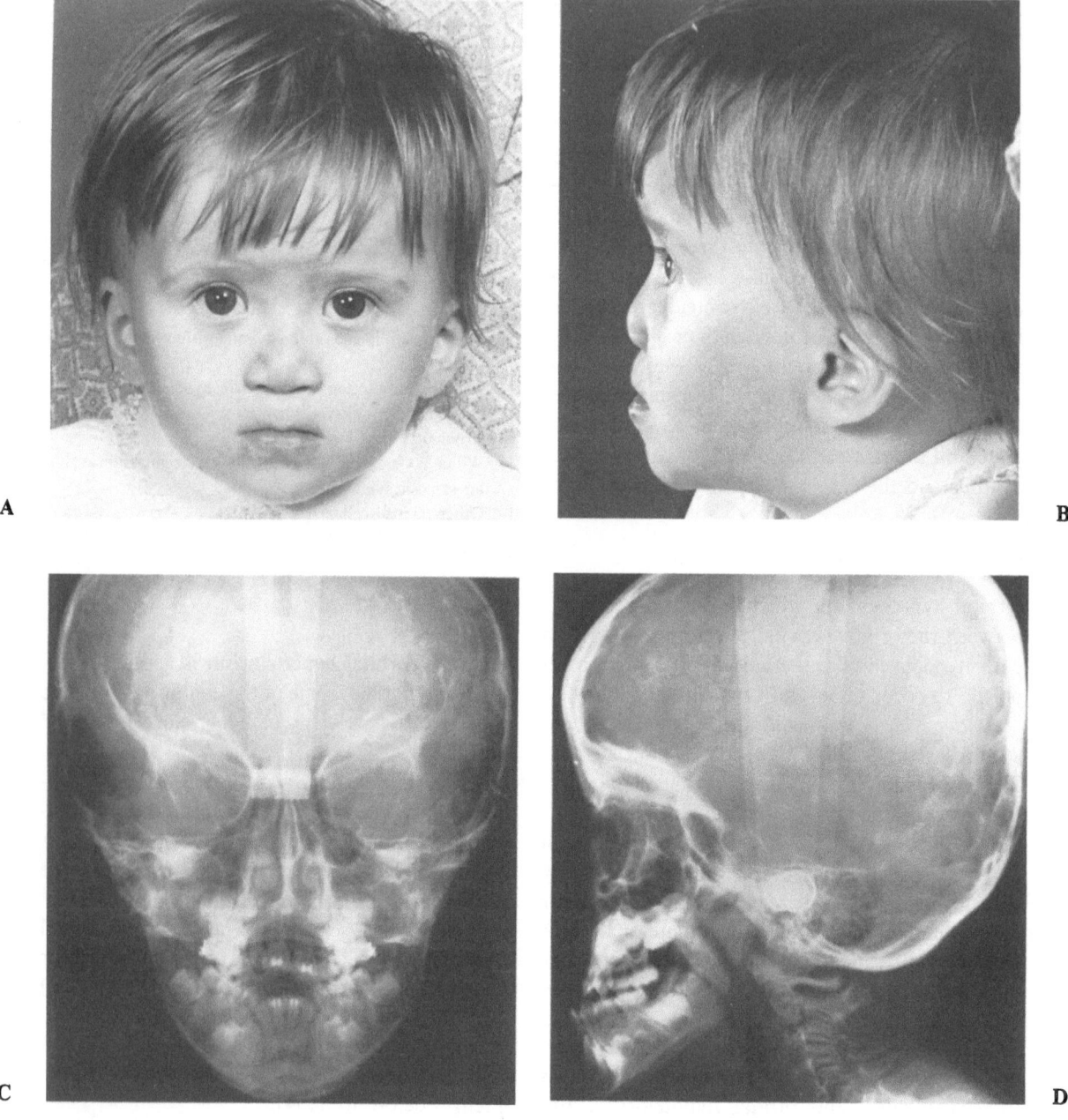

A B

C D

Figure 9.13. A, B. An 18-month-old boy with Binder syndrome. The nose is flat and the midface is mildly retruded. **C, D.** Frontal and lateral cephalometric radio- graphs show mild orbital hypotelorism, a hypoplasic nasal bone, and absence of the nasal spine.

upper lip and (in some cases) the palate, unilateral or bilateral clefting of the alae nasi, lack of formation of the nasal tip, and a widow's peak hairline (33, 77, 123, 237, 254). This malformation complex has been subclassified into four types. The first type is characterized by orbital hypertelorism, broad nasal root, and median nasal groove with absence of the nasal tip (Fig. 9.15). The second type consists of orbitral hypertelorism, broadening of the nasal root, and a deep median facial groove or true clefting of either the nose or the nose and upper lip. There also may be a cleft palate (Fig. 9.16). In the third type, unilateral or bilateral notching of the alae nasi is seen together with orbital hypertelorism and a broad nasal root (Fig. 9.17). The fourth type is a combination of the

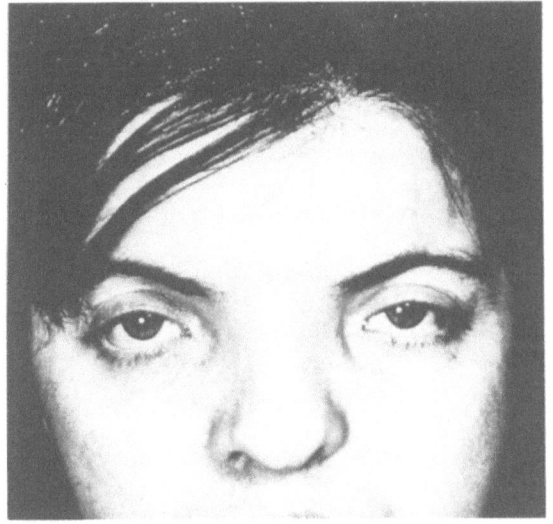

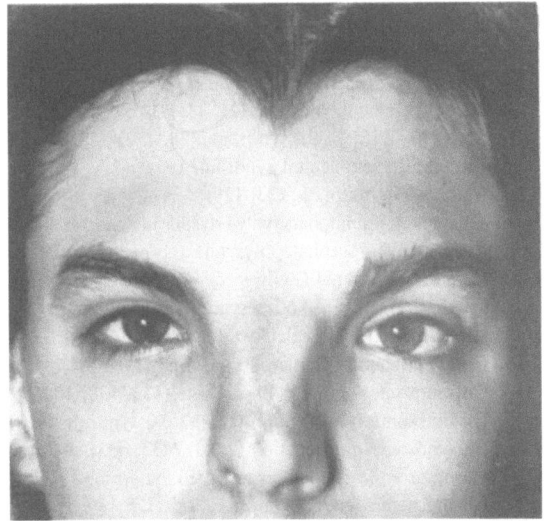

A

A

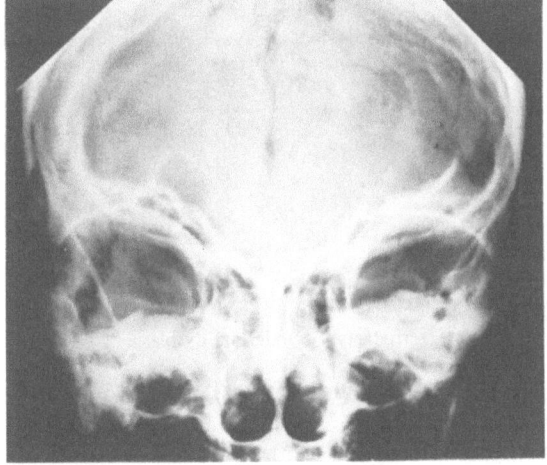

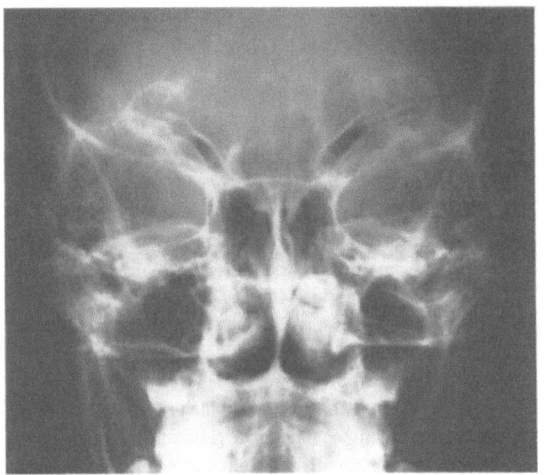

B

B

Figure 9.14. A. A 30-year-old woman with orbital hypertelorism (Greig syndrome). The nasal bridge is wide and flat. **B.** Frontal radiograph showing orbital hypertelorism, depressed cribriform plate, and increased width of the ethmoid sinuses. There are several small lucencies in the frontal bone that are vascular lakes.

Figure 9.15. A. Photograph of a 14-year-old boy with type 1 frontonasal dysplasia with broad nasal root, nasal clefting, and "widow's peak" hairline. **B.** Frontal radiograph showing the orbital hypertelorism and enlarged sinuses.

second and third types (Fig. 9.18) (237). While most cases of frontonasal dysplasia are sporadic, some familial cases have been reported (55). Rarely, epibulbar dermoids have been associated with frontonasal dysplasia (55). When the facial changes of frontonasal dysplasia are mild, extracephalic abnormalities are rare; and, they are more common when the facial changes are severe (77). The frontonasal dysplasia malformation complex should be differentiated from other syndromes in which orbital hypertelorism is present. Radiologic studies will show the presence of orbital hypertel-

orism, and they may reveal an anterior cranium bifidum and obliteration of the frontal sinuses. There often is an accompanying anterior encephalocele. Less frequently, lipomas or teratomas have been associated with frontonasal dysplasia.

There has been a report of a case of frontonasal dysplasia associated with holoprosencephaly. This was in a 3-year-old girl who had orbital hypertelorism, a cleft chin, and CT demonstration of holoprosencephaly (233).

Craniofrontonasal dysplasia probably is an autosomal-dominant syndrome with the facial manifes-

Table 9.6. Conditions associated with increased distance between the eyes

1. Aarskog syndrome (1, 111)
2. Acrodysostosis (229)
3. Apert's syndrome (11, 39, 54, 123)[a]
4. Basal cell nevus syndrome (21, 119, 123)
5. Beckwith-Wiedemann syndrome (28, 172)
6. Brancho-skeleto-genital syndrome (93)
7. Campomelic dysplasia (23, 128)
8. Cardiofacial-pulmonary valve dysplasia syndrome (254)
9. Carpenter (acrocephalopolysyndactyly) syndrome (123, 254)[a]
10. Cerebrohepatorenal (Zellweger) syndrome (70, 270)
11. Cerebral gigantism (Soto's syndrome) (245, 264)
12. Chondrodystrophia calcificans congenita (chondrodysplasia punctata) (123, 174, 247)
13. Chotzen (Saethre-Chotzen) syndrome (123, 254)[a]
14. Chromosome 4$_p$- (Wolf) syndrome (123, 138, 189, 190, 238)
15. Chromosome translocation (1$_p$-; 17q+) syndrome (101)
16. Chromosome translocation (2; 13) (q32; q33) syndrome (105)
17. Chromosome trisomy short arm 10 syndrome (146)
18. Chromosome ring D syndrome (138, 175)
19. Chromosome trisomy 13 syndrome (123, 138, 149)
20. Chromosome 5$_p$- (Cri du chat) syndrome (123, 138, 190)
21. Chromosome 18$_p$, 18$_q$-, 18$_r$ syndromes (138)
22. Chromosome X0 (Turner) syndrome (123, 138)
23. Chromosome 48 XXXX syndrome (138)
24. Chromosome 49 XXXXY syndrome (15, 138, 212)
25. Chromosome 49 XXXXX syndrome (138, 174)
26. Chromosome 47 XXX (Cat's eye) syndrome (123, 138, 254)
27. Chromosome trisomy 14 (D$_2$) syndrome (195)
28. Chromosome partial trisomy 7 syndrome (138, 202)
29. Chromosome trisomy 9 syndrome (17)
30. Chromosome deletion of short arm of 13-15 syndrome (73)
31. Chromosome mosaic (46XY-D, 4 Dr) and (45, XY-D) syndrome (175)
32. Chromosome trisomy 21 (Down) syndrome (123, 138, 254)
33. Cleft lip-palate, lobster claw deformity, nasolacrimal duct obstruction (ectrodactyly ectodermal dysplasia-clefting [EEC]) syndrome (123)
34. Cleft lip-palate and tetraphocomelia (Roberts or Appelt-Gerkin-Lenz) syndrome (122, 123, 138)
35. Cleft lip-palate, ocular hypertelorism, and microtia (HMC) syndrome (37, 123)[a]
36. Cleft lip-palate, cutis gyratum and acanthosis nigricans syndrome (21)
37. Cleft lip-palate and encephalomeningocele syndrome (123)
38. Cleft lip-palate, lid ectropion and ocular hypertelorism syndrome (123)
39. Cleft lip-palate and pseudodiastrophic dwarf syndrome (123)
40. Cleft lip and palate (5, 102, 193)[a]
41. Cleft lip-palate, tetraperomelia, deformed pinna, scarcity of hair, and hypoplastic nipples syndrome (122)
42. Cleidocranial dysplasia (123, 254)
43. Coffin-Lowry syndrome (33, 123)
44. Craniocarpotarsal dysplasia (whistling face or Freeman-Sheldon) syndrome (123, 254)
45. Craniodiaphyseal dysplasia (123)
46. Craniofrontonasal dysplasia (220, 226)
47. Craniometaphyseal dysplasia of Pyle (123, 246, 254)[a]
48. Craniosynostosis, midface hypoplasia, hypertrichasis, and anomalies of the eyes, teeth, heart, and external genitalia syndrome (123)
49. Craniosynostosis, arthrogryposis, and cleft palate (Christian; Andrews-Conneally-Muller) syndrome (123)
50. Craniostenosis, brachydactyly of hands, and absent toes (Herrmann-Opitz) syndrome (123)
51. Craniostenosis, severe symmetrically malformed extremities, and cleft lip-palate (Herrmann-Pallister-Opitz) syndrome (123)
52. Crouzon's disease (craniofacial dysostosis) (123)[a]
53. Cryptophthalmos (Fraser) syndrome (123)
54. Dubowitz syndrome (86, 123)
55. Epicanthus (33)
56. Extra nares (94)
57. F syndrome of acro-pectoro-vertebral dysplasia (126, 127)
58. Facial clefts (79)[a]
59. Facial hemangioma (178)

Table 9.6. (*Continued*)

60. Familial telecanthus-hypospadias-multiple mild malformation syndrome (51, 188, 206)[a]
61. Fetal aminopterin syndrome (138, 225, 254)
62. Fetal face (Robinow-Silverman) syndrome (123, 230)
63. Fetal hydantoin syndrome (33, 123)
64. Fetal trimethadione syndrome (33)
65. Fetal warfarin syndrome (24, 33, 123)
66. Frontal, ethmoidal, or sphenoidal dermoid, lipoma, or teratoma (79)[a]
67. Frontal, ethmoidal, or sphenoidal meningoencephalocele (79)[a]
68. Frontonasal dysplasia (median cleft face syndrome) (55, 79, 108, 123, 210, 237)[a]
69. G syndrome of dyschondroplasia, polysyndactyly, and kewpie doll facies (205)
70. Greig syndrome (125)
71. Hypercalcemia with supravalvular aortic stenosis (254)
72. Hypertelorism with heterotopia of maculas and pseudoexotropia (3)
73. Hypertelorism with inguinal hernia (2, 96)
74. Hypertelorism with iris dysplasia and mental retardation (75)
75. Hydrocephalus (secondary to prenatal causes)[a]
76. Ichthyosis and polysyndactyly (163)
77. Kleeblattschadel (clover leaf skull) (9, 123)[a]
78. Larsen syndrome (256)
79. Leopard syndrome (multiple lentigenes syndrome) (33, 121, 123, 254)
80. Leprechaunism (Donahue syndrome) (33, 254)
81. Lissencephaly syndrome (congenital agyria) (227, 254)
82. Lymphedema and yellow nails (161)
83. Meckel-Gruber Syndrome (33, 123, 254)
84. Megalencephaly (80)
85. Metopism (persistence of the frontal suture) (252)
86. Microblepharon syndrome of small lids, tetrastichiasis, synophrys, and nail dystrophy (262)
87. Mohr syndrome of polysyndactyly, cleft tongue, and micrognathia (OFD syndrome II) (33, 123, 254)
88. Mutilating acropathy (143)
89. Nasal glioma (33)
90. Nasofrontal mucoceles, segmental vitiligo, and porencephaly (253)
91. Noonan syndrome (33, 58, 123, 203, 254)
92. Oculodento-osseous dysphasia (33, 123)
93. Oto-palato-digital (Taybi) syndrome (254)
94. Papillon-league syndrome of oro-digito-facial dysostosis (OFD syndrome I) (33, 123, 254)
95. Pfeiffer syndrome (123, 254)
96. Polydactyly and undescended testes (45)
97. Posttrauma
98. Potter syndrome of renofacial dysplasia (123, 254)
99. Proboscis lateralis (79)
100. Rieger syndrome of iris dysplasia and hypodontia (123, 167, 254)
101. Rubinstein-Taybi (broad thumbs and mental retardation) syndrome (254)
102. Sclerosteosis (33)
103. Sprengel deformity (154)[a]
104. Syndactyly, short neck, microstomia, cutis laxa, and agenesis of the small intestine (200)
105. Ulrich-Feichtiger syndrome (254)
106. Vogt-Waardenburg syndrome (174, 254)[a]
107. Waardenburg syndrome of dystropia canthorum, white forelock, and deafness (33, 123, 263)

[a] Reported in literature as orbital hypertelorism.

tation of frontonasal dysplasia combined with craniosynostosis (usually brachycephaly), as well as other extracranial malformations. Among the extracranial manifestations are webbed neck, dystrophic nails, narrow thoracic inlet, and (occasionally) partial syndactyly (Figs. 9.19 and 9.20) (56, 220, 226, 242).

The fetal face syndrome (*Robinow or Robinow-Silverman-Smith syndrome*) is a disorder consisting of a characteristic face, forearm brachymelia, and hypoplastic genitalia. The face resembles that of a fetus of 8 weeks. Orbital hypertelorism, a bulging forehead, micrognathia, a large neurocranium, and a short upturned nose with anteverted nostrils are seen. The upper extremity has mesomelic brachymelia with disproportionate shortening of forearms (the ulna being shorter than the radius). There is brachymesophalangism and clin-

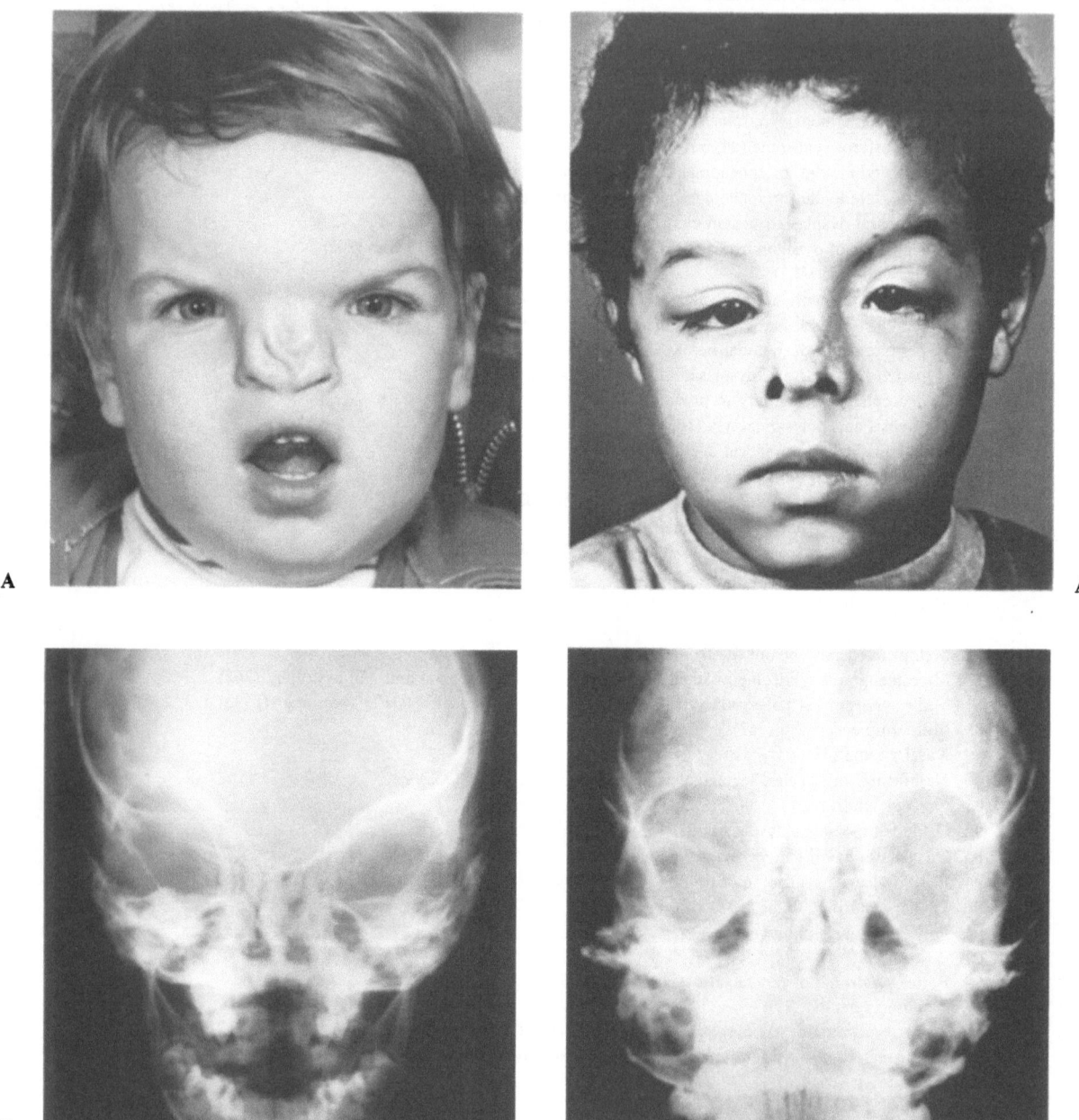

Figure 9.16. A. Two-year-old boy with type 2 frontonasal dysplasia. Note the broad nasal root and the median facial cleft. **B.** Frontal radiograph showing the orbital hypertelorism and enlarged ethmoid sinuses.

Figure 9.17. A. Postsurgical film of 12-year-old boy with frontonasal dysplasia with notching of the alae nasi. **B.** Frontal facial film showing anterior cranium bifidum and orbital hypertelorism with enlarged ethmoid sinuses.

odactyly of the fifth finger; the other phalanges and metacarpals are short. The terminal phalanges of the hands and feet are bifid. Multiple rib anomalies are seen. Scoliosis may be present in association with hemivertebrae, vertebral fusions, and narrow interpediculate distances. This syndrome has genetic heterogeneity, and it has been noted

to be autosomal-dominant and autosomal-recessive (Fig. 9.21) (33, 123, 230, 254).

There are a group of disorders that can be grouped under the term craniotubular bone dysplasias and hyperostoses. The craniotubular dysplasias include Pyle disease, craniometaphyseal dysplasia, craniodiaphyseal dysplasia, frontometa-

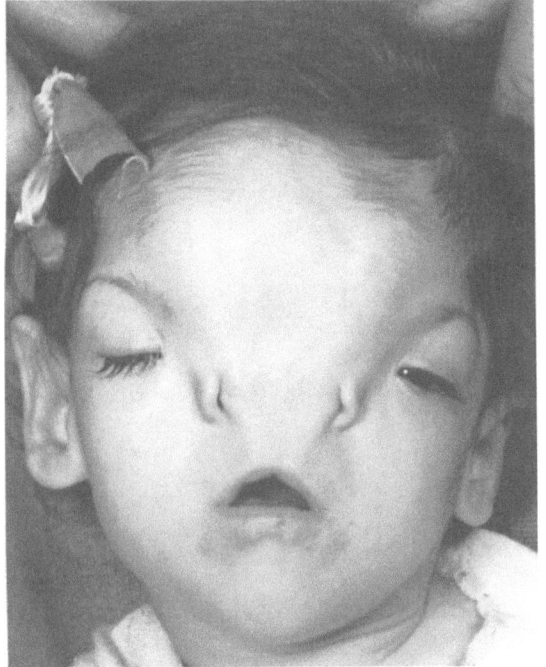

A

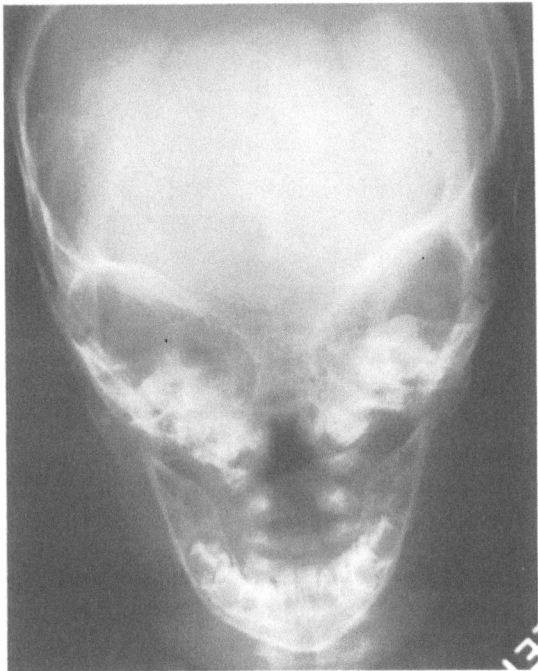

B

C

Figure 9.18. A. Two-year-old girl with type 4 frontonasal dysplasia. Note the marked orbital hypertelorism, the notched upper lip, and the broad midfacial cleft. **B.** Frontal radiograph showing the marked orbital hypertelorism, the bony choanal atresia, and cleft palate. **C.** Computed tomogram showing the midnasal cleft, the absence of a nasal passage, and the marked orbital hypertelorism.

physeal dysplasia, Schwarz-Lelek syndrome, dysosteosclerosis, and oculodentoosseous dysplasia. The craniotubular hyperostoses consist of van Buchem disease, sclerosteosis, congenital hyperphosphatasia, and Camurati-Engelmann disease (120, 123).

Craniometaphyseal dysplasia often is confused with the Pyle metaphyseal dysplasia. In both conditions, there is metaphyseal broadening. However, in craniometaphyseal dysplasia, the metaphyseal widening is less and the craniofacial hyperostosis is more profound. The mode of inheritance of craniometaphyseal dysplasia is unknown; however, it has been reported in autosomal-domi-

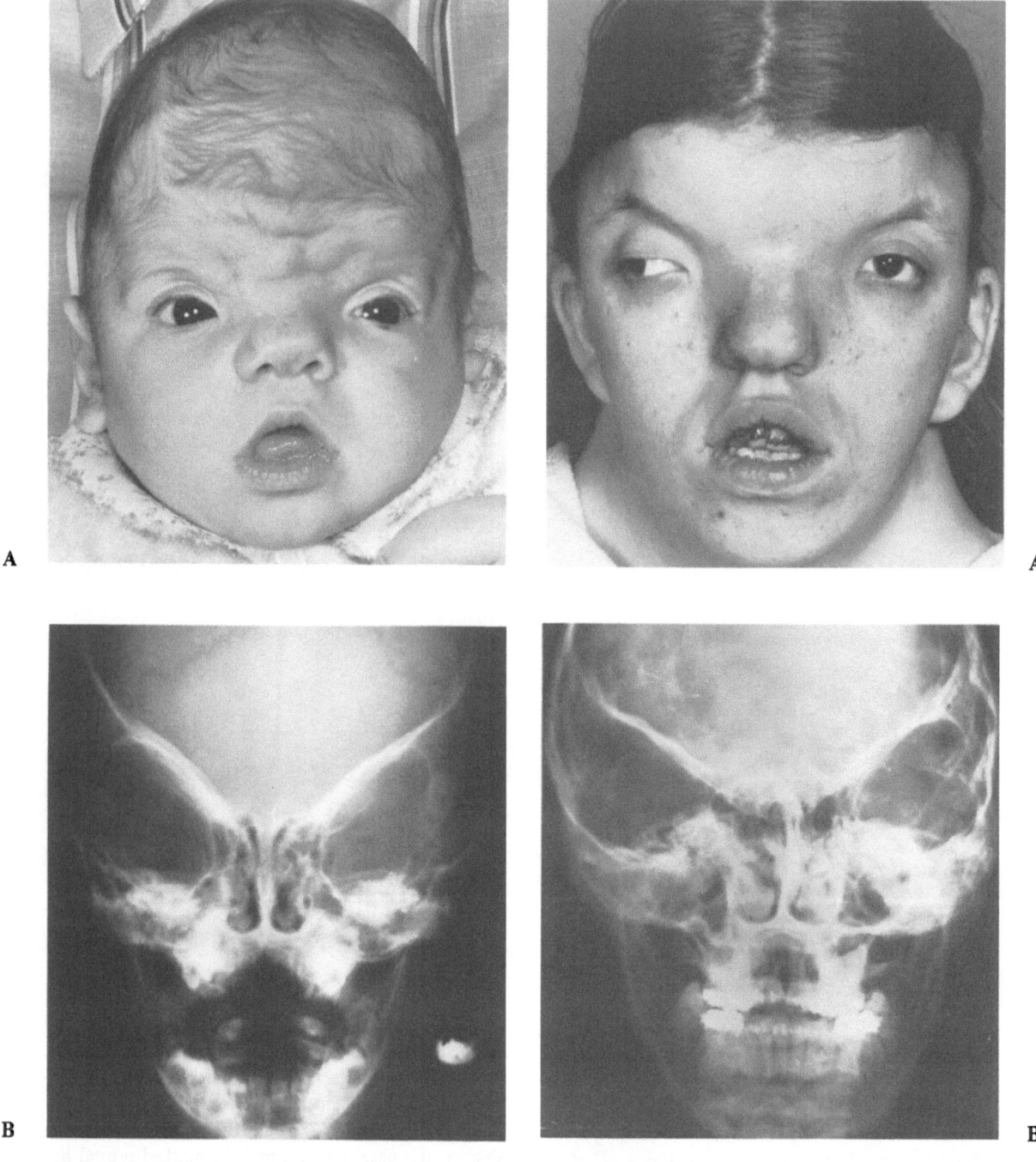

Figure 9.19. A. Two-month-old girl with craniofronto-nasal dysplasia. B. Frontal radiograph showing orbital hypertelorism and harlequin orbit configuration with mild asymmetry.

Figure 9.20. A. A 19-year-old woman with craniofron-tonasal dysplasia. B. Frontal radiograph showing orbital hypertelorism with asymmetric harlequin orbits.

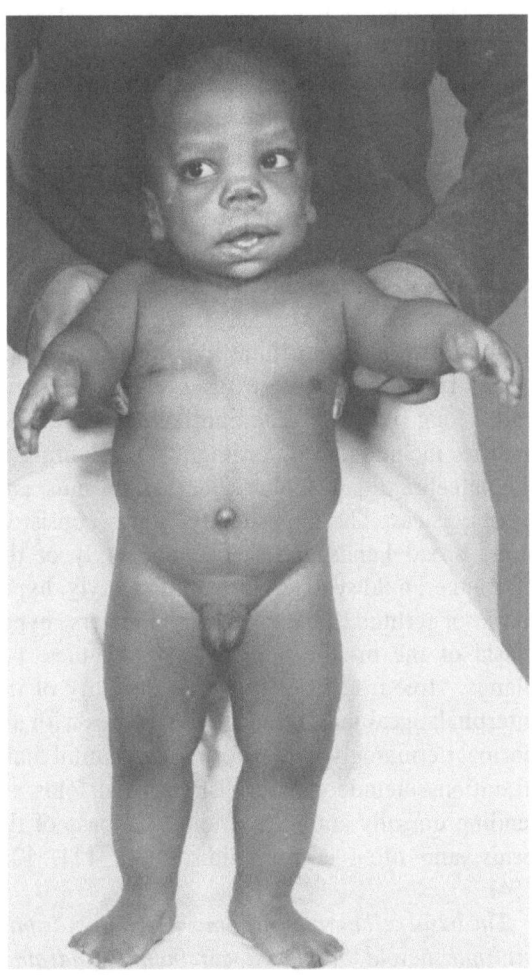

A

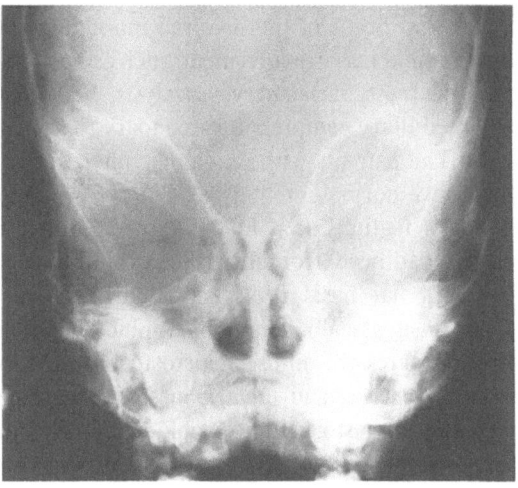

C

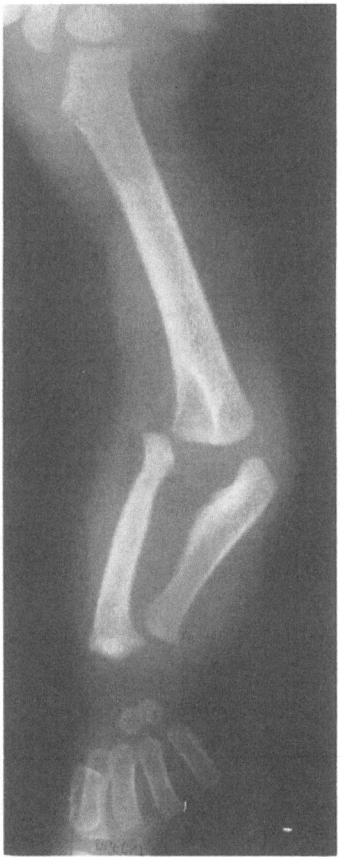

D

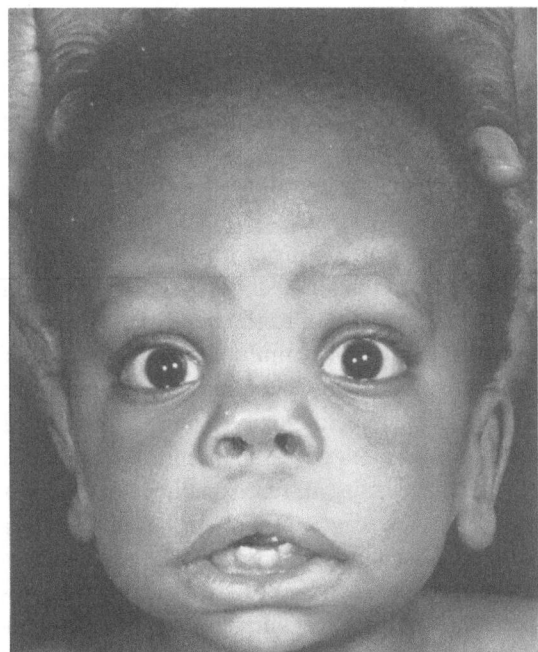

B

Figure 9.21. A, B. Two-year-old boy with the fetal face syndrome. The eyes are widely spaced and the nose is broad. C. This frontal radiograph of the skull shows orbital hypertelorism. D. Radiograph of the upper extremity showing mesomelic brachymelia with disproportionate shortening of the forearm. The ulna is shorter than the radius and the radius is dislocated.

nant and -recessive forms. This disease is evident in infancy. Some of the involved individuals may have cranial nerve involvement, such as optic atrophy, deafness, facial nerve paralysis, hemiplegia, and medullary compression secondary to hyperostosis. The patients with craniometaphyseal dysostosis have normal intelligence. The abnormal craniofacial features seen in this disorder include a large broad head, frontal bossing, orbital hypertelorism, a flat nasal root, and a large mandible ("leontiasis ossea"). The radiographic changes include progressive diffuse hyperostosis of the cranial vault, base, and facial bones. The paranasal sinuses and mastoids may be obliterated. The foramina at the base of the skull and of the orbits may be narrowed by hyperostosis. There is orbital hypertelorism. The tubular bones have flaring and widening of the metaphyses (Fig. 9.22) (48, 123, 141, 246, 254).

Craniodiaphyseal dysplasia probably is an autosomal-recessive disorder. Clinically, it is characterized by severe facial and cranial thickening, distortion, and enlargement (leontiasis ossea). Many patients have growth and mental retardation. Nasal obstruction, deafness, and failure of vision develop along with bony thickening of the skull. Seizures may occur. Radiographically, the skull, facial bones, and mandible become severely sclerotic and hyperostotic. The ribs and clavicles become thickened and sclerotic. The paranasal sinuses and mastoids are obliterated. Hydrocephalus and orbital hypertelorism can be seen. The neural arches of the vertebrae have an increased density. The tubular bones have the shape of a police officer's nightstick and show diaphyseal endostosis (123, 254).

Sclerosteosis is a disease with progressive skeletal deformity that begins in infancy. It is an autosomal-recessive disorder. In this disease, there is an acquired craniofacial dysmorphism with a high, steep forehead, mandibular prognathism, relative midfacial hypoplasia, exophthalmos, and orbital hypertelorism. In many cases, there may be development of deafness, facial nerve paralysis, optic atrophy, reduced visual fields, convergent strabismus, and exophthalmos. Asymmetric cutaneous syndactyly of the middle and index fingers may be present. Radiographically, there is hyperostosis and osteosclerosis of the neurocranium, mandible, ribs, clavicles, pelvis, vertebrae, and tubular bones. The inner acoustic meatus and optic canals may be narrowed. The body of the mandible is greatly thickened and the mandibular angle is greatly obtuse. The tubular bones, in addition to sclerosis, show a lack of diaphyseal modeling. The index finger may have no middle phalanx or just a small triangular bone (delta phalanx) (29, 33, 123, 249, 254).

The Aarskog (facial-digital-genital) syndrome is characterized by short stature, genital abnormalities, and unusual facies. It is probably an X-linked recessive disorder, with partial expression in heterozygotic females. The major facial features include widow's peak, orbital hypertelorism, broad nasal bridge, short nose with anteverted nostrils, and a long philtrum. The ophthalmologic abnormalities include ptoses, antimongoloid slanting of the palpebral fissures, blue sclera, strabismus, and large corneas. The limb manifestations consist of short broad hands and feet, clinodactyly of the fifth finger, mild syndactyly, camptodactyly, hypoplasia of terminal phalanges of the fingers, hypoplasia of the middle phalanges of the toes, pes planus, "tree-frog toes," hyperextensibility of the interphalangeal joints, and simian creases with abnormal dermatoglyphic patterns. The genital manifestations include characteristic scrotal folds extending dorsally and surrounding the base of the penis, and often cryptorchidism (33, 111, 123, 254).

The basal cell nevus syndrome (Gorlin syndrome, multiple nevoid basal cell carcinoma syndrome) probably is an autosomal dominant disorder. The major components of this disorder are multiple nevoid basal cell carcinomas on the exposed and nonexposed skin, jaw cysts, vertebral and rib anomalies, intracranial calcifications, and palmarplantar pits. This syndrome may begin in early childhood. The presence of basal cell carcinoma in a child should be followed to check for other signs of this syndrome. The face has frontal and temporoparietal bossing, with the eyes appearing widely spaced (about 40% have true orbital hypertelorism). In addition to the basal cell carcinomas and the palmar pits, multiple skin lesions (such as milia, cysts, comedones, and cafe-au-lait spots) may be present. Radiologic manifestations include odontogenic cysts of the mandible, rib anomalies (bifid, splayed, absent, fused, rudimentary, and extra), pectus excavatum or carinatum, vertebral anomalies (scoliosis, kyphoscoliosis, and fused spinous processes), and soft-tissue calcifications (especially in the ovary). The skull shows frontal and temporoparietal bosses, lamellar calcification of the falx, bridging of the sella, and (at times) orbital hypertelorism. An increased incidence of medulloblastoma has been seen in families known to have basal cell nevus syndrome. It is possible that the affected child may die before developing the rest of the syndrome (21, 33, 119, 123, 254).

The *branchio-skeleto-genital syndrome* (*Elsahy-Waters syndrome*) probably is an autosomal-recessive disorder that appears to be a midline-clefting disorder, with orbital hypertelorism, cleft palate, pectus excavatum, and hypospadias. In addition, there may be brachycephaly, fusion of the second and third cervical spinous processes, and hypoplasia of the maxilla with relative prognathism (33, 93).

The *cerebrohepatorenal syndrome* (*Zellweger syndrome*) is a severe, usually fatal multisystem disorder that is autosomal-recessive. At birth, there is profound muscular hypotonia, with decreased or absent reflexes and hepatomegaly. A typical craniofacial dysmorphia is manifested by a high bulging forehead, brachyturricephaly, widely open cranial sutures, widened fontanelles, puffy eyelids, ocular hypertelorism, mongoloid slant of the orbital fissures, and epicanthal folds. Also present are Brushfield spots, glaucoma, corneal cloudiness, cataracts, low-set ears, high-arched palate, and micrognathia. The liver is enlarged. Limb anomalies may be seen, such as cubitus valgus, camptodactyly, metatarsus adductus, and talipes equinovarus. Radiologic examination will demonstrate chondral, articular, and periarticular soft calcifications—especially in the patellas at birth, in acetabular areas, and in hyoid bone. The limb anomalies may be demonstrated, such as digital flexion deformities, cubitus valgus, metatarsus adductus, talipes equinovarus, rocker-bottom feet, metatarsus varus, and retarded bone age. The skull will show mild orbital hypertelorism, dolichocephaly, and widened sutures and fontanelles. The cerebral ventricles are dilated. Pathologic examination will show brain dysgenesis (lissencephaly, macrogyria, and polymicrogyria), renal cortical cysts, liver parenchymal damage and fibrosis, and hemosiderosis (33, 70, 123, 254, 270).

Cerebral gigantism (*Sotos syndrome*) is a hereditary disease manifested by advanced height and skeletal maturation beginning in infancy, unusual craniofacial appearance, and mental deficiency. The skull and face show a dolichocephalic macrocranium, prominent forehead, supraorbital ridges, antimongoloid slant of the eyes, ocular hypertelo-

rism, and a prominent jaw. The frontal hairline may have receded. Radiographic manifestations include a large dolichocephalic skull, mild orbital hypertelorism, high-rising orbital roofs, and disproportionately large hands and feet with advanced skeletal maturation. Other changes that have been noted include dilated cerebral ventricles, posteriorly inclined dorsum sella turcica, anterior fontanelle bone, vertebra plana, and kyphosis or kyphoscoliosis (123, 245, 254, 264).

The *Coffin-Lowry syndrome* is a hereditary disorder that may be an X-linked or sex-influenced autosomal-dominant disease. It is characterized by progressive mental and motor deterioration. Craniofacial dysmorphism is manifested by a square forehead, with prominent outer lateral aspects, bitemporal narrowing, thickened supraorbital ridges, down-slanting palpebral fissures, ocular hypertelorism, thickened upper eyelids, broad nasal bridge with thick nasal septum, anteverted nostrils, thick pouting lips, relative prognathism, and large prominent pinnas. Limb abnormalities include large soft hands with hyperextensible thick fingers that taper distally and a short great toe. Radiographic manifestations include thickened facial bones, mild orbital hypertelorism, hyperostosis frontalis, pectus carinatum or excavatum, kyphosis of the dorsal spine, and lumbar gibbous deformity. The hands have drumstick-shaped terminal phalanges with constriction of the adjacent shaft. Other changes that are seen include coxa valga, lower limb discrepancy, and short hallux (33, 123, 254).

Dubowitz syndrome probably is an autosomal-recessive disorder that is manifested by primordial shortness of stature, microcephaly, eczema, mental retardation, and a characteristic face. The facial abnormalities include a high forehead with flat supraorbital ridges, blepharophimosis, canthal hypertelorism, or true orbital hypertelorism. Micrognathia is present. Radiographic changes include mild orbital hypertelorism, retarded bone age, clinodactyly of the fifth finger, preaxial polydactyly, cutaneous syndactyly of the second and third toes, and periosteal hyperostosis of long bones (86, 123, 254).

The *hypertelorism-hypospadias syndrome* (*Opitz syndrome, BBB syndrome*) is a hereditary syndrome that is either autosomally dominant or X-linked. This disorder is characterized by orbital hypertelorism, hypospadias and other urinary tract abnormalities, and mental retardation. Radi-

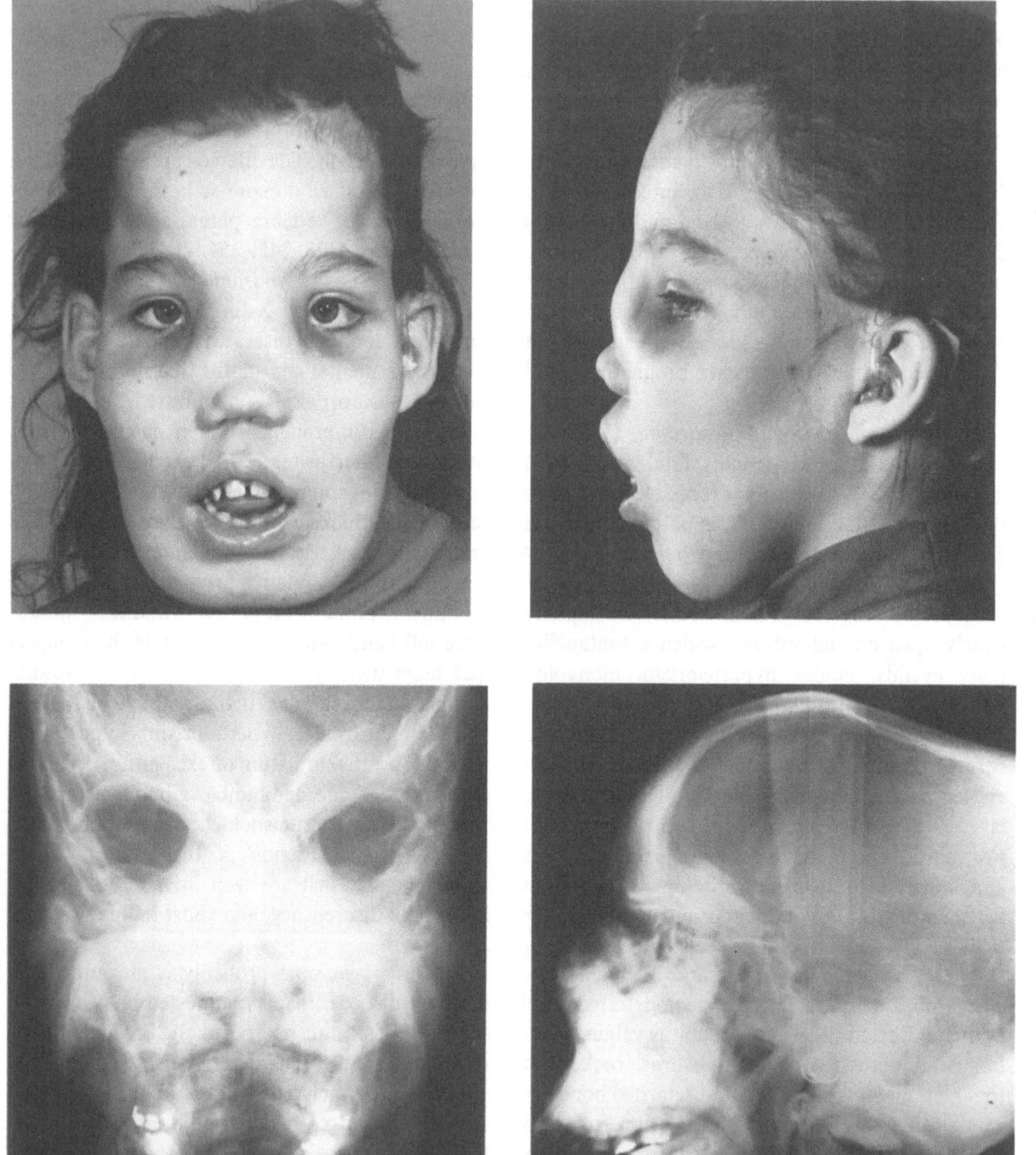

Figure 9.22. A, B. A 10-year-old girl with craniometaphyseal dysplasia. The prominent forehead, bulging nasal bridge, and prominent jaws are secondary to the underlying facial hyperostosis. A hearing aid, present on the left, is used for progressive deafness. **C, D.** Frontal and lateral cephalometric radiographs showing the sclerosis and hyperostosis of the facial bones and the base of the skull, including the petrous bone.

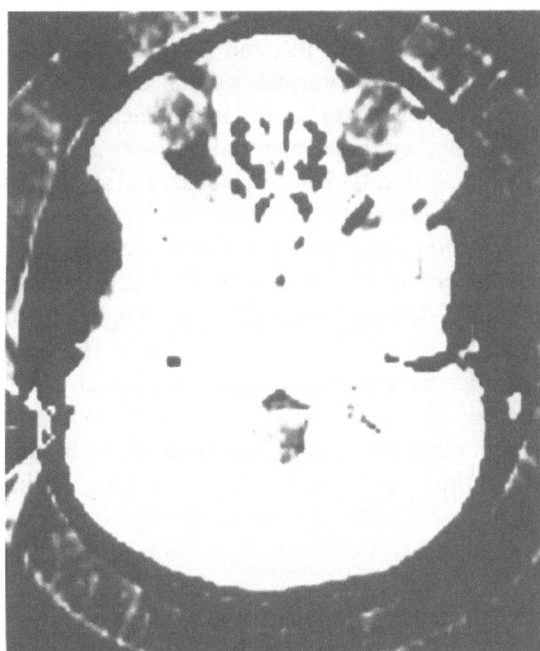

E

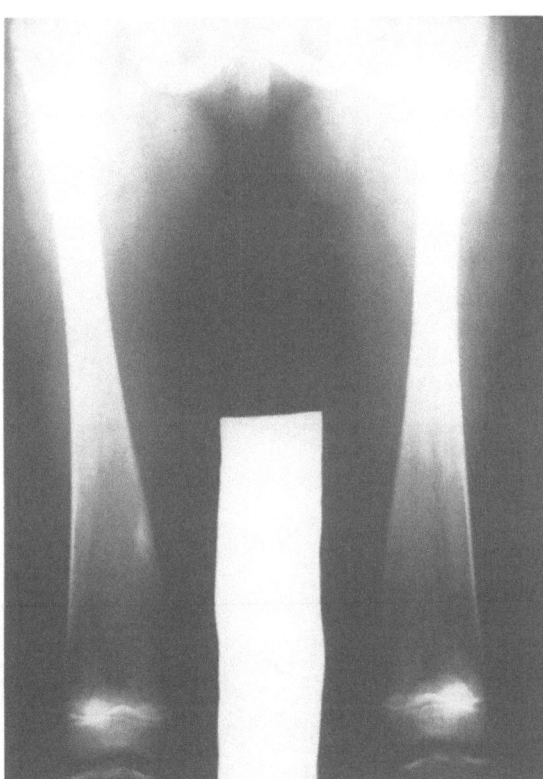

F

Figure 9.22. E. Computed tomogram showing the hyperostosis and sclerosis of bone. The nasal bone is involved with a resulting increase in distance between the orbits. **F.** Frontal radiograph of the femora, which have flared metaphyses resembling an Erlenmeyer flask.

ologic findings include cranial asymmetry and orbital hypertelorism. At times, congenital heart disease, ureteral stenosis, imperforate anus, prognathism, dentigerous cysts, and vertebral anomalies may be seen (33, 123, 254).

Hypertelorism, microtia, and facial clefting syndrome (HMC syndrome, Bixler syndrome) probably is an autosomal-recessive disorder with orbital hypertelorism, cleft lip and palate, microtia, and conductive deafness. Also present may be microcephaly, syndactyly of the second and third toes, shortening of the fifth finger, and hypoplasia of the auditory ossicles (33, 254).

Larsen syndrome is a genetic heterogeneous syndrome characterized by flat facies with a depressed nasal bridge, prominent forehead, dislocations of multiple major joints, and nontapering fingers. Radiographic findings include a flat face with orbital hypertelorism, small skull base, and micrognathia. The spine has abnormal segmentation, flat vertebra, and abnormal curvatures. Congenital joint dislocations, usually bilateral, of major joints (typically, anterior dislocation of the tibia on the femur) are present. The humerus may be short, with hypoplasia of the distal end. Multiple foot deformities are also seen (33, 123, 254).

Leopard syndrome (multiple lentigines syndrome) is an autosomal-dominant disorder with somewhat variable clinical findings. The mnemonic origin of "Leopard" is *l*entigines, *E*CG abnormalities, *o*cular hypertelorism, *p*ulmonary valvular stenosis, *a*bnormal genitalia (hypoplasia), *r*etarded growth, and *d*eafness (sensorineural). A combination of most of these findings usually is sufficient to establish the diagnosis. Radiographic manifestations include a somewhat triangular face, biparietal bossing, orbital hypertelorism, cardiovascular abnormalities, skeletal maturation retardation, abnormal spinal curvature, pectus carinatum or excavatum, winged scapulae, rib anomalies, hypoplastic fifth digit, and Madelung deformity of the wrist (33, 121, 123, 254).

Noonan syndrome (Ullrich syndrome, "male Turner syndrome") is a Turner syndrome-like condition with a normal karyotype. Familial cases have been reported. As in Turner syndrome, the clinical manifestations include short stature, web neck, cubitus valgus, and prominent ears. Cryptorchidism often is present in males. Female cases have rarely been reported. There is an increased incidence of cardiovascular abnormalities, especially pulmonary stenosis. In this condition, the face has a broad forehead, ocular hypertelorism, mild antimongoloid obliquity of the palpebral fissure, ptosis of the eyelids, epicanthal folds, low posterior hairline, and narrow or high-arched palate. Numerous skeletal abnormalities have been described. Radiographic changes include orbital hypertelorism, biparietal foramina, dolichocephaly, microcephaly or macrocephaly, bitemporal bulging, and micrognathia. Skeletal maturation is delayed. The sternal abnormalities are anterior bowing at various levels, elongation of the manubrium, shortness of the body, and premature fusion of ossification centers of the body. The spinal abnormalities include Klippel-Feil syndrome, fusions, and abnormal curvature. Multiple lymphatic anomalies can be present. In the upper extremity, cubitus valgus, congenital dislocations of the radial head, and clinodactyly may be seen (33, 123, 203, 254).

Otopalatodigital syndrome (Taybi syndrome, OPD syndrome) is an X-linked or autosomal-dominant disorder with characteristic facies, conduction deafness, short stature, cleft palate, and bone dysplasia. The craniofacial features are frontal bossing, prominent occiput, prominent supraorbital ridges, orbital hypertelorism, broad nasal root, flat face, antimongoloid slant of the palpebral fissures, microstomia, and cleft palate. There are short broad thumbs and great toes and broad terminal phalanges of the other digits. Radiographic manifestations include a thick dense base of the skull, large supraorbital ridges, steep clivus, delayed closure of the anterior fontanelle, dense middle ear ossicles, and a posterior defect of the neural arch of the vertebrae. Among the abnormalities seen in the limbs are dislocation of the radial heads, coxa valga, lateral bowing of the femur, abnormal carpal and tarsal bones, short thumbs and great toes, and large cone-shaped epiphysis of the distal phalanx of the great toe and thumb (123, 254).

Rubinstein-Taybi syndrome (broad thumbs and toes and mental retardation syndrome, broad thumb-hallux syndrome) is comprised primarily of dwarfism with: 1) mental, motor, and growth retardation; 2) broad thumbs and great toes; and 3) a characteristic face. The craniofacial changes are microcephaly, prominent forehead, antimongoloidal slant of the palpebral fissures, epicanthal folds, mild hypertelorism, a beaked nose with the nasal septum extending below the alae, high-arched palate, abnormally situated ears, and mild micrognathia. Radiographic manifestations are

short, wide terminal phalanx of the thumbs and great toes, short wide-tufted terminal phalanges of the fingers, flared ilia, and delayed skeletal maturation. Other abnormalities that are seen are a large forehead, large anterior fontanelle, parietal foramina, vertebral abnormalities, sternal abnormalities, dislocation of the patellae, and syndactyly (33, 123, 138, 254).

Whistling face syndrome (Freeman-Sheldon syndrome, craniocarpotarsal dysplasia) is an autosomal-dominant disorder characterized by microstomia, flat midface, talipes equinovarus, and ulnar deviation of the fingers. The craniofacial abnormalities are an immobile flat midface, long philtrum, puckered mouth, convergent strabismus, epicanthus, and ouclar hypertelorism. Radio-

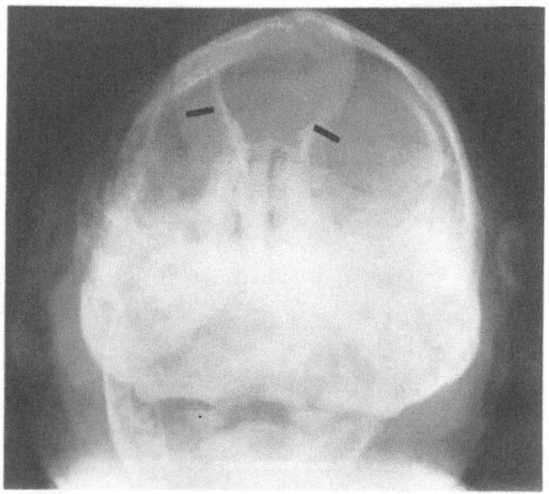

A

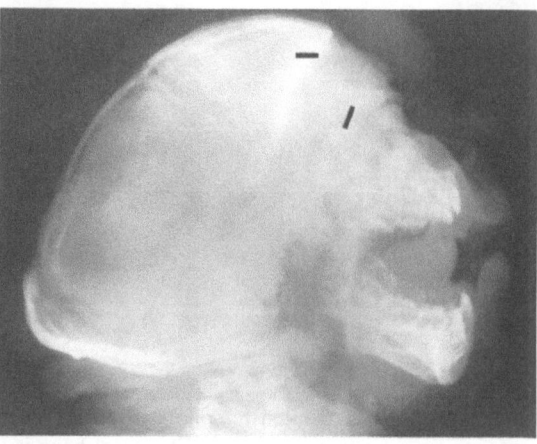

B

Figure 9.23. A, B. Frontal and lateral radiographs of newborn skull showing marked microcephaly and an anterior encephalocele causing a bony defect in the forehead.

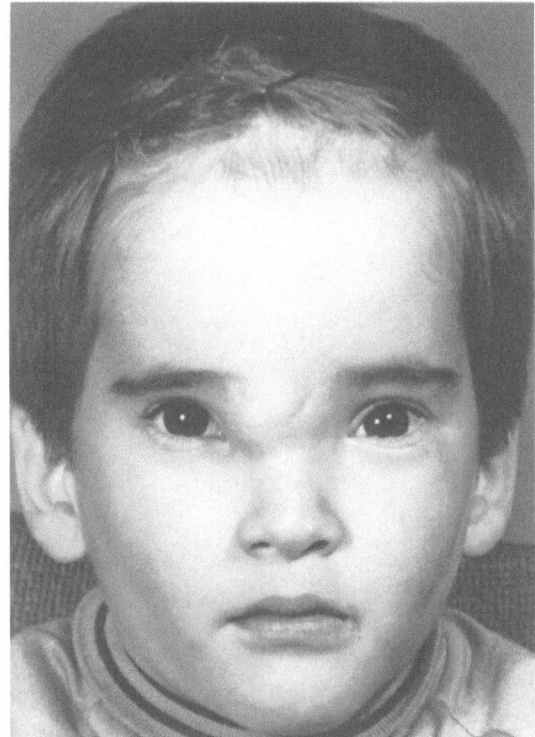

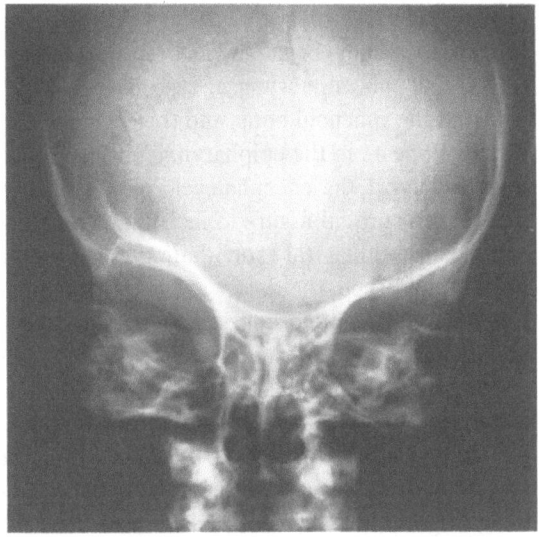

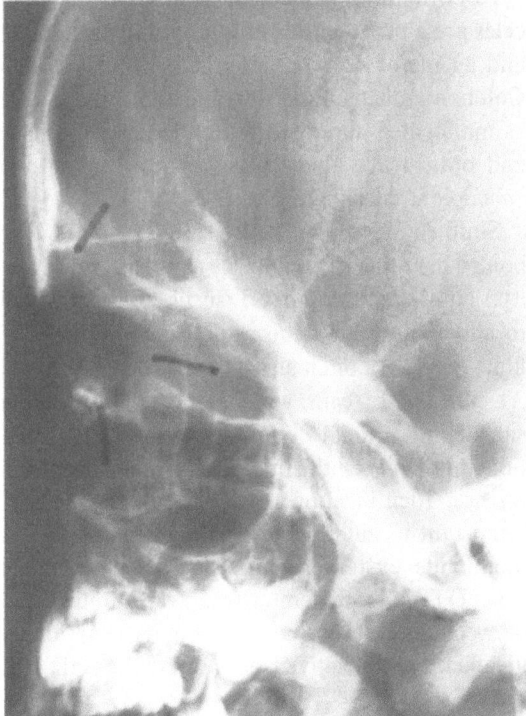

Figure 9.24. A. Four-year-old boy with a frontal encephalocele protruding at the nasal root. **B.** Frontal radiograph showing orbital hypertelorism and enlarged ethmoids. **C.** Lateral radiograph of the skull showing bone defect in the area of the cribriform plate.

graphic manifestations include craniofacial disproportion, dolichocephaly, small malar bones, small mandible, ulnar deviation of the hands, flexed thumbs, club feet, and delayed skeletal maturation with disharmonious maturation of the fingers and carpal bones. Abnormal spinal curvatures may be present (33, 123, 254).

The anterior encephalocele or meningocephalocele is a congenital hernia of meninges, with or without brain tissue, secondary to a midline defect of skull development. It often presents with orbital hypertelorism. While the encephalocele may be found anteriorly in the area of the forehead, nose, or at the base of the skull, most are found posteriorly at the occiput (Figs. 9.23 and 9.24) (159, 217).

The basal type of encephalocele occurs in the area of the cribriform plate or through the sphenoid bone. The mass may be seen in the nasal cavity, nasopharynx, epipharynx, sphenoid sinus, posterior orbit, or pterygopalatine fossa. These encephaloceles may be subdivided into five types (217). The sphenopharyngeal type is seen with a defect in the sphenoid bone, and the encephalocele usually appears in the epipharynx. With the sphenoorbital type, the encephalocele passes through the superior orbital fissure to lie behind the globe, and it causes unilateral exophthalmos. In the sphenoethmoidal type, the defect extends through the sphenoid and ethmoid bones, with the mass often appearing in the posterior nasal cavity. The transethmoidal encephalocele has a defect going through the lamina cribrosa, with the mass appearing in the anterior nasal cavity. The fifth type, the sphenomaxillary, is a theoretic type; to our knowledge, it has not yet been reported clinically (Fig. 9.25) (217).

Abnormalities associated with basal encephaloceles are a broad nasal root, orbital hypertelorism, and an increased biparietal diameter of the skull. Coloboma of the optic disc and exotropia, as well as malformed and distorted optic nerves, chiasm, and optic tracts, have been reported with transsphenoidal encephaloceles (159).

Skull radiographs usually reveal a defect in the bone where the encephalocele exits the cranial cavity. Tomographic and CT scans are more likely to show the bone dehiscence than routine x-ray films, and they often show the nasal mass as well. At times, CT scans will demonstrate the actual site of intracranial communication and the relationships between the intracranial and extracranial disease. Identification of the site of the defect is important in guiding surgical management. A radionuclide cysternogram, using ^{111}In DTPA or ^{99}Tc DTPA, can demonstrate a communication between the cerebrospinal space and the nasal mass if sufficient radioactive tracer enters the stalk (147, 179).

Lesions such as nasal gliomas, dermoid cysts, and other soft-tissue masses occurring at/or near the nasal root must be distinguished from encephaloceles, since they may have similar anatomic abnormalities (e.g., orbital hypertelorism) (123, 254).

Chromosomal Aberrations

The number of normal human chromosomes has been established as 22 pairs of autosomes and one pair of sex chromosomes (X and Y in the male;

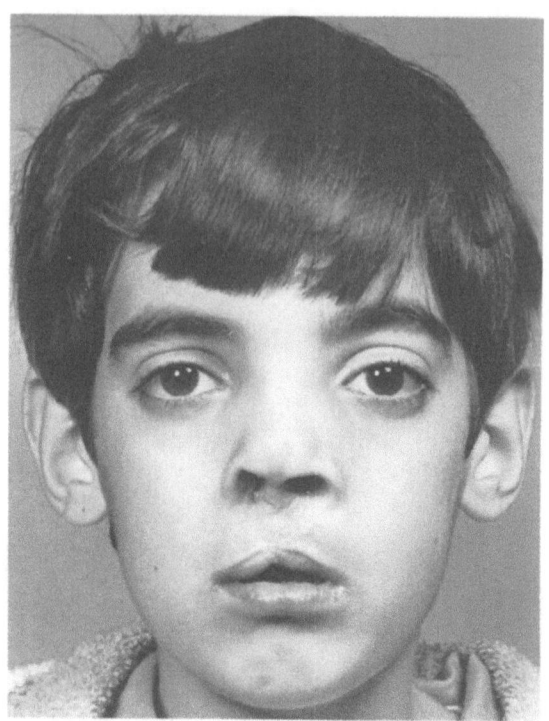

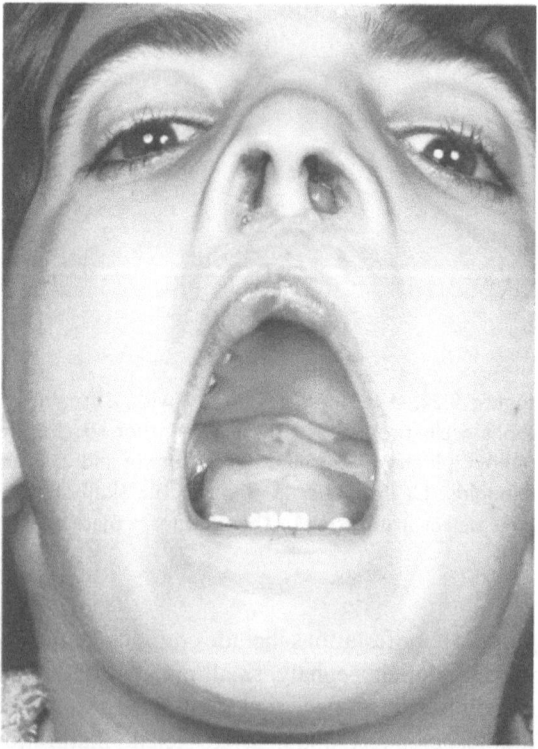

Figure 9.25. **A.** Seven-year-old boy with a sphenoethmoidal encephalocele with orbital hypertelorism and scars of a previous cleft lip repair. **B.** Mass of the encephalocele can be seen in the left nasal passage and bulging the palate.

be seen. This cleft is seen in paramedian craniofacial dysraphia.

Cleft no. 13 (cranial end of cleft no. 1) is situated between the nasal bone and the frontal process of the maxilla. It extends to the frontal bone and olfactory groove. The soft-tissue component is medial to the eyebrow. This cleft may be seen with anterior encephaloceles and marked orbital hypertelorism.

Cleft no. 14 (cranial continuation of cleft no. 0) is seen with median craniofacial dysraphia syndromes.

With the clefts described above, the extent of involvement of the soft and bony tissue is variable. They are rarely affected with equal severity. In general, the facial clefts located between the midline and the infraorbital foramen have less bony deformation than those found lateral to the infraorbital foramen.

Many of the disorders described previously in this chapter may have some form of a craniofacial cleft. This is especially true of the frontonasal dysplasia sequence (cleft no. 0) and the encephaloceles (clefts no. 10 through 14). Other disorders may have an abnormal facial appearance due to clefts alone (possibly from amniotic bands), or they may be part of a genetic disorder such as Treacher-Collins syndrome.

Amniotic band syndrome (*Streeter dysplasia, facial clefts, and congenital ring constrictions or amputations*) is a sporadic disorder manifested by facial clefts, calvarial defects, hydrocephalus, and (at times) more severe abnormalities—such as anencephalus and encephaloceles. Changes seen in the limbs include single- or multiple-ring constrictions (usually distally), varying in severity from minor grooves to total amputation, digital fusion, and club foot deformity. Also present may be gastroschisis, omphalocele, abnormal genitalia, imperforate anus, hypoplastic lungs, and chest deformity (Fig. 9.27) (123, 254).

Unilateral craniofacial microsomia (*hemifacial microsomia, dysostosis otomandibularis, or first and second brachial arch syndrome*) is a sporadic disorder with facial asymmetry of variable degree, microtia, macrostomia, and hypoplasia of the mandibular ramus and condyle. The pinna usually is hypoplastic or absent, and the external auditory canal may be atretic. With the hypoplasia of the maxillary and malar bones on the involved side, the eye may appear to be on a lower level than the eye of the unaffected side; orbital dystopia may

be present. In severe cases, microphthalmia, congenital cystic eye, and coloboma of the iris and choroid may be present (Fig. 9.28) (53, 60).

Goldenhar syndrome (*oculo-auriculo-vertebral syndrome, mandibulofacial dysostosis with epibulbar dermoids*) is considered, by some investigators, to be part of the syndrome complex that includes hemifacial microsomia. Goldenhar syndrome—in addition to the abnormalities seen with hemifacial microsomia—has epibulbar dermoids and/or lipodermoids, various vertebral abnormalities, and (rarely) congenital heart disease (Figs. 9.29 and 9.30) (118, 123, 254).

Mandibulofacial dysostosis (*Treacher-Collins syndrome, Franceschetti-Zwalen-Klein syndrome*) is an autosomal-dominant trait with variable expressivity. It is characterized by a face with downward-sloping palpebral fissures, depressed cheekbones, deformed pinnas, receding chin, and a large fish-like mouth. There often is a preauricular extension of the hairline toward the cheek. The ophthalmologic abnormalities include coloboma of the outer third of the lower eyelid, deficiency of cilia medial to the coloboma, iridial coloboma, possible absence of the lower lacrimal puncta and meibomian glands, and (rarely) microphthalmia. The auditory abnormalities include deformed or atretic pinnas, extra ear tags, blind fistulas, and (at times) absence of the external canal and/or ossicles with resultant conductive deafness. Hypoplasia of the zygoma, malar bones, and mandible occur with variable degrees of severity. Radiographic changes that are seen in the orbit are downward-sloping of the orbit floor, in line medially with a beak-like bony nasal contour, and (often) defective lateral and lower orbital rims. When the defect is present, tomographic studies may show it to be a cleft of variable degree of severity. The greater wing of the sphenoid may be hypoplastic, causing the lateral orbital wall to be defective. The infraorbital foramen may be absent and the lacrimal sac fossa may be larger than normal. The nose often is malformed, with a minimal frontonasal angle, a convex nasal dorsum, and a depressed nasal tip, thus giving the patient a fish-like profile. The paranasal sinuses are small, and the maxillary antra may be absent. Abnormalities of the mandible include a hypoplastic ramus, a more obtuse mandibular angle, a concave undersurface of the horizontal ramus, and antegonial notching. The mandible is shortened relative to body length and ramus height, resulting in both retrusion of the dermatoglyphic findings, skeletal malformations, and abnormal distances between the eyes. A chromosomal disease should be suspected in any patient who has several of the above abnormalities; a karyotype determination should be done.

Some of the ocular changes seen in the chromosomal disorders may be shown by imaging techniques (especially CT). Enophthalmos may be present in trisomy 9, duplication 9p, 11p, 15q, and deletion 18q. Exophthalmos may be seen in duplication 8q and deletion 4p and 9p. Hypertelorism may be seen in duplication 3p, 3q, 4p, 6q, 7q, 9p, 9q, 10q, 11p, 12p, or 20p, and in deletion of 4p, 5p, 11q, 13q, or 18p. Hypotelorism may be seen in: trisomy 13 or 21; duplication 5p, 13q, and 14q; deletion 18p; or ring 22. Mild microphthalmos may be seen in duplication 4q, 10q, or 14q. Severe microphthalmos can be seen in trisomy 13. Retinoblastoma may be seen with deletion 13q (222).

No single abnormality is pathognomonic of any chromosomal disease. For example, cleft lip, epicanthal folds, hypertelorism, webbing of the neck, ptosis, micrognathia, ear anomalies, simian palmar crease, hypogenitalia, lymphedema, and clinodactyly are each associated with several syndromes. The diagnosis of the disorder rests on the pattern of abnormalities present and on the karyotype determination (138).

Trisomy 13 (trisomy D1, Patau syndrome, Bartholin syndrome) has a phenotype that is sufficiently characteristic so that a diagnosis may be made on clinical grounds. The major systemic abnormalities include a low birth weight, failure to thrive, microcephaly, holoprosencephaly with its spectrum of anomalies—including cyclopia, large broad nose, cleft lip and palate, hypotelorism or hypertelorism, low malformed ears, microphthalmia or clinical anophthalmia, long convex finger nails, camptodactyly, fifth finger overlapping the fourth, polydactyly, syndactyly, and rocker-bottom feet. Radiographic changes include microcephaly with a sloping forehead, orbital hypotelorism or hypertelorism, small orbits or (in case of cyclopia) a single orbit, hand and foot abnormalities, hypoplastic ribs, cardiovascular and renal abnormalities, and holoprosencephaly (33, 123, 138, 149, 254).

Trisomy 21 (G1 trisomy syndrome, Down syndrome, mongoloidism) is the best known and probably the most common of the chromosomal diseases. Clinical findings include hypotonia, mental retardation, brachycephaly, large protruding tongue, small nose and ears, narrow palate, congenital heart disease, immunodeficiency, short neck, stubby hands with a single palmar crease, clinodactyly of the fifth digit with hypoplasia of the middle phalanx, and cryptorchidism in males. The characteristic ocular findings are epicanthal folds, mongoloid slant of the palpebral fissure, hypoplasia of the iris, Bushfield spots, myopia, keratoconus, esotropia, cataracts, and blepharitis. Radiographic manifestations include orbital hypotelorism (not hypertelorism, as in older reports), high orbital roofs, brachycephalic microcephaly, hypoplasia of facial bones, short hard palate, high cribriform plate, flared iliac wings with small acetabular angles and iliac index, atlantoaxial subluxation, hypoplastic odontoid process, absent 12th ribs, and two ossification centers for the manubrium. Other changes that are seen are short hands with stubby digits, clinodactyly, variable skeletal maturation, congenital heart disease, and alimentary tract anomalies (especially duodenal atresia or stenosis) (33, 123, 138, 254).

Trisomy 18 (Edwards syndrome, trisomy E) is the third most common autosomal trisomy. Clinical manifestations include a low birth weight, physical and mental retardation, muscular hypertonicity, shield deformity of chest, flexion deformity of fingers (first digit adducted and second digit overlapping the third), and foot deformities. The characteristic facies include an elongated skull with prominent occiput, micrognathia, small triangular mouth with short upper lip, high-arched palate, and low deformed ears. The ocular manifestations include hypertelorism, (but occasionally hypotelorism), small supraorbital ridges, epicanthal folds, ptosis, thick lower lid, microphthalmia, corneal opacities, and glaucoma. Radiographic changes include frontal bossing, prominent occiput, hypoplasia of the mandible and maxilla, 11 pairs of ribs, short sternum, and hand and foot deformities (33, 123, 138, 254).

The "cat-eye syndrome" (Chromosome 22q+) has coloboma of the iris and choroid—and either anal atresia or an imperforate anus. The facial features include orbital hypertelorism, eyes that resemble those of a cat (due to the coloboma), and a small chin (123, 138).

Chromosome deletion 4p− syndrome (Wolf syndrome, Wolf-Hirschhorn syndrome) has clinical signs of mental retardation, seizures, prominent glabella, midline scalp defect, cleft lip and palate, deformed nose, hemangiomas on the forehead, internal hydorcephalus, and cryptorchidism and hy-

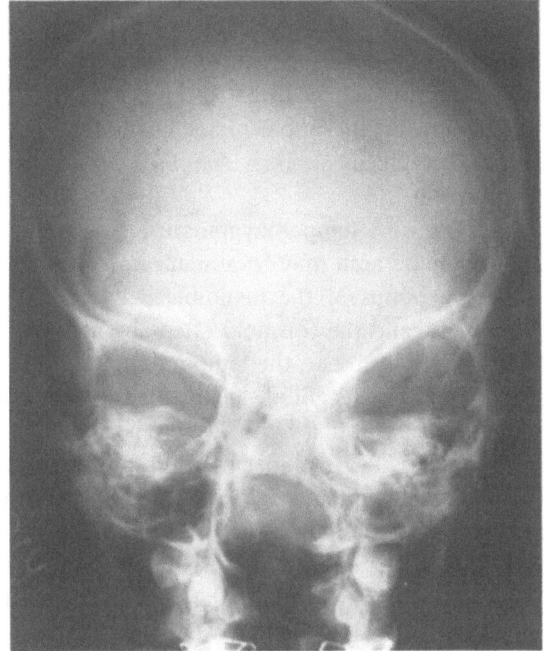

C

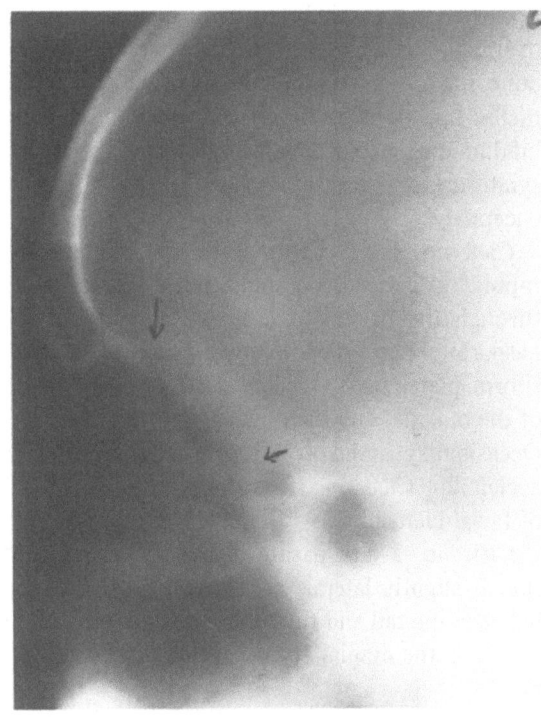

E

D

9.25. C. Frontal radiograph showing orbital hypertelorism and a defect in the nose and palate caused by the encephalocele. **D.** Lateral midline CT Scan showing a defect in the anterior portion of the skull base at the site of exit of the encephalocele. **E.** Brow-up lateral view of a pneumoencephalogram showing the communication of the encephalocele with the cerebrospinal fluid space.

XX in the female); a total of 46. The chromosomes are divided into seven groups based on length and the centromere position: 1) chromosomes 1, 2, and 3 constitute group A; 2) 4 and 5 are group B; 3) 6 to 12 and X are group C; 4) 13 to 15 are group D; 5) 16 to 18 are group E; 6) 19 and 20 are group F; 7) and 21, 22, and Y are group G. The chromosomal abnormalities may be numeric (extra or missing chromosomes) or structural (deletions, rings, or translocations). A nomenclature system has been formulated to describe the human chromosome complement and their departures from the norm. An extra chromosome is indicated by a plus (+) and a missing one by a minus (−); thus 47, XX, +21 is a female trisomy 21. The short arm of a chromosome is "p" and the long one is "q"; hence, 46, XY, 5p− describes a male with a deletion in the short arm of one chromosome 5. A ring is indicated as "r" and translocation as "t" (222).

Ophthalmologic abnormalities are frequently present in patients with chromosomal aberrations. Among the common findings in chromosomal diseases are a low birth weight, failure to thrive, mental retardation, behavioral disorders, congenital heart disease, dental and renal abnormalities, persistent embryonic or fetal hemoglobin, abnormal combinations may be seen: 0–14, 1–13, 2–12, 3–11, and 4–10 (153, 260, 261).

Cleft no. 0 (or 0–14) is a median craniofacial dysraphia, with the cleft going through the frontal bone, the crista galli, the midline of the nose, columella, lip, and maxilla. It is seen with cranium bifidum, median encephalocele, median facial cleft syndrome, frontonasal dysplasia, and holoprosencephaly.

Cleft no. 1 is a paramedian craniofacial dysraphia or paraaxial craniofacial cleft. It passes through the frontal bone along the area of the nasoorbital nerve, the olfactory groove of the cribriform plate, the nasal bone, the frontal process of the maxilla, and the dome of the alar cartilage. Occasionally, it involves the lip and alveolus as a cleft lip. Cleft no. 13 is the cranial equivalent of facial cleft no. 1.

Cleft no. 2 is a paramedian craniofacial cleft that is slightly lateral to cleft no. 1; it is located between the tail and the base of the ala nasi. Cleft no. 12 is the cranial equivalent of the facial cleft no. 2.

Cleft no. 3, the oculonasal cleft, is an orbitomaxillary medial cleft extending through the lacrimal portion of the lower eyelid, the lacrimal gutter, and the frontal process of the maxilla. The inner wall of the antrum often is completely absent. The cleft involves the base of the ala in the nasolabial groove and through the lip and alveolus; orbital dystopia is an example. Cranial cleft no. 11 corresponds with facial cleft no. 3.

Cleft no. 4 is an orbitomaxillary central cleft, which extends vertically through the lacrimal portion of the lower eyelid, the infraorbital ridge, and the orbital floor medial to the infraorbital nerve—and through the antrum and cheek, with exstrophy of the sinus. It then extends through the lip, midway between the philtral crest and the labial commissure. Facial cleft no. 4 corresponds to cranial cleft no. 10.

Cleft no. 5 is an orbitomaxillary lateral cleft that involves the medial third of the lower eyelid, the infraorbital rim, orbital floor, and maxilla lateral to the infraorbital nerve, the antrum, the lip (about ½ inch medial to the corner of the mouth), and (finally) through the alveolus in the premolar area. Microphthalmos is often present. Cranial cleft no. 9 and facial cleft no. 5 are related.

Cleft no. 6 is an intermaxillozygomatic cleft located between the maxilla and the malar bone; it opens the inferior orbital fissure. The posterior portion of the maxilla is short, with a high-vaulted palate and a relative choanal atresia. There is a coloboma of the lower eyelid, between the medial and lateral thirds. A vertical sclerodermal groove is present on the cheek directed towards the labial commissure or the angle of the mandible. This cleft is specifically seen in the Treacher-Collins syndrome.

Cleft no. 7 is a temporozygomatic cleft in which the zygomatic arch may be absent or atretic. The ascending ramus of the mandible is short, with the condyle and the coronoid often absent. When the coronoid is absent, the temporal muscle is absent as well. The height of the maxilla is decreased and the alveolar wall is hypoplastic. The anomalies of the soft tissues include microtia and atrophy or absence of the temporal muscle. The sideburn hair usually is absent in the otomandibular syndrome, and it is divided into two portions in the Treacher-Collins syndrome. Cleft no. 7 is the most lateral of the facial clefts; it is seen in macrostomia and with pretragal enchondromas.

Cleft no. 8 is a frontozygomatic cleft, extending into the greater wing of the sphenoid. It seems to correspond to facial cleft no. 6.

When clefts no. 6, 7, and 8 are found together, they constitute the Treacher-Collins syndrome. Cleft no. 6 is always present in this syndrome. Cleft no. 7 corresponds more specifically to the otomandibular syndrome, and cleft no. 8 corresponds to the Goldenhar syndrome. The three syndromes cited in this paragraph are different aspects of "laterofacial microsomia."

Cleft no. 9 seems to correspond to facial cleft no. 5. It is a superolateral orbital cleft traversing the lateral third of the upper eyelid and the superolateral angle of the orbit.

Cleft no. 10 (equivalent of facial cleft no. 4) is a central superior orbital cleft located at the medial third of the supraorbital rim; it is lateral to the supraorbital nerve. An encephalocele is seen when the cleft extends across the roof of the orbit and the frontal bone. Colobomas of the medial third of the upper eyelid also may be seen.

Cleft no. 11 (equivalent of facial cleft no. 3) is a supermedial orbital cleft, which is seen with coloboma of the medial third of the upper eyelid and sometimes extends to the eyebrow.

Cleft no. 12 (equivalent of facial cleft no. 2) is located medial to the medial canthus. It passes across the lateral mass of the ethmoid and frontal bone. A coloboma of the root of the eyebrow may pospadias in males. The eye abnormalities include colobomas, orbital hypertelorism, and strabismus. Other abnormalities have been described, such as microcephaly, micrognathia, retarded skeletal maturation, club foot, and kyphoscoliosis (33, 123, 138, 189).

Chromosome deletion 5p— syndrome (Cri-du-chat syndrome) is manifested clinically by severe growth and mental retardation, a cat-like cry, round facies, microcephaly, micrognathia, low-set ears, antimongoloid slant of the palpebral fissures, mild orbital hypertelorism, and congenital heart disease (33, 123, 138, 190, 254).

Chromosome 13q— syndrome and chromosome 13r syndrome have similar phenotypes. The clinical picture includes mental and physical retardation, absent or hypoplastic thumbs, congential heart disease, occasional anal atresia, hypospadias, cryptorchidism, hip dislocation, focal lumbar vertebral agenesis, coxa valga, and synostosis of the fourth and fifth metacarpals. The craniofacial manifestations include microcephaly; some have various degrees of holoprosencephaly, prominent nasal bridge, small chin, large low-set ears, and possibly facial asymmetry. The ocular findings include orbital hypertelorism, epicanthal folds, ptosis, microphthalmos, coloboma of the iris, cataract, and retinoblastoma (33, 123, 138).

Chromosome 18p— syndrome, in its mildest form, is manifested by microcephaly, mental retardation, short stature, webbed neck, immunoglobulin abnormalities, midface hypoplasia, deep-set eyes, orbital hypertelorism, epicanthal folds, strabismus, ptosis, and large low-set ears. In its most severe form, this syndrome mimics trisomy 13, with incomplete morphogenesis of the brain, and cebocephaly or cyclopia (33, 123, 138, 254).

Chromosome 18q— syndrome (deGrouchy syndrome) is manifested by a low birth weight, short stature, mental retardation, hypotonia, ligament laxity, club foot, abnormal toe implantation, short thumbs, supernumerary ribs, genital abnormalities, and congenital heart disease. The craniofacial changes are microcephaly, midface hypoplasia, deep-set eyes, prominent antihelix and antitragus of the ears, carp-shaped mouth, narrow ear canals, deafness, and abnormalities of the fundus of the eye (33, 74, 123, 138, 254).

Craniofacial Clefts

Craniofacial clefts are anomalies that result from a failure in normal development. They are charac-

terized by a dehiscence of facial structures that are normally contiguous. While the most common are clefts of the lip and/or palate, the less common clefts (i.e., clefts that coincide with the appositional planes of the primordial facial processes) will be discussed. Currently, the most commonly used classification is that devised by Tessier. This classification incorporates not only surface descriptions of the clefts, but also those of the underlying bony structures (Fig. 9.26). The clefts are numbered from 0 to 14, and they extend along continuous axes through the eyebrows or eyelids, the maxilla, the nostrils, and the lip. The clefts that are directed cephalad, or "northbound," extend through the upper eyelid and are deemed to be "cranial." The caudally directed or "southbound," clefts that pass through the lower eyelid are "facial." A combination of northbound and southbound clefts form the "craniofacial" clefts. The craniofacial clefts follow a well-defined course, and the following

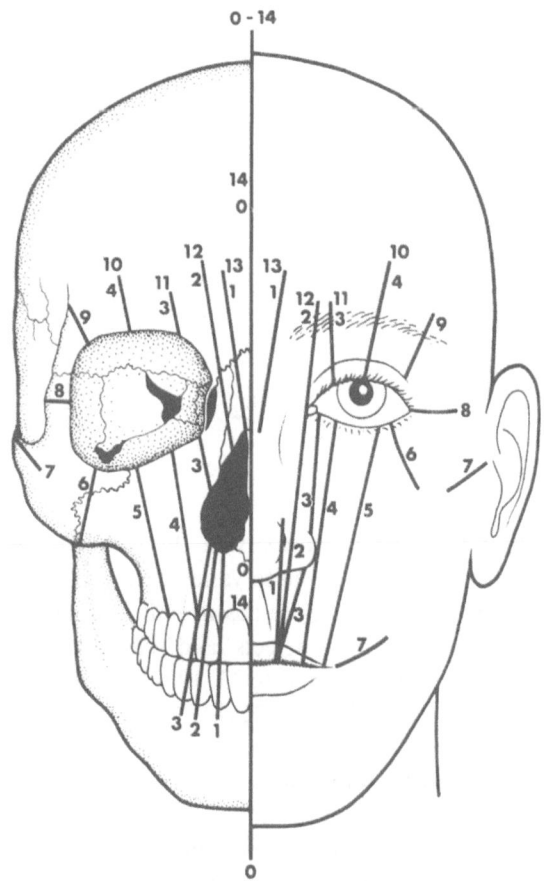

Figure 9.26. Tessier cleft classification (From Tessier [263]).

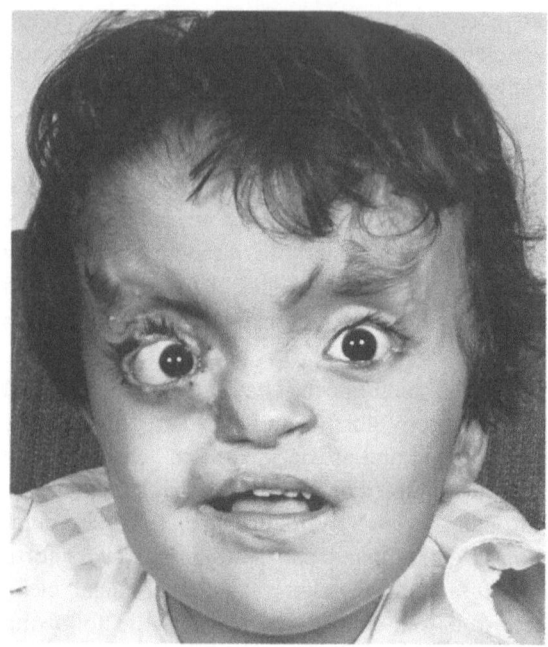

A

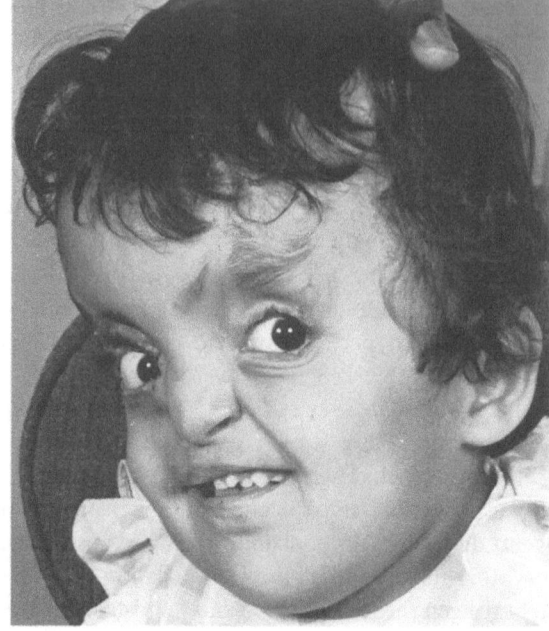

B

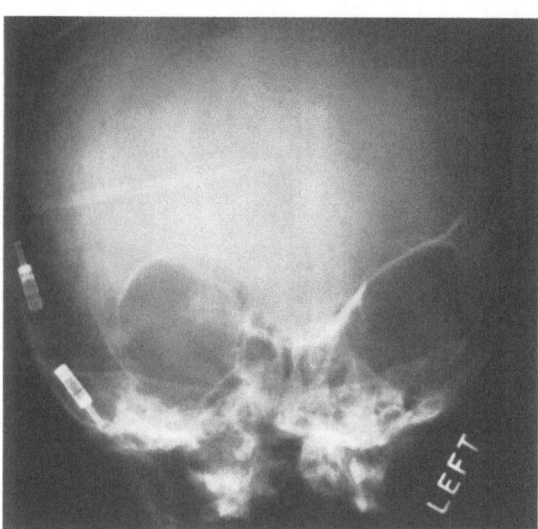

C

Figure 9.27. A, B. Four-year-old girl with orbital hypertelorism and other facial deformities secondary to clefts (Tessier no. 3 and 10 on the left, and 2 and 11 on the right). She also has mild orbital dystopia. Her hands and feet have multiple congenital amputations of parts of fingers and toes, presumably from intrauterine amniotic bands. **C.** Frontal radiograph showing a ventricular shunt tube on the right, orbital hypertelorism with hyperaerated ethmoids, and a depressed cribriform plate. Mild orbital dystopia is also present.

lower face and a convexity of the facial profile. The ear changes are quite variable, ranging from very minimal changes to absent pinna, absent external canal, ossicle defects, and sclerosis of the middle ear (Fig. 9.31) (16, 33, 100, 106, 123, 134, 135, 136, 138, 209, 231, 254).

Skull and Craniosynostosis

The most common developmental abnormalities of the skull involving the orbits are anencephaly and craniosynostosis.

Anencephaly is the most common, serious congenital malformation that is compatible with the completion of pregnancy. It may comprise up to 0.4% of all conceptions in some areas of the world (170). A newborn anencephalic infant usually has a well-formed body, but an absent superior portion of the skull and frontal bone above the orbital ridge (184, 204). As a result, the eyes are at the very uppermost part of the face. The eyes and lids appear to be normal. The orbits are small and shallow, with imperfect roofs. The optic canals may be missing (90). This congenital malformation

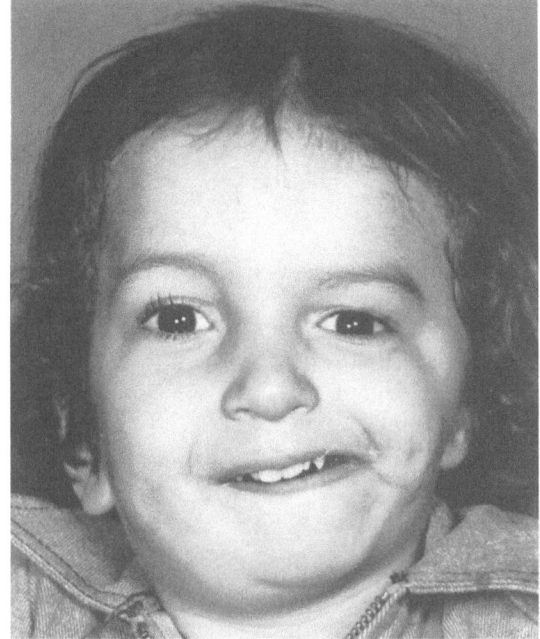

A

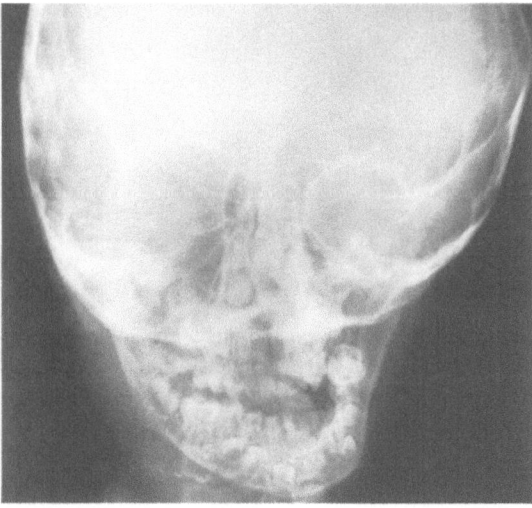

B

Figure 9.28. A. Four-year-old boy with hemifacial microsomia. Note the orbital dystopia, the tilted chin, and small pinna on the involved side. **B.** Frontal radiograph showing the orbital dystopia, hypoplastic mandible and maxilla on the involved side.

is rarely studied with imaging techniques, because it is not compatible with any significant length of life. However, it is important to recognize this disorder in antepartum imaging studies (Figs. 9.32 and 9.33).

Craniosynostosis

Premature fusion of the membranous cranial bones (craniostenosis or craniosynostosis), which causes a skull deformity, may occur as an isolated congenital abnormality, as part of a syndrome of multiple congenital anomalies, or as an acquired deformity shortly after birth (Table 9.7). The closure of a single suture without other anomalies is the most common type of craniostenosis. The sagittal suture is the one most frequently involved, and the coronal and metopic sutures are the next most common. The skull is deformed by craniosynostosis, because normal skull growth perpendicular to the fused suture is inhibited and compensatory skull growth occurs parallel to the suture (138).

The evaluation of suspected craniosynostosis may include routine radiographs, CT scans, and radionuclide studies, in addition to the physical examination. The usual radiographic that is seen is a thin, involved suture with smooth borders, which may be interrupted by bony bridging and sclerosis. However, a distinction must be made between a closed and fused suture. Closed sutures are in close apposition and are difficult to see on a radiograph, but they can resplit if there is subsequent increased intracranial pressure (133). A suture that seems to be open on a radiograph may be fused clinically. This is incomplete transsutural ossification. In this circumstance, the skull is deformed in a shape that would correspond to the physiologically fused suture. In premature craniostenosis, a suture may appear to be open, except for a small segment that is fused. In segmental fusion of a suture, that portion of the suture that has not fused will continue to grow and to deposit bone along the suture lines. The radiographic changes in premature craniostenosis include asymmetry, increased digital markings on the inner table of the skull, increased sharpness and ridging of the sutures, and parasutural sclerosis. Computed tomographic studies of craniosynostosis may disclose both premature closure of cranial sutures and sutures at the craniofacial junction, deformities of the ventricular system of the brain, and deformity of the skull. In some cases of "physiologic closure of the suture," a "sticky suture" may be seen. A "sticky" suture will show a sclerotic margin on only one side of the suture (4, 49). Nuclear medicine studies (skull scintigraphy) have been valuable in the evaluation of craniosynostosis. These studies are done 2.5–3.0 hours after the in-

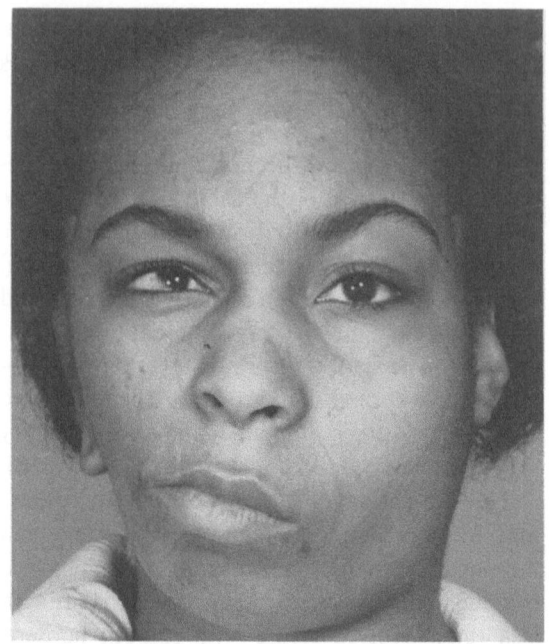

A

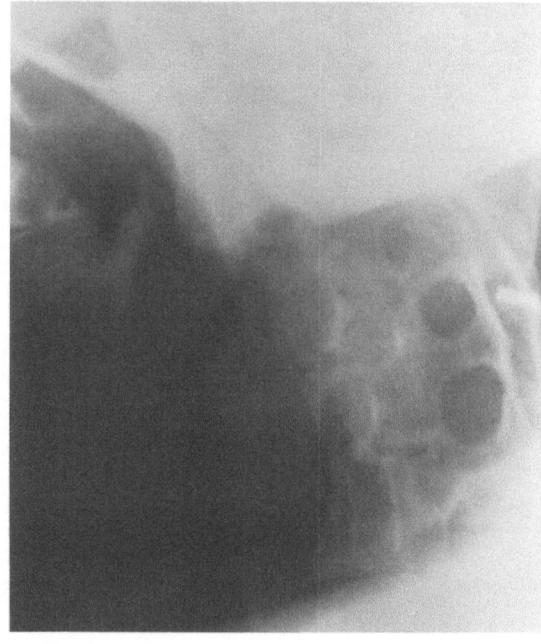

C

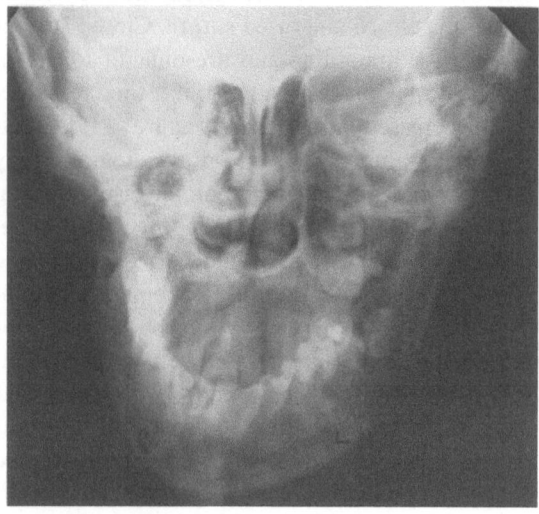

B

Figure 9.29. A. A 15-year-old girl with Goldenhar syndrome. Note the facial asymmetry and the epibulbar dermoid on the involved side. **B.** Frontal radiograph showing the mandibular and maxillary hypoplasia. **C.** Oblique radiograph of the cervical spine showing failure of segmentation and fusion of the posterior neural arches.

jection of Tc 99m methylene diphosphonate (dose, 0.21 mCi/kg or 7.9 mEq/kg). The scans demonstrated four patterns of sutural activity: normal, absent, increased, and wide. Absent activity indicated fused sutures, increased activity indicated fusing hyperactive sutures or sutures reacting to fusion elsewhere, and wide activity indicated split sutures. Thus, this study is helpful when the radiographic studies are abnormal or equivocal (115, 251). Deformity of the orbits is most marked when one or both coronal sutures are closed, with Kleeblattschadel or cloverleaf skull (a rare form of premature craniostenosis), and with trigonocephaly.

Plagiocephaly or rhomboid-shaped head is a moderately common finding at birth. It can be caused by brain malformation, fetal packing problems, torticollis, and (more rarely) by unilateral premature closure of the coronal suture. When plagiocephaly is due to unilateral coronal stenosis, the forward migration of the frontal bone is inhibited, the involved side is flattened, and the normal side has an apparent exaggeration of the frontal boss. The orbit on the involved side is shallow, enlarged, and elliptical, with the superior margin angled sharply upward laterally. The lesser wing of the sphenoid is elevated. The innominate line

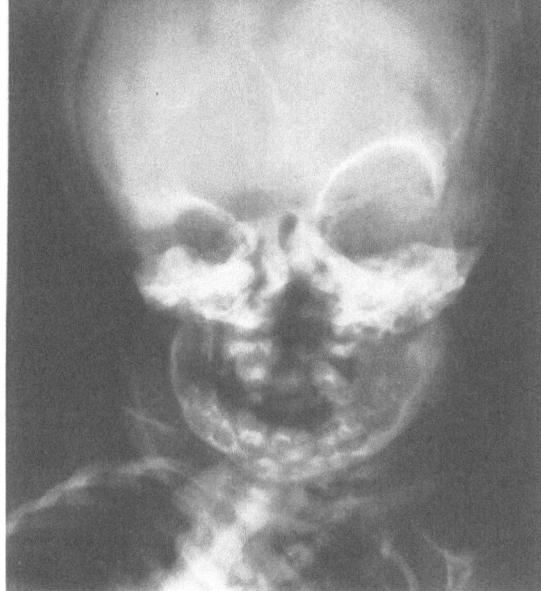

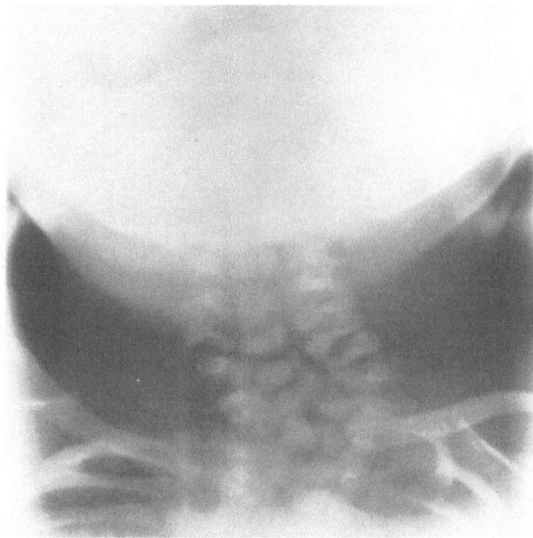

Figure 9.30. A. Frontal radiograph of an infant with Goldenhar syndrome. There is marked unilateral facial hypoplasia, a small orbit on the involved side, and a cleft palate. **B.** Frontal radiograph of the cervical spine showing the abnormalities of the vertebral bodies and associated scoliosis.

of the greater wing of the sphenoid is displaced outward and the nasal septum is inclined obliquely to the involved side (Fig. 9.34) (52, 97, 159, 197).

Brachycephaly or bilateral premature craniostenosis has a shortened front-to-back diameter of the skull, and it may show increased convolutional markings on the inner table of the skull. The orbits

Table 9.7. Craniostenosis

I. Primary (simple, idiopathic, or isolated)
   A. Brachycephaly (short head)—premature bilateral closure of the coronal and/or lamboid sutures
   B. Scaphocephaly (boat head), dolichocephaly (long head)—premature closure of the sagittal suture
   C. Plagiocephaly (oblique head)—unilateral premature closure of the coronal and/or lamboid sutures (may be secondary to torticollis without craniostenosis)
   D. Trigonocephaly (triangular head)—premature closure of the metopic suture
   E. Oxycephaly, acrocephaly, and turricephaly (pointed head)—premature closure of all sutures
II. Secondary
   A. Craniostenosis as a part of known syndromes
     1. Apert syndrome
     2. Armendares syndrome
     3. Baller-Gerold syndrome
     4. Bernat syndrome
     5. Carpenter syndrome
     6. Christian syndrome I
     7. Christian syndrome II
     8. Chromosomal syndromes (3q+, 5p+, 6q+, 7p−, 9p−, 11q−, 13q−)
     9. Craniofacial dyssynostosis
    10. Craniofrontonasal dysplasia
    11. Craniotelencephalic dysplasia
    12. Crouzon syndrome
    13. Elejalde syndrome
    14. Gorlin-Chaudry-Moss syndrome
    15. Kleeblattschadel anomaly
    16. Lowry syndrome
    17. Pfeiffer syndrome
    18. Saethre-Chotzen syndrome
    19. San Francisco syndrome
    20. Sensenbrenner syndrome
    21. Summitt syndrome
    22. Ventruto syndrome
    23. Washington syndrome I
    24. Washington syndrome II
    25. Other miscellaneous syndromes
   B. Craniosynostosis associated with miscellaneous disorders
     1. Fetal aminopterin syndrome
     2. Fetal hydantoin syndrome
     3. Hematologic disorders
     4. Hypophosphatasia
     5. Hyperthyroidism
     6. Idiopathic hypercalcemia
     7. Microcephaly with a small brain
     8. Mucopolysaccharidoses
     9. Rickets and hypophosphatasia
    10. Subsequent to cerebral ventricle shunting

From 57 and 87.

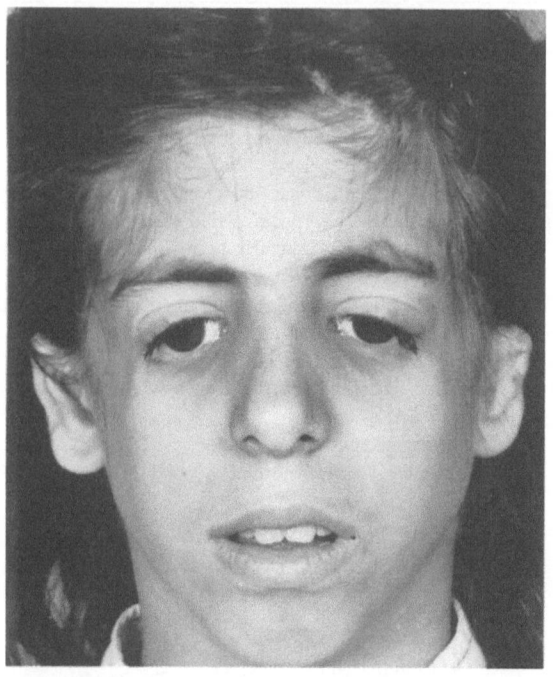

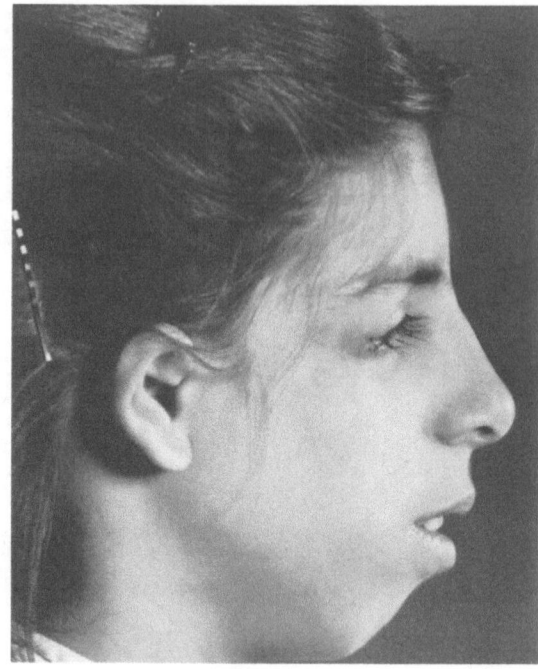

A

B

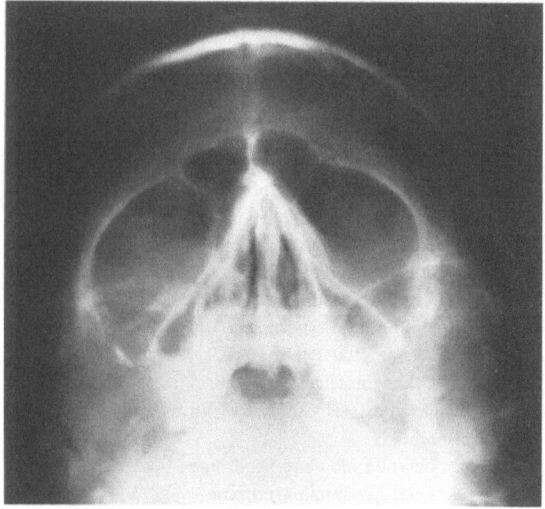

C

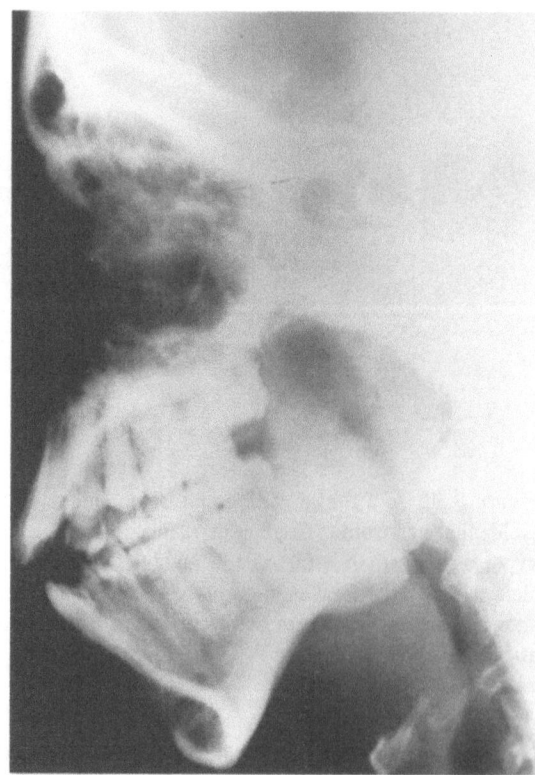

D

Figure 9.31. A, B. A 13-year-old girl with Treacher-Collins syndrome. Note the antimongoloid obliquity of the palpebral fissure, the malar and mandibular hypoplasia, the malformed pinna, the unusual hairline, and absence of lashes on the lower eyelids. **C.** Waters position radiograph showing the "inverted teardrop" shape of the orbit secondary to the hypoplasia of the zygoma and mandible. There is a lateral orbital cleft bilaterally. The midface is pointed and pyramidal in configuration. **D.** Lateral radiograph showing antegonial notching of the mandible and an increased angle between the ascending and horizontal rami.

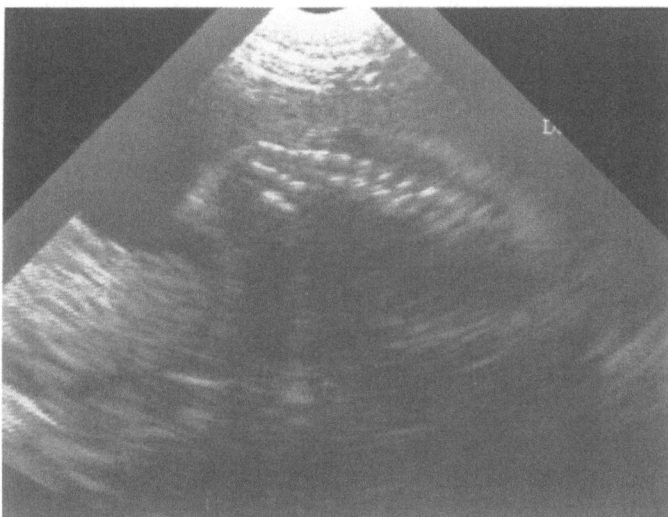
A

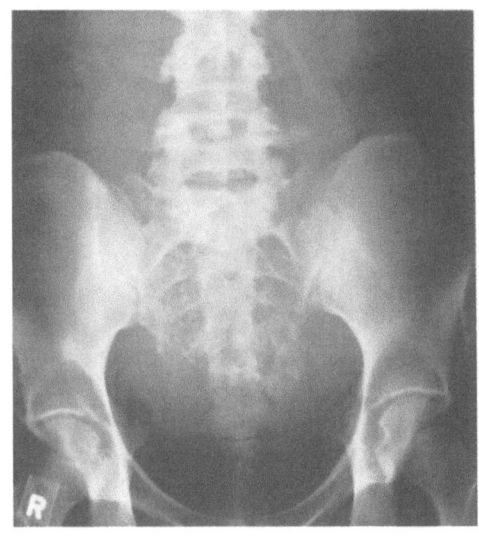
B

Figure 9.32. A. Ultrasound examination of the abdomen of a pregnant woman showing evidence of polyhydramnios and a single intrauterine fetus, but the skull is not present. **B.** Radiograph of abdomen of same patient showing the fetal parts superimposed over the spine; but no fetal skull is present, thus demonstrating an anencephalic fetus.

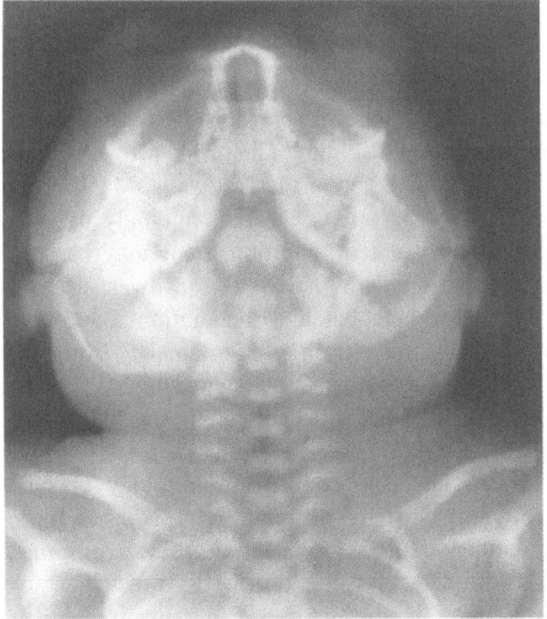
A

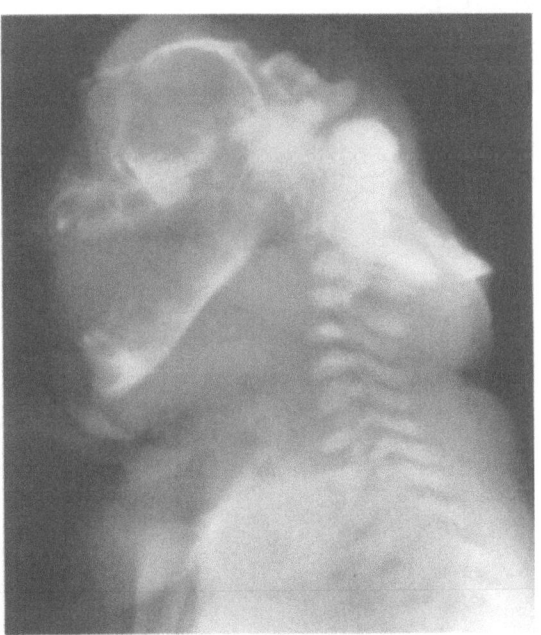
B

Figure 9.33. A, B. Frontal and lateral radiograph of an anencephalic infant. Note the absence of the calvarium and the presence of the base of the skull.

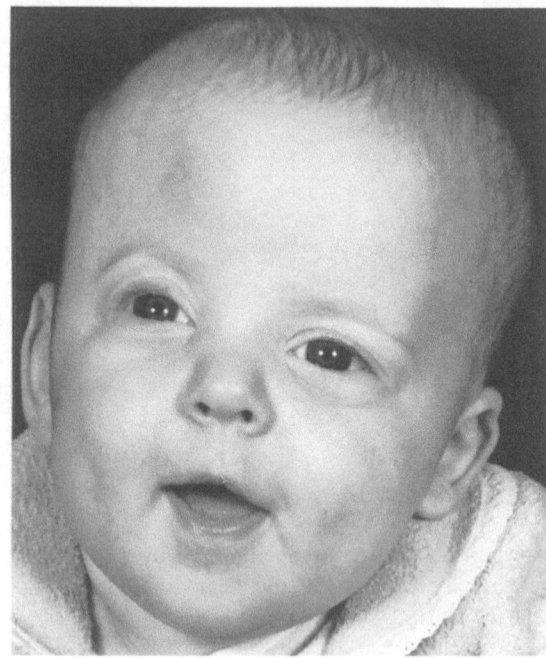

A

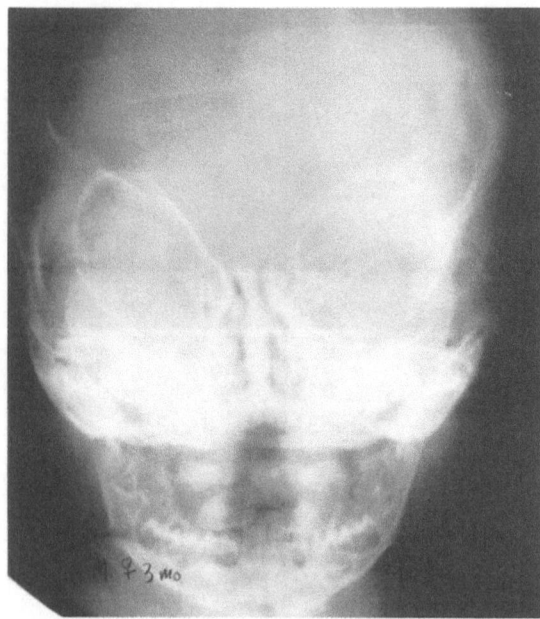

B

Figure 9.34. A, B. Three-month-old girl with plagio-cephaly due to premature unilateral (right) closure of the coronal suture. Note the "harlequin" shape of the right orbit and the tilt of the nasal septum to the in-volved side.

are shallow, elliptical, and enlarged. The shape of the orbit is somewhat diamond-shaped ("harle-quin appearance"), with the superior margins of the roof slanted upward laterally. When the changes of craniostenosis are severe, the optic fora-men may be narrowed and exophthalmos may be seen (Fig. 9.35).

Trigonocephaly (premature closure of the me-topic suture) is characterized by triangular promi-nence of the forehead and by orbital hypotelorism. Radiographic changes that are seen are decreased distance between the medial orbital walls, ovoid orbits with parallel medial walls, poor visualiza-tion of the greater wings of the sphenoid due to their upward pitch, short anterior cranial fossa, and anterior curving of the coronal suture. On the submento-vertex view, the forehead has a keel-shaped angulation and the frontal eminences are flattened (Fig. 9.36) (83).

Kleeblattschadel anomaly (cloverleaf skull) is the name applied to the grotesque trilobed skull that results from congenital hydrocephalus associ-ated with intrauterine synostosis of multiple cra-nial sutures, especially the coronal and lambdoids. This anomaly occurs in variable degrees of sever-ity, and different sutures may be involved in differ-ent patients. The skull deformities are readily seen on radiographic studies. The orbits are very shal-low, with almost absent lateral walls. Marked ex-ophthalmos may be seen. This anomaly may be seen as an isolated condition, or it may be seen in association with thanatophoric dwarfism and other syndromes—such as the amniotic band syn-drome, Apert syndrome, campomelic dwarfism, Carpenter syndrome, Crouzon's syndrome, Pfeif-fer syndrome, and other miscellaneous syndromes (Fig. 9.37) (9, 57, 98, 123, 138, 254).

Since the classification and nosology of syn-dromes associated with craniostenosis is a subject of confusion and misconception, these syndromes should not be classified on the basis of which su-tures are prematurely fused. Different sutures may be affected in different patients with the same syn-drome (57).

Crouzon syndrome (craniofacial dysostosis) usu-ally is an autosomal-dominant disorder that is characterized by premature craniosynostosis, mid-face hypoplasia with shallow orbits, and ocular proptosis. There is considerable variability of ex-pression in this disorder. The shape of the cranium depends on the order and rate of progression of sutural involvement. Brachycephaly is the defor-

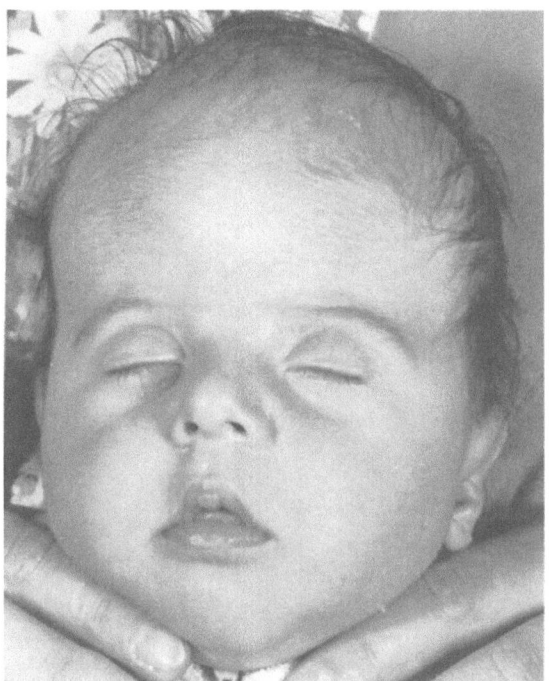

A

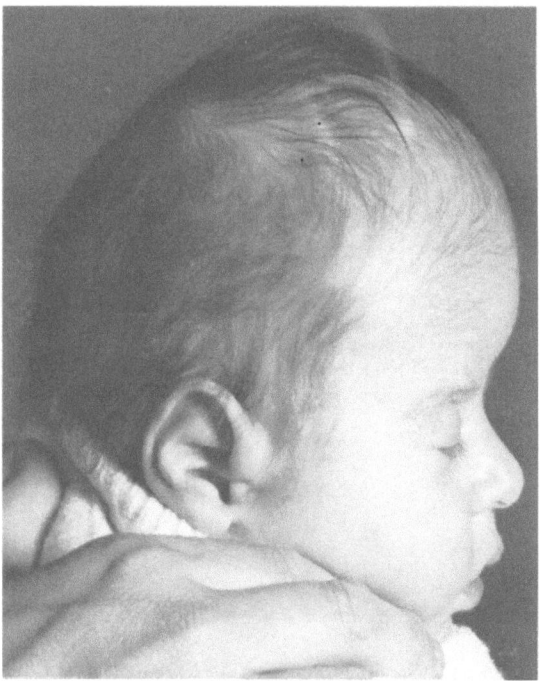

B

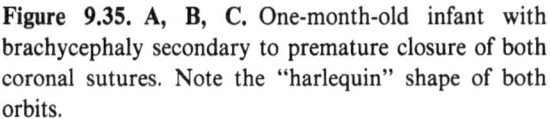

Figure 9.35. A, B, C. One-month-old infant with brachycephaly secondary to premature closure of both coronal sutures. Note the "harlequin" shape of both orbits.

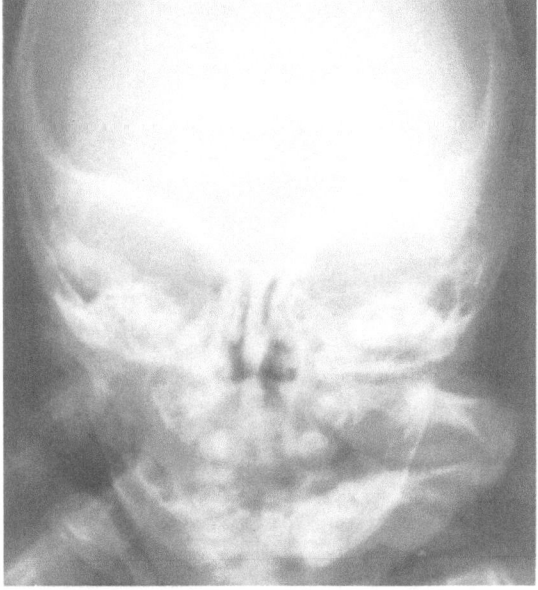

C

mity seen most often, but scaphocephaly, trigonocephaly, and (rarely) Kleeblattschadel deformity have been seen. Midface hypoplasia, relative mandibular prognathism, and a parrot-beaked nose are facial manifestations. The ophthalmic findings include shallow orbits, proptosis, orbital hypertelorism, divergent strabismus, and nystagmus. Optic nerve involvement and abnormalities of the globe rarely have been noted. The nasopharynx is narrowed and hydrocephalus has been reported (Fig. 9.38) (38, 68, 123, 180, 240, 254).

Apert syndrome (acrocephalosyndactyly) is an uncommon, usually sporadic developmental deformity characterized by craniosynostosis (turribrachycephaly), syndactyly of the hands and feet, various ankyloses, and progressive synostosis of the hands, feet, and cervical spine (237). While the skull morphology is said to be similar to that of Crouzon disease, we have noted that the forehead tends to be higher, the eyes slightly less proptotic, the face more asymmetric, and orbital dystopia more common than in Crouzon disease (180, 211, 258). The craniosynostosis of Apert syndrome

usually involves the coronal suture alone, or together with fusion of the sagittal, lambdoid, or squamosal sutures. Hyperbrachycephaly or oxycephaly often is present. Skull radiographs show a high, prominent steep forehead, a flattened frontal bone, and a shortened anterior cranial fossa. The frontal and temporal areas bulge laterally. The frontal sinuses are poorly developed. Orbital hypertelorism is present. As in Crouzon disease, the

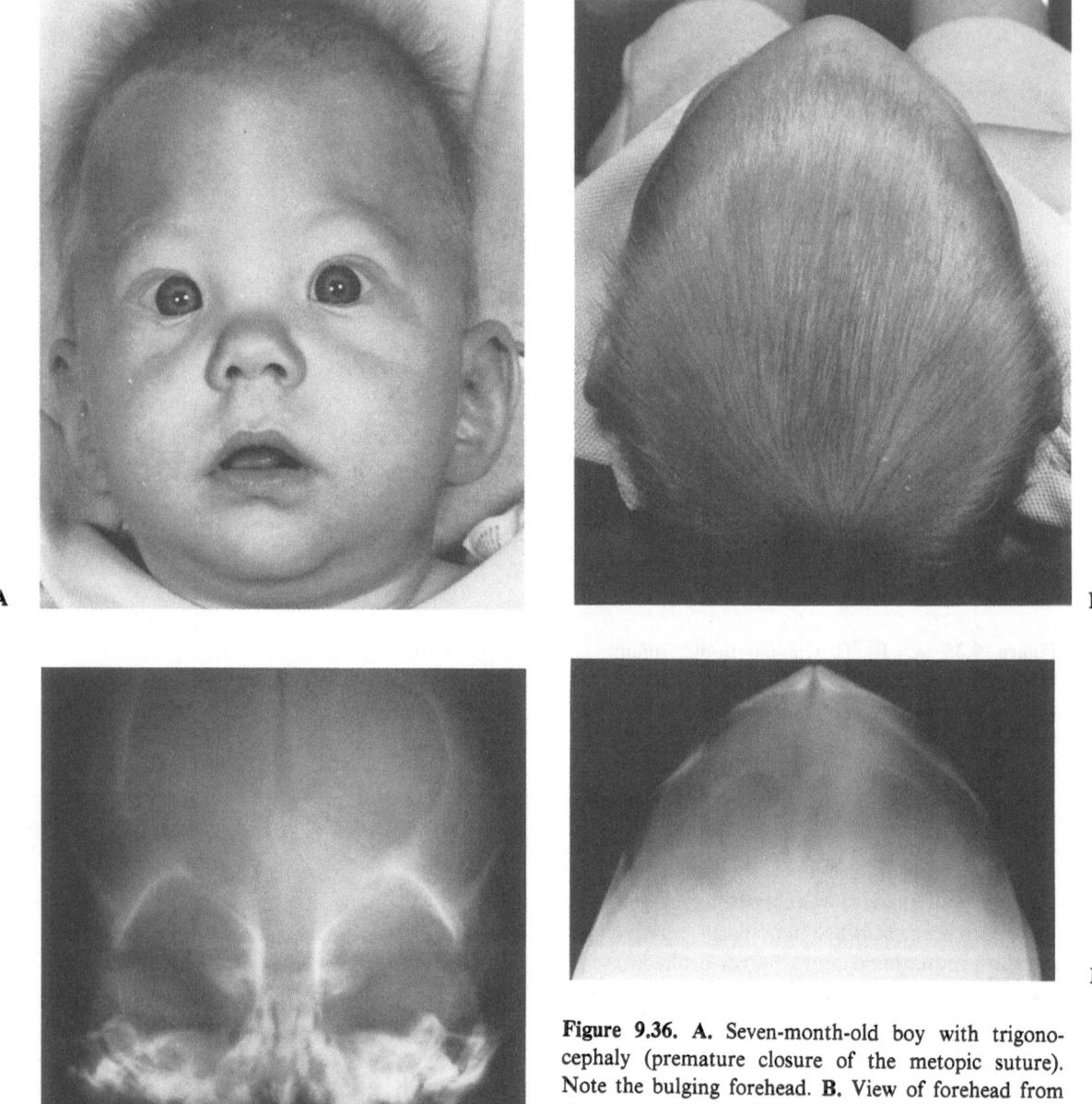

Figure 9.36. A. Seven-month-old boy with trigono-cephaly (premature closure of the metopic suture). Note the bulging forehead. **B.** View of forehead from above, showing the "Keel" shape of the forehead. **C.** Frontal radiograph showing the metopic suture with sclerotic edges and orbital hypotelorism. **D.** Tangential view of the pointed forehead showing the sclerotic edges of the metopic suture.

base of the skull is abnormal with the plane of the clivus more vertical; and the sphenoid plane and cribriform plate are inclined downward and forward. Thus, basilar kyphosis and a constricted nasopharynx are created. The orbital changes are those seen with coronal synostosis, with a harle-quin appearance due to elevation of the roofs and

lateral walls of the orbit. The supraorbital rim is recessed and the infraorbital rim is hypoplastic. Hydrocephalus sometimes is present. The orbits are shallow with resultant exophthalmos. The optic foramina may be narrowed, with optic atrophy being present at times. Strabismus is sometimes present. The facial characteristics may resemble

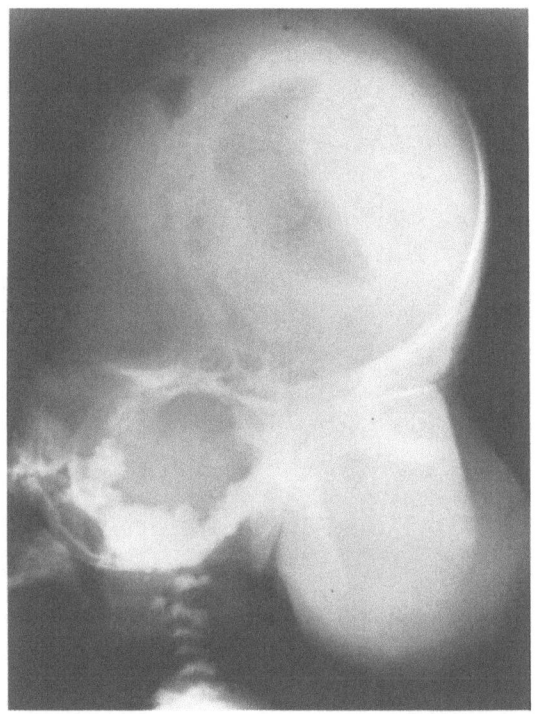

A

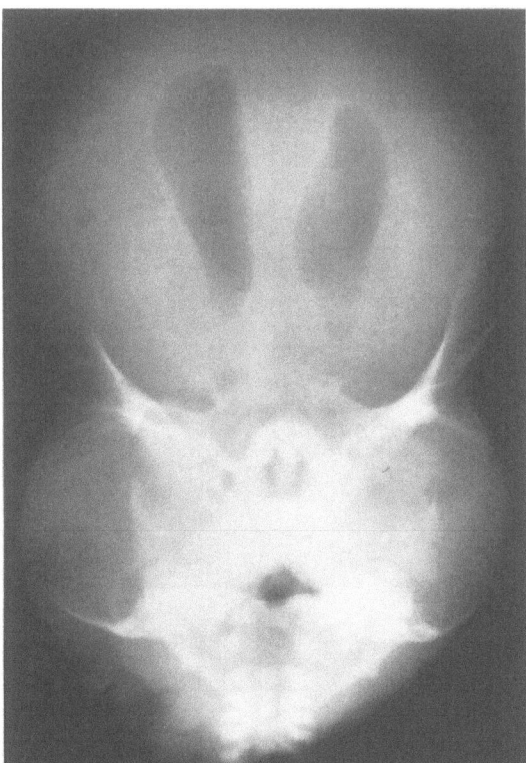

B

those of Crouzon disease, with a hypoplastic middle third of the face, a parrot-beaked nose, relative prognathism, and an open bite. Among the characteristic abnormalities are those seen in the extremities. A middigital hand mass with osseous and soft-tissue syndactyly of digits 2, 3, and 4 is always present. The first and fifth fingers may be joined to the middigital hand mass, or they may be separate. Similar changes usually are present in the feet. Nails of the middigital hand mass may be continuous or partially continuous. Progressive calcification and fusion of the bones of the hands, feet, and cervical spine occur with aging. While the presence of syndactylism definitely separates Crouzon disease and Apert syndrome, other differences have been noted. These include hyperacrobrachycephaly with a bregmatic bump, overhanging of the upper frontal area and a transverse frontal skin furrow, asymmetry of the exorbitism and the ptosis, maximum degree of lateral canthal dystopia, oculomotor paralysis, anterior open bite and cross-bow deformity of the upper lip, cleft palate (often occult), and hyperseborrhea, which are seen in the Apert syndrome (Figs. 9.39 and 9.40) (11, 30, 123, 137, 138, 180, 239, 254, 258).

Pfeiffer syndrome is an autosomal-dominant disorder that somewhat resembles Apert syndrome, but it has less severe abnormalities. It is characterized by craniosynostosis (turribrachycephaly), broad thumbs and great toes, and variable partial soft-tissue syndactyly of the hands and feet. The craniofacial changes include turribrachycephaly with premature closure of the sagittal and coronal sutures, (rarely) Kleeblattschadel, orbital hypertelorism, antimongoloid slope of the palpebral fissures, proptosis, strabismus, maxillary hypoplasia, and (occasionally) facial asymmetry. The skeletal changes include brachymesophalangy of the hands and feet (middle phalanges may be absent at times), trapezoidal or triangular proximal phalanges of the thumb and great toes, radiohumeral and radioulnar synostosis, and symphalangism of the hands and feet. Partial soft-tissue syndactyly may be seen in the hands and feet (Fig. 9.41) (123, 213, 214, 254).

Figure 9.37. A, B. Frontal and lateral views of the skull of one of a set of newborn twins with thanatophoric dysplasia with a Kleebattshadel. A pneumoencephalogram has been done showing the dilated lateral ventricles. Note the trilobar shape of the skull and the relatively small face (Case courtesy of W Berdon, MD, New York, NY).

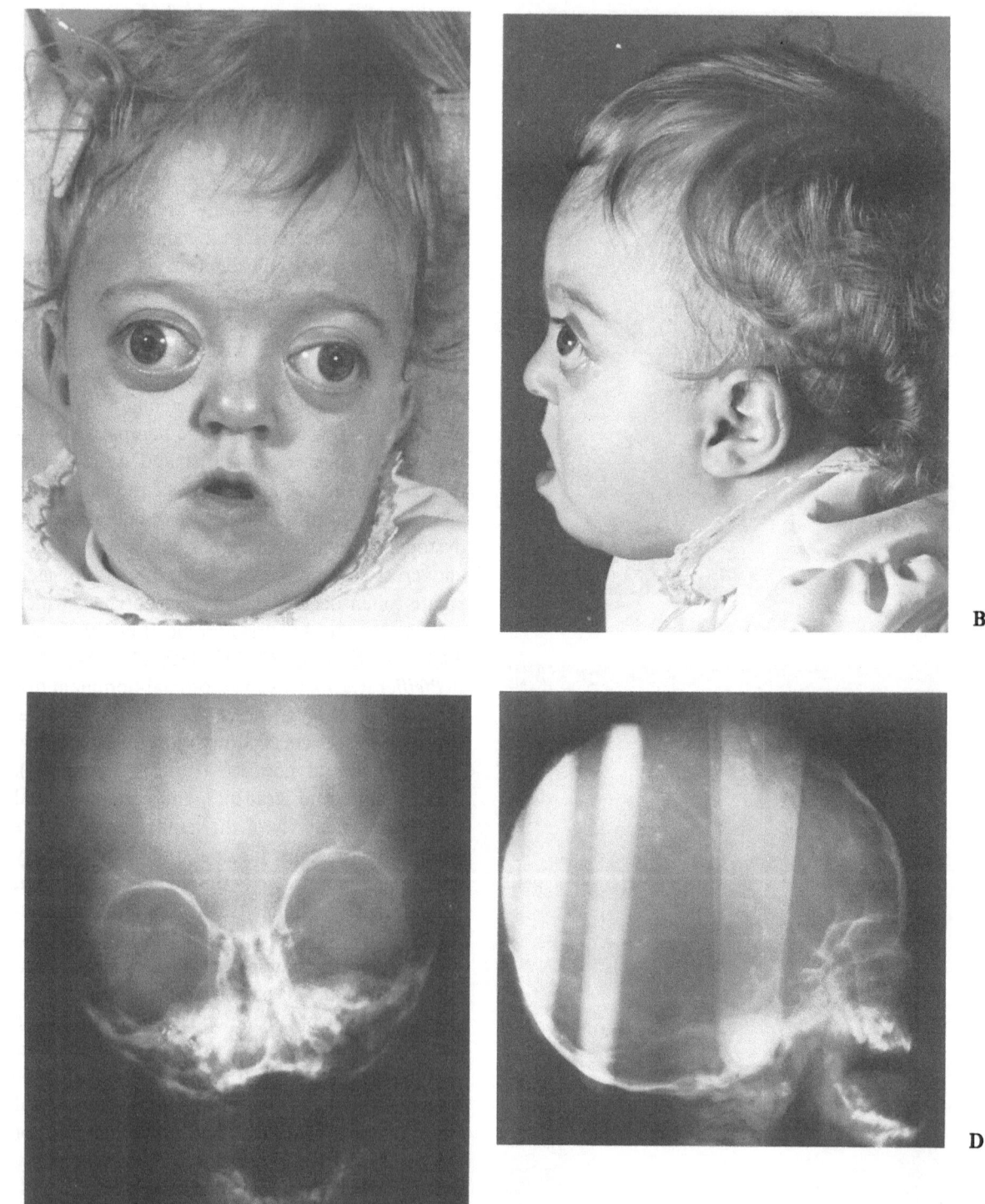

Figure 9.38. A, B. An 18-month-old girl with Crouzon disease. Note the brachycephaly, orbital hypertelorism, exophthalmos, and midface hypoplasia. **C.** Frontal radiograph of the skull showing orbital hypertelorism with a depressed cribriform plate. **D.** Lateral cephalometric radiograph of the skull showing brachycephaly shallow orbits and a retruded hypoplastic midface.

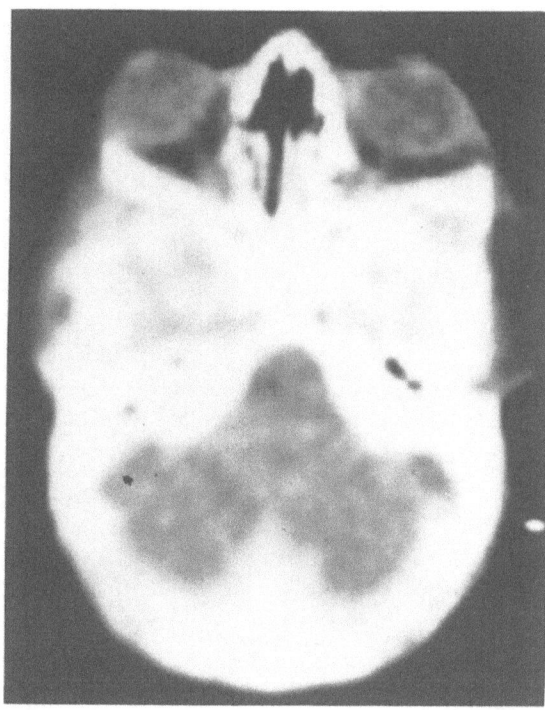

E

Figure 9.38. E. Computed tomogram of the skull showing the exophthalmos and the increased angle between the lateral orbital walls.

Saethre-Chotzen syndrome (acrocephalosyndactyly type 3) is an autosomal-dominant disorder characterized by craniosynostosis, facial asymmetry, mild midface hypoplasia, ptosis of the eyelids, antimongoloid slant of the palpebral fissures, a beaked nose, a low-set frontal hairline, variable brachydactyly, and variable cutaneous syndactyly. Radiographically, a variety of skull shapes may be seen, but the most common is either oxycephaly or brachycephaly. The forehead is flattened. Asymmetric involvement of the cranial sutures results in facial asymmetry with ethmoid and nasal septum deviation. The posterior cranial base is short and is vertically oriented. The anterior cranial fossa is short, the cribriform plate is low, and the shallow orbits are spaced further apart than normal. The nose is beaked and the maxilla is retruded. The fingers are short and wide. Mild cutaneous syndactyly may be present (19, 95, 123, 164, 180, 219, 254).

Carpenter syndrome (acrocephalopolysyndactyly) is an autosomal-recessive disorder characterized by acrocephaly, soft-tissue syndactyly, brachymesophalangy, preaxial polydactyly and syndactyly of the toes, coxa valga, pes varus, congenital heart disease, and hypogonadism. Microcornea and corneal opacities are seen in some patients. Radiographic changes include those of craniosynostosis, brachymesophalangy with soft-tissue syndactyly of the hands, two ossification centers for the proximal phalanx of the thumb leading to duplication of the thumb, and preaxial polydactyly and syndactyly of the feet. Less common findings include coxa valga, genu valgum, pes varus, flared ilia, displaced patella, and congenital heart disease (123, 138, 254, 257).

There are many rare craniostenosis syndromes in addition to the better-known syndromes that have already been described; some of these will be summarized. In all of them, the orbital changes are related to the type of craniostenosis present in the patient.

Craniosynostosis with variable syndactyly and obesity (Summitt syndrome) is an autosomal-recessive syndrome consisting of craniosynostosis (usually acrocephaly), epicanthal folds, strabismus, high-arched palate, variable degrees of syndactyly of the hands and feet, and clinodactyly (123, 250).

Craniosynostosis and radial aplasia (Baller-Gerold syndrome) is an autosomal-recessive syndrome characterized by craniosynostosis (turri-brachycephaly), a steep forehead, high nasal bridge, long philtrum, epicanthal folds, absent or hypoplastic radius, curved ulna, radially deviated hands, missing carpal bones, hypoplastic or absent thumbs, and fusion of the metopic suture with orbital hypotelorism in some patients (Fig. 9.42) (10, 123).

Craniosynostosis and fibular aplasia (Lowry syndrome) probably is an autosomal-recessive disorder, with craniostenosis (coronal and sagittal sutures), absent fibulae, talipes equinovarus, and cryptorchidism (123, 177).

Craniosynostosis with midface hypoplasia, hypertrichosis, and anomalies of the eyes, teeth, heart, and external genitalia (Gorlin-Chaudhry-Moss syndrome) probably is an autosomal-recessive disorder, with craniosynostosis (brachycephaly), hypoplastic maxillary and nasal bones, orbital hypertelorism, hypertrichosis, antimongoloid slope of the palpebral fissures, inability to fully open or close the eyes, upper eyelid colobomas, microphthalmia, and hyperopia. Other changes include patent ductus arteriosus, hypoplasia of the labia majora, and umbilical hernia (123).

Craniosynostosis and radioulnar synostosis (Ber-

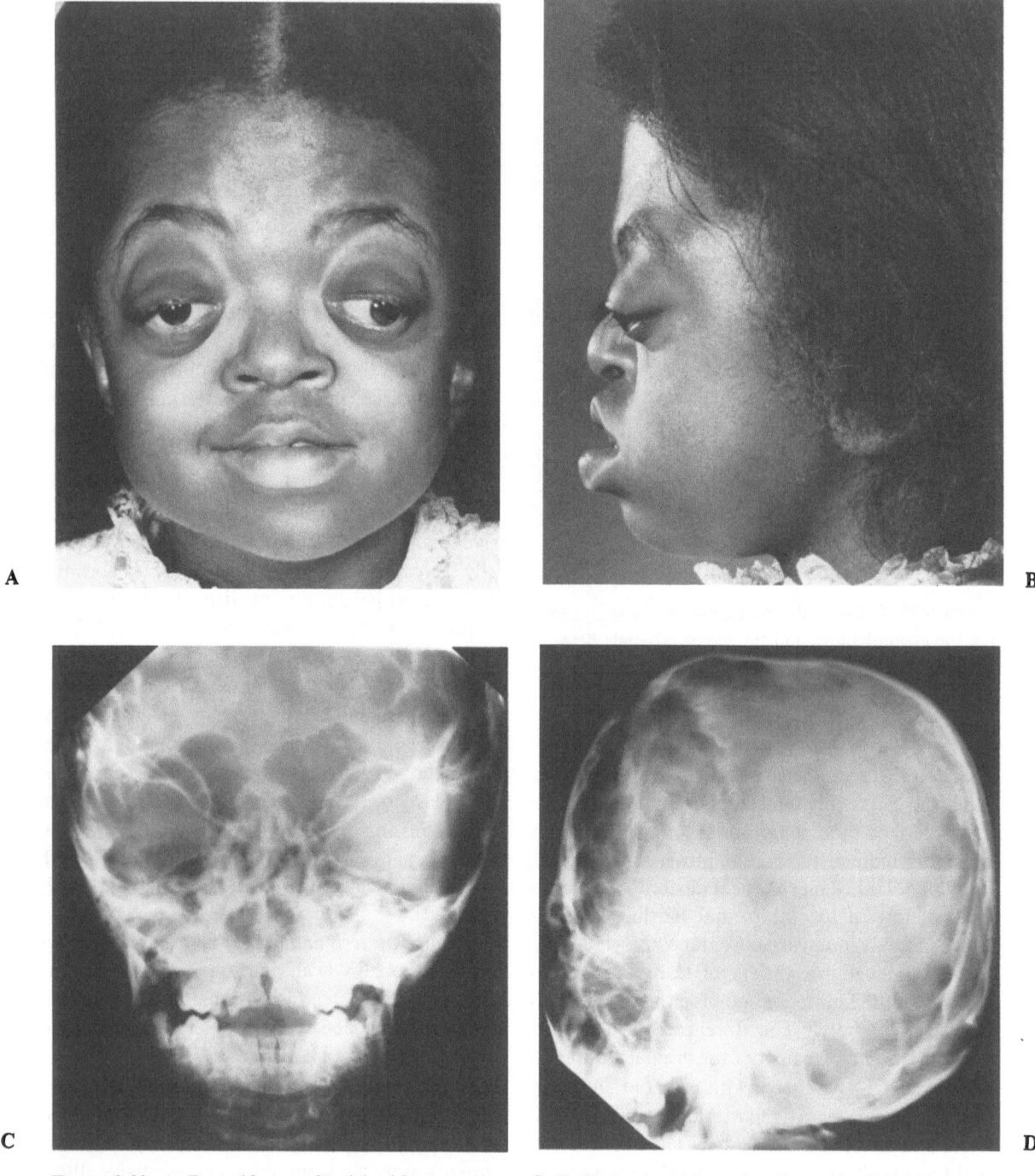

Figure 9.39. A, B. A 10-year-old girl with Apert syndrome. Note the exophthalmos, hypoplastic midface, orbital hypertelorism, and the high brachycephalic skull.

C, D. Frontal and lateral radiographs showing the orbital hypertelorism, brachycephaly, and hypoplastic midface.

ant syndrome) is an autosomal-dominant disorder, with craniostenosis (dolichocephaly) and radioulnar synostosis (34, 123).

Craniosynostosis with dwarfism, retinitis pigmentosa, and other anomalies (Armendares syndrome)

probably is an autosomal-recessive or X-linked recessive disorder, with postnasal growth deficiency, microcephaly, cranial asymmetry, craniostenosis, small face, scant eyebrows, small nose, micrognathia, high-arched palate, ptosis, epicanthal folds,

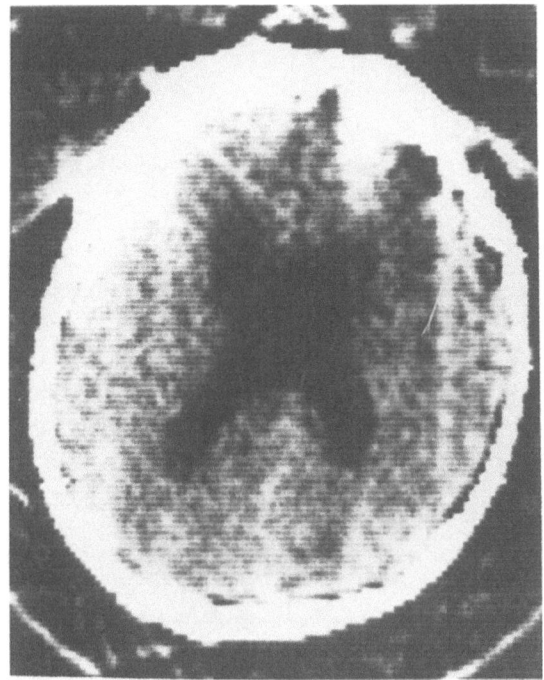

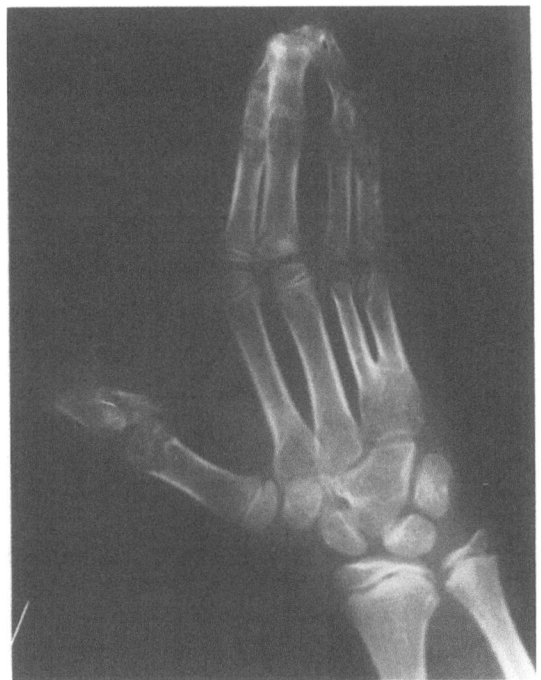

E

F

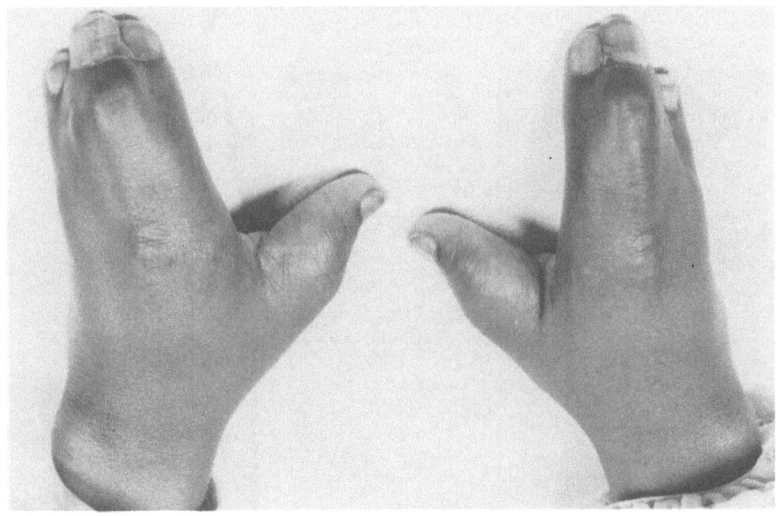

Figure 9.39. E. Computed tomogram showing dilated lateral
ventricles. F, G. Radiograph
and photograph of the hands
showing the syndactyly of the
fingers.

G

retinitis pigmentosa, and short fifth fingers (14, 123).

Phakomatoses

The neurocutaneous diseases are a large group of congenital disorders in which there is involvement of the skin and nervous system. A subgroup is classified as disseminated hereditary hamartomas or phakomatosis—a group of diseases character-ized by phakoi or lentil-shaped birthmarks of the skin and eyes. The phakomatous syndromes are a group of multisystemic dysgenetic features that form recognizable clinical and pathologic entities, with the primary sites of involvement being the nervous system, eyes, and skin. In a given syn-drome, the hamartoma tends to involve predomi-nantly one type of tissue; for example, blood vessels in von Hippel's disease and neural tissue in neurofi-bromatosis. Conditions classified in this group are neurofibromatosis, tuberous sclerosis, Sturge-

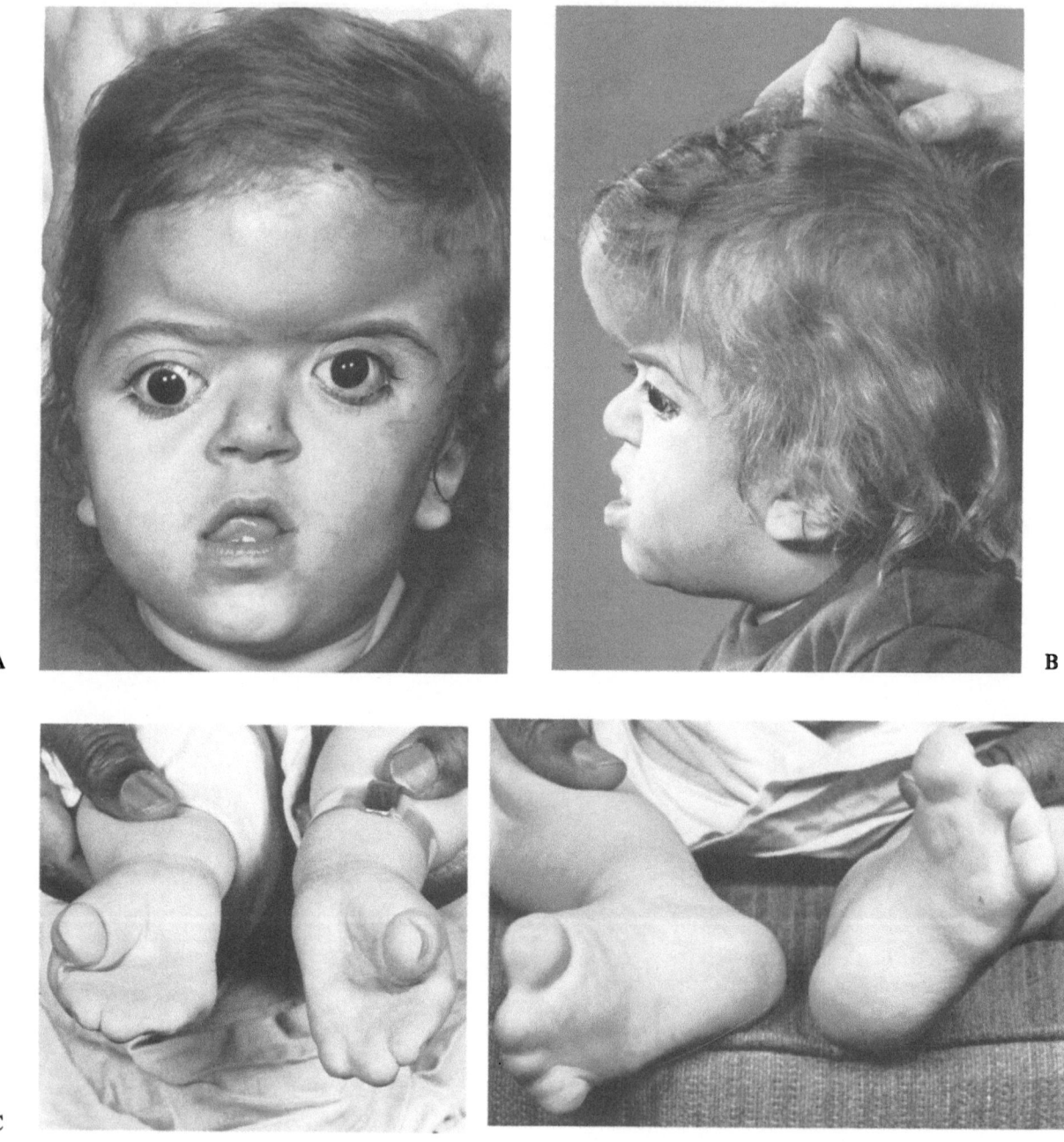

Figure 9.40. A, B. Four-year-old boy with Apert syndrome. Note the brachycephaly, orbital dystopia, exophthalmos, and hypoplastic midface. **C, D.** Photographs of the hands and feet showing the syndactyly.

Weber syndrome, von Hippel's disease, Wyburn-Mason syndrome, and ataxia-telangiectasia (265).

Neurofibromatosis (von Recklinghausen neurofibromatosis) is an autosomal-dominant disorder, with about 50% of the cases being fresh mutations. It is characterized by multiple neurofibromas, cutaneous pigmentation (cafe-au-lait spots), lymphangiomas, hemangiomas, lipomas, skeletal anomalies, and nervous system involvement. This syndrome has protean manifestations that evolve slowly and present in many different ways. Some patients have manifestations of the disorder at birth; over 50% of the patients show signs of the condition by 2 years of age. The skin changes in-

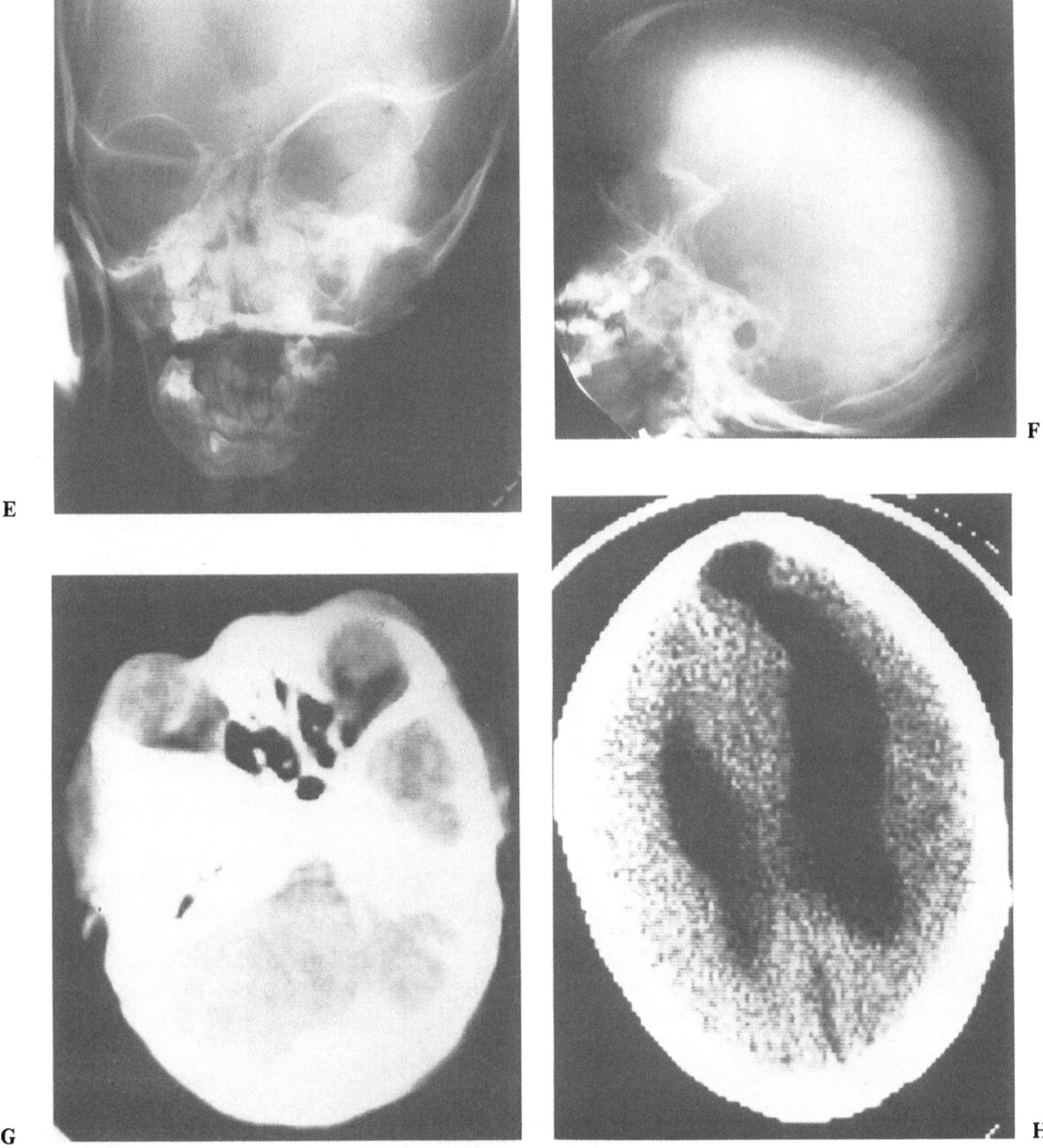

Figure 9.40. E. Frontal radiograph of the skull showing the orbital hypertelorism and the orbital dystopia. **F.** Lateral radiograph showing the brachycephalic skull and the hypoplastic midface. **G.** Computed tomogram showing the orbital hypertelorism and the increased angle between the lateral orbital walls. **H.** Computed tomogram showing dilated lateral ventricles.

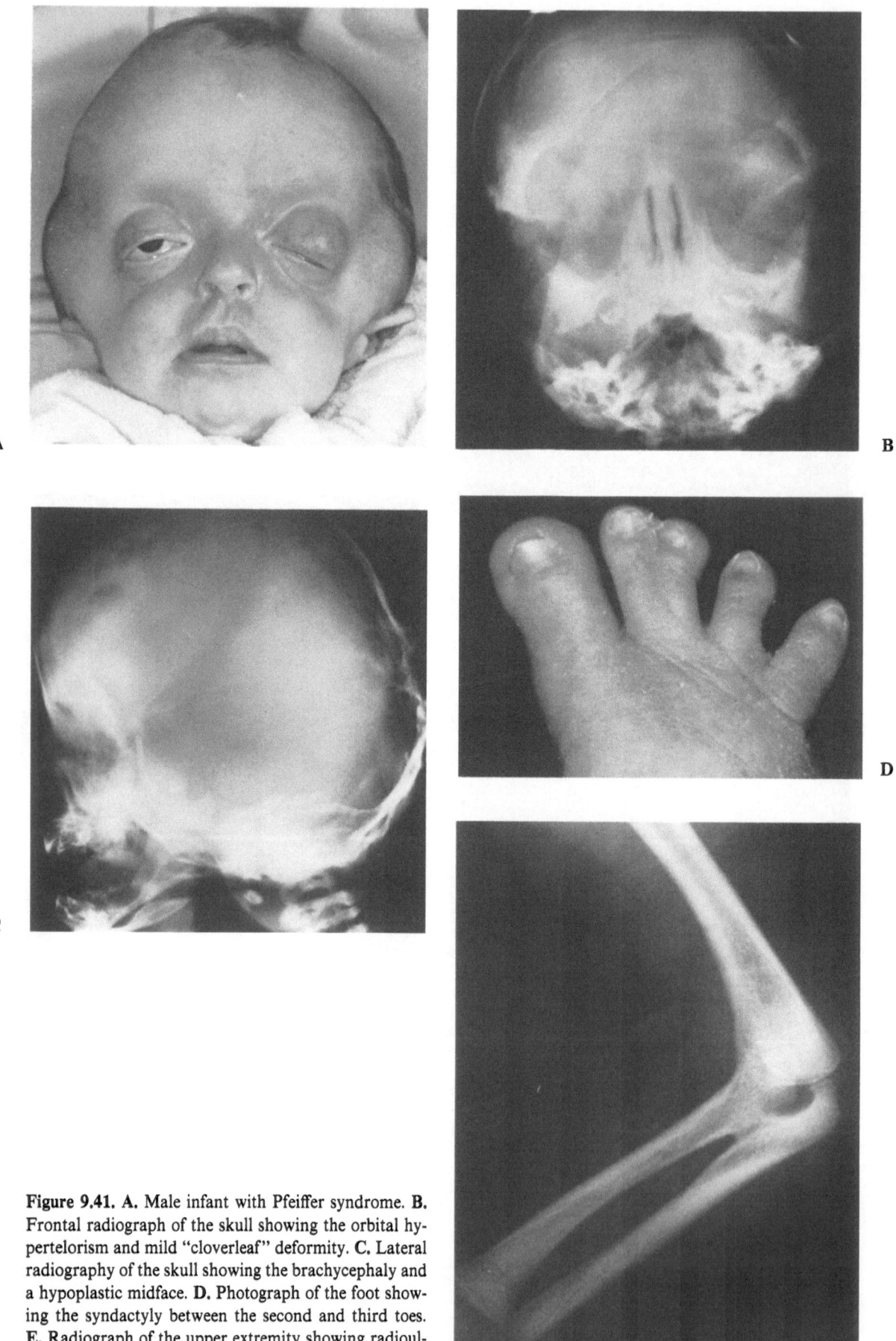

Figure 9.41. A. Male infant with Pfeiffer syndrome. **B.** Frontal radiograph of the skull showing the orbital hypertelorism and mild "cloverleaf" deformity. **C.** Lateral radiography of the skull showing the brachycephaly and a hypoplastic midface. **D.** Photograph of the foot showing the syndactyly between the second and third toes. **E.** Radiograph of the upper extremity showing radioulnar synostosis.

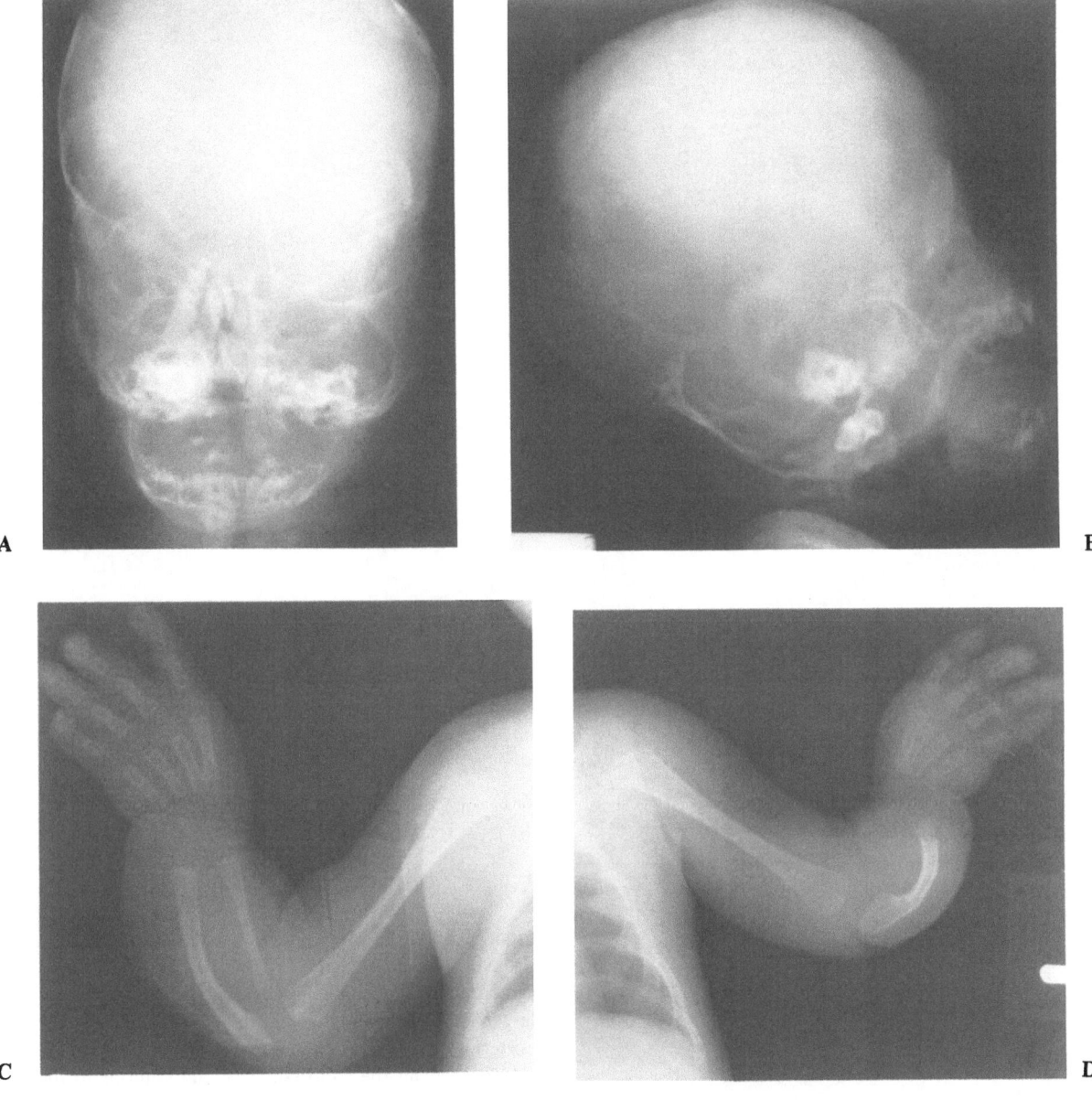

Figure 9.42. A, B. Frontal and lateral radiographs of the skull showing turribrachycephaly in an infant with Baller-Gerold syndrome (craniosynostosis-radial aplasia). **C, D.** Radiographs of the upper extremities showing absent thumbs. A hypoplastic radius is shown on the right and an absent radius is on the left.

clude nodular tumors, pigmented hairy nevi, and cafe-au-lait spots. The presence of six or more cafe-au-lait spots greater than 1.5 cm in diameter should arouse suspicion of neurofibromatosis (67). Other skin manifestations are various types of tumors and elephantoid overgrowth of skin and soft tissues. There are many skeletal abnormalities, including bowing of limbs, kyphoscoliosis, skull and orbit defects, regional hypertrophy, pseudoarthroses, subperiosteal erosions due to pressure from neurofibromas in adjacent tissues, cystic lesions in bone (sometimes due to neurofibromas; at times, no cause is found), partial absence of limbs, pressure defects in spinal canal due to dural ectasia, and other occasional anomalies; megacephaly may be present. Tumors may be present at birth or may at any time later in life. These tumors (mostly neurofibromas) involve practically every organ in the body, including the brain, spinal cord, stomach, intestine, kidney, bladder, larynx,

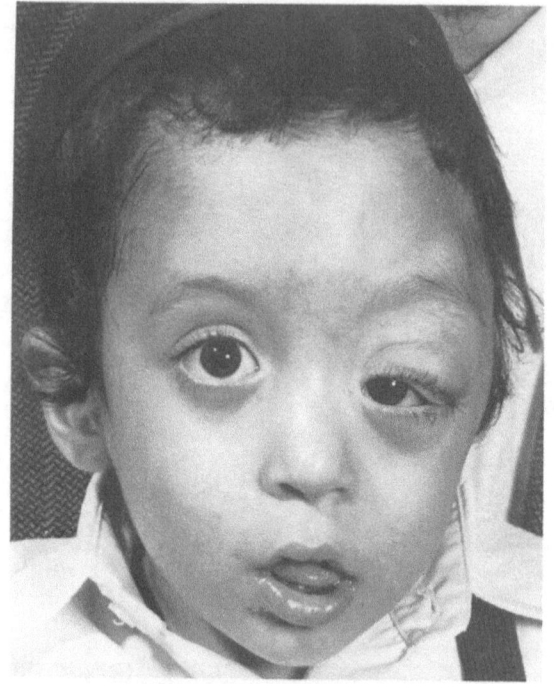

A

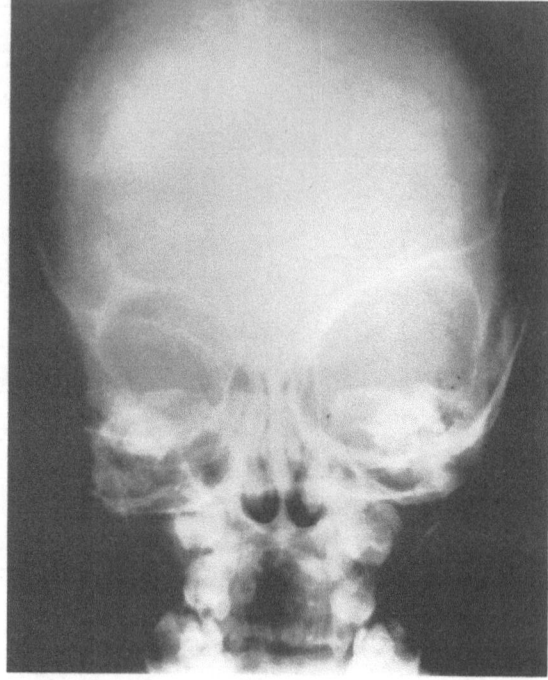

B

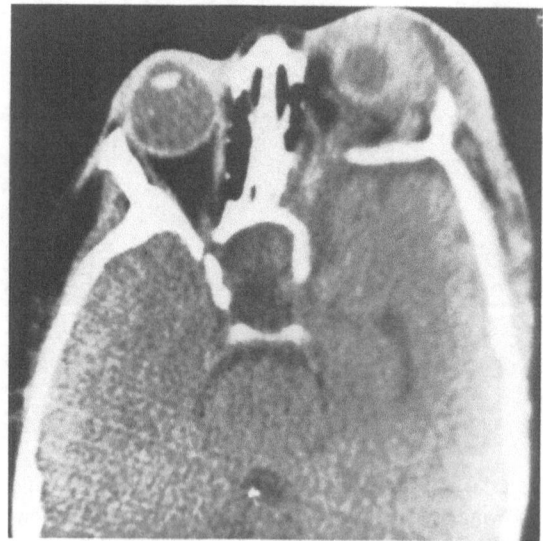

C

Figure 9.43. A. Four-year-old boy with neurofibromatosis. Note the displacement of the left eye. **B.** Frontal radiograph of the skull showing the left orbit to be enlarged and an absence of the bony structures of the posterior orbit. **C.** Computed tomographic study of the orbits, showing the soft-tissue swelling anterior to the left orbit, defects in the left sphenoid, and anterior displacement of the left eyeball secondary to herniation of the brain through the sphenoid defect.

and heart. In the central nervous system, schwannomas, meningiomas, gliomas, astrocytomas, ependymomas, and neuromas of the cranial nerves (especially optic and acoustic) are often found. The ophthalmologic abnormalities seen with this condition include Lisch spots of the iris, neurofibromas of the eyelids, intraorbital tumors producing exophthalmos and oculomotor palsies, phakoma, congenital glaucoma, fibroma of the iris, corneal opacity, optic gliomas, and optic atrophy. Radio-

graphic changes include erosions of the skull, enlarged foramina, bone defects (especially in posterior and superior orbital walls), enlarged orbit, macrocranium, macrencephaly, hydrocephalus, psammomatosis calcifications in the temporal horns of the brain, brain tumors, cranial nerve neuromas, and enlargement of both optic foramina and orbital fissures with and without neuromas. The defects in the orbital walls may permit brain herniation into the orbit and may produce pulsat-

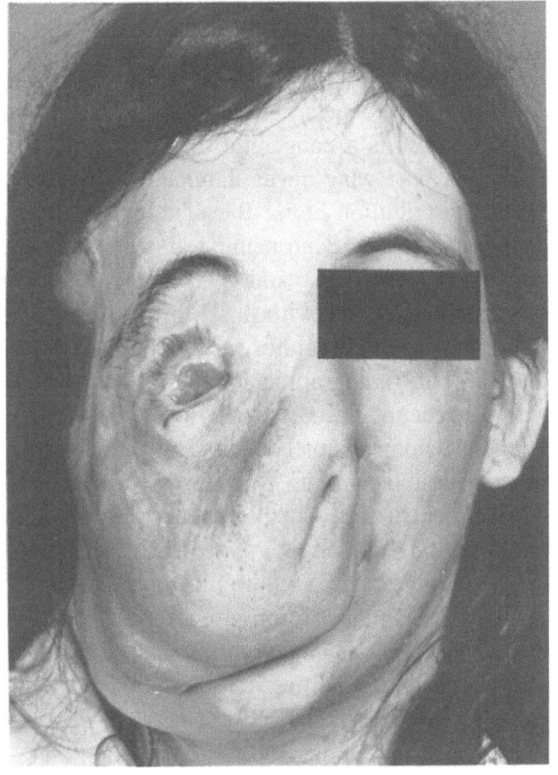

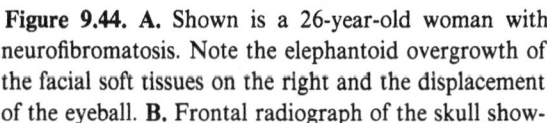

A

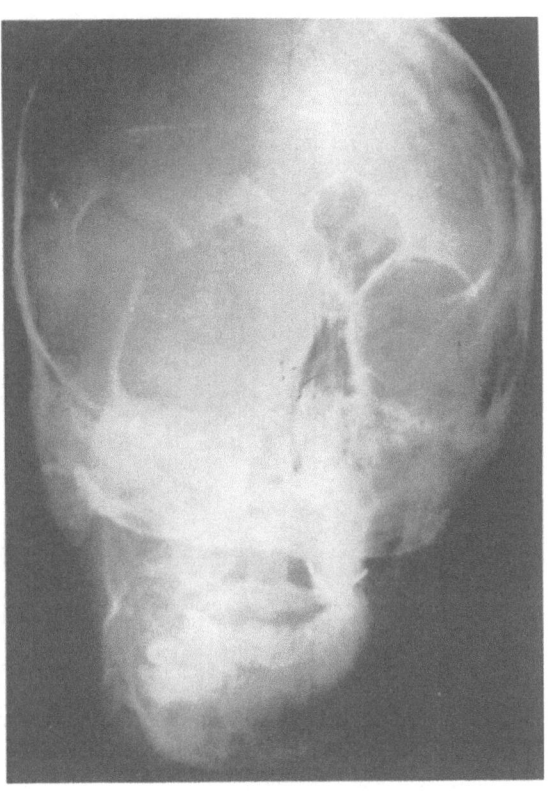

B

Figure 9.44. A. Shown is a 26-year-old woman with neurofibromatosis. Note the elephantoid overgrowth of the facial soft tissues on the right and the displacement of the eyeball. **B.** Frontal radiograph of the skull show-ing an enlarged orbit on the right with absence of the posterior wall. Also note the indentation on the right side of the mandible.

ing exophthalmos. Many changes are seen in the skeletal system, including pressure defect from soft-tissue tumors, pseudoarthrosis, kyphoscoliosis, enlargement of the intervertebral foramina, posterior notching of the vertebral bodies from dural ectasia, intramedullary tumors, local overgrowth, and bone sclerosis. Changes may be seen in almost every organ secondary to tumors, especially neurofibromas. Computed tomographic studies are valuable for showing brain tumors, cranial nerve gliomas and neuromas, and lesions involving the eye and orbit (Figs. 9.43 and 9.44) (36, 41, 47, 66, 72, 107, 123, 138, 139, 142, 145, 160, 234, 254, 266).

Tuberous sclerosis (Bourneville-Pringle syndrome, epiloia) is an autosomal-dominant disorder with variable expressivity and many fresh mutations. It is characterized by skin lesions (especially sebaceous adenomas), cerebral tubers, and retinal phakomas. Many patients with this disease are mentally retarded. Epilepsy is a common present-ing complaint. Many skin lesions are seen; the most common being adenoma sebaceum (angiofibromas) of the face. Other cutaneous lesions are "shagreen patches", cafe-au-lait spots, ash leaf-shaped depigmented macules, leathery skin in the lower trunk, and subungual fibromas. Visceral hamartomas can be seen, especially in the kidneys (angiomyolipomas). Rhabdomyomas of the heart and hamartomas of the liver and lungs have been reported. The ophthalmologic signs include: 1) retinal phakomas (flat or nodular, warty, mulberry-shaped, whitish or yellowish hyaline-like masses near the papilla); 2) oval or round, flat, nonvascular whitish plaques of variable size in the retina (retinal spots); and 3) retinal angiomas. Radiologic changes demonstrate brain calcification, which apears as the patient ages. This takes place in cortical tubers and ventricular nodules. These masses may be homogeneous with irregular contours or vermicular and annular with central radiolucent area. Computed tomography will confirm the diag-

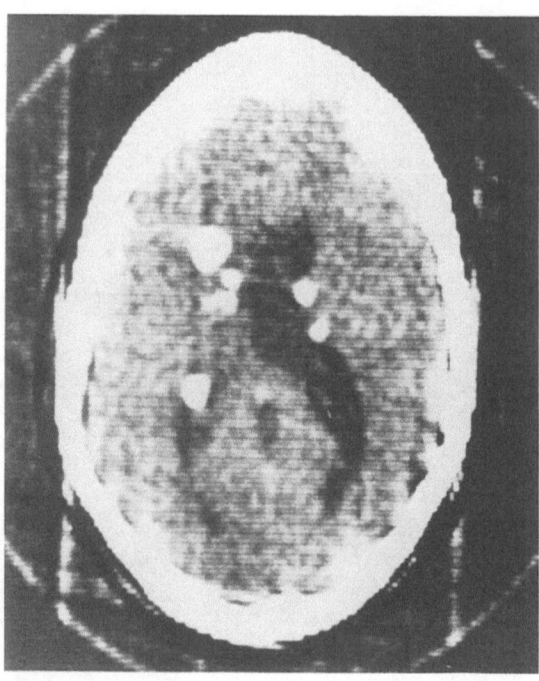

Figure 9.45. Computed tomogram of an adult with tuberous sclerosis showing calcification in the cortical tubers and ventricular nodules.

nosis of tuberous sclerosis by showing the subependymal calcification; it can detect the disease in asymptomatic relatives. The cortical tubers have a density higher than that of the brain on the CT scan, and they are not usually enhanced by contrast media. Hydrocephalus in some patients may be shown to be due to obstruction by tumors. Also, the CT scan may show low-density areas within the deep-white matter and cortical and subcortical areas. Exophytic retina tumors, such as angiomas, may be seen on the CT scan. The pneumoencephalogram demonstrates cerebral atrophy and ventricular nodules, with the characteristic candle-guttering appearance. Radiographic findings in the skeleton include patchy, localized sclerotic densities in the skull, vertebrae, pelvis, and long bones. Cyst-like changes may be seen in the phalanges, metatarsals, and metacarpals. Localized periosteal thickening along the shafts of the tubular bones, rib expansion and sclerosis, exostoses, and enostoses may be detected. In the chest, interstitial reticular infiltrates, a "honeycomb" appearance of a lung, pulmonary cysts, lymphangioma, spontaneous pneumothorax, and cardiac tumors may be noted. Renal tumors (angio-

myolipomas), cysts, and rarely) renal cell carcinoma may be found (Fig. 9.45) (18, 46, 50, 104, 107, 113, 123, 124, 138, 140, 171, 182, 187, 236, 254, 265).

Sturge-Weber syndrome (encephalotrigeminal angiomatosis) is a congenital disorder characterized by a port wine nevus flammeus of the face, with a distribution along the first branch of the trigeminal nerve, leptomeningeal angiomatosis, convulsive disorders, and glaucoma. The eye changes that are seen with this disorder are choroidal angioma, buphthalmos, glaucoma, and hemianopia. The radiographic manifestations include a smaller hemicranium on the involved side, enlarged vascular channels of the skull, the characteristic double-contour "gyriform" intracranial calcification in subcortical areas (usually parietal and occipital), dilated lateral ventricle of the brain on the involved side, and brain atrophy; with vascular studies, manifestations are arterial occlusion, capillary or venous angiomatous stains, and various venous abnormalities. The intracranial calcifications are rarely seen before 2 years of age, but they subsequently develop. Most are unilateral, but bilateral intracranial calcifications are seen. The CT scan shows the calcification earlier than routine X-ray films. With the use of contrast media, there is enhancement of the leptomeningeal angiomas (Figs. 9.46 and 9.47) (6, 64, 107, 123, 254, 265, 267, 268).

Hippel-Lindau syndrome (von Hippel-Lindau syndrome) is an autosomal-dominant disorder with incomplete penetrance. It consists of a combination of central nervous system and ocular hemangioblastomas, cysts within the solid organs of the abdomen, polycythemia, and neoplasms of the kidney, adrenal, and sympathic chains. It is usually recognized in the third, fourth, and fifth decades. Most patients present with symptoms related to cerebellar, cerebral, or spinal cord lesions. The ocular findings vary, depending on the stage of the disease. Retinal hemangioblastoma (or hemangioma) is first seen as a mural nodule on ophthalmoscopic examination. The tumor size varies, and it usually lies adjacent to a large afferent artery and efferent vein. When the tumor has a cystic component, retinal detachment and increased ocular pressure occur. Hemorrhage and uveitis may be present. Retinal hemangioblastoma may calcify or even ossify. If a massive macular exudate develops, the resulting picture may resem-

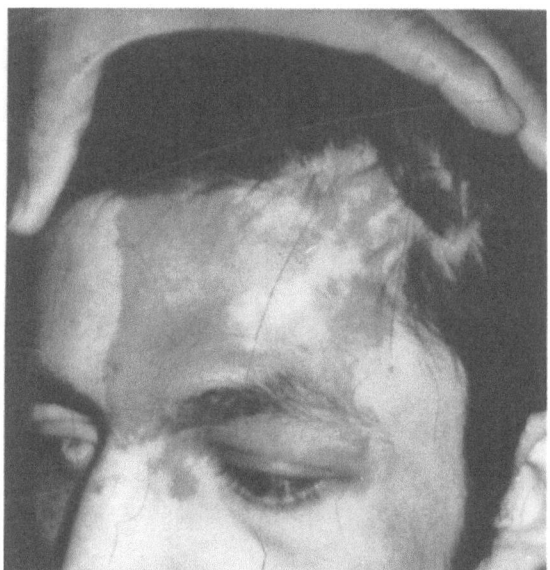
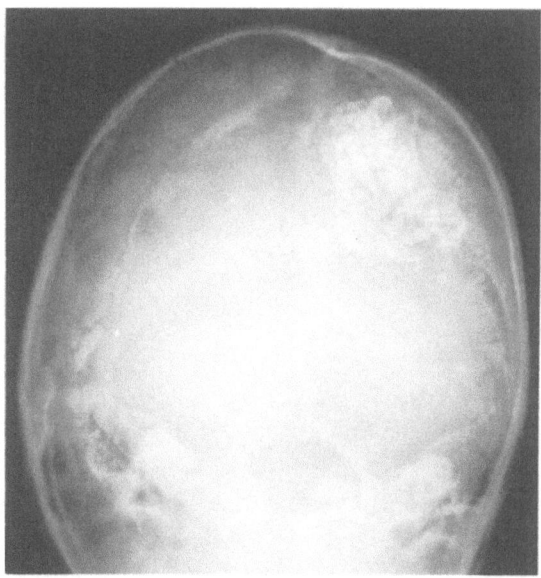

A

B

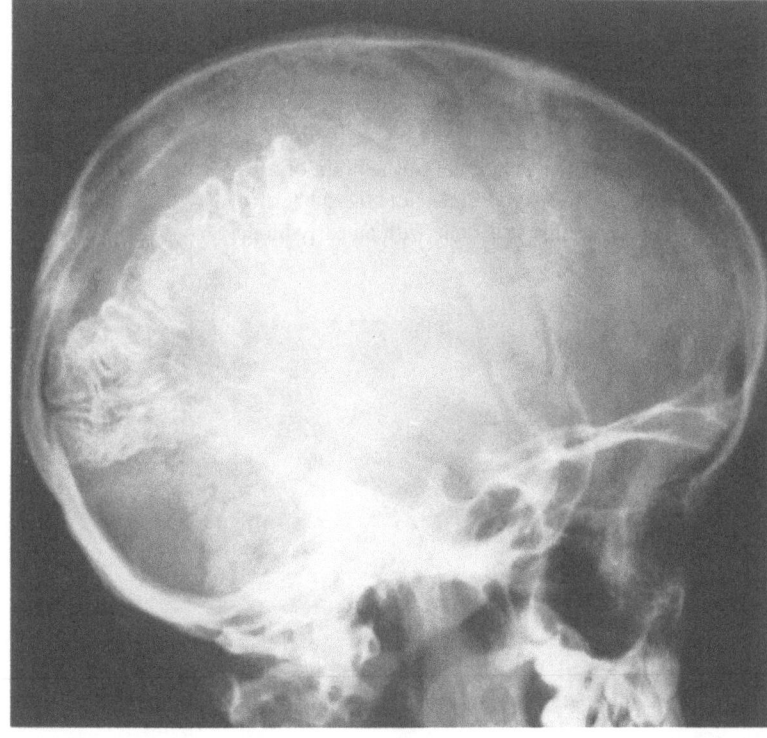

Figure 9.46. A. Photograph of patient with Sturge-Weber syndrome. Note the nevus flammeus (port wine strain) in the area of the distribution of the first branch of the trigeminal nerve. **B, C.** Skull radiographs showing the typical double-contour "gyriform" calcifications.

C

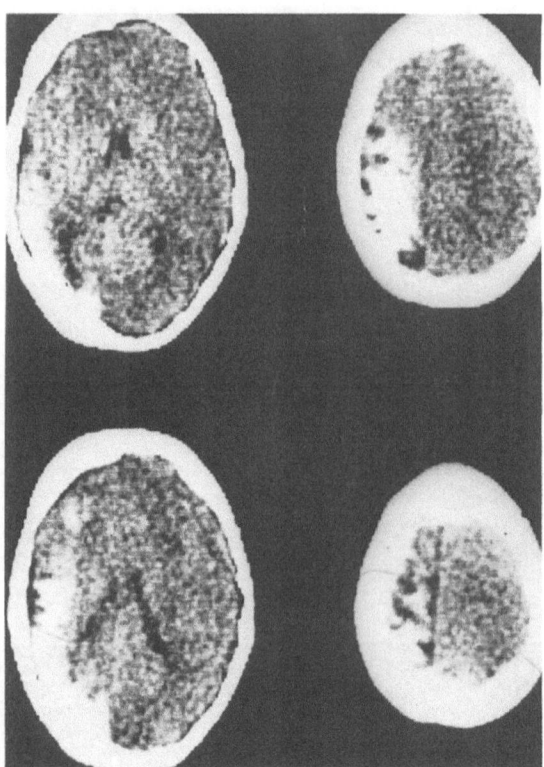

Figure 9.47. Computed tomogram of the brain of a patient with Sturge-Weber syndrome. Note the subcortical calcifications. This study was done with an early model CT scanner.

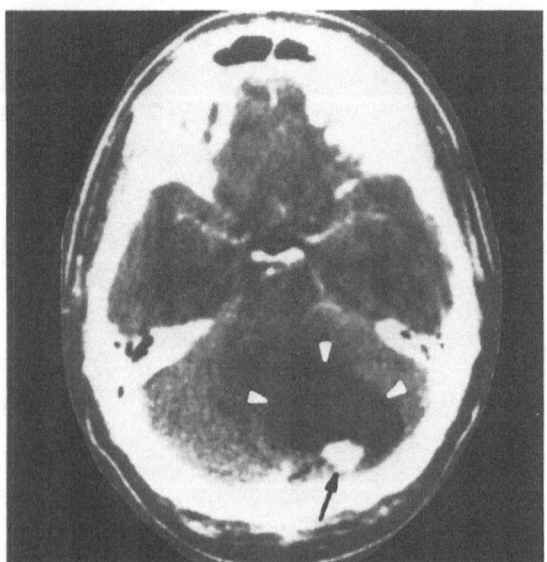

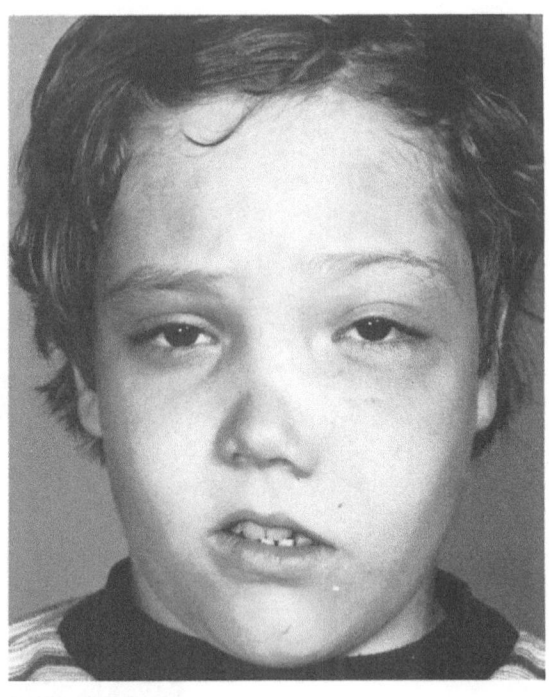

A

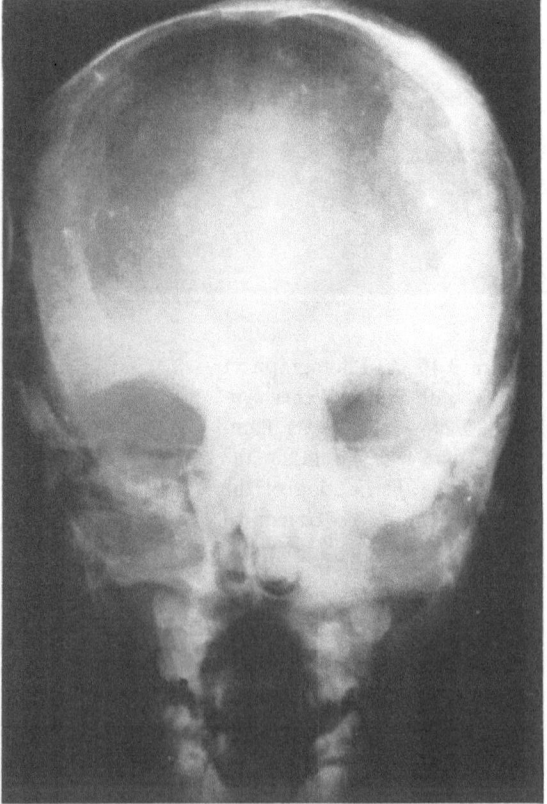

B

Figure 9.48. Computed tomogram in a patient with von Hipple-Lindau syndrome, taken after an injection of contrast media. In the posterior fossa, the axial CT scan shows a large hemangioblastoma (cyst) in the left cerebellar hemisphere (arrowhead). Enhancement of the dural nodule is present (black arrow).

Figure 9.49. A. A 10-year-old boy with fibrous dysplasia. Note the swelling about the left side of the face. **B.** Frontal radiograph showing sclerosis of the bones of the left side of the face and skull. Note the small left orbit.

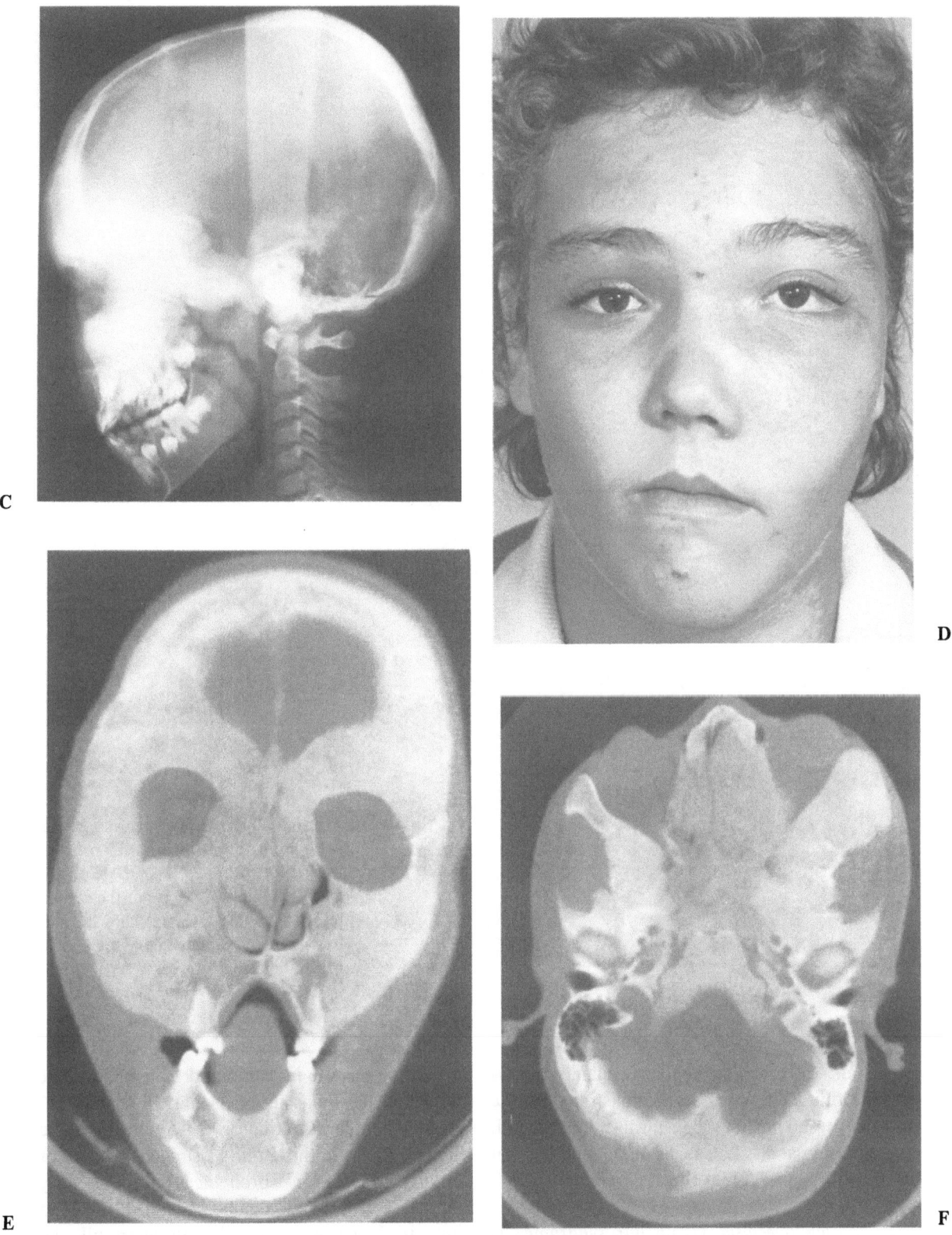

Figure 9.49. C. Lateral radiograph taken at same time as **B. D.** Photograph of patient 4 years later. **E, F.** A CT scan at 14 years of age showing the progression of the craniofacial involvement.

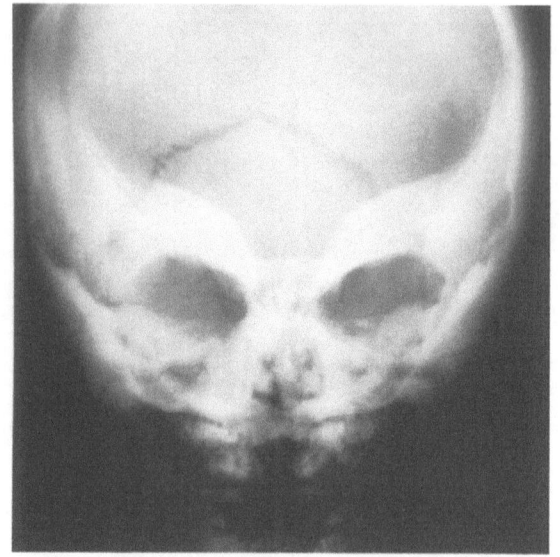

A

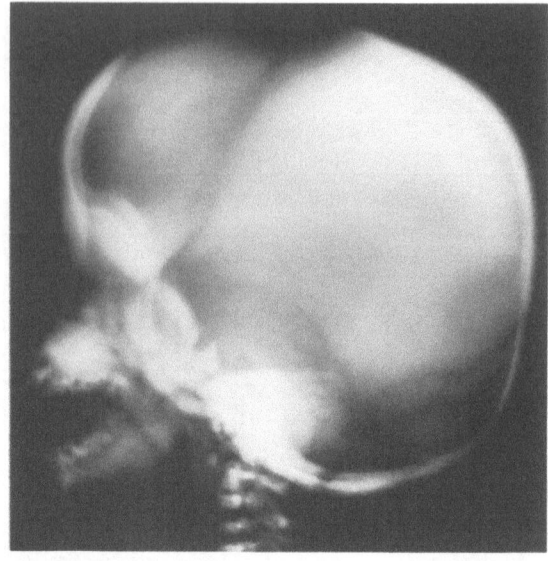

B

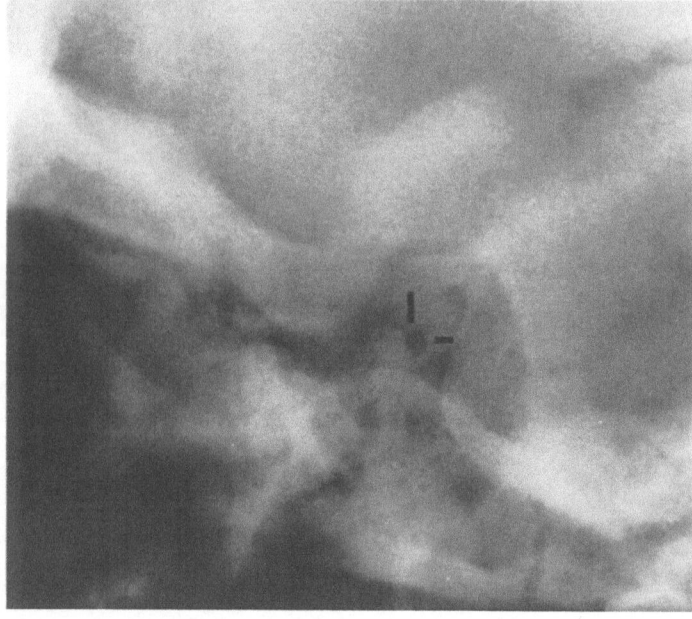

C

Figure 9.50. A, B. Frontal and lateral radiographs of an infant with osteopetrosis. Note the sclerosis of the skull and face with relative sparing of the mandible. **C.** Optic foramen view showing narrowing of the optic canal. This patient had optic atrophy.

ble Coats' disease. The radiologic manifestations are the tumors and masses demonstrated at the various sites. They may be shown by ultrasound, angiography, and CT. Calcifications may be seen in the orbit and/or brain (Fig. 9.48) (65, 107, 254, 265).

Ataxia-telangiectasia (Louis-Bar syndrome) is an autosomal-recessive disorder. It appears in early childhood, with progressive cerebellar ataxia, ocular and cutaneous telangiectases, immunologic deficiencies, absent or deficient thymus gland, and

a predisposition to infection and malignancy. The characteristic ocular finding is marked telangiectasia of the bulbar conjunctiva. The radiographic changes seen are those due to sinusitis, recurrent pulmonary infections, bronchiectasis, pulmonary fibrosis, lack of thymic shadow, deficient lymphoid tissue in the nasopharynx and pulmonary hili, cerebral atrophy, and the imaging changes associated with neoplastic lesions (33, 44, 107, 138, 254, 265).

Wyburn-Mason syndrome (Bonnet-Lechaume-Blanc syndrome) is characterized by the associa-

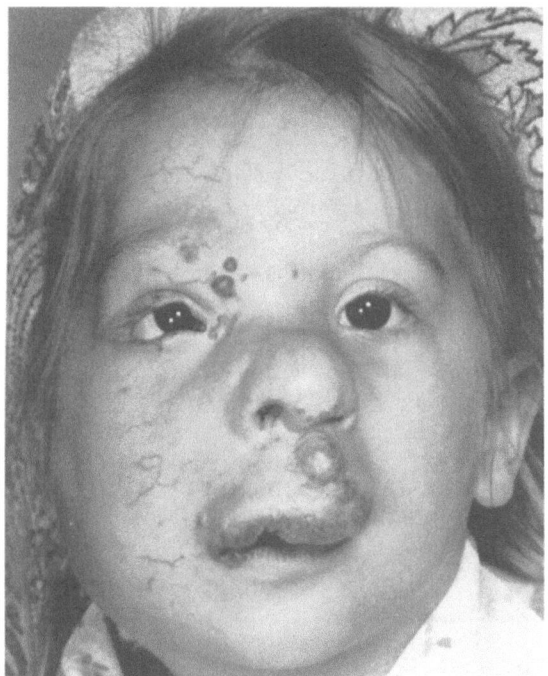 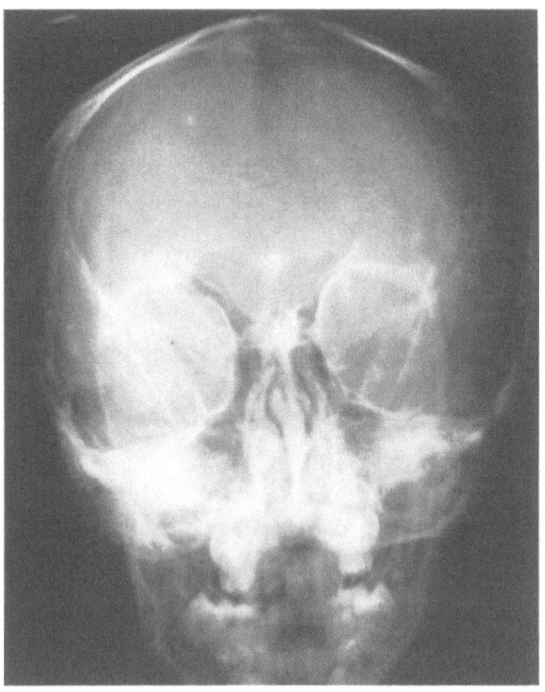

Figure 9.51. A. Three-year-old girl with regressing facial hemangiomas. **B.** Frontal skull radiograph showing orbital hypertelorism.

tion of a cirsoid (racemose) aneurysm of the retina, a juxtamesencephalic or juxtathalamic cerebral cirsoid aneurysm (often in continuity with the retinal lesion), and a cutaneous angioma (nevus flammeus) in the trigeminal area of one side of the face (12, 107, 272).

Miscellaneous Disorders

Fibrous dysplasia is a disorder that usually begins during childhood. It is characterized by the replacement of normal bone undergoing physiologic lysis by an abnormal proliferation of fibrous tissue. It may involve a single bone (monostotic) or any number of bones (polyostotic). There is a predilection for the long bones, but any bone may be involved. Areas of skin pigmentation (cafe-au-lait spots) may be present. The most severe form of the disorder is the McCune-Albright syndrome, which consists of polyostotic fibrous dysplasia, cutaneous pigmentation, and precocious puberty. The face and orbits usually are normal; but when one or more of the facial bones is involved, the face and orbit may be grossly distorted and asymmetric. The skull is involved in 50% of patients

with polyostotic fibrous dysplasia and about 20% of patients with the monostotic form. Common sites of skull involvement are the frontal, sphenoid, maxillary, and ethmoid bones, with the occipital and temporal bones being involved less often. Radiographic changes include lucent and sclerotic areas in bone. The sclerotic changes predominate in the skull (especially in the base and sphenoid wings). Radiolucent lesions may be associated with widened diploic spaces (expanding in an outward direction with the inner table being undisturbed). Silent or asymptomatic cranial lesions may progress to cause either visual impairment due to narrowing of the optic canal or hearing loss due to temporal bone changes. Downward displacement of the orbital contents can be the result of the gross deformity and asymmetry of the skull. The involvement of the bony orbital walls can lead to a decrease in the size of the orbit ("small orbit sign") (Fig. 9.49) (26, 71, 91, 109, 114, 123, 132, 148, 152, 173, 218, 254, 256).

Osteopetrosis (Albers-Schoenberg disease, marble bone disease) is a disorder with variable degrees of severity. It is autosomal-recessive in the malignant type and autosomal-dominant in the benign

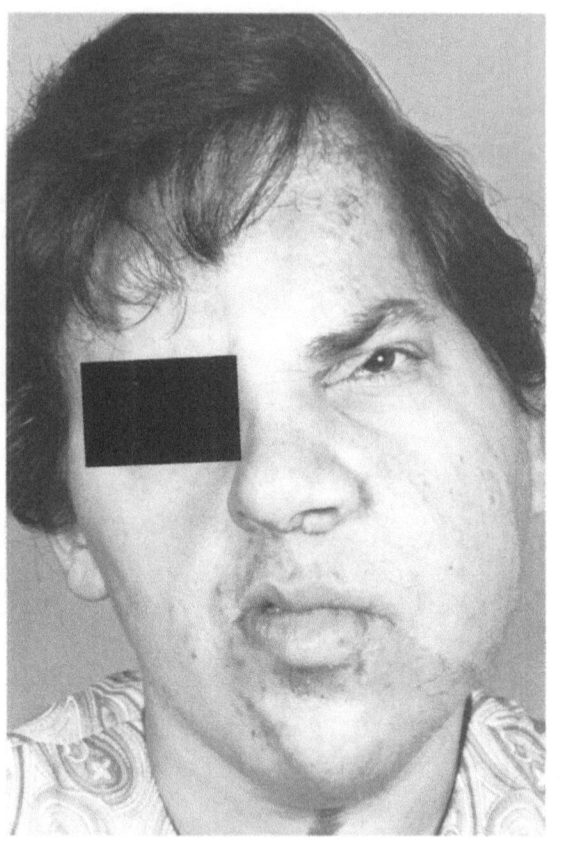

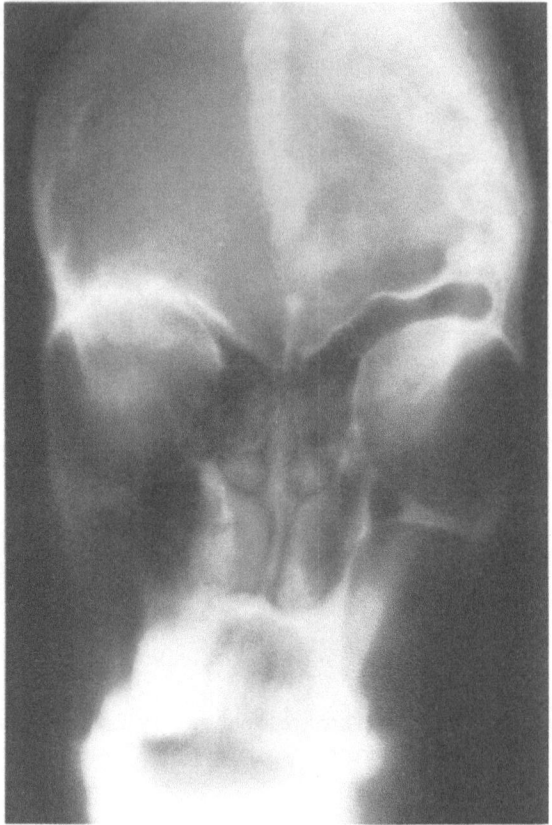

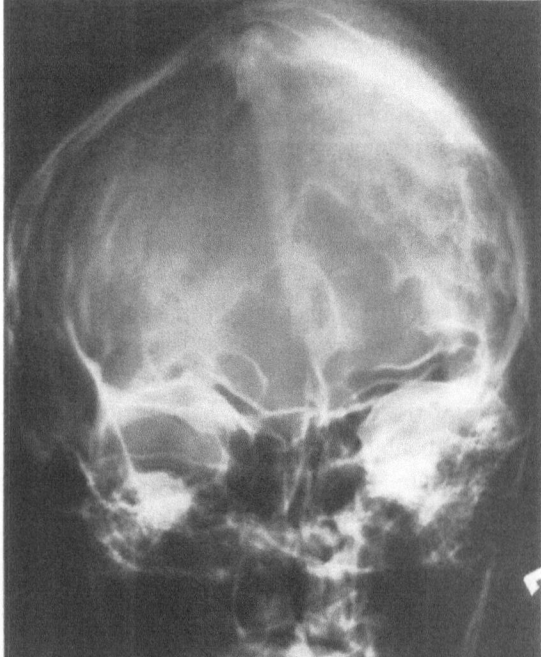

Figure 9.52. A. A 28-year-old woman with hemangio-lymphangioma causing overgrowth of the left side of the face. **B, C.** Frontal radiograph and tomogram of face and skull, showing the bone overgrowth and orbital hypertelorism.

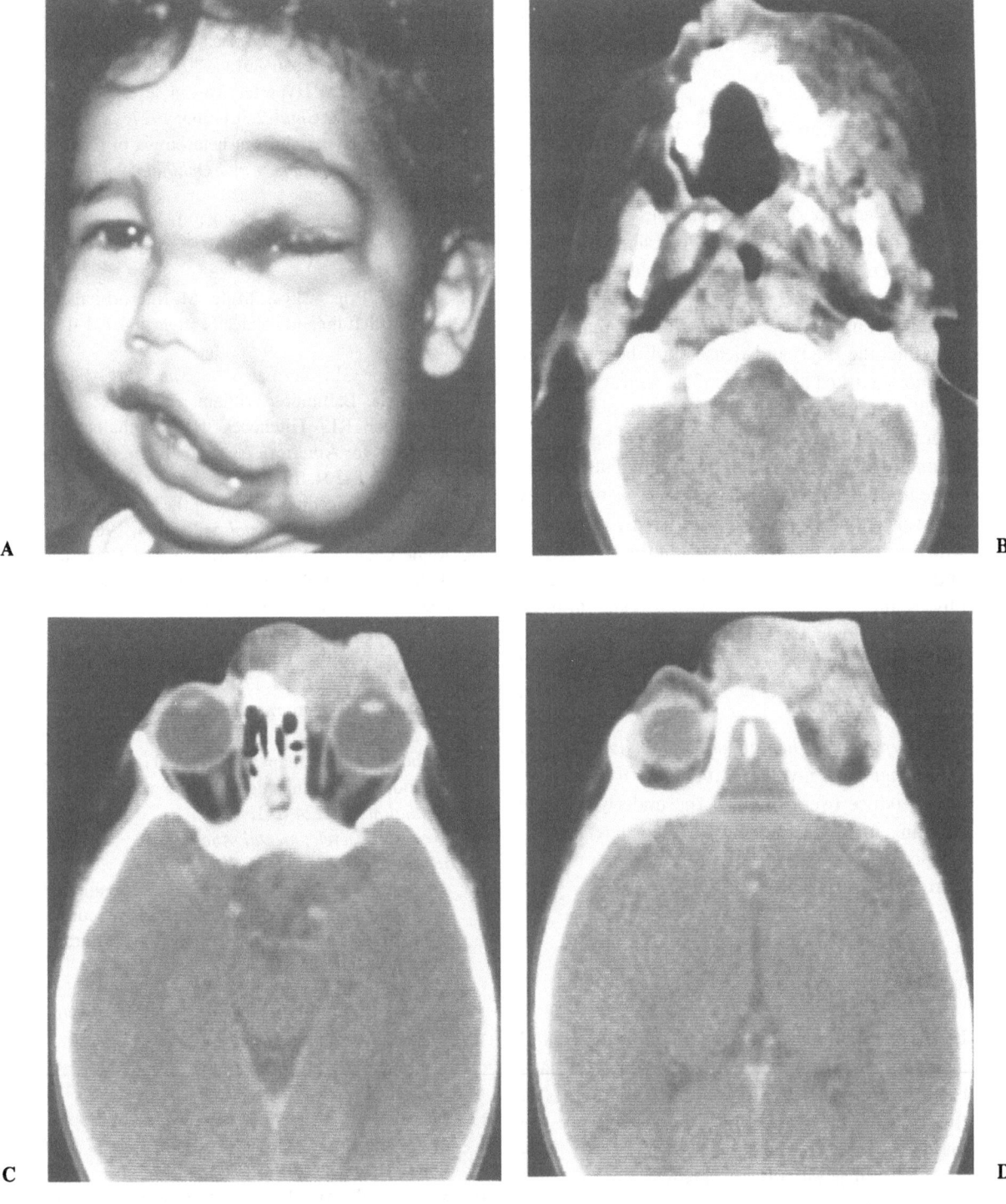

Figure 9.53. A. 17-month-old boy with progressive swelling of left side of face since birth. **B.** CT showing facial involvement with lymphangioma at level of the maxilla. **C.** CT showing the lymphangioma in front and medial to the globe displacing it downward and laterally. A deformity of the nasal bone is also present. **D.** CT showing the lymphangioma above the globe. Used with permission.

form. In newborn infants, it presents with anemia, pancytopenia, jaundice, hepatosplenomegaly, infections, and (possibly) early death. In the infantile form, a majority of the patients have optic atrophy and may have retinal degeneration. In older patients, cranial nerve palsies, progressive deafness, blindness, fractures, anemia, and osteomyelitis may be seen. The adult or benign form may be asymptomatic, but fractures and osteomyelitis may occur. Other reported abnormalities that are seen with osteopetrosis are choanal atresia, hypertelorism, flattened nose, renal tubular acidosis, vitamin D-resistant rickets, hypocalcemia, hyperphosphatemia, and tetany. The radiologic manifestations include thick and dense skull bones, which are most marked at the base. The neural foramina usually are narrowed, resulting in cranial palsies with blindness, deafness, and hydrocephalus. The paranasal sinuses are small or absent. The skeletal radiographic changes include either a uniformly dense skeleton or a generalized increase in density, with alternate radiolucent bands in the metaphyses and diaphyses of long bones, splaying of metaphyses and rib ends, "bone within bone" appearance, pathologic fractures, osteomyelitis, "sandwich" appearance of vertebral bodies, and delayed skeletal maturation (Fig. 9.50) (138, 151, 155, 254).

Hemangiomas, hemangiolymphangiomas, and lymphangiomas involving the face, if extensive, may produce overgrowth of the underlying bone resulting in facial deformity, which may be grotesque. Hemihypertrophy of the face also may be seen (Figs. 9.51, 9.52, 9.53).

Summary

In this chapter, many, but not all, of the congenital disorders that may involve the eye and orbit have been discussed briefly. The number of reports of these disorders is unending; therefore, only the major ones were discussed. The diagnosis of these disorders must include the history and physical findings. The imaging studies help by defining the abnormal anatomy, and thereby can aid in treatment planning. Currently, if we wish to show the anatomy of the globe and the orbital contents, CT scanning is used. Magnetic resonance imaging shows great promise for the future.

References

1. Aarskog D: A familial syndrome of short stature associated with facial dysplasia and genital anomalies. *J Pediatr* 77:856–861, 1970.
2. Abernethy DA: Hypertelorism in several generations. *Arch Dis Child* 2:361–365, 1927.
3. Acers TE: Hypertelorism, heterotopia of maculas and pseudo-exotropia. *Am J Ophthal* 59:494–495, 1965.
4. Adam RU, Lee SH, Truex RC Jr: Computed tomography in primary craniosynostosis. *CT* 4:125–131, 1980.
5. Aduss H, Pruzansky S, Miller M: Interorbital distance in cleft lip and palate. *Teratology* 4:171–182, 1971.
6. Alexander GL, Norman RM: *The Sturge-Weber Syndrome.* Baltimore, Williams & Wilkins, 1960.
7. Alexander RL, Hitchcock HP: Cephalometric standards for American Negro children. *Am J Orthod* 74:298–304, 1978.
8. Allen JC: Congenital absence of the lacrimal punctum. *J Pediatr Ophthalmol* 5:176–178, 1968.
9. Angle CR, McIntire MS, Moore RC: Cloverleaf skull: Kleeblattschadel deformity syndrome. *Am J Dis Child* 114:198–202, 1967.
10. Anyane-Yeboa K, Gunning L, Bloom AD: Baller-Gerold syndrome, craniosynostosis-radial aplasia syndrome. *Clin Genet* 17:161–166, 1980.
11. Apert ME: De l'acrocephalosyndactylie. *Bull Mem Soc Med Hop (Paris)* 23:1310–1330, 1906.
12. Archer DB, Deutman A, Ernest JT, et al: Arteriovenous communications of the retina. *Am J Ophthalmol* 75:224–241, 1973.
13. Arey LB: *Developmental Anatomy,* ed 6. Philadelphia, WB Saunders, 1970.
14. Armendares S, et al: A newly recognized inherited syndrome of dwarfism, craniosynostosis, retinitis pigmentosa, and multiple congenital malformations. *J Pediatr* 85:872–873, 1974.
15. Atkins L, Connely JP: XXXXY sex-chromosome abnormality. *Am J Dis Child* 106:514–519, 1963.
16. Axellson A, Brolin I, Engstrom H, et al: Dysostosis mandibulo-facialis. *J Laryngol Otol* 87:575–592, 1963.
17. Baccichetti C, Tenconi R: A new case of trisomy for the short arm of a No. 9 chromosome. *J Med Genet* 10:296–299, 1973.
18. Barmeir EP, Price HI, Danziger A: The value of computed tomography in tuberous sclerosis. *S Afr Med J* 57:583–585, 1980.
19. Bartsocus CS, Weber AL, Crawford JD: Acrocephalosyndactyly type 3: Chotzen's syndrome. *J Pediatr* 77:267–272, 1970.
20. Beard C: Congenital and hereditary abnormalities

·of the eyelids, lacrimal system, and orbit, in *Symposium on Surgical and Medical Management of Congenital Anomalies of the Eye*. Transactions of the New Orleans Academy of Ophthalmology, St Louis, CV Mosby, 1968.

21. Becker MH, Kopf AW, Lande A: Basal cell nevus syndrome: Report of four cases and review of the literature. *Am J Roentgenol* 99:817–825, 1967.

22. Becker MH, McCarthy JG, Genieser NB, et al: A proposed classification for craniofacial malformations. *Birth Defects* 10(7):171–175, 1974.

23. Becker MH, Finegold M, Genieser NB, et al: Campomelic dwarfism. *Birth Defects* II(6): 113–118, 1975.

24. Becker MH, Genieser NB, Finegold M, et al: Chondrodysplasia punctata. Is maternal warfarin therapy a factor? *Am J Dis Child* 129:356–359, 1975.

25. Becker MH, McCarthy JG, Chase N, et al: Computerized axial tomography of craniofacial malformations. *Am J Dis Child* 130:17–20, 1976.

26. Becker MH, Genieser NB, Goldman A: Tumorlike lesions, in Ranniger K: *Bone Tumors. Encyclopedia of Medical Radiology*. Berlin, Heidelberg, New York, Springer-Verlag, 1977, vol 5, part 6.

27. Beckerman BL: Lacrimal anomalies in anhidrotic ectodermal dysplasia. *Am J Ophthalmol* 75:728–730, 1973.

28. Beckwith JB: Macroglossia, omphalocele, adrenal cytomegaly, gigantism, and hyperplastic visceromegaly. *Birth Defects* 5(2):188–196, 1969.

29. Beighton P, Cremin BJ: *Sclerosing Bone Dysplasias*. Berlin, Springer-Verlag, 1980.

30. Beligere N, Harris V, Pruzansky S: Progressive bony dysplasia in Apert syndrome. *Radiology* 139:593–597, 1981.

31. Bell W, Van Allen M: Agenesis of the corpus callosum with associated facial anomalies. *Neurology (Minneap)* 9:694–698, 1959.

32. Ben-Hur N, Ashur H, Musseri M: An unusual case of median cleft lip with orbital hypotelorism—a missing link in the classification. *Cleft Palate Jr* 15:365–368, 1978.

33. Bergsma D: *Birth Defects Compendium*, ed 2. New York, Alan R Liss, 1979.

34. Berant W, Berant N: Radioulnar synostosis and craniosynostosis syndromes. *Birth Defects* II(2): 137–189, 1973.

35. Binder KH: Dysostosis maxillo-nasalis, ein arhinencephalar missbildungskomplex. *Dtsch Zahnarztl Z* 17:438–444, 1962.

36. Binet EF, Kieffer SA, Marin HS, et al: Orbital dysplasia in neurofibromatosis. *Radiology* 93:829–833, 1969.

37. Bixler D, Christian J, Gorlin R: Hypertelorism, microtia, and facial clefting: A new inherited syndrome. *Birth Defects Orig Art Series* 5(2):77–81, 1969.

38. Bixler D, Spivack J, Bennett J, et al: The ectrodactyly-ectodermal dysplasia-clefting (EEC) syndrome. *Clin Genet* 3:43–51, 1971.

39. Blank CE: Apert's syndrome (a type of acrocephalosyndactyly): Observations on a British series of thirty-nine cases. *Ann Hum Genet* 24:151–164, 1960.

40. Boniuk M: Eyelids, lacrimal apparatus, and conjunctiva. *Arch Ophthalmol* 88:91–105, 1972.

41. Borberg A: Clinical and genetic investigations in tuberous sclerosis and Recklinghausen's neurofibromatosis. *Acta Psychiatr Neurol* 71(Suppl):11–239, 1951.

42. Brill CB, Hsu LYF, Hirschhorn K: The syndrome of ectrodactyly ectodermal dysplasia and cleft lip and palate: Report of a family demonstrating a dominant inheritance pattern. *Clin Genet* 3:295–302, 1972.

43. Broadbent BH Sr, Broadbent BH Jr, Golden WH: *Bolton Standards of Dentofacial Developmental Growth*. St Louis, CV Mosby, 1975.

44. Brown LR, Coulam CM, Reese DF: Ataxia-telangiectasia (Louis-Bar syndrome). *Semin Roentgenol* 11:67–70, 1976.

45. Bunge R, Bradbury J: Two unilaterally cryptorchid boys with spermatogenic precocity in the descended testes, hypertelorism and polydactyly. *J Clin Endocrinol* 19:1103–1109, 1959.

46. Burck U, Langenstein I: CAT scan findings in clinically healthy relatives of tuberous sclerosis patients. *Eur J Pediatr* 135:117–118, 1980.

47. Burrows EH: Bone changes in orbital neurofibromatosis. *Br J Radiol* 36:549–561, 1963.

48. Carlson DH, Harris GBC: Craniometaphyseal dysplasia. *Radiology* 103:147–151, 1972.

49. Carmel PW, Luken MG, Ascherl GF: Craniosynostosis, CT evaluation of skull base and calvarial deformities. *Neurosurgery* 9:366–372, 1981.

50. Cassidy SB, Pagon RA, Pepin M, et al: Family studies in tuberous sclerosis. *JAMA* 249:1302–1309, 1983.

51. Christian J, Bixler D, Blythe S, et al: Familial telecanthus with associated congenital anomalies. *Birth Defects Orig Art Series* 5(2):82–85, 1969.

52. Clarren SK: Plagiocephaly and torticollis, etiology, natural history and helmet treatment. *J Pediat* 98:92–95, 1981.

53. Coccaro PJ, Becker MH, Converse JM: Clinical and radioscopic variations in hemifacial microsomia. *Birth Defects* 11(2):314–324, 1975.

54. Cohen MM Jr, Gorlin RJ, Berkman MS, et al: Facial variability in Apert type acrocephalosyndactyly. *Birth Defects* 7(7):143–152, 1971.

55. Cohen M, Sedano H, Gorlin R, et al: Frontonasal

dysplasia (median cleft face syndrome): Comments on etiology and pathogenesis. *Birth Defects Orig Art Series* 7(7):117–119, 1971.

56. Cohen MM Jr: Craniofrontonasal dysplasia, in O'Donnel JJ, Hall BD (eds): *Penetrance and Variability in Malformation Syndromes.* New York, Alan R. Liss, For The National Foundation—March of Dimes. 15(5B):85–89, 1979.

57. Cohen MM Jr: Craniosynostosis and syndromes with craniosynostosis: Incidence, genetics, penetrance, variability, and new syndrome updating. *Birth Defects* 15(5B):13–63, 1979.

58. Collins E, Turner G: The Noonan syndrome—a review of the clinical and genetic features of 27 cases. *J Pediatr* 83:941–950, 1973.

59. Converse JM, Smith B, Strong JO: Defects of the lacrimal apparatus, in Converse JM (ed): *Reconstructive plastic surgery.* Philadelphia, WB Saunders, 1964.

60. Converse JM, Coccaro PJ, Becker MH, et al: On hemifacial microsomia. The first and second branchial arch syndromes. *Plast Reconstr Surg* 51:268–279, 1973.

61. Converse JM, McCarthy JG Wood-Smith D: Orbital hypotelorism, pathogenesis, associated faciocerebral anomalies, surgical correction. *Plast Reconstr Surg* 56:389–395, 1975.

62. Costaras M, Pruzansky S, Broadbent BJ Jr: Bony interorbital distance (BIOD), head size, and level of the cribriform plate relative to orbital height: I. Normal standards for age and sex. *J Craniofac Genet Develop Biol* 2:5–18, 1982.

63. Costaros M, Pruzansky S: Bony interorbital distance (BIOD), head size, and level of the cribriform plate relative to orbital height: II. Possible pathogenesis of orbital hypertelorism. *J Craniofac Genet Develop Biol* 2:19–34, 1982.

64. Coulam CM, Brown LR, Reese DF: Sturge-Weber syndrome. *Semin Roentgenol* 11:55–60, 1976.

65. Coulam CM, Brown LR, Reese DF: Hippel-Lindau syndrome. *Semin Roentgenol* 11:61–66, 1976.

66. Crowe FW, Schull WJ, Neeb JV: *A Clinical, Pathological and Genetic Study of Multiple Neurofibromatosis.* Springfield, Ill, Charles C Thomas, 1948.

67. Crowe FW, Schull WJ: Diagnostic importance of cafe-au-lait spot in neurofibromatosis. *Arch Intern Med* 91:758–766, 1953.

68. Crouzon O: Dysostose cranio-faciale hereditaire. *Bull Soc Med Hop* (*Paris*) 33:545–555, 1912.

69. Currarino G, Silverman F: Orbital hypotelorism, arhinencephaly, and trigonocephaly. *Radiology* 74:206–217, 1960.

70. Danks DM, Tippett P, Adams C, et al: Cerebrohepatorenal syndrome of Zellweger *J Pediatr* 86:382–387, 1975.

71. Daves ML, Yardly JH: Fibrous dysplasia of bone. *Am J Med Sci* 234:590–606, 1957.

72. Davidson KC: Cranial and intracranial lesions in neurofibromatosis. *Am J Roentgenol* 98:550–556, 1966.

73. De Grouchy J, Salmon C, Salmon D, et al: Deletion of the short arm of a 13–15 chromosome, hypertelorism and HPO haptoglobin phenotype in the same family. *Ann Genet Paris* 9:80–85, 1966.

74. De Grouchy J: The 18p-, 18q- and 18r syndromes. *Birth Defects Orig Art Series* 5(5):74–87, 1969.

75. De Hauwere R, Leroy J, Adriaenssens K, et al: Iris dysplasia, orbital hypertelorism, and psychomotor retardation: A dominantly inherited developmental syndrome. *J Pediatr* 82:679–681, 1973.

76. Dekaban AS: Tables of cranial and orbital measurements, canial volume, and derived indexes in males and females from 7 days to 20 years of age. *Ann Neurol* 2:485–491, 1977.

77. De Myer W: The median cleft face syndrome. *Neurology* 17:961–971, 1967.

78. De Myer W, Zeman W: Alobar holoprosencephaly (arhinencephaly) with median cleft lip and palate: clinical, electroencephalographic and nosologic considerations. *Confin Neurol* (*Basel*) 23:1–36, 1963.

79. De Myer W: The median cleft face syndrome. Differential diagnosis of cranium bifidum occultum, hypertelorism, and median cleft nose, lip and palate. *Neurology* 17:961–971, 1967.

80. De Myer W: Megalencephaly in children. *Neurology* 22:634–643, 1972.

81. De Myer W: Median facial malformations and their implications for brain malformations. *Birth Defects Orig Art Series* 11(7):155–181, 1975.

82. De Myer W: Neurologic evaluation, associated forebrain maldevelopment, and orbital hypotelorism, in Converse JM, McCarthy JG, Wood-Smith D (eds): *Symposium on Diagnosis and Treatment of Craniofacial Anomalies.* St Louis, CV Mosby, 1979.

83. Dominguez R, Oh SK, Bender T, et al: Uncomplicated trigonocephaly. *Radiology* 140:681–688, 1981.

84. Downs WB: Variations in facial relationships: Their significance in treatment and prognosis. *Am J Orthod* 34:812, 1948.

85. Drummond RA: A determination of cephalometric norms for the Negro race. *Am J Orthod* 54:670–682, 1968.

86. Dubowitz V: Familial low birthweight dwarfism with an unusual facies and skin eruptions. *J Med Genet* 2:12–17, 1965.

87. Duggan CA, Keever EB, Gay BB: Secondary craniosynostosis. *Am J Roentgenol* 109:277–293, 1970.

88. Duke-Elder S, Wybar KC: *System of Ophthalmology: The Anatomy of the Visual System.* St Louis, CV Mosby, 1961, vol II.

89. Duke-Elder S, Cook C: *System of Ophthalmology: Normal and Abnormal Development. Part I, Embryology.* St Louis, CV Mosby, 1963, vol III.

90. Duke-Elder S, Cook C: *System of Ophthalmology: Normal and Abnormal Development. Part 2, Congenital Deformities.* St Louis, CV Mosby, 1963, vol III.

91. Edeiken J, Hodes RJ: *Roentgen Diagnosis of Diseases of Bone.* Baltimore, Williams & Wilkins, 1967.

92. Ehlers N: Crytophthalmos with orbitopalpebral cyst and microphthalmos. *Acta Ophthalmol* 44:84–94, 1966.

93. Elsahy NI, Waters WR: The branchio-skeletogenital syndrome. A new hereditary syndrome. *Plast Reconstr Surg* 58:542–550, 1971.

94. Erich JB: Nasal duplication. Report of case of patient with two noses. *Plast Reconstr Surg* 29:159–166, 1962.

95. Evans CA, Christiansen RL: Cephalic malformation in Saethre-Chotzen syndrome. *Radiology* 121:399–403, 1976.

96. Falchi G, Gerlini F: Ipertelorismo di Greig. *Lattante* 30:202–215, 1959.

97. Faure C, Bonamy P, Rambert-Misset C: Craniostenosis from premature unilateral fusion of the coronal suture. *Ann Radiol* 10:32–42, 1967.

98. Feingold M, O'Conner JF, Berkman M, et al: Kleeblattschadel syndrome. *Am J Dis Child* 118:589–594, 1969.

99. Feingold M, Bossert W: Normal values for selected physical parameters: An aid to syndrome delineation. *Birth Defects Orig Art Series* (10):1–16, 1974.

100. Fernandez AO, Ronis ML: The Treacher-Collins syndrome. *Arch Otolaryngol* 80:505–520, 1964.

101. Ferrari I, Hering S: Case report: reciprocal translocation, t(1p–; 17q+), in a patient with multiple anomalies. *Birth Defects Orig Art Series* 5(5):132–135, 1969.

102. Figalova P, Hajnis K, Smahel Z: The interocular distance in children with clefts before the operation. *Acta Chir Plast (Praha)* 16:65–77, 1974.

103. Firmin F, Coccaro PJ, Converse JM: Cephalometric analysis in diagnosis and treatment planning of craniofacial dysostoses. *Plast Reconstr Surg* 54:300–311, 1974.

104. Fitz CR, Harwood-Nash DCF, Thompson JR: Neuroradiology of tuberous sclerosis in children. *Radiology* 110:635–642, 1974.

105. Forabosco A, Dutrillaux B, Tont G, et al: Translocation equilibree t(2; 13) (q32; q33) familiare et trisomie 2q partielle. *Ann Genet* 16:255–258, 1973.

106. Franceschetti A, Klein D: The mandibulo-facial dysostosis, a new hereditary syndrome. *Acta Ophthalmol* 27:141–224, 1949.

107. Francois J: Ocular aspects of the phakomatoses, in Vinken PJ, Bruyn GW: *Handbook of Clinical Neurology: The Phakomatoses.* New York, American Elsevier Publishing Co, Inc, 1972, vol 14, chap 22.

108. Freund M: Hypertelorisme et autres malformations congenitales dans une famille. *Genet Hum* 21:237–278, 1973.

109. Fries JW: The roentgen features of fibrous dysplasia of the skull and facial bones. *Am J Roentgenol* 77:71–88, 1957.

110. Frosini R, Papini M, Campana G, et al: Contribution of computerized tomography to the study of severe congenital ocular dysplasias. *Ophthalmologica (Basel)* 183:72–76, 1981.

111. Furukawa C, Hall B, Smith D: The Aarskog syndrome. *J Pediatr* 81:1117–1122, 1972.

112. Garcia CJ: Cephalometric evaluation of Mexican Americans using the Downs and Steiner analyses. *Am J Orthod* 68:67–74, 1975.

113. Garrick R, Gomez MR, Hauser OW: Demyelination of the brain in tuberous sclerosis: computed tomography evidence. *Mayo Clin Proc* 54:685–689, 1979.

114. Gass JDM: Orbital and ocular involvement in fibrous dysplasia. *South Med J* 58:324–329, 1965.

115. Gates GF, Dore EK: Detection of the craniosynostosis by bone scanning. *Radiology* 115:665–671, 1975.

116. Gerald B, Silverman F: Normal and abnormal interorbital distances, with special reference to mongolism. *Am J Roentgenol* 95:154–161, 1965.

117. Goldberg MF: Waardenburg's syndrome with fundus and other anomalies. *Arch Ophthalmol* 76:797–810, 1966.

118. Goldenhar M: Associations malformations de l'oeil et de l'oreille, en particulier le syndrome dermoide epibulbar-appendices auriculaires-fistula auris congenita et ses relations avec la dysostose mandibulofaciale. *J Genet Hum* 1:243–282, 1952.

119. Gorlin RJ, Vickers RA, Kellin E, et al: The multiple basal cell nevi syndrome. An analysis of a syndrome consisting of multiple nevoid basal cell carcinoma, jaw cysts, skeletal anomalies, medulloblastoma, and hyporesponsiveness to parathormone. *Cancer* 18:89–104, 1965.

120. Gorlin RJ: Genetic craniotubular bone dysplasias and hyperostoses. *Birth Defects* 5(4):79–95, 1969.

121. Gorlin R, Anderson R, Blaw M: Multiple lentigines syndrome. *Am J Dis Child* 117:652–662, 1969.

122. Gorlin R, Cervenka J, Pruzansky S: Facial clefting and its syndromes. *Birth Defects Orig Art Series* 7(7):3–49, 1971.

123. Gorlin RJ, Pindborg JJ, Cohen MM Jr: *Syndromes of the Head and Neck,* ed 2. New York, McGraw-Hill, 1976.

124. Green GJ: The radiology of tuberose sclerosis. *Clin Radiol* 19:135–147, 1968.

125. Greig D: Hypertelorism. A hitherto undifferenti-

ated congenital deformity. *Edinb Med J* 31:560–593, 1924.

126. Gros C, Sacrez R, Levy J, et al: Hypertelorisme avec malformations cranio-faciales encephaliques et vertebrales multiples. *J Radiol Electrol* 44:635–638, 1963.

127. Grosse F, Hermann J, Opitz J: The F-form of acro-pectorovertebral dysplasia: The F-syndrome. *Birth Defects Orig Art Series* 5(3):48–63, 1969.

128. Hall BD, Spranger JW: Campomelic dysplasia. *Am J Dis Child* 134:285–289, 1980.

129. Hamilton WJ, Boyd JD, Mossman HW: *Human Embryology: Development of Form and Function*, ed 3. Baltimore, Williams & Wilkins, 1962.

130. Hansman C: Growth of interorbital distance and skull thickness as observed in roentgenographic measurements. *Radiology* 86:87–96, 1966.

131. Harley RD: Pediatric Ophthalmology, ed 2. Philadelphia, WB Saunders, 1983, chap 2.

132. Harris WH, Dudly HR, Barry JR: The natural history of fibrous dysplasia. *J Bone Joint Surg* 44A:207–233, 1962.

133. Harwood-Nash DC: Coronal synostosis, in Rogers LF (ed): *Disorders of the Head and Neck Syllabus. Second Series*. Chicago, American College of Radiology, 1977.

134. Herberts G: Otological observations on the Treacher-Collins syndrome. *Acta Otolaryngol* 54:457–465, 1962.

135. Herring SW, Rowlatt UF, Pruzansky S: Anatomical abnormalities in mandibulofacial dysostosis. *Am J Med Genet* 3:225–259, 1979.

136. Hinds EC, Kent JN: *Surgical Treatment of Developmental Jaw Deformities*. St Louis, CV Mosby, 1972.

137. Hogan GR, Bauman ML: Hydrocephalus in Apert's syndrome. *J Pediatr* 79:782–787, 1971.

138. Holmes L, Moser H, Halldorsson S, et al: *Mental Retardation. An Atlas of Diseases with Associated Physical Abnormalities*. New York, Macmillan, 1972.

139. Holt JF, Wright EM: Radiologic features of neurofibromatosis. *Radiology* 51:647–663, 1948.

140. Holt JF, Dickerson WW: The osseous lesions of tuberous sclerosis. *Radiology* 58:1–7, 1952.

141. Holt JF: The evolution of cranio-metaphyseal dysplasia. *Ann Radiol (Paris)* 9:209–224, 1966.

142. Holt JF: Neurofibromatosis in children. *Am J Roentgenol* 130:615–639, 1978.

143. Hozay J: Sur une dystrophie familiale particuliere. *Rev Neurol* 89:245–258, 1953.

144. Hsia YE, Vanitha-Appadorai BM, Roy Breg W, et al: Chromosomal abnormality (46xx, 3p+) in a case of Meckel syndrome. *Birth Defects* 10(8):19–25, 1974.

145. Hunt JC, Pugh DG: Skeletal lesions in neurofibromatosis. *Radiology* 76:1–20, 1961.

146. Hustimix W, Terhaar B, Scheres J, et al: Trisomy for the short arm of chromosome No. 10. *Clin Genet* 6:408–415, 1974.

147. Jaffe B, Welch K, Strand R, et al: Cerebrospinal fluid rhinorrhea via the fossa of Rosenmuller. *Laryngoscope* 86:903–907, 1976.

148. Jaffe HL: Fibrous dysplasia of bone. *Bull NY Acad Med* 22:588–604, 1946.

149. James W, Belcourt C, Atkins L, et al: Trisomy 13–15. *Radiology* 92:44–49, 1969.

150. Jarmas AL, Weaver DD, Ellis FS, et al: Microcephaly, microphthalmia, falciform retinal folds, and blindness. *Am J Dis Child* 135:930–934, 1981.

151. Johnston CC Jr, Lavy N, Lord T, et al: Osteopetrosis. *Medicine* 47:149–167, 1968.

152. Kanthak FF, Hamm WG, Yaru CP: Fibrous dysplasia of facial bones. *Plast Reconstr Surg* 15:41–55, 1955.

153. Kawamoto HK Jr: The kaleidoscopic world of rare craniofacial clefts. *Clin Plas Surg* 3:529–572, 1976.

154. Keats T: Ocular hypertelorism (Greig's syndrome) associated with Sprengel's deformity. *Am J Roentgenol* 110:119–122, 1970.

155. Keith CG: Retinal atrophy in osteopetrosis. *Arch Ophthalmol* 79:234–241, 1968.

156. Kennedy RE: The effect of early enucleation on the orbit in animals and humans. *Am J Ophthal* 60:277–306, 1965.

157. Khudr G, Olding L: Cyclopia. *Am J Dis Child* 125:120–122, 1973.

158. Kirk RC: Developmental anomalies of the lacrimal passages. *Am J Ophthal* 42:227–232, 1956.

159. Kirkpatrick JA, Capitanio MA: Radiology of the orbit in infancy and childhood. *Rad Clin North Am* 10:143–166, 1972.

160. Klatte EC, Franken EA, Smith JA: The radiographic spectrum in neurofibromatosis. *Semin Roentgenol* 11:17–33, 1976.

161. Kleinman P: Congenital lymphedema and yellow nails. *J Pediatr* 83:454–456, 1973.

162. Korchmaros L: Contralateral rhinostomy for dacryocystitis due to facial malformation. *Acta Ophthalmol* 50:390–391, 1972.

163. Korting G, Ruther H: Ichthyosis vulgaris und akro-faciale dysostose. *Arch Belg Derm Syph* 197:91–104, 1954.

164. Kreiborg S, Pruzansky S, Paskayan H: The Saethre-Chotzen syndrome. *Teratology* 6:287–294, 1972.

165. Ladenheim J, Metrick S: Congenital microphthalmos and cyst. *Am J Ophthal* 41:1059–1962, 1956.

166. Laestadius N, Aase J, Smith D: Normal inner canthal and outer orbital dimensions. *J Pediatr* 74:465–468, 1969.

167. Langdon J: Rieger's syndrome. *Oral Surg* 30:788–795, 1970.

168. Langman J: *Medical Embryology*, ed 2. Baltimore, Williams & Wilkins, 1969.

169. La Piana FG: Management of occult atretic lacrimal puncta. *Am J Ophthal* 74:332–333, 1972.

170. Leck J, Rogers SC: Changes in the incidence of anencephalus. *Br J Prevent Soc Med* 21:177–180, 1967.

171. Lee BCP, Gawlew J: Tuberous sclerosis: Comparison of computed tomography and conventional neuroradiology. *Radiology* 127:403–407, 1978.

172. Lee FA: Radiology of the Beckwith-Wiedemann syndrome. *Radiol Clin North Am* 10:261–276, 1972.

173. Leeds N, Seaman WB: Fibrous dysplasia of the skull and its differential diagnosis. *Radiology* 78:570–583, 1962.

174. Leiber B, Olbrich G: *Die klinischen Syndrome.* Munich, Urban & Schwarzenbert, 1972.

175. Lejeune J, Lafourcade J, Berger R, et al: Le Phenotype Dr; Etude de trois cas de chromosomes D en anneau. *Ann Genet (Paris)* 2:79–87, 1968.

176. Lowe R: The eyes in mongolism. *Br J Ophthal* 33:131–174, 1949.

177. Lowry RB: Congenital absence of the fibula and craniosynostosis in sibs. *J Med Genet* 9:227–229, 1972.

178. MacGillivray R: Hypertelorism with unusual associated anomalies. *Am J Ment Defic* 62:288–291, 1957.

179. McKusick KA, Malomud L, Korrdela P: Radionuclide cisternography. *J Nucl Med* 14:933–934, 1973.

180. Mafee MF, Valvassoro GE: Radiology of the craniofacial anomalies. *Otolaryngol Clin North Am* 14:939–988, 1981.

181. Mahindra S, Dalgit R, Jamwal N, et al: Lateral nasal proboscis. *J Laryngol Otol* 87:177–181, 1973.

182. Maki Y, Enomoto T, Maruyama H, et al: Computed tomography in tuberous sclerosis. *Brain Development* 1:38–48, 1979.

183. Mann I: *Developmental Abnormalities of the Eye.* London, Cambridge University Press, 1937.

184. Mann I: *Developmental Abnormalities of the Eye,* ed 2. Philadelphia, JB Lippincott, 1957.

185. Mann I: *The Development of the Human Eye,* ed 3. London, British Medical Association, 1964.

186. Marsh JL, Gado M: Surgical anatomy of craniofacial dysostoses: Insights from CT scans. *Cleft Palate J* 19:212–221, 1982.

187. Medley BE, McLeod RA, Houser OW: Tuberous sclerosis. *Semin Roentgenol* 11:35–54, 1976.

188. Michaelis E, Mortier W: Association of hypertelorism and hypospadias—the BBB-syndrome. *Helv Paediatr Acta* 27:575–581, 1972.

189. Miller JQ: Mental retardation and hypertelorism in chromosome deletion studies. *Neurology* 23:1141–1146, 1973.

190. Miller O, Warburton D, Breg W: Deletions of group B chromosomes. *Birth Defects Orig Art Series* 5(5):100–105, 1969.

191. Ming-Kuang GG: Cephalometric standards of Steiner analysis established on Chinese children. *J Formosan Med Assn* 70:97–102, 1971.

192. Miura F, Inoue N, Suzuki K: Cephalometric standards for Japanese according to the Steiner analysis. *Am J Orthod* 51:288–295, 1965.

193. Moss M: Hypertelorism and cleft palate deformity. *Acta Anat* 61:547–557, 1965.

194. Munro IR, Das SK: Improving results in orbital hypertelorism correction. *Ann Plastic Surg* 2:499–507, 1979.

195. Murken J, Bauchinger M, Palitzsch D, et al: Trisomie D_2 bei einem 2½ jahrigen Madchen (47, XX, 14+). *Humangenetik* 10:254–268, 1970.

196. Mustarde JC: Epicanthus and telecanthus. *Br J Plast Surg* 16:346–356, 1963.

197. Nathan MH, Newman A: The skewed nasal septum. A pathognomonic sign of premature unilateral coronal suture stenosis. *Br J Radiol* 43:139–141, 1970.

198. Newton TH, Potts DG (eds): *Radiology of the Skull and Brain.* St. Louis, CV Mosby, 1971, vol 1, book 1.

199. Newton TH, Potts DG: *Radiology of the Skull and Brain. The Skull.* St Louis, CV Mosby, 1971, vol 1, book 2.

200. Niederle J: Dunndarmagenesie mit multiplen Fehlbildungen. *Arch Kinderheilk* 179:187–193, 1969.

201. Nishirmura H, Takano K, Tanimura T, et al: Normal and abnormal development of human embryos. First report of the analysis of 1,213 intact embryos. *Teratology* 1:281–290, 1968.

202. Noel B, Moffett J, Nantors Y, et al: Contribution to the identification of the small supernumerary submetacentric chromosome in Cat's eyes syndrome. *J Genet Hum* 21:23–32, 1973.

203. Noonan J: Hypertelorism with Turner phenotype. A new syndrome with associated congenital heart disease. *Amer J Dis Child* 116:373–380, 1968.

204. Norman AP: *Congenital Abnormalities in Infancy,* ed 2. Oxford, Edinburgh, Black 2311 Scientific Publications, 1971.

205. Opitz J, Frias J, Gutenberger J, et al: The G syndrome of multiple congenital anomalies. *Birth Defects Orig Art Series* 5(2):95–101, 1969.

206. Opitz J, Summitt R, Smith D: The BBB syndrome. Familial telecanthus with associated congenital anomalies. *Birth Defects Orig Art Series* 5(2):86–94, 1969.

207. Pashayan H, Pruzansky S, Putterman A: A family with blepharo-naso-facial malformation syndrome. *Am J Dis Child* 125:389–393, 1973.

208. Patten BM: *Human Embryology,* ed 3. New York, McGraw-Hill, 1968.

209. Pavsek EJ: Mandibulofacial dysostosis (Treacher Collins syndrome). *Am J Roentgenol* 79:598–602, 1958.

210. Peterson M, Cohen M, Sedana H, et al: Comments on fronto-nasal dysplasia, ocular hypertelorism and dystopia canthorum. *Birth Defects Orig Art Series* 7(7):120–124, 1971.

211. Peterson SJ, Pruzansky S: Palatal anomalies in the syndromes of Apert and Crouzon. *Cleft Palate J* 11:394–403, 1974.

212. Pfeiffer R: Beitrag zum Erscheinungsbild der XXXXY-constitution. *Z Kinderheilk* 87:356–369, 1962.

213. Pfeiffer RA: Dominant erbliche akrocephalosyndakylie. *Z Kinderheilk* 90:301–320, 1964.

214. Pfeiffer RA: Associated deformities of the head and hands. *Birth Defects* 5(3):18–34, 1969.

215. Pico G: Congenital anomalies of the lacrimal system, in Veirs ER (ed): *The Lacrimal System: Proceedings of the First International Symposium.* St Louis, CV Mosby, 1970.

216. Pico G, Townsend W: Congenital and developmental anomalies of the orbit, in Duane TD (ed): *Clinical Ophthalmology.* Hagerstown, Harper & Row, 1976, vol 2, chap 30.

217. Pollock JA, Newton TH, Hoyt WF: Transsphenoidal and transethmoidal encephaloceles. *Radiology* 90:442–453, 1968.

218. Pritchard JE: Fibrous dysplasia of the bones. *Am J Med Sci* 222:313–332, 1951.

219. Pruzansky S, Pashayan H, Kreiborg S, et al: Roentgencephalometric studies of the premature craniofacial synostosis: Report of a family with the Saethre-Chotzen syndrome. *Birth Defects* 11(2):226–237, 1975.

220. Pruzansky S, Costaras M, Rollnick BR: Radiocephalometric finding in a family with craniofronto-nasal dysplasia. *Birth Defects Orig Art Series* 18(1):121–138, 1982.

221. Pryor H: Objective measurement of interpupillary distance. *Pediatrics* 44:973–977, 1969.

222. Punnett HH, Harley RD: Genetics in pediatric ophthalmology, in Harley PD (ed): *Pediatric Ophthalmology,* ed 2. Philadelphia, WB Saunders, 1983.

223. Putterman A: Treatment of epiphora with absent lacrimal puncta. *Arch Ophthalmol* 89:125–127, 1973.

224. Putterman M, Pashayan H, Pruzansky S: Eye findings in the blepharo-naso-facial malformation syndrome. *Am J Ophthalmol* 76:825–831, 1973.

225. Reich E, Cox RP, Becker MH, et al: Recognition in adult patients of malformations induced by folic-acid antagonists. *Birth Defects Orig Art Series* 14(6B): 139–160, 1978.

226. Reich EW, Cox RP, McCarthy JG, et al: A new heritable syndrome with frontonasal dysplasia and

227. Reznik M, Alberca-Serrano R: Familial form of hypertelorism associated with lissencephalia with the clinical picture of a form of mental retardation associated with epilepsy and spastic paraplegia. *J Neurol Sci* 1:40–58, 1964.

associated extracranial anomalies (abstract), in Littlefield JW (ed): *Fifth International Conference on Birth Defects.* Amsterdam, Excerpta Medica, 1977.

228. Riolo ML, Moyers RE, McNamara JA, et al: *An Atlas of Craniofacial Growth.* Ann Arbor, Center for Human Growth and Development, University of Michigan, 1974.

229. Robinow M, Pfeiffer RA, Gorlin RJ, et al: Acrodysostosis: A syndrome of peripheral dysostosis, nasal kypoplasia and mental retardation. *Am J Dis Child* 121:195–203, 1971.

230. Robinow M, Silverman F, Smith H: A newly recognized dwarfing syndrome. *Am J Dis Child* 117:645–651, 1969.

231. Rogers BO: Berry-Treacher Collins syndrome: A review of 200 cases. *Br J Plast Surg* 17:109–137, 1964.

232. Rogers BO: Rare craniofacial deformities, in Converse JM (ed): *Reconstructive Plastic Surgery: The Head and Neck.* Philadelphia, WB Saunders, 1964, vol III.

233. Roubicek M, Spranger J, Wende S: Frontonasal dysplasia as an expression of holoprosencephaly. *Eur J Pediatr* 137:229–251, 1981.

234. Salvolini U, Pasquini U, Babin E, et al: Von Recklinghausen's disease and computed tomography. *J Belg Radiol* 61:313–318, 1978.

235. Schauerte EW, St-Albin PM: Progressive synostosis in Apert's syndrome (acrocephalo-syndactyly) with description of roentgenographic changes in feet. *Am J Roentgenol* 97:67–73, 1966.

236. Schwartz PI, Beards JA, Maris PJG: Tuberous sclerosis associated with a retinal angioma. *Am J Ophthalmol* 90:485–488, 1980.

237. Sedano H, Cohen M, Jirasek J, et al: Frontonasal dysplasia. *J Pediatr* 76:906–913, 1970.

238. Sedano H, Look R, Carter C, et al: B group short-arm deletion syndromes. *Birth Defects Orig Art Series* 7(7):89–97, 1971.

239. Seelenfreund M, Gartner S: Acrocephalosyndactyly (Apert's syndrome). *Arch Ophthal* 78:8–11, 1967.

240. Shiller JG: Craniofacial dysostosis of Crouzon. A case report and pedigree with emphasis on heredity. *Pediatrics* 23:107–112, 1959.

241. Siedband G: Roentgen-study of the development of the frontal sinus and the interorbital distance in the half-axial view during infancy and childhood. *Ann Paediatr (Basel)* 206:175–187, 1966.

242. Slover R, Sujansky E: Frontonasal dysplasia with coronal craniosynostosis in three sibs, in O'Donnell JJ, Hall BD (eds): *Penetrance and Variability in*

Malformation Syndromes. New York, Alan R. Liss for the National Foundation—March of Dimes, BD: OASXV (5B) 1979, pp 75–83.

243. Smith B, Valauri AJ: Anophthalmia and microphthalmia, in Converse JM: *Reconstructive Plastic Surgery.* Philadelphia, WB Saunders, 1964, vol II.

244. Smith DW: *Recognizable Patterns of Human Malformation.* Philadelphia, WB Saunders, 1970.

245. Sotos JF, Dodge PR, Muirhead D, et al: Cerebral gigantism in childhood. *N Engl J Med* 271:109–116, 1964.

246. Spranger J, Paulsen K, Lehmann W: Die kraniometaphysare dysplasie (Pyle). *Z Kinderheilk* 93:64–79, 1965.

247. Spranger JW, Opitz JM, Bidder U: Heterogeneity of chondrodysplasia punctata. *Humangenetik* 11:190–212, 1971.

248. Steiner CC: Cephalometrics in clinical practice. *Angle Orthod* 29:8–29, 1959.

249. Sugiura Y, Yasuhara T: Sclerosteosis. *J Bone Joint Surg* 57A:273–276, 1975.

250. Summitt RL: Recessive acrocephalosyndactyly with normal intelligence. *Birth Defects* 5(3):35–38, 1969.

251. Tait MV, Gilday DL, Ash JM, et al: Craniosynostosis correlation of bone scans, radiographs and surgical findings. *Radiology* 133:615–621, 1979.

252. Tan K: The metopic fontanelle. *Am J Dis Child* 124:211–214, 1972.

253. Tay C: Porencephaly, nasofrontal mucoceles, hypertelorism and segmental vitiligo. Report of a new neurocutaneous disorder. *Singapore Med J* 11:253–257, 1970.

254. Taybi H: *Radiology of Syndromes and Metabolic Disorders,* ed 2. Chicago, Year Book Publishers, 1983.

255. Taylor WO: Effect of enucleation of one eye in childhood on subsequent development of the face. *Trans Ophthal Soc* 59:361–371, 1939.

256. Tchang SPK: The small orbit sign in supraorbital fibrous dysplasia. *J Can Assoc Radiol* 24:65–69, 1973.

257. Temtamy SA: Carpenter's syndrome: Acrocephalopolysyndactyly. An autosomal recessive syndrome. *J Pediatr* 69:111–120, 1966.

258. Tessier P: The definite plastic surgical treatment of the severe facial deformities of craniofacial dysostosis, Crouzon's and Apert's diseases. *Plast Reconst Surg* 48:419–442, 1971.

259. Tessier P: Orbital hypertelorism. I. Successive surgical attempts, material and methods. Causes and mechanisms. *Scand J Plast Reconstr Surg* 6:135–155, 1972.

260. Tessier P, Callahan A, Mustarde JC, et al: *Symposium on Plastic Surgery in the Orbital Region.* St Louis, CV Mosby, 1976.

261. Tessier P, Hervouet F, Lekieffre M, et al: *Plastic Surgery of the Orbit and Eyelids.* New York, Paris, Masson, 1981.

262. Tost M: Beitrag zur hereditaren Mikroblepharie *Wiss Z Univ Rostock 18 Math-Nat Reihe* 9:1107–1108, 1969.

263. Ulivelli A, Silenzi M: Hypertelorism and Waardenburg's syndrome. *Helv Paediat Acta* 24:123–126, 1969.

264. Villaverde M, Da Silva J: Soto's syndrome—hypertelorism, antimongoloid slant of eye, and high arched palate complex. *J Med Soc New Jersey* 68:805–808, 1971.

265. Vinken PJ, Bruyn GW: *Handbook of Clinical Neurology: Congenital Malformations of the Brain and Skull.* Amsterdam, New York, Oxford, North Holland Publishing Co, 1977, vol 31, part II.

266. Von Recklinghausen FD: *Uber die multiplen Fibrome der Haut und ihre Beziehung zu den multiplen Nueromen: Festschrift fur Rudolf Virchow.* Berlin, August Hirshwald, 1882.

267. Wagner EJ, Rao KCVG, Knipp HC: CT angiographic correlation in Sturge-Weber syndrome. *Computed Tomography* 5:324–327, 1981.

268. Welch K, Naheedy MH, Abroms IF, et al: Computed tomography of Sturge-Weber syndrome in infants. *J Comput Assist Tomogr* 4:33–36, 1980.

269. Whitnall SE: *Anatomy of the Human Orbit and Assessory Organs of Vision,* ed 2. London, Toronto, New York, Oxford University Press, 1932.

270. Williams JP, Secrist L, Fowler GW, et al: Roentgenographic features of the cerebro-hepatorenal syndrome of Zellweger. *Am J Roentgenol* 115:607–610, 1972.

271. Wolff E: *Anatomy of the Eye and Orbit,* ed 6. Philadelphia, Toronto, WB Saunders, 1968.

272. Wyburn-Mason R: Ateriovenous aneurysm of mid-brain and retina, facial naevi and mental changes. *Brain* 66:163–203, 1943.

273. Zide B, Grayson B, McCarthy JG: Cephalometric analysis. *Plast Reconstr Surg* 68:816–823, 1981.

274. Zizmor J, Lombardi G: *Atlas of Orbital Radiography.* Birmingham, Aescalysius Pub, 1973.

10
Evaluation of Exophthalmos and Thyroid Ophthalmopathy

THADDEUS S. NOWINSKI and JOSEPH C. FLANAGAN

Exophthalmos is a condition that is often seen by ophthalmologists. A thorough physical examination is not sufficient to establish a specific diagnosis and its etiology. Diagnostic imaging, especially computed tomography (CT), is especially helpful in the study of orbital disease; its use helps to avoid unnecessary surgical explorations.

While the terms exophthalmos and proptosis have been used interchangeably, the term proptosis (Greek meaning fall forward) is defined as a forward displacement or bulging. Exophthalmos is an abnormal prominence of one or both eyes, which usually is secondary to orbital inflammation, tumor, vascular disorder, or thyroid ophthalmopathy (Graves' disease). The most common cause of unilateral and bilateral exophthalmos is thyroid ophthalmopathy (4, 5, 6, 12).

A number of clinical entities may simulate exophthalmos. Pseudoexophthalmos is either the simulation of an abnormal prominence of the eye or a true prominence that is not secondary to orbital inflammation, tumor, or vascular disorder (Table 10.1). Many causes of pseudoexophthalmos may be eliminated by a thorough ocular history and physical examination.

A detailed history can give many clues to the etiology of exophthalmos. The patient's age probably is the most important single factor (Table 10.2). Duration and rate of progression of symptoms are also important. Rapidly progressing orbital disease generally signifies infection, acute inflammation, or malignancy, whereas chronic inflammations or benign tumors tend to progress slowly. The presence of constitutional symptoms may point to an endocrine abnormality or pseudotumor.

The medical history should exclude the presence of tumors elsewhere in the body, since metastases

Table 10.1. Pseudoexophthalmos

Enlarged globe
Myopia
Buphthalmos
Congenital cystic eye
Eyelid or palpebral-fissure asymmetry
Lid retraction
Ptosis
Seventh-nerve palsy
Postsurgical effect
Extraocular muscle abnormality
Weakness
Paralysis
Shallow or asymmetric bony orbits
Contralateral enophthalmitis
Metastatic breast carcinoma
Orbital floor fracture
Congenital bone defect

of the breast or malignant melanoma of the skin may occur years after initial treatment. Heavy cigarette smoking may raise suspicion of a lung carcinoma, which may metastasize to the orbit before discovery of the primary lesion. Past trauma may have resulted in a carotid-cavernous fistula or formation of a blood cyst. A history of sinus disorders may herald sinusitis, extension of a tumor, or expansion of a mucocele. Exophthalmos may be associated with a systemic syndrome (Table 10.3).

Orbital Disorders Associated with Exophthalmos in Adults and Children

There are many causes of unilateral exophthalmos in childhood, including cellulitis, benign tumors, malignant tumors, and idiopathic inflammatory pseudotumor. Orbital cellulitis, usually extending

Table 10.2. Common Orbital Disorders Associated with Exophthalmos

Children	Adults
Orbital cellulitis	Graves' ophthalmopathy
Dermoid and epidermoid cysts	Pseudotumor
Capillary hemangioma	Cavernous hemangioma
Rhabdomyosarcoma	Lacrimal gland tumors
Pseudotumor	Sinus mucocele
Graves' ophthalmopathy	Secondary tumor invasion
Optic nerve glioma	Metastatic breast and lung carcinoma
Neurofibroma	Meningioma
Metastatic tumors	Carotid-cavernous fistula
Neuroblastoma	Fibrous histiocytoma
Ewing's sarcoma	Lymphoma
Leukemia	Systemic vasculitis
Lymphangioma	Lymphangioma
	Neurofibroma
	Cellulitis
	Encephalocele

Table 10.3. Syndromes Associated with Exophthalmos

Albright	Gruber
Apert	Hallermann-Streiff
Basedow	Hand-Schuller-Christian
Bloch-Sulzberger	Hollenhorst
Bonnet-Dechaume-Blanc	Hurler
Caffey	Hutchinson
Carotid artery-cavernous sinus fistula	Kasabach-Merritt
Craniocleidodysostosis	Letterer-Siwe
Crouzon	Melkersson-Rosenthal
Dejean	Mobius
DeLange	Noonan
Diencephalic epilepsy	Paget
Engelmann	Siegrist
Extreme hydrocephalus	Silverman
Feer	Sphenocavernous
Foix	Turner
Foramen lacerum	Von Recklinghausen
	Wegener

Modified from Geeraets WJ: *Ocular Syndromes.* Philadelphia, Lea & Febiger, 1976.

Table 10.4. Evaluation of Exophthalmos

Pseudoexophthalmos
History
   Age-common orbital disorders
      Children
      Adults
   Duration, rate of progression
   Medical history
Ocular examination
   General habitus
   Exophthalmometry
   Orbital mass
   Lids
   Pulsations—palpation and auscultation
   Motility—forced duction
Systemic examination
Systemic screening
   Chest x-ray film
   CBC, ESR
   Vanillylmandelic acid, normetanephrine
   Radioimmunoassays T4 and T3, T3 resin uptake
Orbital studies
   Plain x-ray films, tomography, xeroradiography
   Arteriography
   Venography
   Thermography, radionuclide scanning
   Ultrasonography
   CT Scanning
   Biopsy and special histopathologic techniques

from adjacent paranasal sinuses probably is the most common cause of unilateral exophthalmos in childhood (see Table 10.2 and Chapters 11 and 15).

Many of the common etiologies of adult exophthalmos are similar to those in children, with a few important differences. In adults in the United States, the leading cause of both unilateral and bilateral exophthalmos is Graves' ophthalmopathy.

There are many causes of exophthalmos that should be differentiated from Graves' ophthalmopathy. These include benign and malignant tumors, pseudotumors, vascular malformation, and inflammatory conditions (see Table 10.2 and Chapters 11 and 15).

Orbital Disease Evaluation

A complete ocular examination is fundamental in the work-up of proptosis (Table 10.4). The general habitus of the face, skull, and orbits should be observed. A method of documenting the presence and amount of exophthalmos by an objective means is provided by a Hertel-type exophthalmometer (Fig. 10.1). Reference measurements are taken for each eye from the lateral orbital rim to the apex of the anterior corneal surface. Although the upper limit of the normal range often is stated to be 20 mm, this is arbitrary because racial and even familial differences often influence the size. However, the opposite eye should be very similar, and an asymmetry of more than 2 mm between the two eyes is suggestive of unilateral exophthalmos. If the proptosis is more than 6–7 mm between the eyes (which rarely occurs in Graves' ophthalmopathy or pseudotumor), an or-

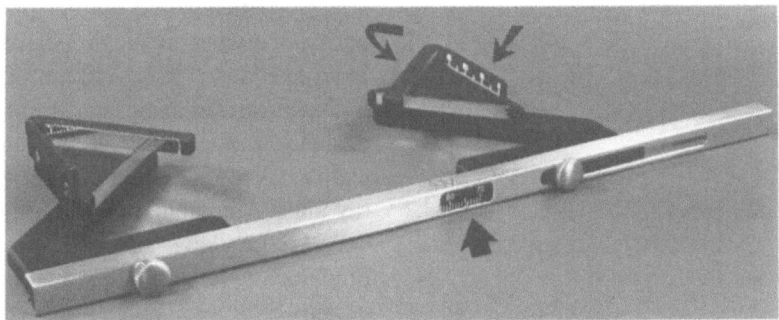

Figure 10.1. Hertel exophthalmometer. Measurements are made on each side, from the lateral orbital rim to the anterior corneal surface, by viewing a millimeter scale through a set of mirrors. The prominence of both eyes is measured simultaneously. The distance between the orbital rims is also recorded at each visit as a reference for future serial measurements.

bital mass should be suspected. Even if a patient is found to have pseudoexophthalmos, it is appropriate to examine the orbits carefully and to obtain baseline studies for future reference.

Lid abnormalities are seen in many disorders, including Graves' ophthalmopathy, capillary hemangioma, plexiform neurofibroma, and metastatic disease.

Palpation of a mass and its anatomic location may suggest a diagnosis, especially in the lacrimal gland area. If a mass is palpable and exophthalmos exists, part of the mass *must* lie behind the equator of the globe. The mass should be characterized as hard, wormy, flunctuant, reducible, shotty, or rubbery. There exists an overall tendency for tumors, idiopathic inflammatory pseudotumors, and cysts of the orbit to occur in the upper quadrants. Resistance to manual palpation of the globes suggests Graves' ophthalmopathy or retrobulbar tumor.

Pulsations of the globe may indicate an arteriovenous communication, as in a carotid-cavernous fistula, a bony abnormality with a meningoencephalocele after previous surgery, or with sphenoid maldevelopment (neuorfibromatosis). An ocular bruit may exist in a carotid-cavernous fistula or an extensively vascularized orbital tumor. A rapid change of proptosis with different positions of the head suggests an orbital varix, arteriovenous fistula, or meningoencephalocele.

Evaluation of the extraocular muscle motility is of primary importance. Restrictions of motion are seen in Graves' ophthalmopathy and pseudotumor as part of the inflammatory process. They also may exist if a space-occupying mass involves the globe. A forced duction test is a simple and

essential method for evaluating a restriction of motility. After adequate topical anesthesia, the globe is mechanically manipulated in all positions of gaze. The opposite eye is used as a control, if needed. Restriction of movement of the globe indicates a mechanical etiology, possibly secondary to an inflammatory process (Fig. 10.2). Absence of restriction may indicate a muscular or neurogenic etiology of the motility problem. Intraocular pressure should be measured in primary gaze and upgaze. Elevation on upgaze is commonly seen in Graves' ophthalmopathy and in other inflammatory conditions that cause inferior rectus restriction.

A complete general medical examination should be performed on every patient with exophthalmos. A few relevant points should be emphasized, although some orbital disorders may be related to multisystemic involvement.

After the general habitus and vital signs are examined, a thorough skin evaluation should be performed. Cafe-au-lait spots, malignant melanoma, erythema nodosum, or skin lesions may indicate systemic disease or malignancy. Breast evaluation in women and chest radiography in every patient may detect signs of a previously unnoticed malignancy. Lymphadenopathy, although very nonspecific, should be noted. Palpation and auscultation of the thyroid gland is essential. Speculum examination of the nares and turbinates may reveal signs of chronic sinusitis. Abdominal masses, especially in children, should be investigated with suspicion of neuroblastoma or another tumor. A thorough neurologic examination should be done in each patient.

A hematologic survey may show evidence of

selected patients, and lumbar puncture should be considered when meningeal signs suggest a neurologic disorder.

Diagnostic imaging studies are helpful in the evaluation of exophthalmos. Some patients with exophthalmos show an abnormality on plain x-ray films. A combination of Caldwell, Waters, lateral, axial or base, and optic canal projections is fundamental in orbital evaluation. The presence of bony erosions, an abnormal sella, unusual calcification, and other abnormalities may suggest an etiology for the orbital disorder. Tomography, in selected cases, may further define bony defects that are seen on initial studies. Arteriography via carotid artery injection can be used if a vascular lesion is suspected. Orbital venography may be helpful in the diagnosis of varices and cavernous sinus thrombosis (see Chapter 5). Other very important diagnostic tools are ultrasonography and CT scanning.

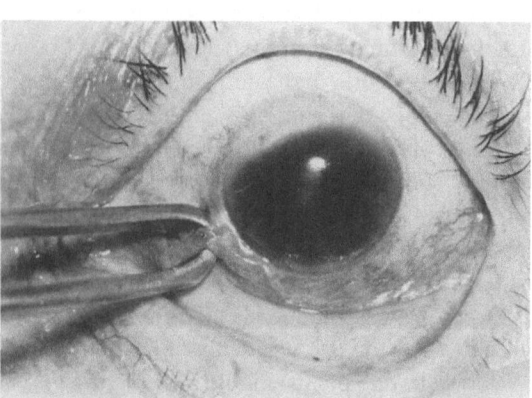

Figure 10.2. Forced duction test. Local anesthesia is accomplished by using topical cocaine (**A**). (**B**) Muscle forceps are used to manipulate the globe in the direction of the clinical deficit; in this patient, an abduction abnormality is present. Mechanical restriction is indicated if difficulty of forced rotation is encountered. Both eyes are tested for comparison.

leukemia, lymphoma, infection, or a systemic disease. The sedimentation rate may be elevated in pseudotumor and systemic vasculitis. Assays of vanillylmandelic acid (VMA) and normetanephrine should be done in children with suspected neuroblastoma or pheochromocytoma. Primary screening tests of thyroid function should be done. Tumor-secreted blood factors may be studied in

Graves' Ophthalmopathy

Graves was not the first to describe thyroid ophthalmopathy, but he did give one of the earliest accounts of the causal relationship between the clinical ocular manifestations and swelling of the thyroid. In 1835, he described a patient in whom ". . . the eyeballs were apparently enlarged, so that when she slept or tried to close her eyes, the lids were incapable of closing. When the eyes were open, the white sclerotic could be seen . . . all around the cornea (3).

Graves' disease probably is best defined clinically as a multisystem disease of unknown etiology characterized by one or more of three clinical entities: hyperthyroidism with diffuse hyperplasia of the gland, infiltrative ophthalmopathy, and infiltrative dermopathy (pretibial myxedema) (14, 21). Ophthalmic Graves' disease is the term used to describe the ocular changes that may occur with this disorder.

The ocular changes of Graves' disease do not always correlate in time or severity with the thyroid disease. Although most patients with Graves' ophthalmopathy have hyperthyroidism, the ocular manifestations may occur before, at the time of, or after the discovery of the thyroid abnormalities. In addition, a significant number of hyperthyroid patients have no signs or symptoms suggestive of ocular involvement.

Table 10.5. Evaluation of Graves' Disease

History
Orbital and ocular physical examination
  NO SPECS
  Forced-duction test
  Exophthalmometer readings
Systemic physical examination
Primary thyroid tests
  T4 radioimmunoassay
  T3 radioimmunoassay
  T3 resin uptake
  TSH
Secondary thyroid tests
  TRH (infusion)
Radiologic evaluation
  Plain x-ray films of the orbit
  CT Scanning
    Axial—CAT
    Coronal—CCT
  Ultrasound A and B

TSH, thyroid-stimulating hormone; TRH, thyrotropin-releasing hormone; CAT, computed axial tomography; CCT, computed coronal tomography.

Evaluation of Graves' Ophthalmopathy

A detailed history, as in any orbital disorder, can often give many clues to the diagnosis (Table 10.5). Especially important are complaints of weight change without change of diet, palpitations, changes in hair character, tremor, and lethargy. Nervousness, depression, headaches, change of bowel habits, and muscle weakness also may be present. Ocular complaints usually include staring, eyelid swelling, or diplopia. Although a definite etiologic relationship between Graves' ophthalmopathy and hyperthyroidism has not been estab-

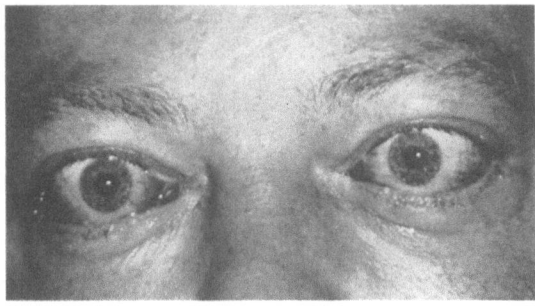

Figure 10.3. Early Graves' ophthalmopathy with hypervascularity and congestion of the conjunctival and episcleral vessels over the insertions of the rectus muscles. Diplopia was also present.

lished, the two are commonly associated. One third of all patients with Graves' disease have a family history of Graves' disease or thyroid disorders. Women between 20–45 years of age are most commonly affected.

The most commonly used classification of the eye changes in Graves' disease is that of the American Thyroid Association (Table 10.6) (18, 19, 21). Although some investigators feel it has little clinical value, we find it to be useful as a guide for evaluating and following our patients with thyroid ophthalmopathy. Even though the seven classes of eye changes do not necessarily occur in a progressive manner, multiple-class involvement often is simultaneous in severely affected patients (Figs. 10.3 through 10.6).

Class 0 includes those patients with hyperthyroidism who have no signs of ophthalmopathy. Diffuse thyroid gland enlargement is present, as well as tachycardia, systolic hypertension, and hy-

Table 10.6. Classification of Stages in Orbital Graves' Disease

Class	Definition
0	No signs or symptoms
1	Only signs, no symptoms (signs limited to upper lid retraction and stare, with or without lid lag and proptosis)
2	Soft-tissue involvement (symptoms and signs)
3	Proptosis
4	Extraocular muscle involvement
5	Corneal involvement
6	Sight loss (optic nerve involvement)

From Werner SC: Classification of the eye changes of Graves' disease. *J Clin Endocrinol* 29:782, 1969.

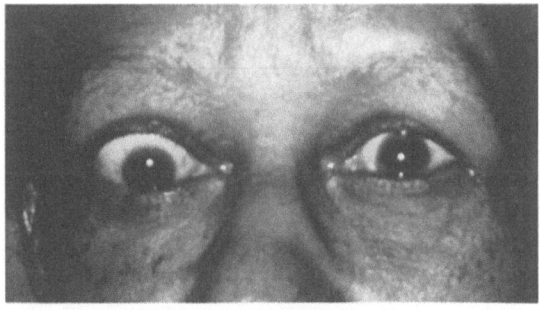

Figure 10.4. Asymmetric clinical involvement with unilateral exophthalmos, inferior rectus restriction, and soft tissue swelling. Bilateral lid retraction (more prominent on the right) is also present.

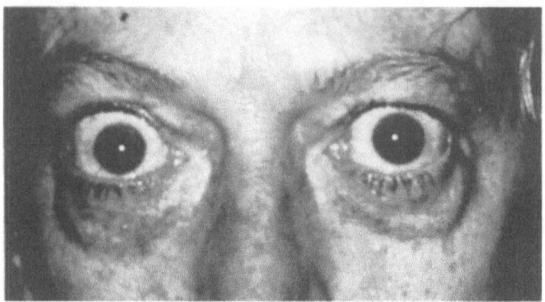

Figure 10.5. Bilateral exophthalmos and stare are present, both of which are exaggerated by lid retraction and soft-tissue edema. The patient had pain and loss of vision O.D. over 2 weeks due to mechanical compression of the optic nerve by the enlarged extraocular muscles converging at the orbital apex.

perreflexia. Lymphadenopathy, proximal skeletal myopathy, splenomegaly, osteoporosis, and hypercalcemia may be discovered.

Classes 1 and 2 occur together and should not be separated. Many eyelid changes have been described; the most common is upper lid retraction (Table 10.7). Although they are not pathognomonic, these eyelid findings are highly suggestive of Graves' ophthalmopathy (Table 10.8). A striking feature of the eye signs in this disorder is their asymmetry. Unilateral involvement often is detected clinically, but further investigation reveals bilateral involvement. Tearing, eyelid edema, chemosis, epibulbar vascular congestion, photophobia, and lagophthalmos are frequently described. A number of nonspecific soft-tissue findings also have been described (Table 10.9). Proptosis up to and including 22 mm also is included here. Eyelid

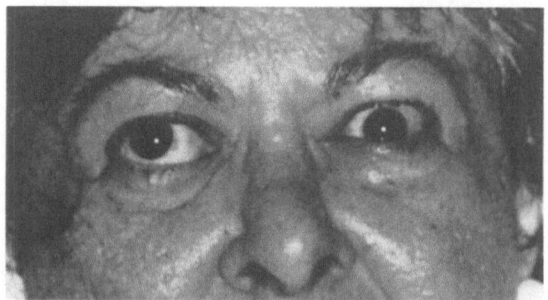

Figure 10.6. Patient with exophthalmos O.D. and bilateral lid retraction. The attempted gaze to the right shows motility restriction of both eyes. Forced duction confirmed the bilateral restriction as being mechanical in etiology.

Table 10.7. Causes of Lid Retraction

Graves' ophthalmopathy
Parinaud's dorsal midbrain syndrome
Hydrocephalus
Third-nerve aberrant regeneration
Unilateral ptosis with overactivity of contralateral levator
Potassium-related periodic paralysis
Cirrhosis of the liver
Chronic systemic corticosteroid therapy

retraction may simulate exophthalmos, but exophthalmometer readings usually are normal.

Class 3 includes patients with a minimum of 22 mm of proptosis in either eye. This class rarely appears as a separate finding without other signs of ophthalmopathy. Bilateral involvement, although many times asymmetric, usually is demonstrated. Asymmetry of more than 6 mm of proptosis is unusual.

Class 4 includes clinical manifestations of extraocular muscle involvement. Muscle enlargement is an important and constant finding in Graves' ophthalmopathy. There may be a range from minimal enlargement of a few muscles in Classes 1 and 2 to enormous enlargement of multiple muscles in severe forms. Functionally, the enlarged muscles initially contract normally. However, as a result of chronic inflammation, they become fibrotic and unable to relax, resulting in restriction of motility. The patient complains of diplopia, and involvement presents as an underaction of the antagonist muscle, which is not supported by a forced duction test. In severe and massive muscle involvement, there may be total loss of contractile properties. The inferior rectus often is the first muscle involved and simulates a double elevator palsy. As with the levator superior rectus complex, it may become more extensively enlarged than the other muscle. However, the involvement of the levator superior rectus complex is difficult to demonstrate clinically. Medial rectus involvement is common, and can mimic a sixth-nerve palsy. A variable amount of proptosis usually accompanies extraocular muscle involvement, but no

Table 10.8. Eyelid Signs of Thyroid Ophthalmopathy

Retraction of upper or lower eyelid (Dalrymple)
Lag of upper eyelid on downgaze (von Graefe)
Restriction of downward traction on upper eyelid (Grove)
Increased pigmentation of eyelids (Jellinek)
Tremor of closed eyelids (Rosenbach)

Table 10.9. Assorted Signs of Thyroid Ophthalmopathy

Absence of forehead wrinkling on upward gaze (Joffroey)
Infrequent blinking (Stellwag)
Poor fixation on lateral gaze (Suker)
Weakness of convergence (Moebius)
Dilation of pupil with weak epinephrine solution (Loewi)
Jerky pupillary contraction to consensual light (Lowen)
Increased intraocular pressure or upgaze

absolute correlation exists. An increase of intraocular tension on upgaze is common, and it may be demonstrated clinically in many patients early in the course of their disease (2).

Class 5 should be reserved for corneal involvement that can threaten vision. Corneal necrosis and perforation may occur in the patient with lagophthalmos.

Class 6, which is the most acute and severe form, involves sight loss caused by optic nerve involvement. It is not caused by direct involvement of the nerve or meninges, but by compression of the optic nerve by the swollen "bellies" of the extraocular muscles converging near their origin at the orbital apex. Congestive signs and symptoms always precede visual loss, but their rate of progression may be variable.

A thorough history and physical examination must be augmented by a few select laboratory studies. Thyroxine (T4) and triiodothyronine (T3) are the major circulating hormones of the thyroid. Radioimmunoassay of these hormones is a readily available and highly accurate screening method. Measurement of T3 resin uptake further delineates the abnormality. Occasionally, measurement of thyroid-stimulating hormone (TSH) levels from the pituitary gland is done to confirm the T4 and T3 results.

Thyrotropin-releasing hormone (TRH) is the hypothalamic regulatory factor controlling the release of TSH from the pituitary gland. An assay of TRH is more costly and time-consuming; it should be reserved for those patients in whom diagnostic suspicion is high despite normal values from the primary thyroid function tests. Remember, however, that a well-defined group of patients who have clinical manifestations of Graves' disease and normal thyroid function test results does exist.

The diagnosis of Graves' ophthalmopathy by case history, physical examination, and primary thyroid blood tests is accurate in classic cases. Both CT scanning and ultrasound are useful adjuncts

in diagnosis and evaluation of the extent of the orbital involvement. Plain x-ray films of the orbit rarely show abnormalities, but they should be done to exclude other orbital disorders. A CT scan of the orbits should be done even when the clinical diagnosis of Graves' disease is apparent.

CT Scanning in Thyroid Ophthalmopathy

A CT scan of the orbits in thyroid ophthalmopathy has been studied since the introduction of the EMI Mark I head scanner in 1972 (1, 7–10, 15–17). Each new generation of scanner with improved resolution has further delineated the findings in Graves' disease. Computed axial tomographic (CAT) scans and computed coronal tomographic (CCT) scans used together enable three-dimensional study of the extraocular muscles, globe, orbital bones, vascular system, paranasal sinuses, and intracranial structures. Contrast enhancement, image reversal, and narrow-density window techniques can further outline tumors, inflammations, blood vessels, and foreign bodies.

Enlargement of the extraocular muscles is the most important and constant finding on a CT scan in Graves' ophthalmopathy. New-generation scanners allow definition of all extraocular muscles whose normal maximal thickness is 2.8 mm to less than 1 mm at the tendinous insertion. Some degree of exophthalmos usually accompanies the muscle enlargement. Although a mass lesion may be suspected when orbital involvement is asymmetric, CT scanning commonly reveals bilateral extraocular muscle involvement, thus obviating

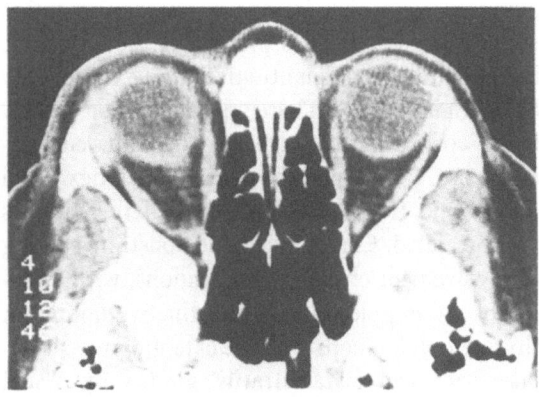

Figure 10.7. Axial scan of ventral orbit demonstrating involvement of the horizontal rectus muscles, with sparing of their tendons. Note the bilateral lacrimal gland enlargement.

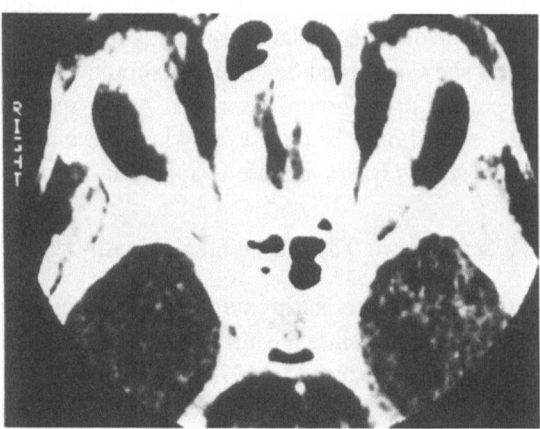

Figure 10.8. Axial scan of dorsal orbit showing bilateral enlargement of superior rectus-levator muscle complexes.

unnecessary surgical exploration. Extraocular muscle enlargement can range from minimal or no involvement in Classes 1 and 2 to enormous multiple involvement in more severe forms. Some patients with laboratory proven hyperthyroidism have CT scans showing only proptosis without observable extraocular muscle enlargement. (Figs. 10.7 through 10.11).

The inferior rectus is the initial and most common muscle involved. The inferior rectus and the levator superior rectus complex may become more extensively enlarged than other muscles. These are difficult to evaluate on CAT scans, but CCT scans visualize these muscles accurately. These scans may prove to be valuable in detecting early changes of these muscles in mild Graves' disease.

Medial and lateral rectus muscle enlargements are common findings on a CT scan. An ophthalmopathy index, which is a numeric representation of the various eye signs present, is used by some investigators as a quantitative guide to severity of ophthalmopathy. There appears to be a grossly linear correlation between medial rectus enlargement on CT scans and the ophthalmic index. Both diffuse and fusiform enlargement of the muscles is appreciated. Coronal views demonstrate sparing of involvement of the muscle tendons, with swelling of the muscle bellies—a distinctive finding in thyroid ophthalmopathy. The extent of muscle enlargement can be arbitrarily graded by visual means. A general trend exists for the largest muscle to be present in patients with the highest ophthalmopathy index and vice versa. However,

prediction of the degree of clinical involvement from the CT appearance is very uncertain.

Although clinical signs and symptoms may appear to be confined to one orbit, CT scanning usually reveals bilateral muscle involvement, which suggests inflammation rather than a neoplasm as the etiology. Occasionally, the greater degree of muscle enlargement is present in the eye having the lesser amount of clinical proptosis. In rare cases, involvement by clinical and CT examination may be purely unilateral. The CT scan may also be of value in diagnosing Graves' disease in patients with eye symptoms, but no systemic symptoms. The CT scans of these patients may show enlarged muscles, but no exophthalmos. When proptosis is present, scans through the midorbit provide the best visualization of the amount of proptosis.

The radiodensity of orbital fat is normal in Graves' disease. Any changes in fat are secondary and insignificant. Anterior displacement of the orbital septum is caused by the pressure of the enlarging orbital content, but the proptosis is not due to water accumulation in the orbital fat, as was once proposed.

No optic nerve, meningeal, or perineural connective tissue inflammation is consistently found

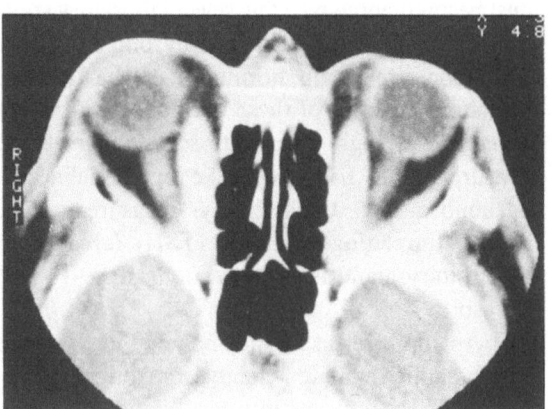

Figure 10.9. Axial scan of patient with bilateral proptosis showing enlargement of the horizontal rectus muscles. Note the massive enlargement of the medial rectus muscles. Pressure exerted on the lamina papyracea of the ethmoid bones has resulted in both a medial bowing of the structures and the resulting "coke bottle" or "wasp waist" appearance. Also note the mechanical compression produced in the area of the optic nerves at the orbital apex by the enlarged muscles converging at their origins.

in thyroid ophthalmopathy. A small amount of optic nerve sheath swelling and prominence may occur secondary to mechanical compression, when congestive orbital involvement of the apex causes decreased vision.

The lacrimal gland and superior ophthalmic vein are consistently involved in Graves' disease. Their increased visualization on CT scanning may be due to inflammatory changes of the gland or may be secondary to congestive changes of the retrobulbar orbit. In general, enlargement of the lacrimal gland correlates with the severity of extraocular muscle enlargement.

The lamina papyracea of the ethmoid bone is the thinnest bone of the orbit. Enlargement of the medial rectus muscle belly may cause medial bowing of this structure, which is a form of spontaneous orbital decompression. Displacement of both orbital medial walls in severe Graves' ophthalmopathy may form a "wasp-waisted" or "Coca-Cola bottle" contour appearance on the CT scan.

The soft tissue of the orbit may become edematous and inflamed in Graves' disease. This may be seen on the CT scan as thickening and increased densities of the soft tissues, and it often is enhanced

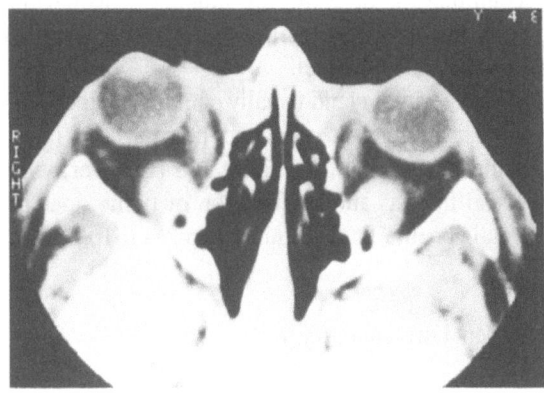

Figure 10.11. Axial scan of ventral orbit demonstrating simulation of bilateral orbital masses resulting from the enlarged inferior rectus muscles. Coronal scans usually clarify the etiology in confusing cases.

following contrast media injection. Prominent vascular channels may be seen within the orbital fat, but these are not a prominent feature.

Recent evidence suggests that all of the associated findings—including proptosis, bowing of the lamina papyracea, venous engorgement from stasis secondary to orbital venous compression, conjunctival and lid swelling, and lacrimal gland enlargement—probably are secondary to extraocular muscle enlargement (17).

Extensive histologic study of Graves' ophthalmopathy has failed to detect a specific etiologic agent to account for the pathophysiology of the orbital abnormalities (11, 13, 17). Grossly, the extraocular muscles are firm, rubbery, and enlarged up to five times their normal size. The damage is caused by infiltration of the endomysium by lymphocytes and plasma cells and by the associated edema. Early in the process, these cells usually grow near blood vessels. The cause of this cell migration is unknown. This infiltrate leads to the activation of fibroblasts and to production of acid mucopolysaccharides, which is nonspecific and rather late finding.

The muscle fibers show no signs of primary degeneration. Alteration of muscle cells seems to be secondary to the inflammatory infiltrate. Electromyographic studies appear to be normal during the early stages. The inflammatory edema and activation of fibroblasts lead to fibrosis and to permanent structural alterations. Increased muscle densities are seen, resulting from enlargement of the muscles and the inflammatory edema; not from

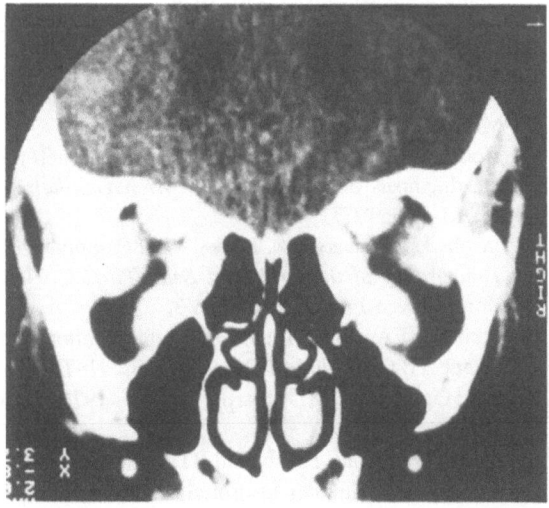

Figure 10.10. Coronal scan of midretrobulbar area showing massive enlargement of multiple rectus muscles. Note the huge "hamburger patty" appearance on coronal scans of the congested muscles. The inferior rectus muscles are enlarged and are bulging medially to blend with the lateral rectus muscles. Note encroachment of the optic nerve on the right by massively enlarged muscle bellies. The patient had pain and loss of vision on that side.

accumulation of water or mucopolysaccharides, which have lower densities than muscle. The tendons are not inflamed.

The lacrimal gland usually contains an increased number of lymphocytes and plasma cells in the connective tissue septa and acini. However, widespread fibrosis and obliteration of tissue does not usually occur. The orbital fat appears to be normal.

B-Scan Ultrasonography

Ultrasonography of the orbit has been valuable in the study of Graves' ophthalmopathy (5, 9, 20). Immersion B-scan ultrasonography provided the first reliable method for demonstrating retrobulbar abnormalities. B-scan (intensity-modulated) ultrasonography provides a two-dimensional view that resembles an anatomic cross-section. B-scan findings in Graves' disease have been predominantly qualitative. Accentuation of the temporal wall of the orbit, thickening of the extraocular muscles, erosion of retrobulbar fat, and perineural inflammation have been reported. However, many of these findings were poorly defined and lacked diagnostic accuracy. Despite its limitations, B-scan ultrasonography may be able to demonstrate orbital abnormalities in early Graves' ophthalmopathy. A-scan (time-amplitude) ultrasonography produces one-dimensional images composed of vertical spikes representing acoustic interfaces. An experienced observer often can obtain reliable histologic information from this noninvasive test. A-scan ultrasonography may quantitatively measure each rectus muscle with reproducible accuracy. It may show bilateral orbital involvement in cases in which the diagnosis is uncertain.

Conclusion

Although newer generation CT scanners have replaced ultrasound in most baseline studies of thyroid ophthalmopathy, the two are not mutually exclusive; each can give valuable information. The familiarity of the observer with each technique may determine which yields the most useful information. The role of MRI in Grave's ophthalmopathy is not yet well defined. The majority of patients with enlarged extraocular muscles have Graves' disease. However, muscle enlargement is not pa-

thognomonic, and it may also be seen in pseudotumor, carotid-cavernous fistula, and some metastatic tumors (see Chapters 4, 5, and 11) (11, 12, 15, 17).

Acknowledgment

Special thanks to Robert Sergott, M.D. for providing some of the clinical photographs.

References

1. Enzmann D, Marshall WH, Rosenthal AR, et al: Computed tomography in Graves' ophthalmopathy. *Radiology* 118:615–620, 1976.
2. Gamblin GT, Harper DG, Galentine P, et al: Prevalence of increased intraocular pressure in Graves' disease—evidence of frequent subclinical ophthalmopathy. *N Engl J Med* 308:420–424, 1983.
3. Graves RJ: Clinical lectures. *London Med Surg J* 7:516, 1835.
4. Grove AS: Evaluation of exophthalmos. *N Engl J Med* 292:1005–1013, 1975.
5. Grove AS: Orbital disease: Examination and diagnostic evaluation. *Ophthalmology* 86:854–863, 1979.
6. Hall R, Kirkham K, Doniach D, et al: Ophthalmic Graves' disease. *Lancet* 375–378, 1970.
7. Hilal SK: Computed tomography of the orbit. *Ophthalmology* 86:864–870, 1979.
8. Hilal SK, Kreps SM, Trokel SL: Diseases of the orbit: computerized tomography, in Duane TD (ed): *Clinical Ophthalmology II: The Orbit.* Hagerstown, MD, Harper & Row, 1976, chap 23.
9. Hodes BL, Weinberg P: A combined approach for the diagnosis of orbital disease. *Arch Ophthalmol* 95:781–788, 1977.
10. Jacobs L, Weisberg LA, Kinkel WR: *Computerized Tomography of the Orbit and Sella Turcica.* New York, Raven Press, 1980, chap 3.
11. Jakobiec FA, Jones IS: Orbital inflammations, in Duane TB (ed): *Clinical Ophthalmology II: The Orbit.* Hagerstown, MD, Harper & Row, 1976, chap 35.
12. Jones IS, Jakobiec FA, Nolan BT: Patient examination and introduction to orbital disease, in Duane TB (ed): *Clinical Ophthalmology II: The Orbit.* Hagerstown, MD, Harper & Row, 1976, chap 21.
13. Kroll AJ, Kuwabara T: Dysthyroid ocular myopathy. *Arch Ophthalmol* 76:244–257, 1966.
14. Sergott RC, Glaser JS: Graves' ophthalmopathy, a clinical and immunologic review. *Surv Ophthalmol* 26:1–21, 1981.
15. Trokel SC, Hilal SK: Recognition and differential diagnosis of enlarged extraocular muscles in com-

puted tomography. *Am J Ophthalmol* 87:503–512, 1979.

16. Trokel SC, Hilal SK: Submillimeter resolution CT scanning of orbital diseases. *Ophthalmology* 87:412–417, 1980.

17. Trokel SC, Jakobiec FA: Correlation of CT scanning and pathologic features of ophthalmic Graves' disease. *Ophthalmology* 88:553–564, 1983.

18. Werner SC: Classification of the eye changes of Graves' disease. *J Clin Endocr* 29:982–984, 1969.

19. Werner SC: Modification of the classification of the eye changes of Graves' disease. *Am J Ophthalmol* 83:725–727, 1977.

20. Werner SC, Coleman DJ, Franzen LA: Ultrasonographic evidence of a consistent orbital involvement in Graves' disease. *N Engl J Med* 290:1447–1450, 1974.

21. Werner SC: *The Thyroid. A Fundamental and Clinical Text.* New York, Harper & Row, 1971, pp 535–543.

11
Orbital Tumors

Mark C. Ruchman, Mary A. Stefanyszyn, Joseph C. Flanagan, Carlos F. Gonzalez and Melvin H. Becker

There are many tumors that involve the orbit. Some of them are malignant and others are benign. Primary tumors may arise from any of the orbital components. Secondary tumors may involve the orbit from adjacent structures, such as the parana-sal sinuses, the eyeball, the intracranial structures, and the eyelids; or they may be metastatic lesions from distant structures. (Table 11.1). Inflammations, pseudotumors, and vascular lesions also appear as mass lesions in the orbit.

The evaluation of a suspected orbital tumor includes a thorough clinical history, physical examination, and imaging studies (routine radiographs, tomography, ultrasonography, computed tomography [CT], and Magnetic Resonance Imaging [MRI], as well as vascular studies in selected cases). CT scanning yields the most information for diagnosis and management of a given lesion. Lesions of the orbit and its contents have a tendency to localize in a specific area of the orbit, such as in the globe, intraconal area, muscle, extraconal area, and extraorbital area (see Table 2.1).

Table 11.1. Orbital tumors

Neurogenic
  Meningioma
  Juvenile pilocytic astrocytoma-glioma
  Neurofibroma
  Neurilemmoma
Vascular
  Cavernous hemangioma
  Lymphangioma
  Hemangiopericytoma
  Capillary hemangioma
Vascular malformations
  Orbital varix
  Arteriovenous fistulae
  Aneurysms
Lacrimal gland tumors
Choristomas
  Teratoma
  Dermoid
Mesenchymal tumors
  Lipoma
  Fibrous histiocytoma
  Rhabdomyosarcoma
Secondary orbital tumors
  Mucocele
  Carcinoma from sinuses, nose, or nasopharynx
  Carcinoma from eyelids
  Intraocular tumors with orbital extension
    Retinoblastoma
    Malignant melanoma
  Metastatic disease
Inflammations and lymphomas
  Pseudotumor
  Reactive lymphoid hyperplasia
  Lymphoma

Meningioma

Meningioma usually is a slow-growing tumor that arises from arachnoid cells. Histologically it can be classified into three types. In the meningoepitheliomatous type, the cells are in a solid sheet-like arrangement. The transitional or mixed-cell meningioma has cells in a circular or whirl-like configuration (Fig. 11.1) (16, 36). The central core of these whirl-like configurations may calcify forming psamomma bodies. The third type is characterized by multiple capillary sites, blood spaces, and is known as angioblastic meningioma.

While most meningiomas occur inside the calvarium, they are also seen in the orbit—either as a primary neoplasm or as an extension from an anterior or middle cranial fossa meningioma. When the tumor is primary in the orbit, it arises

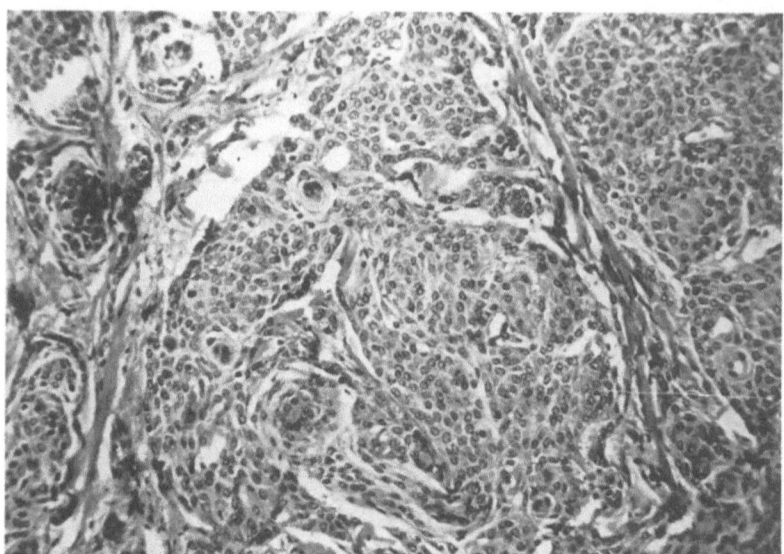

Fig. 11.1. A hematoxylin and eosin preparation of a transitional cell-type meningioma. Notice circular or whirl-like configuration of the tumoral cells.

from arachnoid cells of the optic nerve sheath, ectopic arachnoid cells, or the meninges attached to the orbital wall and optic canal. Intraorbital meningiomas are most frequently seen in middle-aged women (16). However, when seen in patients in their third decade or younger, there usually is an association with neurofibromatosis (20, 35, 82).

Clinical manifestations of optic nerve sheath meningiomas include visual loss, proptosis, optic atrophy, papilledema, scotomatous field defects, and motility disorders. If the tumor arises elsewhere in the orbit or paraorbital structures, proptosis and disturbed ocular motility are the primary complaints.

Optic sheath meningioma is intraconal and usually is not contiguous with the orbital bone. It produces orbital bone changes only when the tumor extends into the optic foramen, causing enlargement of the foramen and hyperostosis. Both CT scanning and orbital ultrasonography are the ideal imaging techniques for demonstrating these tumors. Meningiomas of the optic nerve sheath are characteristically seen on a CT scan as symmetric fusiform, or an excrescent optic nerve enlargement (69, 76). Meningiomas tend to be slightly hyperdense, and enhancement after intravenous (IV) injection of contrast media is often seen. If the process has primarily involved the optic nerve sheath preserving the nerve, the nerve will be seen as a central lucency. The appearance of this lucency, which is best seen after injection of contrast media, has been described as a "railroad

track sign" or "tramtracks sign" on the axial section and as a "donut sign" in the coronal section (Fig. 11.2) (69). However, intraorbital optic nerve sheath enlargement on CT scanning can be produced by a variety of neoplastic and nonneoplastic processes (18). The central lucency is most frequently found in optic sheath meningiomas; it is less commonly seen in cases of optic perineuritis, perineural hematomas, and perineural metastasis. It is absent in papilledema and optic nerve gliomas; in these conditions, the optic nerve cannot be differentiated from the tumor. Calcification is seen occasionally. Optic foramen enlargement may be produced by an optic nerve sheath meningioma, as well as by other intraconal lesions, such as glioma, hemangioma, and neurofibroma. If a vascular lesion is considered in the differential diagnosis, ultrasonography is slightly better than CT scanning due to its dynamic features (5). Orbital venography and ophthalmic arteriography are of limited value in evaluating optic nerve sheath meningioma, since the vascular displacement, abnormal vessels, or tumor stain seen in sphenoid wing meningioma, are absent in optic sheath meningiomas.

Treatment of intraorbital meningioma is controversial (1). Since the tumor and the enclosed optic nerve share the same blood supply, tumor resection usually will result in blindness. However, Mark (58) has reported some success in resecting small meningiomas immediately behind the globe. Most ophthalmic surgeons prefer conservative management; they will resect tumors only in already blind

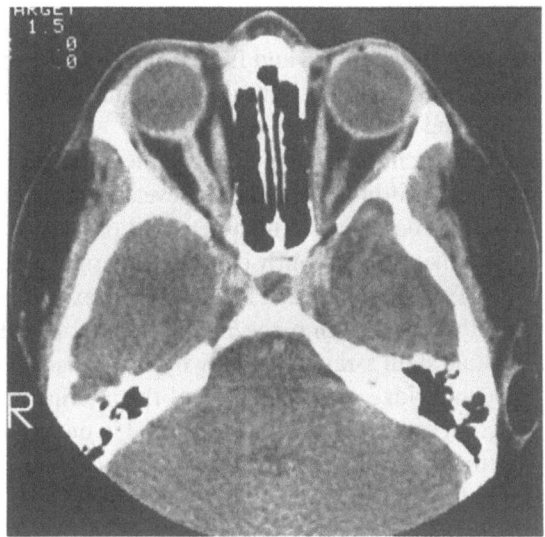

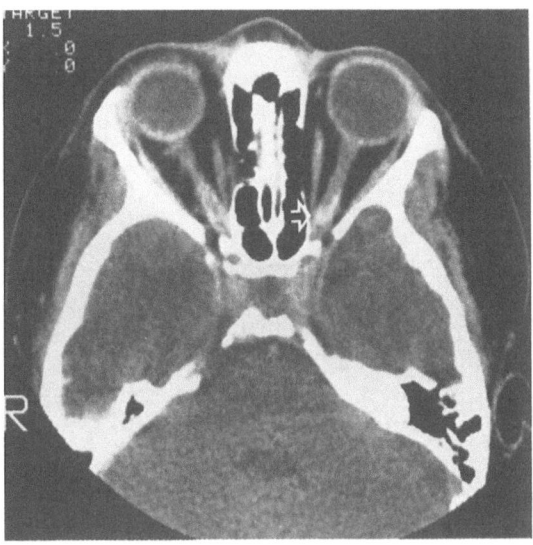

Fig. 11.2A. Optic nerve sheath meningioma. A 32-year-old woman with progressive visual loss in the right eye. An Axial CT scan shows diffuse thickening of the optic nerve sheath on the involved side. After contrast injection, enhancement of the tumor surrounding the lower density optic nerve can be seen (railroad track sign.)

Fig. 11.2B. Axial CT scan of same patient (slightly different section) demonstrates a radiodense plaque-like mass surrounding the posterior portion of the optic nerve in the clinically uninvolved left eye (open arrow). This was an optic nerve sheath meningioma.

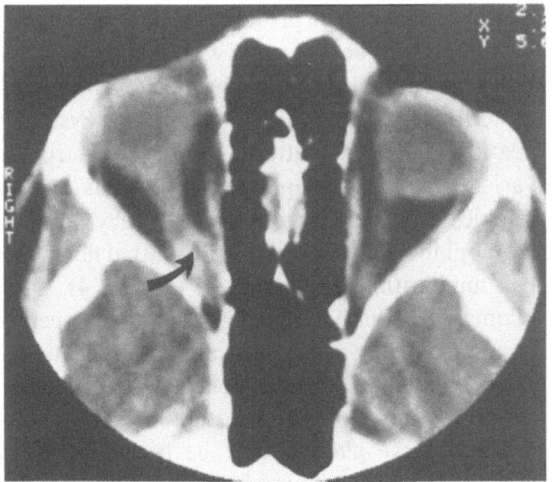

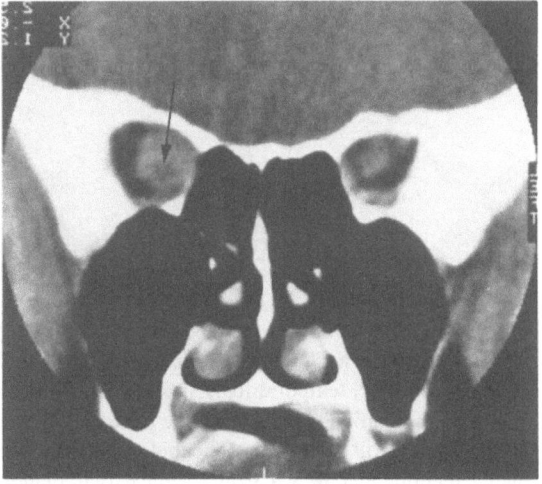

Fig. 11.2C Optic nerve sheath meningioma on another patient. Axial CT scan. A 42-year-old patient with progressive loss of vision in the right eye. There is enlargement of the optic nerve with a clearly seen "railroad" sign (arrow) in the orbital apex.

Fig. 11.2D. Coronal view on the same patient (posterior orbital level) showing the "donut" sign (arrow). (Courtesy of Robert Peyster, Philadelphia).

eyes to prevent intracranial spread. Smith has reported improved vision after radiation therapy (72).

The second type of meningioma related to the orbit is the intraorbital extension of an intracranial tumor, especially from the sphenoid ridge (see also Chapter 15). En-plaque meningioma of the sphenoid wing may cause proptosis and temporal fossa fullness, without orbital apex signs, by directly infiltrating the posterior bony wall of the orbit.

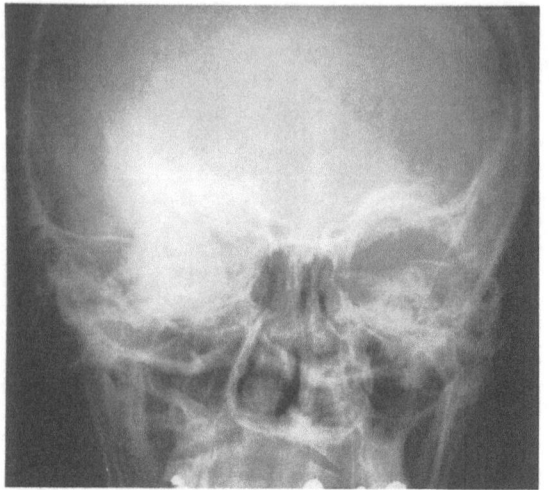

A

B

Fig. 11.3A. Sphenoid ridge meningioma. A plain X-ray film of the skull in a 57-year-old woman presenting with right eye swelling, temporal fossa swelling, and proptosis. The examination reveals extensive sclerotic changes in the right orbit and right sphenoid wing from enplaque meningioma. **B.** CT scan of same patient demonstrates diffuse thickening of right sphenoid wing, anterior displacement of the right lateral rectus muscle (open arrow) and right exophthalmus produced by the tumor.

If the tumor encroaches on the superior orbital fissure or the optic canal, proptosis, unilateral loss of vision, optic atrophy, and unilateral scotomatous field defects can occur. If the meningioma extends medially into the parasellar region, the anterior clinoid process and the sella turcica may

be destroyed; and the symptoms are related to the chiasmatic involvement. Meningioma of the anterior cranial fossa and frontal region may indirectly produce visual symptoms secondary to mass effect and intracerebral edema.

A CT scan of a sphenoid ridge meningioma involving the orbital apex usually reveals a thickened sphenoid bone and a high-density homogeneous tumor that is significantly enhanced after the injection of contrast media. The lesion may extend inside the orbit or into the middle fossa, or both. Routine skull x-ray films show hyperostosis of the sphenoid ridge. Arteriography of the internal and external carotid arteries is very useful in determining the vascular supply of this tumor (Fig. 11.3) (see also Figs. 2.27, 5.7, 13.28–13.31).

Optic Nerve Glioma

Gliomas of the optic nerve are the most common benign orbital neoplasms found in children (73). The tumor is composed of proliferating astrocytes and oligodendrocytes within the substance of the nerve. Pathologically, three different patterns of tumor growth can be present (73). The optic nerve may appear to be enlarged, with glial hypercellularity and less orderly arrangement. The second pattern encountered is myxomatous or cystic-appearing. The third pattern—fibrous or astrocytic variant—consists of spindle-shaped cells and resembles a juvenile astrocytoma. Intracytoplasmic eosinophilic inclusions called Rosenthal fibers may be found within the astrocytes (Fig. 11.4). Optic gliomas of adulthood differ from those seen in childhood. The adult tumors are usually histologically malignant astrocytomas or glioblastomas, which appear in middle-aged adults. (44)

Optic nerve gliomas may be found anywhere along the optic nerve or chiasm. Some pathologists consider the intraorbital optic nerve gliomas as a separate group from the intracraneal variety. They all present with visual loss. When the glioma is predominantly intraorbital, visual loss usually is associated with proptosis. Nonspecific visual field defects, optic nerve papilledema, or atrophy, with Marcus-Gunn pupillary reaction may also be present. When the glioma is predominantly intracranial, visual loss may be associated with hydrocephalus and diabetes insipidus. (30) The association of optic nerve gliomas and neurofibromatosis is well known. When optic nerve glio-

Fig. 11.4. Hematoxylin and eosin preparation of a glioma, fibrous or astrocystic type, with prominent Rosenthal fibers.

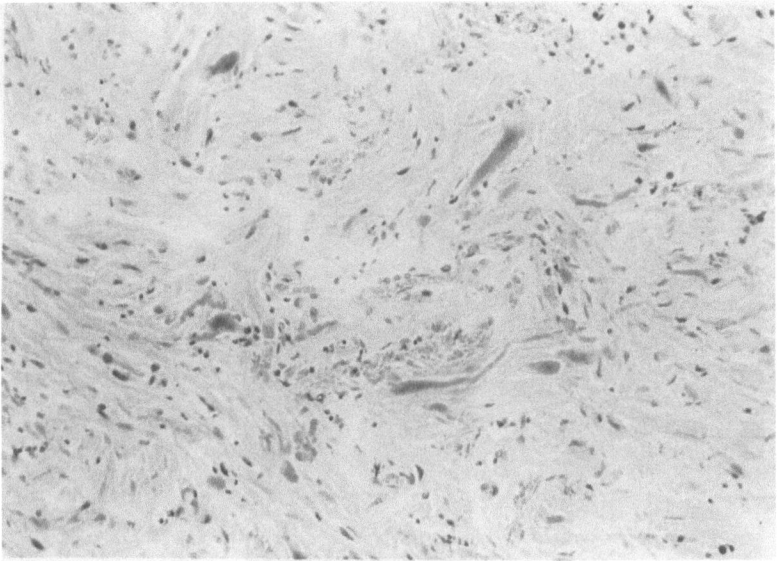

mas are bilateral, one should suspect the diagnosis of neurofibromatosis (44, 56, 66).

The CT scan appearance of orbital nerve gliomas is closely related to the tumor's pattern of growth. Since the tumors arise from glial cells within the nerve, they may expand the nerve by longitudinal, circumferential, or eccentric growth. Therefore, the CT scan appearance of the optic nerve is tubular, fusiform, or eccentric (lobulated) (69). Since the tumor is usually confined by the stretched dura, the margins usually remain well defined and smooth (69). The CT density of an optic glioma is homogeneous and close to the density of the normal optic nerve (45, 66). There is no clear separation between tumor and nerve on CT or ultrasonography (Fig. 11.5) (5). These features help to differentiate optic nerve gliomas from optic nerve sheath meningiomas, which are usually denser; they also can be easily separated from the optic nerve and are characterized by a central lucency within the tumor (tramtrack appearance). (69)

Enhancement of optic gliomas after IV injection of contrast material varies from imperceptible to moderate, but it is generally less intense than in meningiomas, neurofibromas, metastatic lesions, and other lesions that may mimic optic gliomas (45). Calcifications occasionally are seen (66). Bilateral optic nerve tumors are most commonly found in neurofibromatosis (45, 66). Extension of the tumor into the optic canal can be demonstrated by CT scanning and/or conventional polytomography (70). Metrizamide cisternography may aid in detecting a subtle involvement of the intracranial optic nerve, chiasm, and optic tracts (65).

Intraorbital optic gliomas have to be differentiated from other tumors involving the optic nerve (mainly meningiomas of the optic nerve sheath) and other neoplasms that grow in a nearby area, such as neurofibromas, hemangiomas, metastasis, leukemia, and retinoblastoma in children. Nonneoplastic enlargement of the optic nerve sheath occurs with papilledema, where the enlargement is apparently due to dilatation of the subarachnoid space that is continuous with the optic nerve sheath (12, 29, 57). Metrizamide entering the optic nerve sheath during cisternography can be used to confirm the dilation of the sheath's subarachnoid space. Uniform enlargement and contrast enhancement of the optic nerve is also seen with optic papillitis and retrobulbar neuritis due to both edema and increased vascularity. (41) Retrobulbar neuritis can be clinically distinguished by multiple short periods of remissions, and it is usually associated with multiple sclerosis (4, 41). Optic nerve/sheath enlargement also has been reported in orbital pseudotumor, toxoplasmosis, tuberculosis, sarcoidosis, central retinal vein thrombosis, and traumatic hematoma (52, 55, 75, 77, 78).

Computed tomography has been a major advance in the diagnosis of optic nerve gliomas. Prior to the development of CT scanning, orbital involvement was detected by the less precise modali-

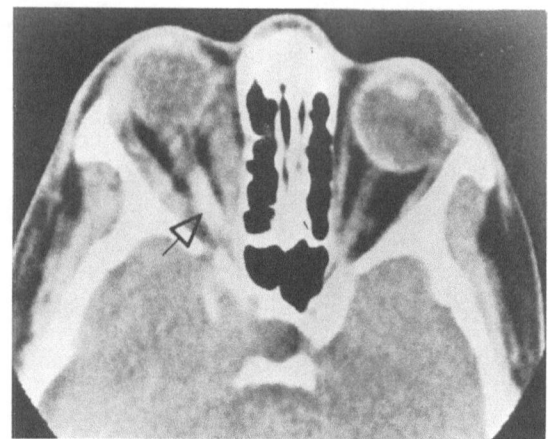

A

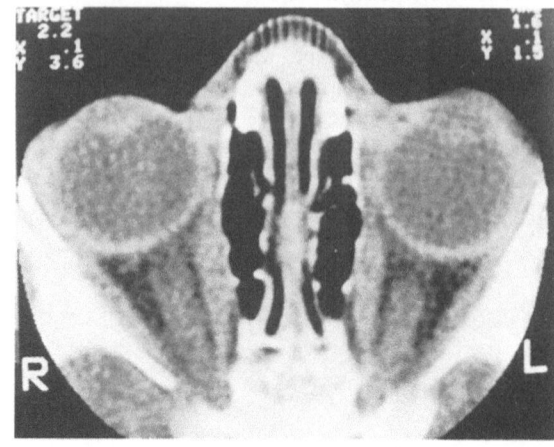

B

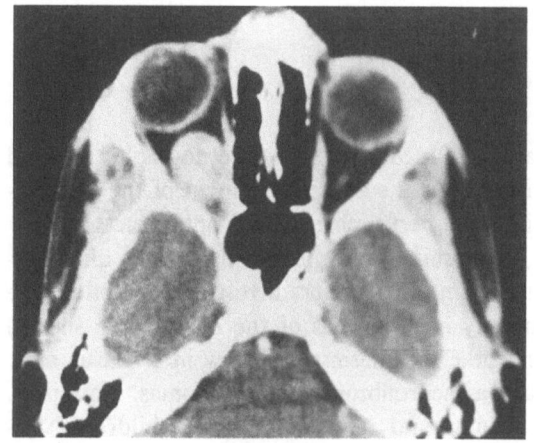

C

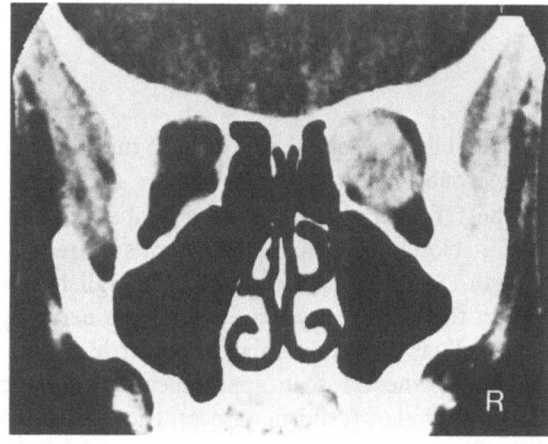

D

Fig. 11.5A. Calcified optic nerve glioma. A 13-year-old patient with neurofibromatosis. There is thickening and calcification of the optic nerve (arrow), along with sphenoid dysplasia and distortion of the sella. **B.** Bilateral optic nerve gliomas in an 11-year-old patient without neurofibromatosis. Notice the diffuse enlargement of both optic nerves. **C.** Optic nerve glioma. A 10-year-old girl with poor vision in the right eye, exotropia, and proptosis. An axial CT scan after contrast injection shows a well-circumscribed homogeneous mass lesion intrinsic to the right optic nerve. This pattern of tumor growth is also seen in other intraconal lesions, such as cavernous hemangiomas, neurofibromatosis, and meningiomas. **D.** Optic nerve glioma, coronal view. Notice the lesion is homogeneous without a "donut" sign. A and B from Gonzalez CF, Grossman CB, Masdeu JC: *Head and spine imaging.* New York, Wiley Medical, 1985.

ties of ultrasound (see Fig. 4.9), venography, and air contrast orbitography; intracranial involvement had to be documented by pneumoencephalography and polytomography.

The resolution of CT scanning has been so far superior to that of magnetic resonance imaging (MRI) (see Fig. 8.12). However, the recent development and use of orbital coils in MRI imaging of the orbit is making this modality the procedure of choice to study diseases of the optic nerve (5A). With MRI, the optic nerve glioma shows similar intensity characteristics of the normal optic nerve. Optic nerve sheath meningiomas yield a slightly stronger signal on both spin echo and saturation recovery.

With the current trend toward the conservative management of this tumor, serial CT and/or MRI scans are excellent means of following tumor growth. Radical surgery is reserved for progressive growing tumors. The management of gliomas of the optic nerve and chiasm remains controversial. Hoyt (43) believes that conservative management is indicated for the benign slow-growing tumors. Orbital surgery is indicated to debulk the tumor in a blind proptotic eye. Intracranial surgery usually is limited to shunting for hydrocephalus (73).

Wright (83), however, has defined a subpopulation of patients whose gliomas undergo rapid (rather than indolent) growth (associated with a lower incidence of neurofibromatosis). If these rapidly progressive tumors remain confined to the optic canal and orbit, then full surgical excision is attempted. If the chiasm is involved, tumor excision is not possible. Lloyd (56) believes that intraorbital gliomas usually should be removed through a lateral orbitotomy regardless of the growth pattern. Radiation therapy is not considered to be helpful (30).

Amputation Neuroma, Neurofibroma, and Neurilemmoma

Neurogenic tumors of peripheral nerve origin arise as proliferations of connective tissue elements, such as Schwann cells.

Amputation neuroma occurs following injury or amputation of a nerve. The Schwann cells start to form potential sheaths, and axons follow; however, as there is no guide to indicate which way to grow, the regenerating nerve becomes a coiled nodule of disorganized neural tissue. An amputation neuroma can occur following enucleation, and it can be mistaken for a recurrent tumor. Although benign, these tumor-like nodules can be painful or can cause extrusion of a prosthesis.

Neurofibromas can occur as solitary orbital tumors or, more frequently, as a part of a generalized neurofibromatosis (von Recklinghausen disease). The plexiform neurofibroma usually presents in childhood. It usually involves the eyelid. It can be associated with severe craniofacial anomalies. The neurofibroma can involve the orbit as it intertwines between muscles, nerves, blood vessels, and any other orbital structures along the way, thereby making dissection very difficult—if not impossible. Neurilemmomas or Schwannomas are composed

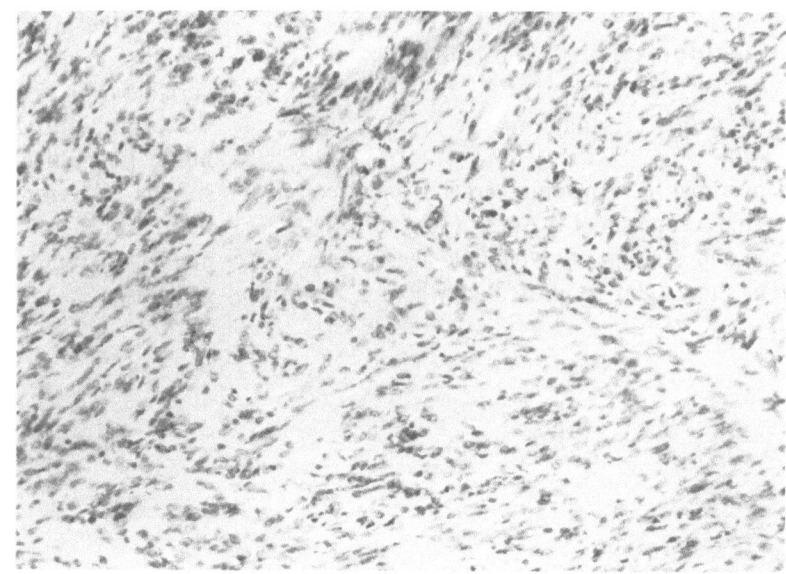

A

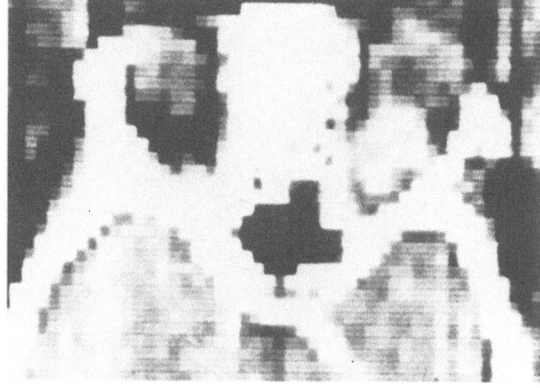

B

Fig. 11.6A. Hematoxylin and eosin preparation of an Antoni-A type neurilemmoma, showing interlacing bundles of spindle-shaped cells surrounding acellular spaces. Neurilemmoma, which have a more haphazard arrangement with areas of necrosis and microcytoid degeneration, are called Antoni-B type. **B.** Plexiform neurofibroma. An axial CT scan after contrast injection reveals an intraconal retrobulbar mass lesion in a 43-year-old woman with proptosis, papilledema, and diminished visual acuity of the left eye. This is an old CT scan.

capsulated. Histologic examination reveals long, spindle-shaped palisading cells surrounding acellular spaces (Fig. 11.6A).

Intraorbital neurofibromas and neurilemmomas are seen on CT scans as homogeneous mass lesions with distinct borders. The tumors may be intraconal, extraconal, or extraorbital, involving the preseptal soft tissue, the eyelids, and the temporal fossa. These tumors usually have higher attenuation than optic gliomas, with a density similar to that of meningiomas. Moderate-to-significant enhancement is seen after contrast injection (Fig. 11.6B) (31, 33, 42). Plexiform neurofibromas involving the orbital apex can be easily confused with optic gliomas or meningiomas. In neurofibromatosis, this tumor can be found in association with partial dysplasia or aplasia of the sphenoid bone, which allows herniation of the middle fossa structures into the orbit causing proptosis of the globe.

Vascular Orbital Tumors

Cavernous Hemangiomas

Cavernous hemangiomas are the most common benign neoplasm of the orbit (36) (68) (81). They occur most frequently in middle-aged women (34). The tumor may be located anywhere in the orbit.

Cavernous hemangiomas in the eyelid may present as palpable mass lesions. Tumors in the muscle cone may present with proptosis and blurred vision due to direct pressure on the optic nerve or retina. Tumors located immediately behind the eye may indent the globe, causing choroidal folds and tumor-induced anisometropic hyperopia. The rate of tumor growth is slow. Pain is rarely part of the clinical picture, except when proptosis causes lagophthalmos and corneal exposure. The gross pathology of cavernous hemangiomas is an encapsulated tumor with a rubbery or spongy quality. Since they are independent of the general circulation, they often can be shelled out with little bleeding. The tumor is composed of blood-filled, sinusoid-like spaces lined by thin, attenuated epithelium (Figs. 11.7A and 11.7B).(40)

On the CT scan, these lesions appear as sharply marginated soft-tissue densities that are slightly hyperdense with respect to the optic nerves and extraocular muscles. (80) The lesions are more frequently seen in the intraconal space lateral to the optic nerve, and occasionally in the orbital apex (Figs. 11.7C and 11.7D) (see Fig. 2.21). They may contain calcifications (see Fig. 2.25) and may have variable degrees of enhancement due to the very slow intratumoral circulation. The CT scan is highly suggestive of the diagnosis, but it is not specific. Cavernous hemangiomas may be confused with neurofibromas, lymphangiomas, lacrimal gland tumors, metastatic lesions, and other growths.

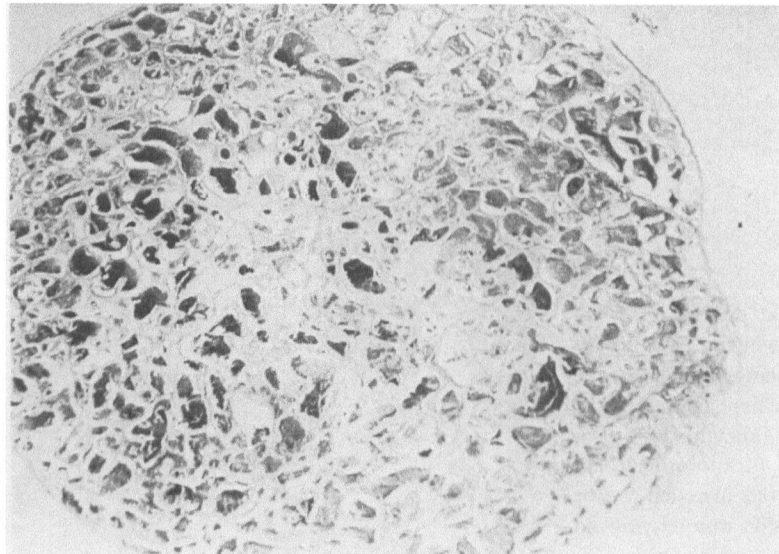

Fig. 11.7A. Hematoxylin and eosin preparation of cavernous hemangioma demonstrates multiple sinusoid-like, blood-filled spaces.

Fig. 11.7B. Hematoxylin and eosin preparation demonstrating blood-filled sinusoid line by thin, attenuated endothelium.

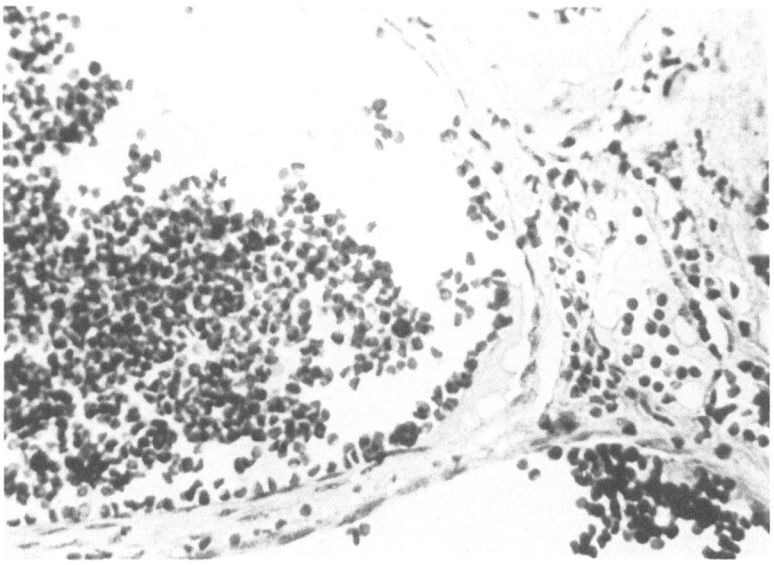

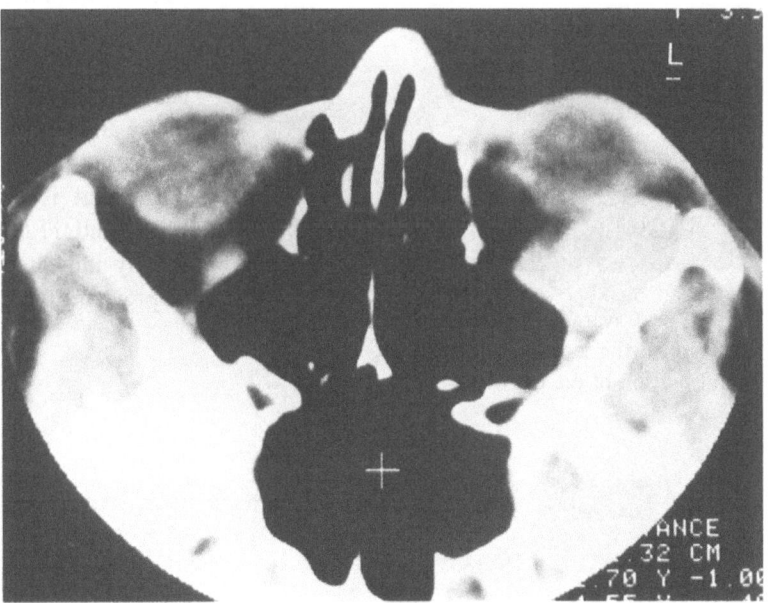

Fig. 11.7C. Cavernous hemangioma of the left orbit. A 36-year-old woman with progressive left eye proptosis and blurred vision. There was a rounded mass palpated along the infratemporal orbital mass. Funduscopic examination shows choroidal folds. An axial CT scan after contrast injection at the lower orbital level reveals a well-circumscribed mass lesion with sharply delineated borders located in the lateroposterior portion of the left orbit. Medial anterior displacement of the left globe by the mass is shown.

Orbital expansion is a common finding in plain x-ray films of the orbit. Phleboliths also can be observed (71). Orbital ultrasound is a useful examination for patients whose CT scan suggests a cavernous hemangioma (14, 21). On B-mode examination, the tumor has well-delineated anterior border echoes with good sound transmission (Fig. 11.7E). A-mode ultrasonography demonstrates moderate internal reflectivity (Fig. 11.7F) that is considered to be characteristic of this orbital tumor. Prior to CT scanning, arteriography or venography was used for the diagnosis of this tumor (81). Interestingly, these examinations indicate a tumor presence only indirectly by showing displacement of the normal orbital vasculature. Despite their obvious vascular origin, cavernous hemangiomas (as opposed to capillary hemangiomas of childhood) are low-flow systems that are independent of the systemic circulation. Thus, they behave on angiography as avascular masses and do not "light up" or "blush," with the exception of an occasional small pool of contrast media in the area of the tumor (see Fig. 5.4) (22). Partial opacification of cavernous hemangiomas with orbital venography have been reported (2). Both arteriography and venography have been largely supplanted by CT scanning and ultrasound in the evaluations of patients with this disease.

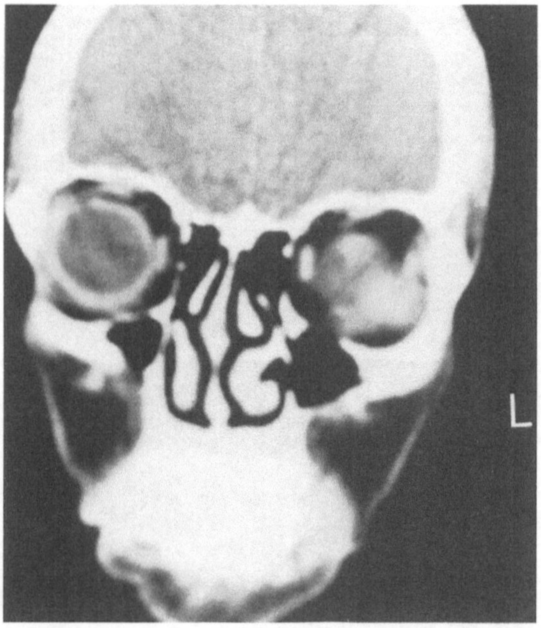

Capillary Hemangioma

Capillary hemangiomas are tumors of early childhood, with a tendency to grow for 6 or more months and then to involute (49). These "strawberry nevi" of childhood, when present on the eyelid, can occlude the pupillary axis and cause amblyopia. In the orbit, they can involve the retrobulbar space and can cause proptosis. Microscopically, the tumor is composed of benign endothelial cells surrounding small, capillary-sized vascular spaces—most of which become occluded with age (Fig. 11.8A). On the CT scan, these lesions are usually well-marginated extraconal lesions that enhance after IV contrast injection (Fig. 11.8B). Angiography usually reveals an extensive capillary blush that is characteristic of the lesion (Figs. 11.8C and 11.8D) (see Fig. 5.3) (22). Treatment is only indicated for severe cosmetic blemish or to prevent amblyopia.

Fig. 11.7D. Cavernous hemanigoma, direct coronal section. Notice the location of the tumor in the inferior lateral portion of the left orbit.

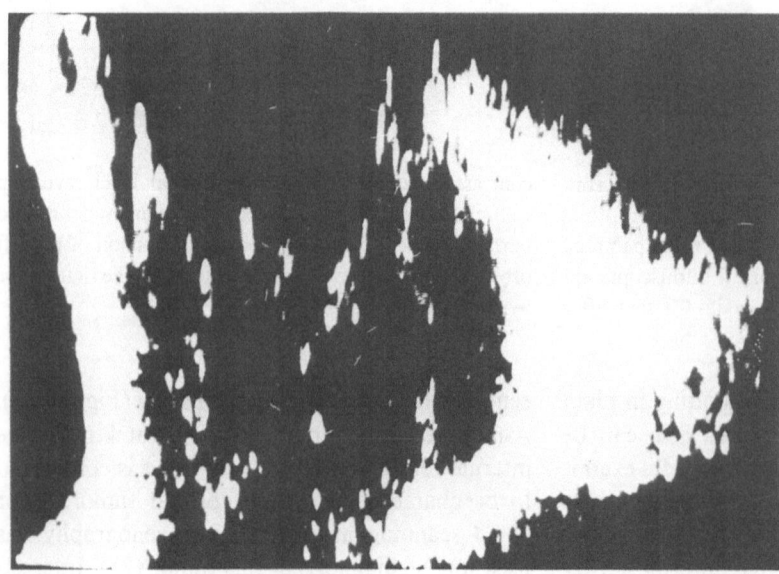

Fig. 11.7E. B-mode ultrasonogram of a cavernous hemangioma demonstrates sharply delineated border echoes with good sound transmission.

Fig. 11.7F. A-mode ultrasonography of cavernous hemangioma demonstrating moderate internal reflectivity.

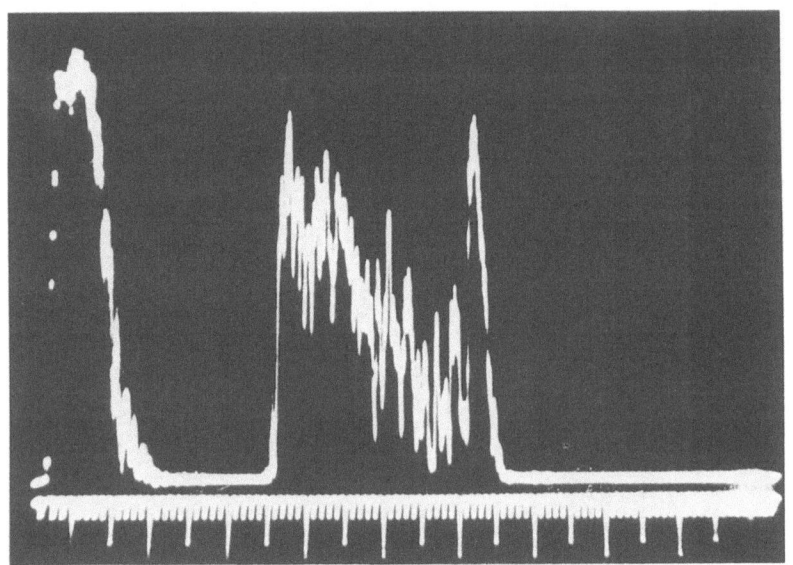

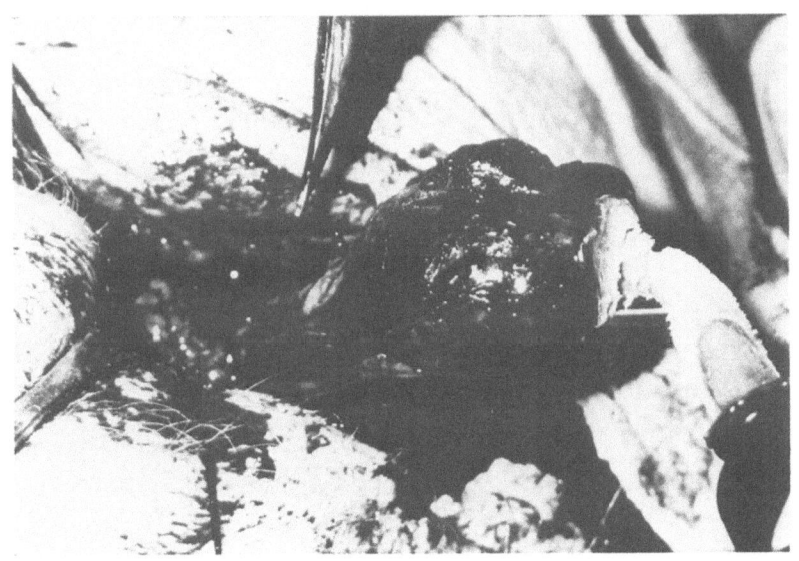

Fig. 11.7G. Cavernous hemangioma removed from the patient's left orbit.

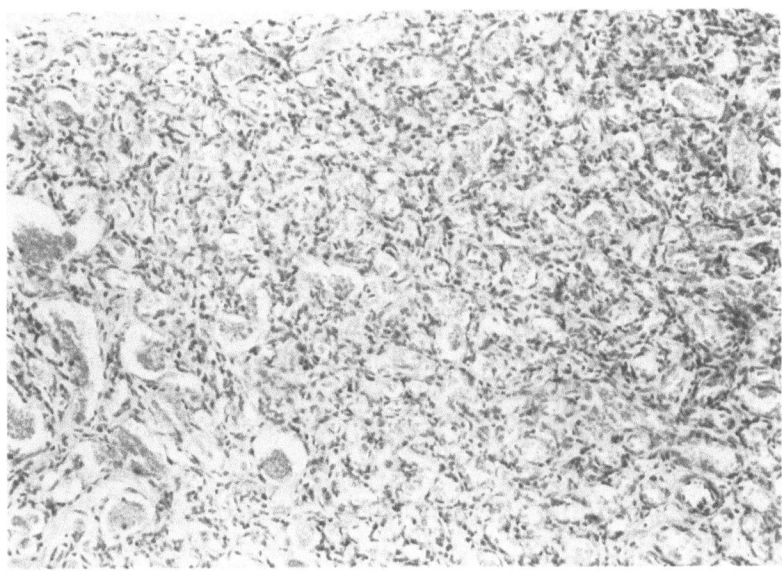

Fig. 11.8A. Hematoxylin and eosin preparation of a capillary hemangioma. Note capillary-sized channels formed by endothelial cells and filled with blood.

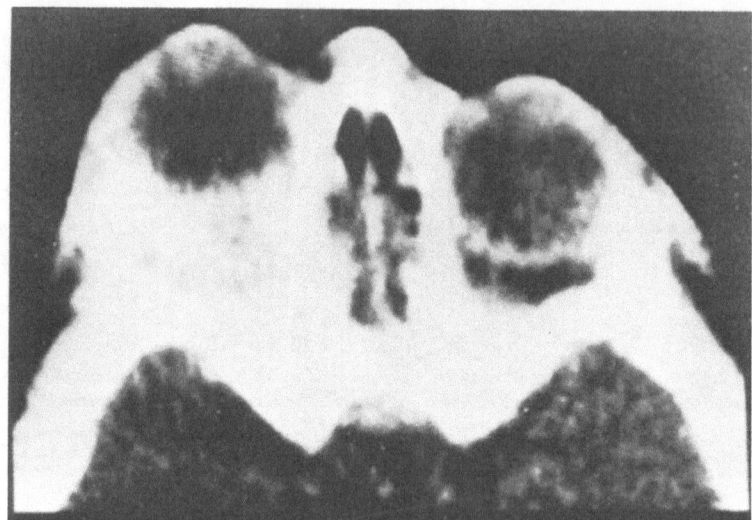

Fig. 11.8B. Contrast-enhancement CT scan demonstrating marked proptosis. There is a mass that involves the entire retrobulbar space with profound enhancement (capillary hemangioma).

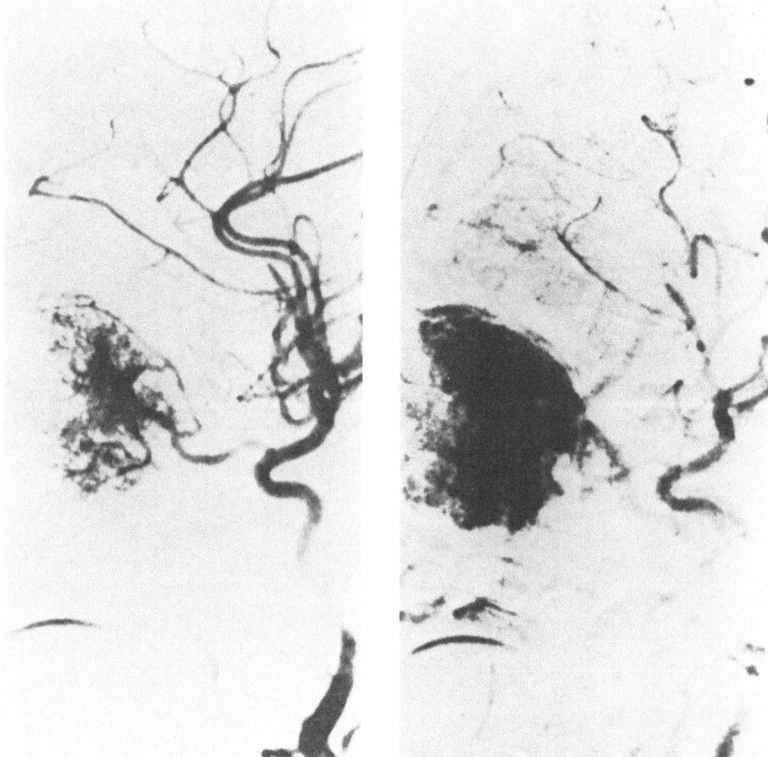

Fig. 11.8C. Lateral view from a carotid arteriogram of a capillary hemangioma demonstrates an intense orbital vascular blush occurring in the early arterial phase. The ophthalmic artery is enlarged. **D.** The blush becomes more intense in the capillary phase. No arteriovenous shunting is present (Courtesy of Hammerschlag SB, Hesselink JR, Weber AL: *Computed Tomography of the Eye and Orbit.* Norwalk, CT, Appleton-Century-Crofts, 1983).

Lymphangioma

Lymphangiomas occur in the orbits of children and young adults. They continue to increase in size, causing protrusion of the globe, swelling of the eyelids, conjunctiva, pain, and blurring of vision. Hemorrhage in a lymphangioma can occur spontaneously or with mild trauma, causing a sudden increase in proptosis. These tumors contain lymphoid tissue that can increase during various systemic infections, resulting in intermittent increases in proptosis. Lymphangiomas usually are not nonencapsulated and infiltrate orbital tissue,

thereby making resection more difficult. Histologic examination reveals numerous lymph-filled spaces lined by endothelium and surrounded by fibrous septae with foci of benign lymphoid tissue in the stroma (Fig. 11.9A). The CT scan shows a nonencapsulated heterogeneous mass lesion that may involve the intraconal or extraconal spaces (Fig. 11.9B). In the extraconal location, they are commonly seen medial to the optic nerve—a feature that helps in the differentiation of these tumors, with cavernous hemangiomas that are usually lateral to the optic nerve (21). On ultrasonography, tumors, cavernous hemangiomas, and lymphangi-

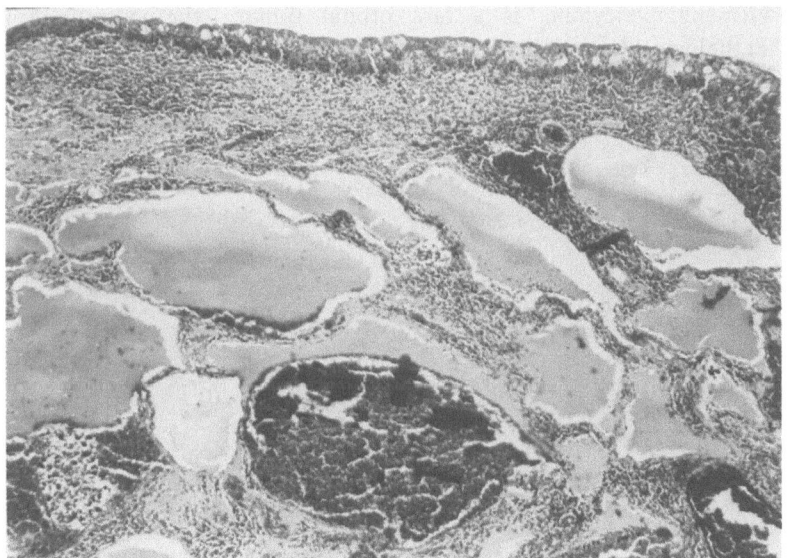

Fig. 11.9A. Hematoxylin and eosin preparation of a lymphangioma. The endothelium lines vascular spaces, which are filled with lymph or blood and surrounded by lymphoid tissue.

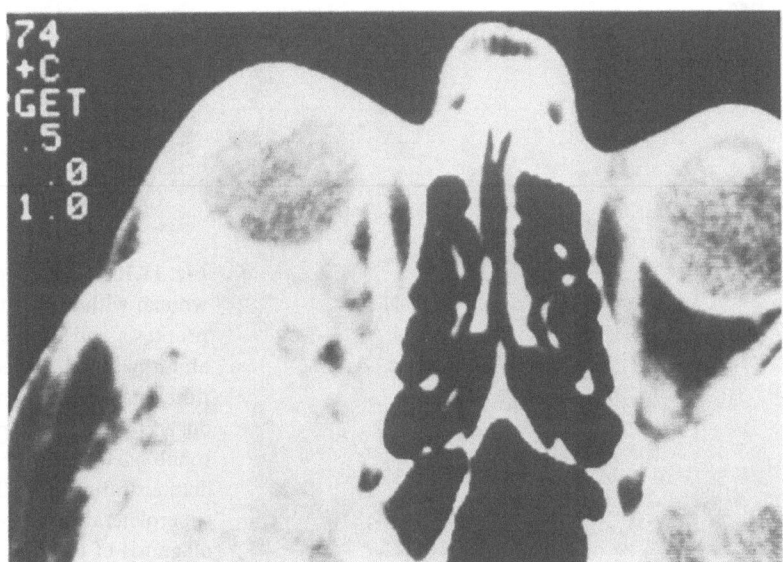

Fig. 11.9B. Lymphangioma of the right orbit. An axial CT scan after contrast injection reveals an irregular, heterogeneous mass lesion with ill-defined margins involving both the intraconal and extraconal spaces.

omas tend to have well-defined anterior border echoes with good sound transmission and moderate internal reflectivity. On MRI, the high-signal intensity on the T2-weighted intensity images probably result from the partially cystic nature of this lesion; they help to differentiate it from edematous infiltrative processes of the retrobulbar fat, such as orbital pseudotumor (see Fig. 8.10). Although lymphangiomas and cavernous hemangioma are proliferations of vascular elements, they tend to behave on angiography as avascular mass lesions and on venography only to the extent that they deflect normal orbital venous channels.

Hemangiopericytoma

Hemangiopericytoma is a rare orbital tumor. Pathologically these tumors are composed of plump pericytes surrounding a rich capillary network. The biological behavior of this tumor cannot be predicted on the basis of its histologic appearance (48). It has many similarities with cavernous hemangioma of the orbit. Hemangiopericytoma presents as a slowly progressive mass lesion in the orbit that develops in a period of 1–2 years. If the tumor is located within the muscle cone, it may present with proptosis and blurred vision. However, the tumor may also present as a mass along the orbital rim. Radiographically, the tumor cannot be distinguished from the more benign cavernous hemangioma. Computed tomography of both tumors typically demonstrates a well-circumscribed encapsulated mass lesion (Fig. 11.10). Hemangiopericytomas are usually intraconal, but they may involve the extraconal space as well. The density of these tumors is usually higher than the normal density of the optic nerve and rectus muscles. Enhancement is usually seen. Erosion of the underlying bone may occur. Magnetic resonance imaging shows relative high signal intensity

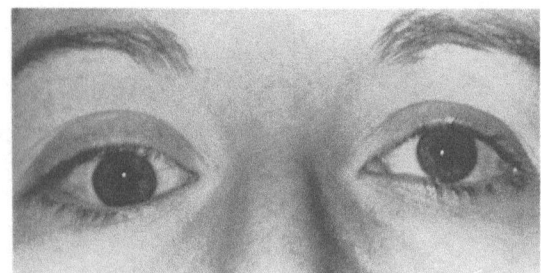

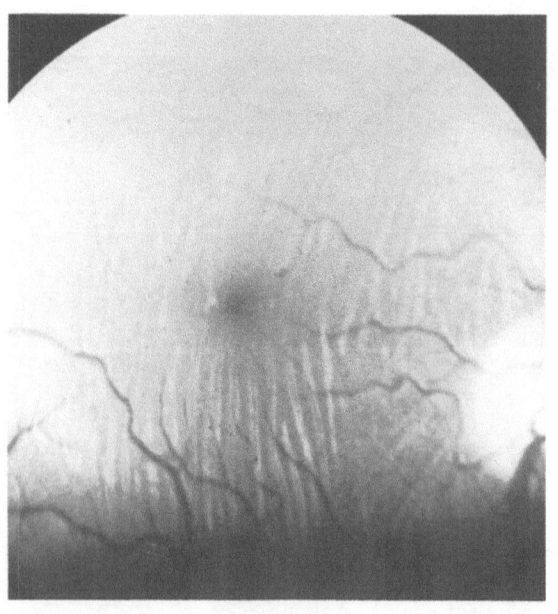

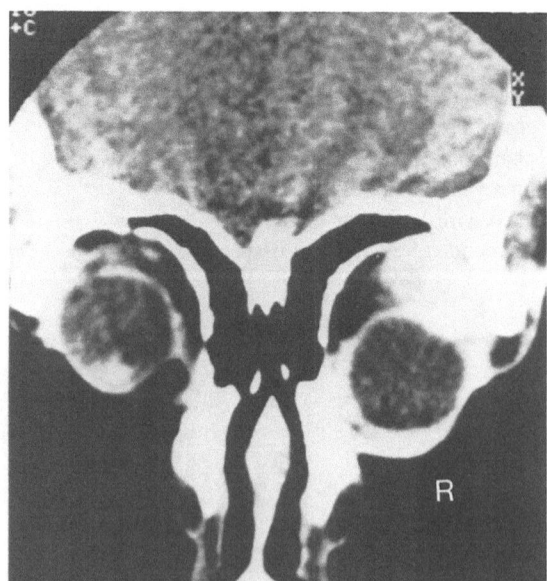

Fig. 11.10A. Hemangiopericytoma. A 30-year-old white woman with a 1-year history of progressive visual loss, proptosis and dysplasia in the right eye, shown on an abnormal funduscopic examination. B. Picture of a funduscopic examination, showing chorioretinal striae produced by the hemangiopericytoma. C. A CT scan, coronal view, of the orbit after contrast injection demonstrating a well-defined enhancing lesion in the superolateral aspect of the right orbit. The pathologic diagnosis of the tumor was hemangiopericytoma.

on T2-weighted images (see Fig. 8.11). A dense homogeneous stain is seen on selective carotid angiography.

Any orbital tumor that seems to be clinically consistent with cavernous hemangioma rarely may be a potentially malignant hemangiopericytoma. Since tumor recurrence may be related to incomplete excision, a complete en-bloc resection should be done in any tumor believed to be a cavernous hemangioma.

Vascular Malformations

Although they are not real neoplasms, vascular malformations must be considered in the differential diagnosis of orbital tumors. Intraorbital extensions of carotid-ophthalmic aneurysms, arteriovenous fistulas and varices, and extraorbital carotid-cavernous fistulas can present with features of a primary orbital tumor.

Orbital Varix

An orbital varix is a congenital benign proliferation of venous elements that become increasingly symptomatic with age; it presents with intermittent proptosis and pain. The proptosis may be pulsating. The pain is typically quite severe and results from diffuse vascular engorgement. Symptoms commonly occur in the morning after patients have been in the recumbent position during sleep. However, this is not always true, and the acute onset of orbital symptoms may occur at any time of day.

Orbital varices often involve the superior and inferior ophthalmic veins, both of which have a large component in the muscle cone. Enhancement is marked after IV injection of contrast media. The CT scan may be normal, without provocative tests such as Valsalva maneuver or compression of the jugular vein. After the provocative test, the distended varices appear as sharply marginated intraconal masses. (10) Orbital venography, however, is still of value for demonstrating these lesions (Fig. 11.11) (6).

Since orbital varices tend to be diffuse processes, rather than focal tumefactions, surgical excision involves significant risk. It is rarely possible to completely excise or clip off these multichannelled vascular anomalies; thus, surgical intervention is reserved only for the most debilitating form of the disease. Even in this circumstance, a resection

of the varix often is subtotal and usually is limited to the more anterior manifestations of the venous anomaly. (26)

Carotid-Cavernous-Fistulae

The orbital manifestations of carotid-cavernous fistulae are typically seen after major head trauma although it may occur spontaneously. There is a sudden arterialization of the orbital venous plexus, which results in a characteristic conjunctival hyperemia without inflammation. This is often associated with significant chemosis. The elevation in episcleral venous pressure may result in a secondary open-angle glaucoma. Proptosis is constant. On the CT scan, a carotid-cavernous fistula is characterized by an enlarged superior ophthalmic vein and cavernous sinus and proptosis. Carotid angiography is necessary to demonstrate the lesion, which is characterized by rapid filling of a very dilated superior ophthalmic vein, with poor perfusion of the intracranial carotid artery branches (Fig. 11.12). Obliteration of the fistulae with a detachable balloon catheter is the present treatment of choice.

Lacrimal Gland Tumors

Fifty percent of the tumors in the lacrimal gland region are epithelial in nature and 50% are lymphoid or inflammatory lesions (38). The most common epithelial neoplasm of the lacrimal gland is the benign mixed tumor, followed by adenoid cystic carcinoma, malignant mixed tumor, adenocarcinoma, mucoepidermoid carcinoma, and other rare tumors. (74)

A benign mixed tumor of the lacrimal gland generally presents as a painless mass in the lacrimal fossa of more than 1 year's duration. It is usually seen in the third or fourth decade. A history of recent pain in association with increased tumor size is the clinical correlate of the histologic transformation of the mass from a benign mixed tumor to a malignant mixed tumor. Malignant mixed tumors and adenoid cystic carcinomas usually present as a rapidly progressive painful mass lesion in the lacrimal fossa.

On microscopic examination, mixed tumors of the lacrimal gland contain both secretory and ductal elements and vary greatly, even in different parts of the same tumor. Tubular structures that

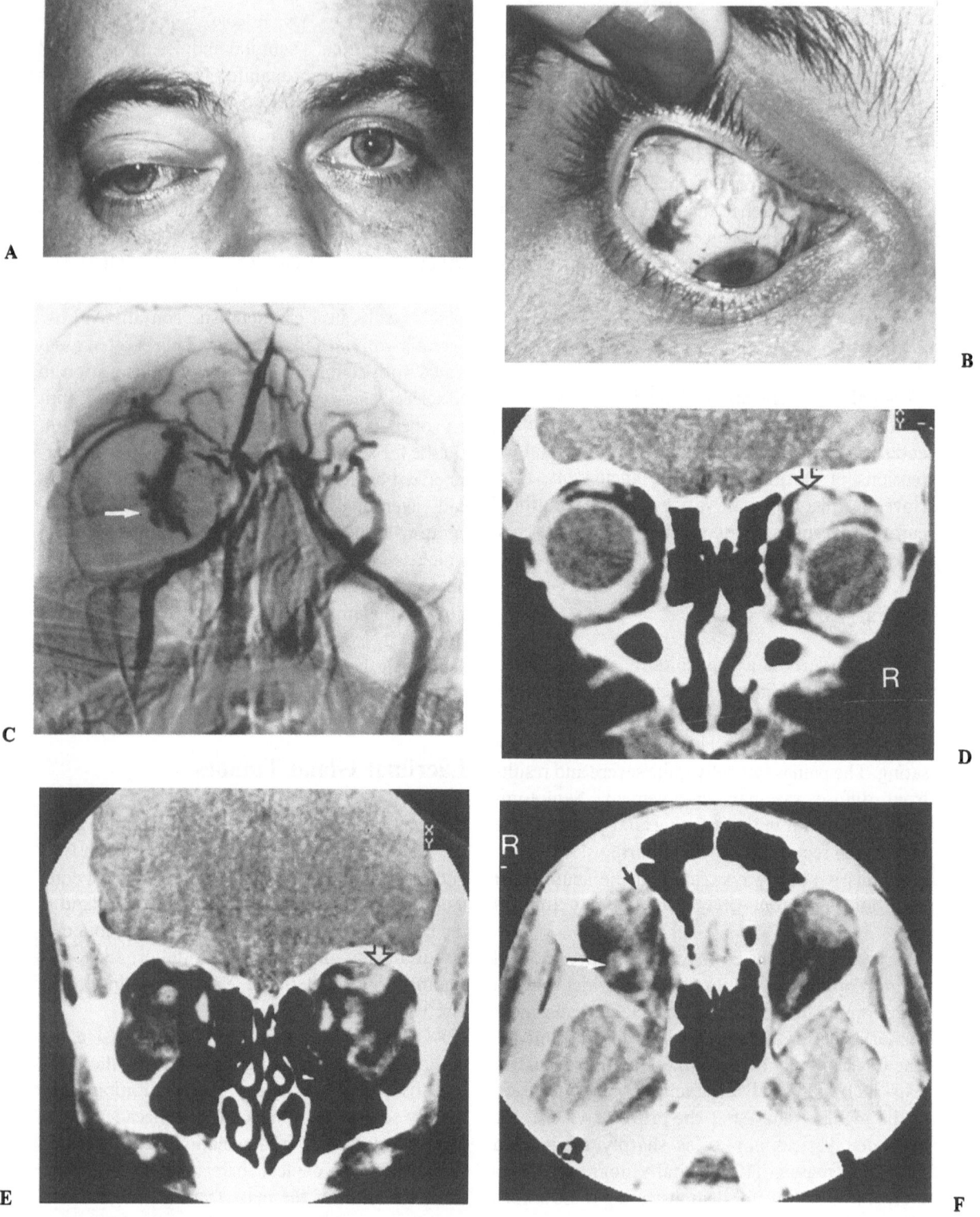

Fig. 11.11A. Orbital varix. A 35-year-old man with intermittent acute orbital syndrome of pain and proptosis for 11 years. **B.** The same patient as in A. Note the vascular dilatation of superior conjunctiva of the right eye. **C.** Presurgical venogram documenting orbital varix of the right side (arrow). **D.** A CT scan, coronal view. Irregular high-density, soft-tissue abnormality in the superior medial aspect of the right orbit outside the muscle cone (arrow). Enhancement was seen after contrast injection. **E.** A CT scan. Posterior coronal section in the same patient as in **D** showing the location of the lesions outside the muscle cone (arrows). **F.** Axial CT scan section of another patient taken in the superior aspect of the orbit showing the irregular, elongated soft-tissue mass extending posteriorly outside the muscle cone (arrow) (Courtesy of Robert Peyster, M.D., Philadelphia).

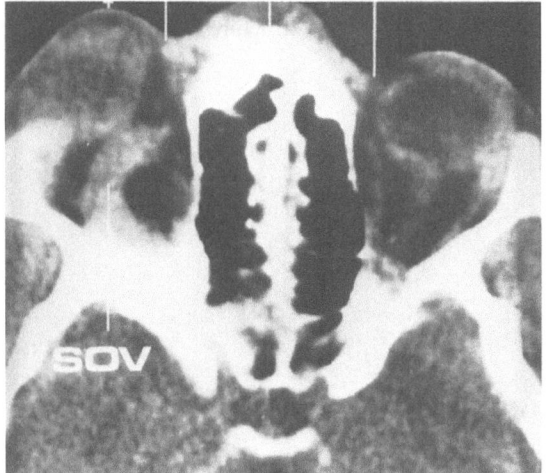

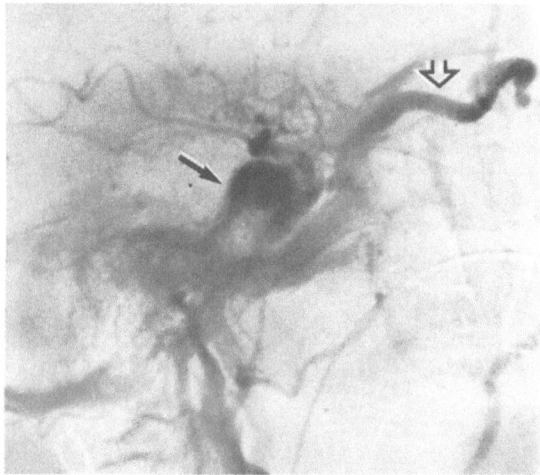

Fig. 11.12. Arteriovenous fistula. **A.** CT scan, axial view. Marked dilatation of the superior ophthalmic vein (sov) due to a carotid arteriovenous fistula. **B.** Selective carotid arteriogram demonstrating the carotid-cavernous fistula (solid arrow) and the significant dilatation of the superior ophthalmic vein (open arrow).

anastamose in an irregular fashion lie in a myxoid, fibrous, or cartilaginous stroma (Fig. 11.13A). The ducts or tubes are lined by a double layer of epithelial cells; the inner layer is thought to secrete mucus and the outer layer to give rise to a myxoid or fibrous stroma. A malignant mixed tumor contains areas resembling a benign mixed tumor, along with areas of adenocarcinoma. Adenoid cystic carcinoma has a "Swiss cheese" appearance, as aggregates of poorly differentiated small-packed cells contain cystic spaces lie in a hyalinized stoma (Fig. 11.13B).

Plain skull x-ray films of benign mixed tumors may show a pressure defect in the bone of the superotemporal portion of the orbit as a marker of long-standing mass effect on adjacent bone. The CT appearance of benign mixed adenomas is variable. Usually, the tumor presents as a well-defined extraconal lesion in the superior lateral aspect of the orbit that displaces the globe medially and inferiorly (Figs. 11.13C, 11.13D, 11.13E, and 11.13F). Proptosis may be apparent. Bone erosion may be present. The tumors usually have a homogeneous high density that enhances after contrast media injection. Calcifications may be seen, but they usually are microscopic and are found only on pathologic examination. If the tumor has cystic components, it may be irregular and may not enhance. When the tumor enlarges, it usually extends posteriorly, displacing the muscle cone medially and the globe anteriorly.

Malignant tumors, on the other hand, are irregular, poorly defined lesions that infiltrate and destroy the bone and other orbital structures. Malignant epithelial tumors also may extend outside the orbit into the infratemporal fossa or the intracranial cavity. Plain skull x-ray films usually show bony destruction of the superolateral orbital rim (Fig. 11.13H). Calcification and bone sclerosis may also be present. On CT examination, adenoid cystic carcinoma has an attenuation similar to that of soft-tissue density, and it shows moderate enhancement after IV contrast media injection (Fig. 13.23). Malignant mixed tumors, on the other hand, usually have a higher attenuation than soft tissue, and they show marked enhancement after contrast media injection (Figs. 11.13G, 11.13H, and 11.13I) (38) (see Fig. 4.10).

The lymphoid inflammatory lesions (pseudotumor) are seen on CT scanning as diffuse homogeneous gland enlargements that are indistinguishable from other lacrimal gland tumors or orbital cellulitis (Fig. 11.13J). Ultrasonography may be more accurate in differentiating inflammatory disease from solid tumors, and thus can be helpful in these cases (38).

Choristomas

Orbital choristomas are congenital tumors composed of elements that are normally not present in the orbit. Dermoid cysts, epidermoid cysts, and teratomas comprise this group of orbital tumors.

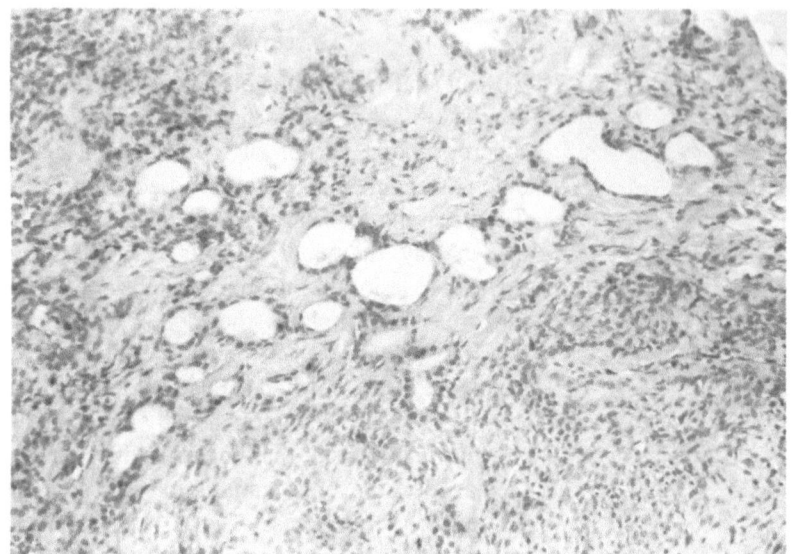

Fig. 11.13A. Hematoxylin and eosin preparation of a benign mixed tumor showing tubular structures and a fibrous stroma.

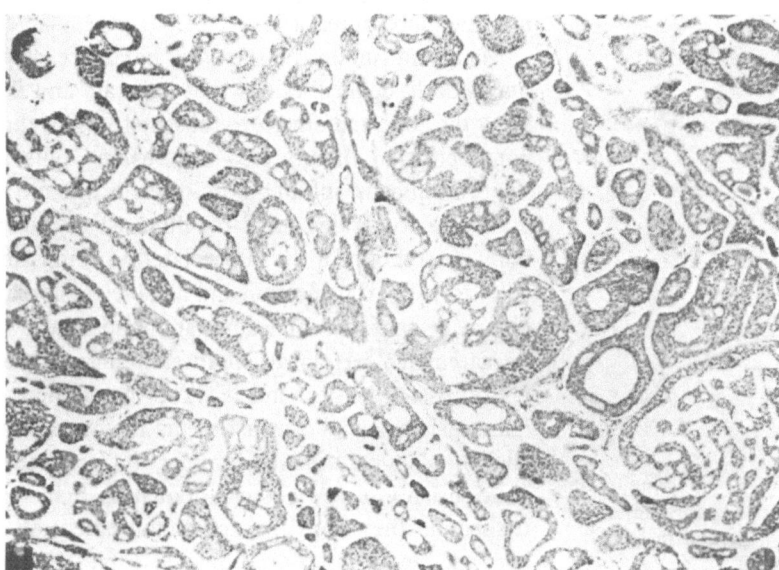

Fig. 11.13B. Hematoxylin and eosin preparation of adenoid cystic carcinoma displaying the characteristic "Swiss cheese" pattern.

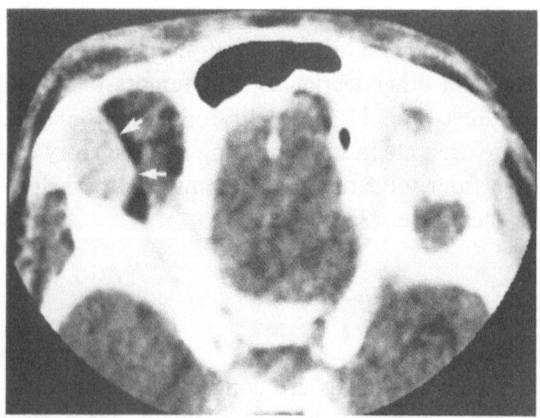

C

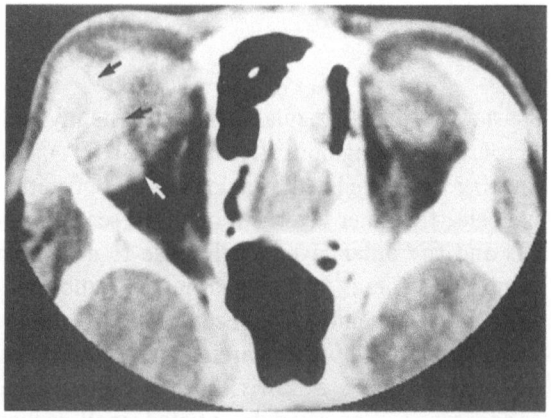

D

Fig. 11.13C, D. A CT scan of a benign mixed tumor, axial sections. A large, homogeneous, sharply defined mass is seen in the right lacrimal fossa (arrows).

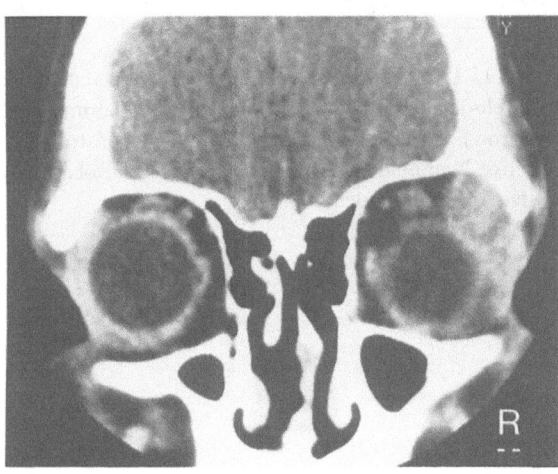
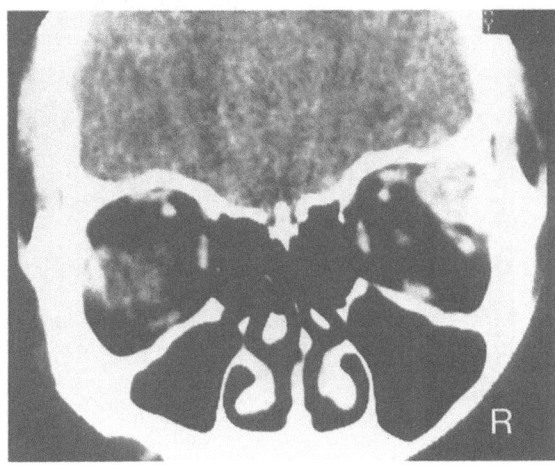

E   F

Fig. 11.13E, F. A CT scan of a benign mixed tumor, coronal sections. The mass is shown displacing the globe and the lateral rectus muscle medially and inferiorly (Courtesy of Robert Peyster, M.D., Philadelphia).

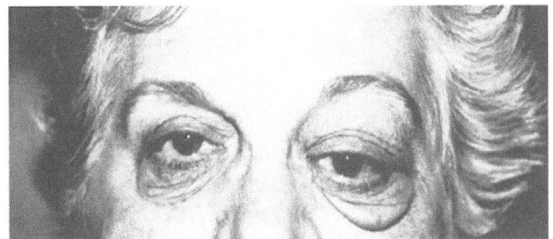

G

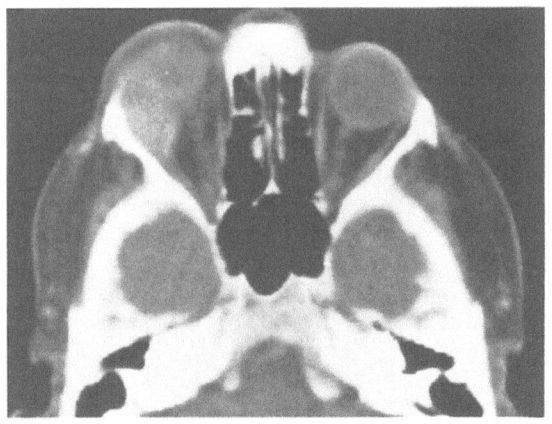

I

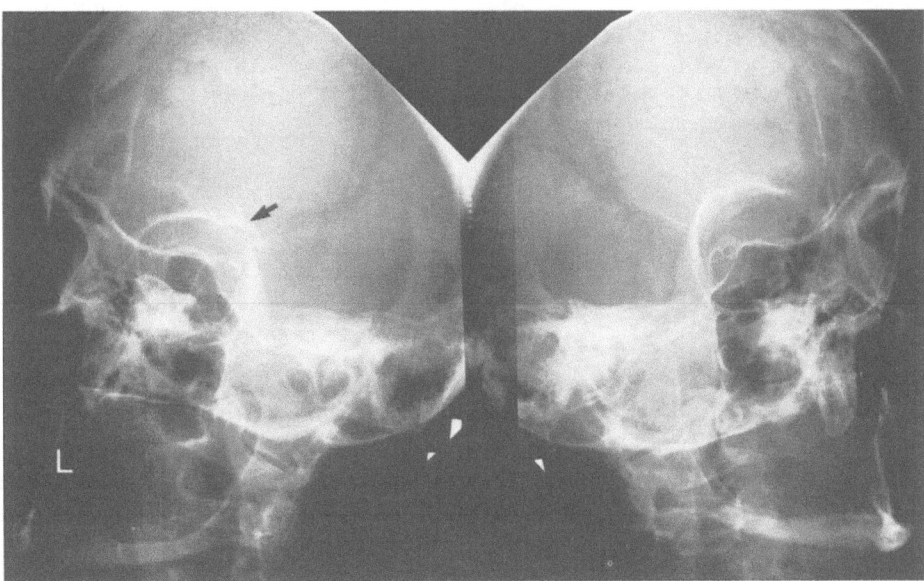

H

Fig. 11.13G. Malignant mixed tumor of the lacrimal gland. Shown is a 65-year-old woman presenting with a history of swelling in the superolateral aspect of the left eye. **H.** Plain skull radiographs from the patient in **G** demonstrate sclerosis and bone erosion in the supra-lateral aspect of the left orbit (arrow). **I.** A CT scan of the patient in **G** demonstrates a soft-tissue mass intrinsic to the lacrimal gland in the lacrimal fossa of the left orbit, with anterior and medial deviation of the left globe.

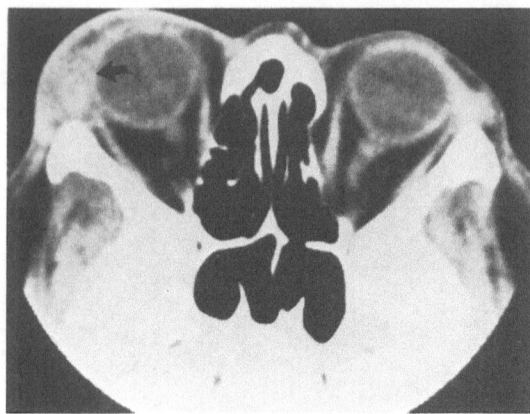

Fig. 11.13J. A CT scan of another patient demonstrates a well-defined soft-tissue mass in the right lacrimal fossa (arrow). The histiologic examination demonstrated reactive lymphoid hyperplasia (Courtesy of Robert Peyster, M.D., Philadelphia).

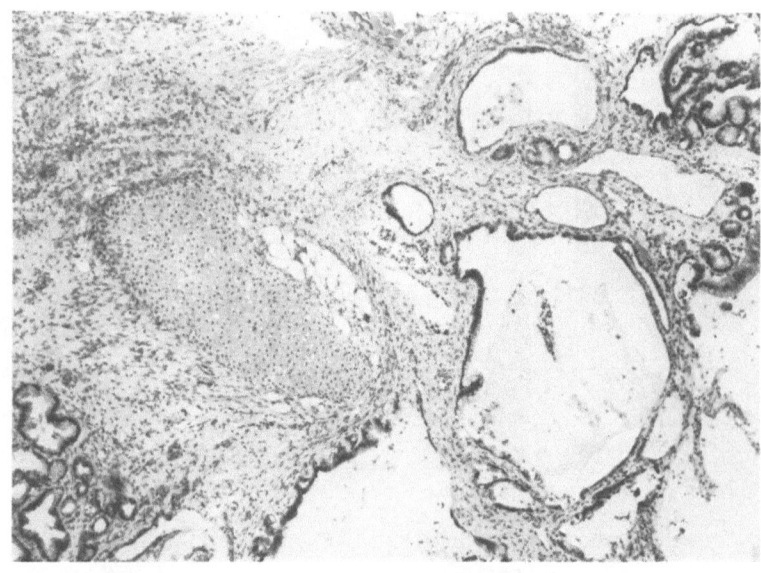

Fig. 11.14A. Hematoxylin and eosin preparation demonstrating an orbital teratoma characterized by enteric-type epithelium. Note an island of cartilage on the left.

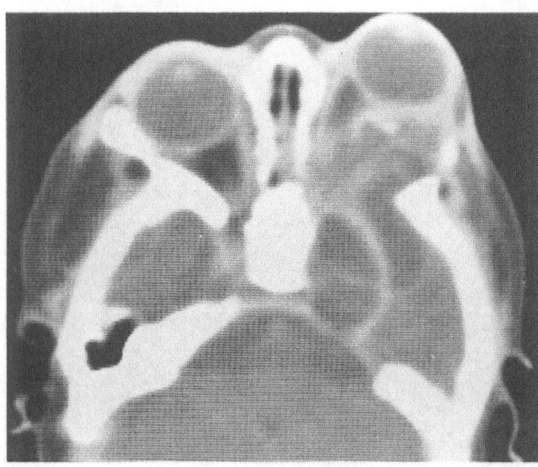

Fig. 11.14B. A CT scan of a teratoma with right orbital and intracranial involvement. An axial CT scan shows a defect in the left sphenoid bone and a heterogeneous, retrobulbar, multicystic mass lesion extending into the temporal lobe.

Fig. 11.15A. Hematoxylin and eosin preparation of a dermoid. Note the sebaceous glands present in the wall of the cyst.

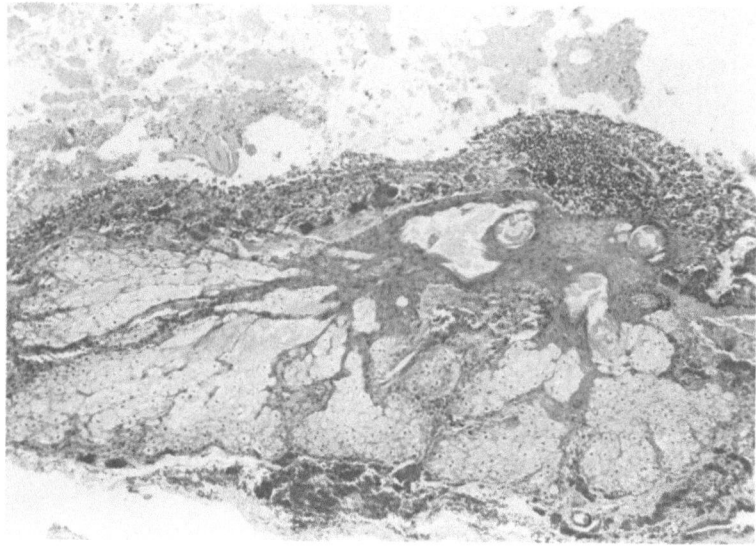

Teratoma

Teratomas are first noted at birth or shortly thereafter resulting in exophthalmos, with stretching of the eyelids and enlargement of the palpebral fissure. Teratomas contain tissue from all three germinal layers (Fig. 11.14A) and have a heterogeneous appearance on a CT scan, as they may contain calcified high-density areas as well as low-density cysts and fat (Fig. 11.14B) (3). The cystic structures may be the result of mucin-secreting enteric mucosa or epidermoid cysts.

Dermoid

Dermoid cysts are tumors arising from the epithelial rests, which involve the periorbital tissues as well as the orbit. Dermoid cysts contain keratin, epithelial debris, sebaceous material, hair, and oily liquids. Two presentations in the orbit are common. In young children, they appear as superficial, small mass lesions with a marked predilection for the superotemporal orbital rim, often with osseous involvement. In older children and adults, dermoids may present as deep orbital tumors. These tumors typically present as painless mass lesions of long duration. All can cause contoured bony deformity by a chronic pressure effect. The histologic examination of dermoid tumors is characterized by the presence of a mix of keratinized and nonkeratinized epithelium, sebaceous gland, and hair follicles (Fig. 11.15A). (46) On CT scanning, a dermoid is seen as a smooth, extraconal, clearly defined cystic tumor with a low-density center that usually contains materials with fatty density (Figs.

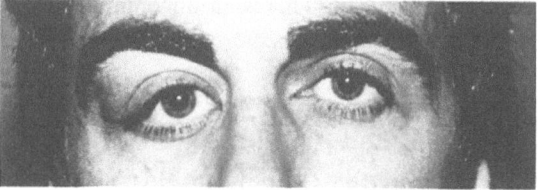

Fig. 11.15B. Deep orbital dermoid. A 41-year-old man presented for evaluation of painless swelling, of many years duration, in the superotemporal aspect of the right orbit. Note the S-shaped contour deformity of the right upper eyelid and the deviation of the globe down and in.

11.15B and 11.15C) (Fig. 2.20, 13.15–13.17) (38). The rim of the cyst is thin and enhances after IV injection of contrast media (33). On plain x-ray films, dermoid may produce a sharply marginated defect in the orbital rim with a sclerotic border. On MRI, the tumors are recognized because they yield the same signal intensity as retrobulbar fat (Fig. 8.7).

Although pathologically, these tumors always contain sebaceous material, the CT scan may not always be hypodense and may have (on occasions) attenuation closer to that of muscle. In those cases where the tumors are situated in the lacrimal gland area (a common location for dermoid), the differentiation from lacrimal gland tumors can be very difficult. The CT scan is invaluable for establishing the correct diagnosis. Benign mixed tumors tend to be homogeneous, while deep orbital dermoids are more likely to have a structure that is heterogeneous with multiple areas of low attenuation. Dermoids also frequently have a "tail" that extends

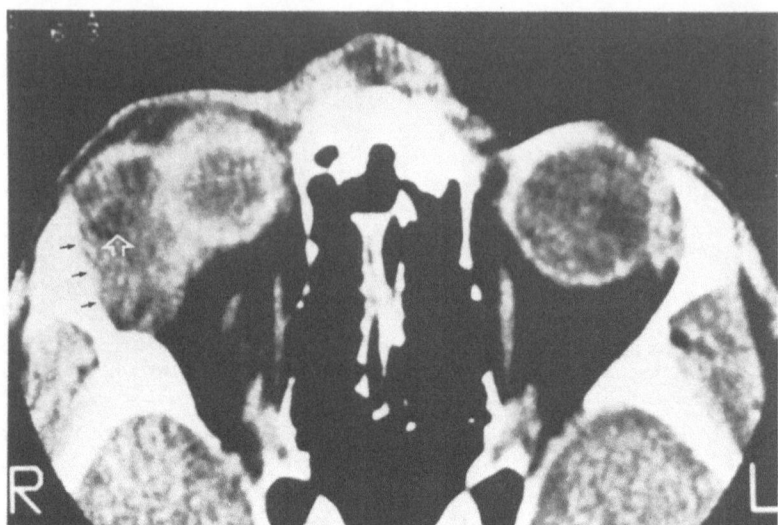

Fig. 11.15C. Right orbital dermoid. A CT scan after contrast injection reveals a well-defined, but heterogeneous, mass lesion in the right lateral portion of the orbit displacing the globe medially and forward. Note the associated bony erosion produced by the tumor (solid black arrows), and the fat density within the tumor (open arrow).

deep into the orbit. This is an uncommon finding in benign mixed tumors.

Mesenchymal Tumors—Fatty, Fibrous, and Muscle

Lipoma and Liposarcoma

Lipomas are composed of groups of mature fat cells that are separated by fibrovascular septae. These tumors may occur in the retrobulbar position of the orbit, in the soft tissue of the eyelids,

or in the soft tissues around the orbit. Proptosis, enlargement of the eyelids, and bulging of the periorbital soft tissues are common clinical manifestations of these tumors. Histologically, they do not differ from normal orbital fat. On CT scanning, the tumors appear as circumscribed masses of low density (fat density). Their appearance is usually similar to that of dermoids with fat density. Liposarcomas are rare in the orbit.

Fibrous Histiocytoma

Fibrous histiocytomas occur in middle-aged patients and present as slowly evolving proptosis.

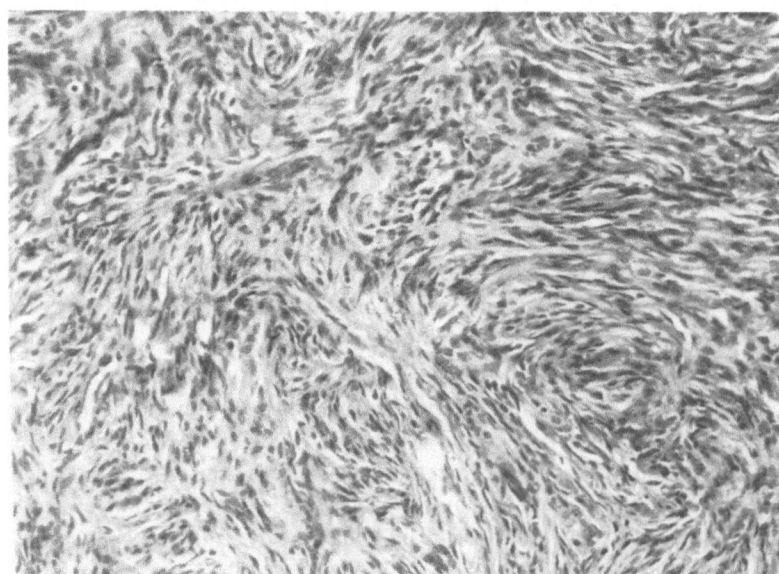

Fig. 11.16A. A hematoxylin and eosin preparation of a benign fibrous histiocytoma displaying a storiform pattern of spindle-shaped fibroblast- and histiocyte-like cells.

Fig. 11.16B. Hematoxylin and eosin preparation of a malignant fibrous histiocytoma. Note the bizarre, multinucleated giant cell and nuclear pleiomorphism.

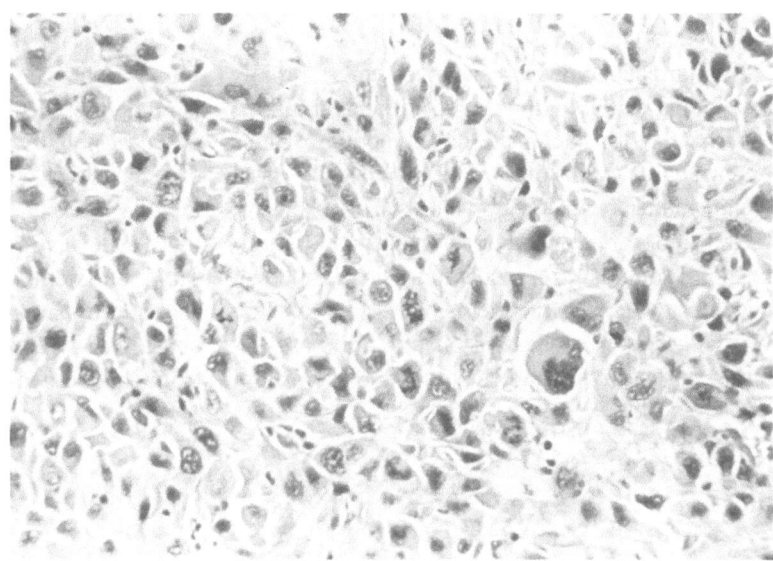

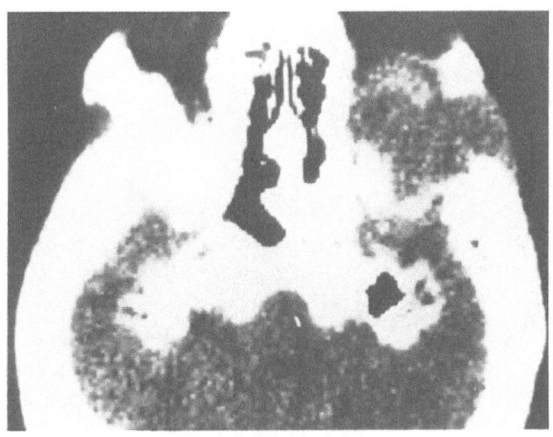

Fig. 11.16C. Axial CT scan showing marked bony thickening secondary to Paget's disease, involving the calvarium, orbits, and base of the skull. There is marked destruction of the lateral and posterior wall of the left orbit produced by a malignant fibrous histiocytoma.

In a series of 150 fibrous histiocytomas, Font and Hidayat reported that patients endured their symptoms for an average of 29 months before initial surgery was performed (28). Patients with malignant variants had a much more rapid course, with a duration of symptoms of less than 4 months. Histologically, benign fibrous histiocytomas consist of spindle-shaped, fibroblast-like cells and plump histiocyte-like cells that intertwine to form a storiform pattern (Fig. 11.16A). Malignant fibrous histiocytomas are distinguished by nuclear pleiomorphism, bizarre multinucleated giant cells,

areas of hemorrhage necrosis, and increased mitotic activity (Fig. 11.16B).

Most benign fibrous histiocytomas are well circumscribed; however, they are not well encapsulated and can be locally aggressive. On CT scans, these tumors are usually well-defined, homogeneous mass lesions seen in the intraconal or extraconal compartments, or both. Contrast enhancement is moderate to marked (Fig. 11.16C). A selective carotid angiogram usually shows a characteristically homogeneous stain (17). Complete surgical excision is occasionally difficult, and recurrences may evolve. Malignant fibrous histiocytomas are very aggressive locally, and they lead to death by intracranial invasion or by metastatic complications.

Rhabdomyosarcoma

Orbital tumors of muscle origin most commonly include rhabdomyosarcoma and (rarely) leiomyoma and leiomyosarcoma. In the pediatric age group, rhabdomyosarcoma probably is the most common primary malignant orbital tumor. It arises from the embryonic mesenchyme and can be divided histologically into four types: embryonal, alveolar, botryoid, and pleiomorphic or differentiated. (50) The embryonal form is most common; it consists of rhabdomyoblasts with large hyperchromic nuclei and variable amounts of cytoplasm. Occasional cells have a strap or ribbon of cytoplasm that may contain cross-striations (Fig. 11.17A). The alveolar form has the worst prognosis and consists of rhabdomyoblasts arranged in an alveolar-like pattern (Fig. 11.17B).

Orbital rhabdomyosarcomas present as rapidly developing exophthalmos, subconjunctival masses associated with chemosis, or lid nodules. Sinus or intranasal extension can be heralded by nasal stuffiness and recurrent nosebleeds. On CT scans, these tumors are seen as large homogeneous lesions in the retrobulbar area, including both extraconal and intraconal compartments. These tumors are very aggressive, and extension into the nasal sinuses, nasopharynx, and the brain and periorbital soft tissues is commonly seen (Figs. 11.17C and 11.17D) (84). Extensive bone destruction is usually found. Enhancement after contrast media injection is moderate. Distal hematogeneous metastases occur occasionally. Local recurrence after surgical excision is seen, at times. The differential diagnoses include leukemia, other more rare sarcomas, and metastatic neuroblastoma. In children exhibiting rapid unilateral ptosis or conjunctival swelling, rhabdomyosarcoma and neuroblastoma should be considered. Neuroblastoma may be distinguished from rhabdomyosarcoma by its relatively high at-

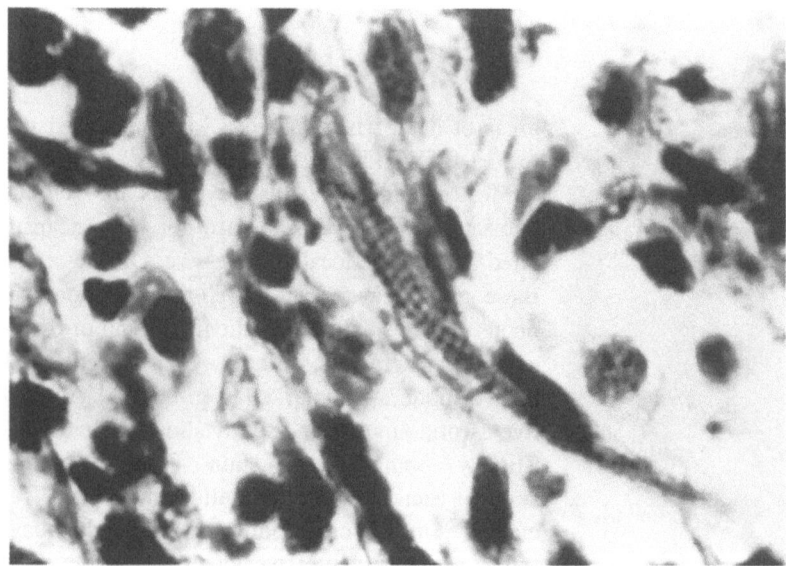

Fig. 11.17A. PATH stain of an embryonal rhabdomyosarcoma demonstrating a strap cell with cross-striations.

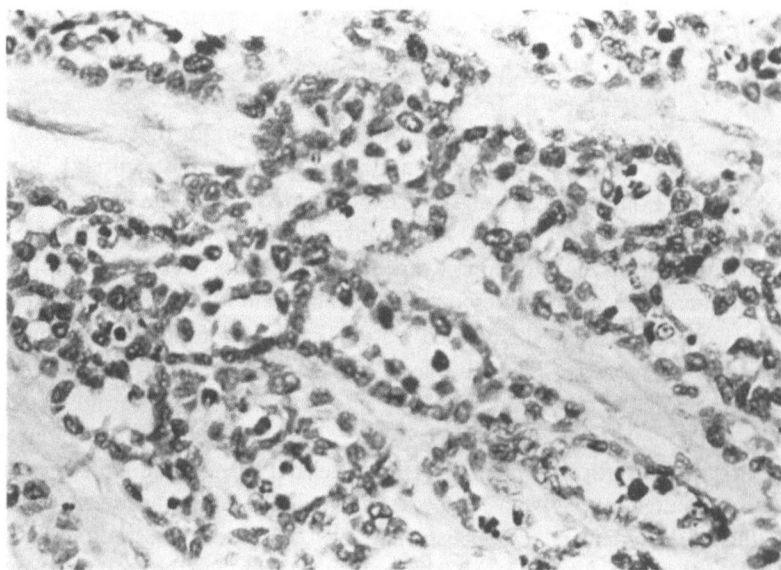

Fig. 11.17B. Hematoxylin and eosin preparation of an alveolar rhabdomyosarcoma. Septa divide the tumor into alveolar compartments.

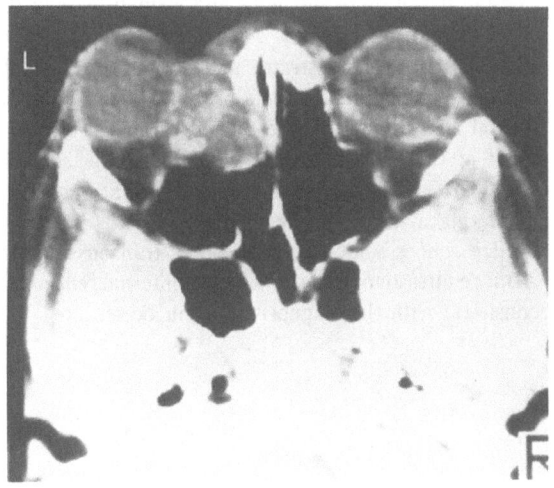

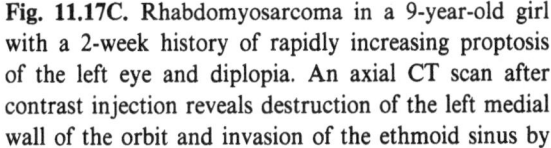

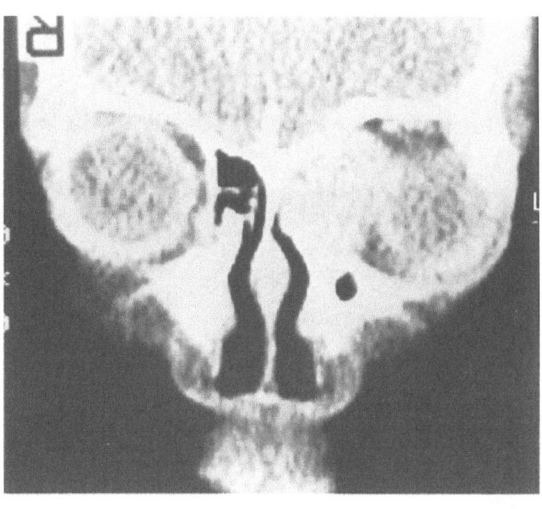

C

D

Fig. 11.17C. Rhabdomyosarcoma in a 9-year-old girl with a 2-week history of rapidly increasing proptosis of the left eye and diplopia. An axial CT scan after contrast injection reveals destruction of the left medial wall of the orbit and invasion of the ethmoid sinus by an enhanced, irregular mass lesion. **D.** A CT scan, coronal view, of the same patient showing the irregular tumor margin with invasion of the ethmoid sinus. Mild contrast enhancement is also present.

tenuation value, as seen in the CT examination, and a lack of preseptal extension (a common finding in rhabdomyosarcoma) (54). While rhabdomyosarcoma can mimic hemangioma or lymphangioma, the vast majority of rhabdomyosarcomas develop more rapidly than the two vascular lesions. Until the advent of chemotherapy, the prognosis of this disease was grave despite heroic excenteration procedures. Treatment with vincristine, adriamycin, and cyclophosphamide and local radiation has increased the survival greatly (59, 60).

Secondary Orbital Tumors

Tumors and Pseudotumors from Paranasal Sinuses, Nasal Cavity, and Nasopharynx

Orbital extension of a neoplasm arising in the paranasal sinuses and paraorbital structures often is responsible for orbital symptoms (see also Chapter 13). (62) The tumors gain access to the orbit through the various foramina and fissures that provide interconnections between the orbit and the sinuses and other regions. For example, benign tumors arising in the infratemporal (angiofibromas) and pterygopalatine fossa (neurofibromas) have access to the orbit through the inferior orbital fissure.

Mucocele

Mucoceles of the paranasal sinuses are cyst-like structures lined with a pseudostratified, columnar epithelium resulting from inflammatory diseases of the sinus. They may impinge on the orbit. Mucoceles usually have characteristic plain x-ray film findings that are manifested by expanded opacified sinuses with preservation of the bony margins. Erosion of the bone without the extensive destruction of malignant tumors and sclerosis of the bony margins also can occur. The CT scan is more accurate in delineating the extent of the lesions (see Fig. 2.24) (39, 64). The involved sinus is usually filled with homogeneous material that has an attenuation similar to the density of the brain; however, the density may change, depending on whether the mucocele contains clear mucous or the thick viscous material of the infected pyocele (Fig. 11.18). Normally, no enhancement can be seen after contrast media injection; however, in acutely infected mucopyoceles, an enhanced capsule may be seen. Ultrasonography is a valuable supplementary test, since mucoceles have characteristic findings, such as an excellent sound transmission and a low internal reflectivity that readily distinguishes them from other orbital and paraorbital tumors (Figs. 11.18C and 11.18D) (see Fig. 4.8). Clinically, mucoceles located in the frontal

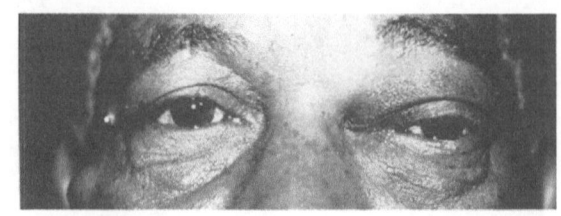

A

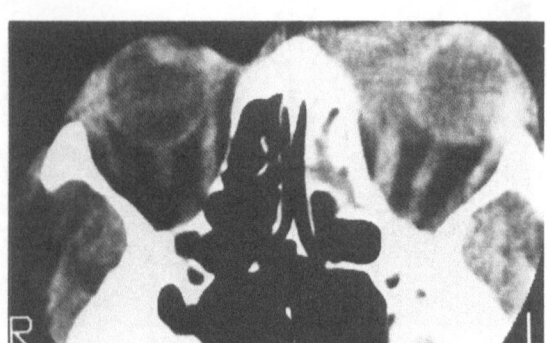

B

Fig. 11.18A. Left frontal sinus mucocele. A 66-year-old man presenting with a 6-month history of swelling of his left upper eyelid. On examination, he had a down-and-out deviation of the globe and a small mass in the superonasal orbital rim. **B.** An axial CT scan after contrast injection demonstrates an extraconal soft-tissue mass extending into the left orbit from the adjacent frontal and ethmoid sinuses. There is lateral displacement of the globe. There is clouding of the ethmoid sinus. **C.** B-mode ultrasonogram of a frontal sinus demonstrating a large cyst-like structure, with delineated border echoes and excellent sound transmission. **D.** A-mode ultrasonogram showing low internal reflectivity consistent with the diagnosis of a mucocele.

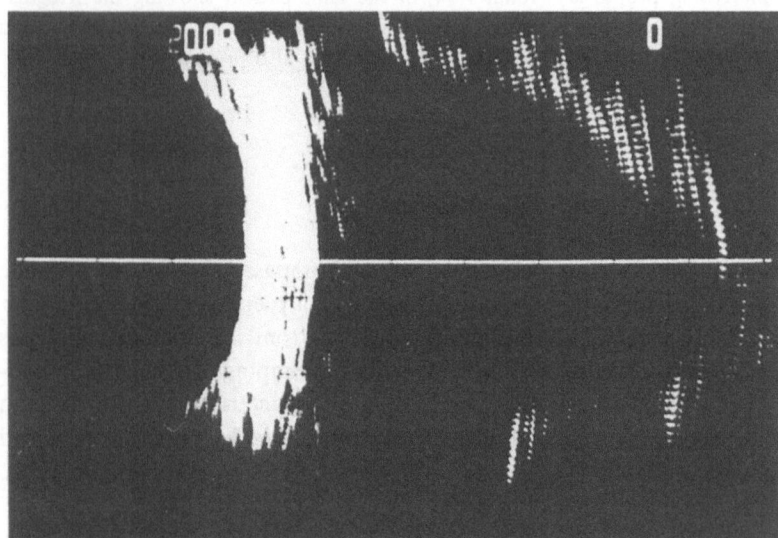

C

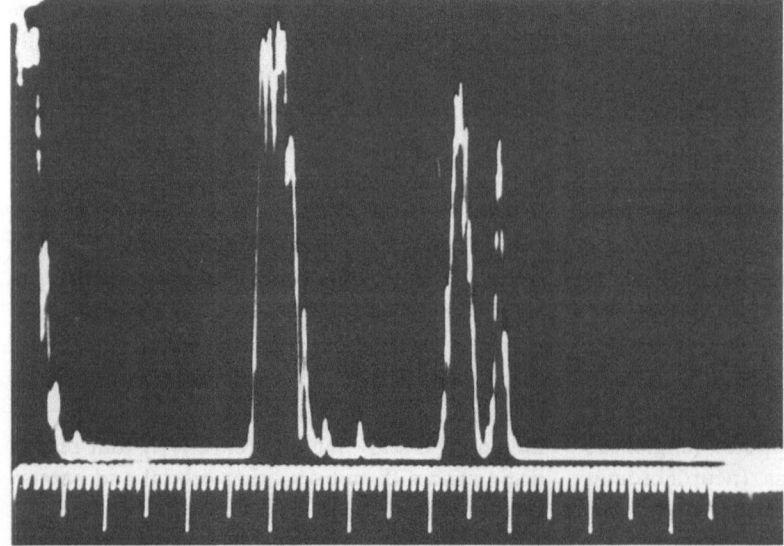

D

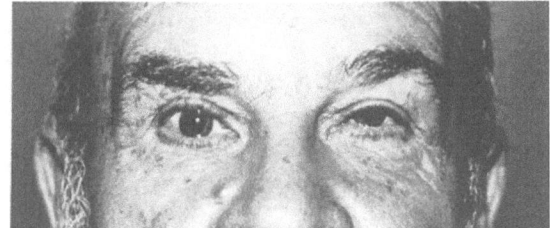

A

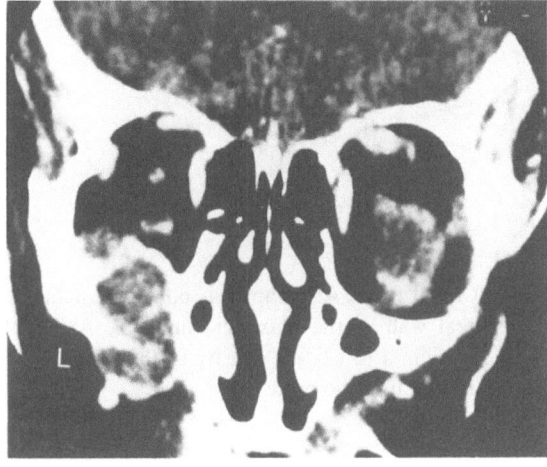

C

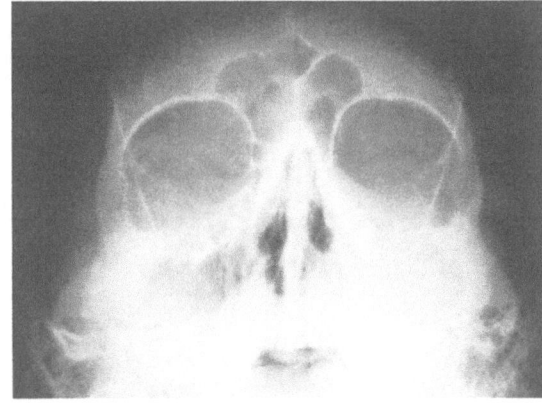

B

Fig. 11.19A. Left maxillary sinus mucocele. A 62-year-old man with a 3-month history of swelling of the left lower eyelid, numbness, and dysplasia. On examination, the globe was deviated upward and a mass was palpated in the inferior left orbital rim. **B.** Plain skull radiograph demonstrating loss of the left inferior orbital rim and clouding of the left maxillary sinus. **C.** A CT scan coronal section documenting opacification of the left maxillary sinus, with a soft-tissue mass eroding through the floor of the left orbit.

sinuses frequently present with orbital signs related to interference with levator and superior oblique muscle function.

Although mucoceles are more common in the frontal and ethmoidal sinuses, they also occur in the maxillary sinus and present with inferior orbital signs (see Chapters 13 and 15) (Fig. 11.19, 13.6–13.8).

Sinus Malignancies

Malignant tumors invade the orbit by bone destruction. Of the malignant neoplasms invading the orbit, 80% are epithelial; the remaining 20% include tumors such as esthesioneuroblastoma, rhabdomyosarcoma, other rare sarcomas, malignant melanoma, lymphomas, and adenocarcinoma (15). Squamous cell carcinoma, which is the most common malignant epithelial neoplasm of the sinuses invading the orbit, often presents with no symptoms or is manifested only as sinusitis. Only later does the tumor presents with orbital symptoms. Clouding of the sinus and bone destruction can be detected early on plain x-ray films and on

tomograms of the orbit and sinuses (Fig. 11.20). The CT scan will demonstrate the extensions of the tumor mass and the soft tissues around the lesion. The CT scan is also helpful in determining the extent of the tumor for treatment planning and follow up (13.18, 13.19, 13.22).

Basal cell, squamous cell, and sebaceous carcinomas of the eyelids, if neglected, can invade the orbit. Of the three types, basal cell carcinoma is the most frequent tumor of the eyelids and ocular adnexa. Basal cell carcinomas located in the medial canthus or of the morpheaform diffusely infiltrating histologic type present special problems as they are deeply invasive. Invading through the cutaneous structures of the medial canthus, the carcinoma may gain entry to the sinuses and threaten the intraorbital contents. In these circumstances, radial surgery (including orbital exenteration and ethmoidectomy) may be necessary. In evaluating patients with suspected deep involvement due to surface malignancy, CT scanning is an invaluable means of documenting penetration into the orbit and sinuses (11.21, 14.1–14.3). This facilitates treatment planning (see Chapter 14).

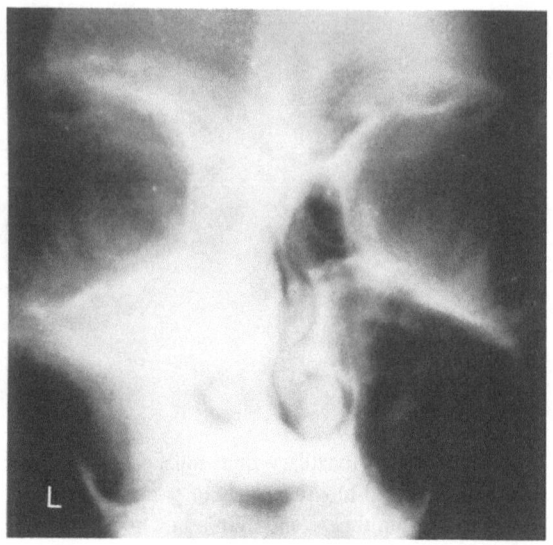

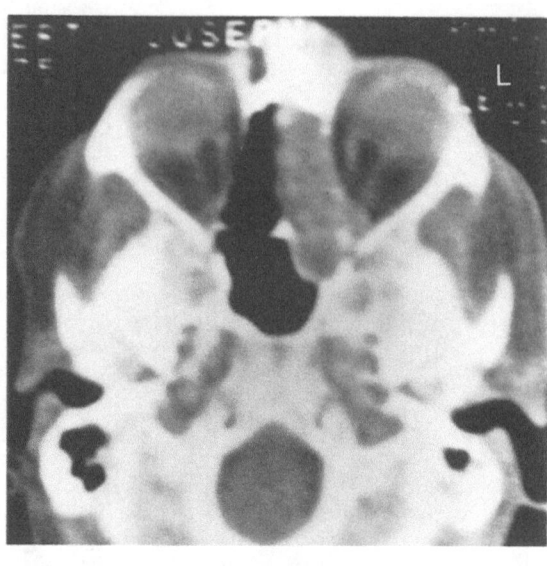

Fig. 11.20A. Squamous cell carcinoma of the right ethmoid sinus. A 38-year-old man presenting with nasal congestion and epictaxis. Plain skull X-ray film shows opacification of the ethmoid and maxillary sinus and the left nasal fossa. Also shown is bone destruction of the lateral wall of the maxillary sinus. **B.** Axial CT scan revealing a soft-tissue density in the left ethmoid sinus eroding into the orbit.

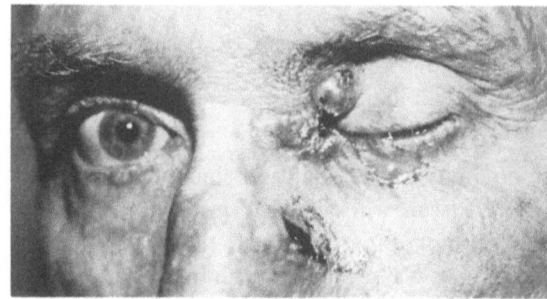

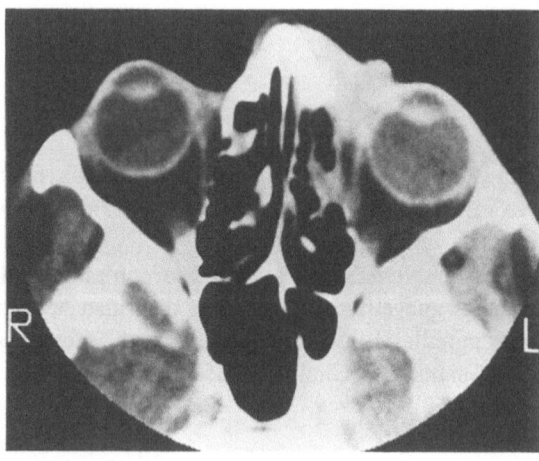

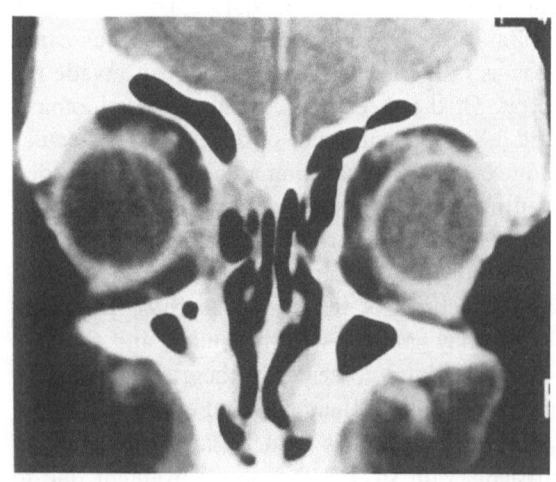

Fig. 11.21A. Basal cell carcinoma of the left medial canthus and upper eyelid. A 65-year-old man presenting with a recurrent cutaneous mass lesion along the inner aspect of the left upper eyelid. **B.** A CT scan axial projection documenting a soft-tissue mass lesion in the inner aspect of the left upper eyelid. Shown are erosion of the tumor into the left ethmoid sinus and the orbit and infiltration along the left medial rectus muscle. **C.** A CT scan, coronal view, documenting loss to the medial wall of the left orbit due to this infiltrating malignancy arising in the left upper eyelid.

Intraocular Tumors with Orbital Extension

Retinoblastoma

Retinoblastoma is the most common intraocular childhood malignancy. The tumor is autosomal-dominant in 60% of the cases. (36, 66) Retinoblastoma may have multicentric origins, and it is bilateral in some patients. Clinical manifestations of retinoblastoma include leukoria, strabismus, poor vision, and orbital inflammation (9). Retinoblastoma is usually diagnosed by ophthalmoscopy. The differential diagnosis includes multiple diseases (Table 11.2). Retinoblastomas are usually intraocular (Figs. 11.22A and 11.22B), but they can expand into the vitreous, perforate the sclera, and invade the orbital tissues; or extend posteriorly, following the optic nerve into the chiasmatic region and beyond. Distant hematogeneous metastasis may also occur (23, 36). The histology of retinoblastoma is similar to medulloblastoma and neuroblastoma, showing uniform lines of densely stained cells with rosette and pseudorosette formation (Fig. 11.22C).

In children with retinoblastoma, CT scans should be performed to rule out possible intraorbital or intracranial extension. On CT scans, retinoblastoma is characterized by single or multiple irregular masses arising in the posterior or lateral wall of the globe. (Figs. 11.22B and 11.22D) (13, 19). Calcification is present in many of the cases (42). If the tumor invades the sclera, then scleral enhancement is seen when contrast media is used. Posterior extension of the tumor is manifested by a thick optic nerve and/or a chiasmatic lesion (Fig. 11.22E and 11.22F). The density of the tumor is usually higher than the normal optic nerve, and enhancement after IV injection of contrast media has been noted.

Intraorbital extention of retinoblastoma is seen when the tumor is neglected (Figs. 11.22G and 11.22H). Recurrence of retinoblastoma can occur in the orbit after enucleation, especially when extrascleral extension has been present originally. Radiation-induced sarcoma should be considered if a tumor recurrence is found. The location and extent of this tumor also can be defined by CT scanning.

Retinoblastomas are well visualized with ultrasonography; appearing as fungating lesions with variable patterns due to necrosis, calcium deposits, associated vitreous debris, and retinal detachment. On MRI, retinoblastomas exhibit shorter T1 and T2 relaxation times that are similar to the melanomas and other intraocular tumors. A significant shortcoming of MRI in the diagnosis of these tumors is the failure to delete punctate calcifications (Fig. 8.6). On CT scan and MRI the differential diagnosis is usually limited to Coat's disease and other calcifying pathology of the globe such as toxoplasmosis, histoplasmosis, and calcified angiomatous masses (45).

If diagnosed early and properly treated, retinoblastoma may have a significant cure rate (see Chapter 17) (9) (67) (85). When spread of the tumor has already occurred, the prognosis is worse.

Table 11.2. Lesions confused with retinoblastoma

1. Anomalous optic disc
2. Anterior dislocated lens with secondary glaucoma
3. Coats' disease and other angiomatoses of the retina
4. Coloboma of the choroid and optic disc
5. Congenital cataract
6. Congenital corneal opacity
7. Cysts in a remnant of the hyaloid artery
8. Developmental retinal cyst
9. Glioma of the retina
10. Hematoma under retinal pigment epithelium
11. High myopia with advanced chorioretinal degeneration
12. Juvenile retinoschisis
13. Juvenile xanthogranuloma
14. Larva granulomatosis (*Toxocava canis*)
15. Medullation of nerve fiber layer
16. Metastatic endophthalmitis
17. Norrie's disease
18. Oligodendeoglioma of the retina
19. Organization of intraocular hemorrhage
20. Persistent primary vitreous
21. Retinal detachment due to choroidal or vitreous hemorrhage
22. Retinal dysplasia (massive retinal fibrosis)
23. Retrolental fibroplasia
24. Retrolental membrane associated with Bloch-Sulzberger syndrome (incontinentia pigmenti)
25. Rhematogenous and falciform retinal detachment
26. Secondary glaucoma
27. Toxoplasmosis
28. 13–15 Trisomy
29. Uveitis in secondary retinal detachment

Coats' Disease

Coats' disease (isolated retinal telangiectasia) begins as a circumscribed area of relatively flat, telangiectatic proliferation on the retinal surface.

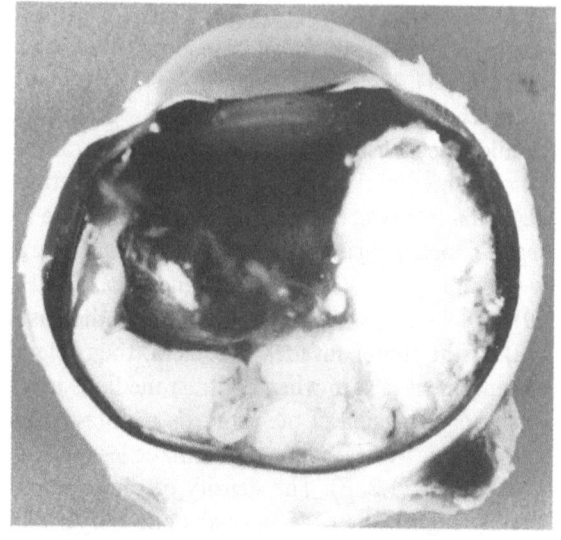

A

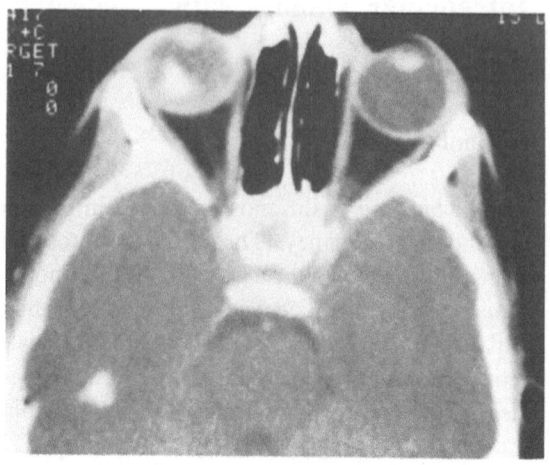

B

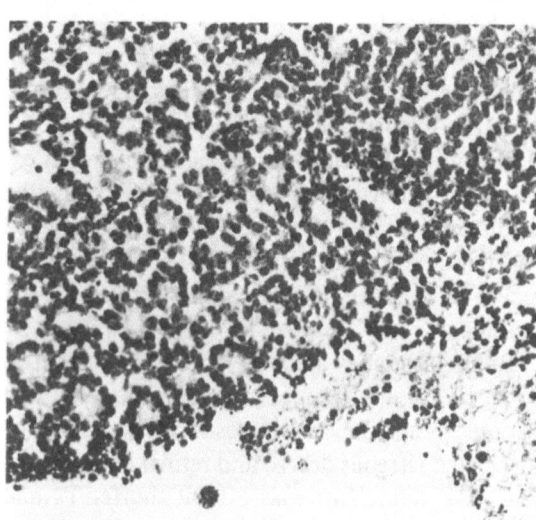

C

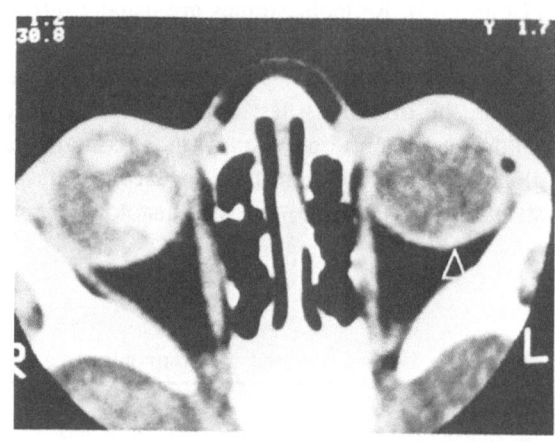

D

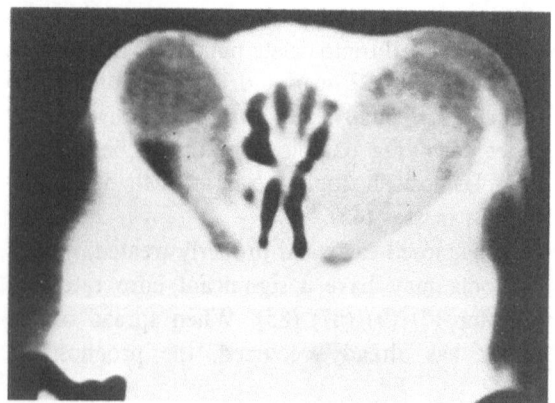

E

Fig. 11.22A. Intraocular retinoblastoma, anatomic section. The calcified tumor is seen in the posterior portion of the globe (Courtesy of JA Shields, M.D., Wills Eye Hospital, Philadelphia, PA). **B.** A CT scan of the same patient showing the calcified mass lesion in the posterior portion of the right globe. **C.** A hematoxylin and eosin preparation of an intraocular retinoblastoma showing uniform lines of densely stained cells with rosette and pseudorosette formation. **D.** An axial CT scan showing bilateral intraocular retinoblastoma. The intraocular area of increased density in the posterior part of the right globe is shown. A small area of thickening and increased density in the posterior portion of the left globe corresponds to a second retinoblastoma (open arrowhead). **E.** Bilateral intraorbital and extraorbital retinoblastomas shown on an axial CT scan. The homogeneous area of increased density extends into the left globe and retrobulbar area. A sharply marginated tumor is also seen in the right retrobulbar region.

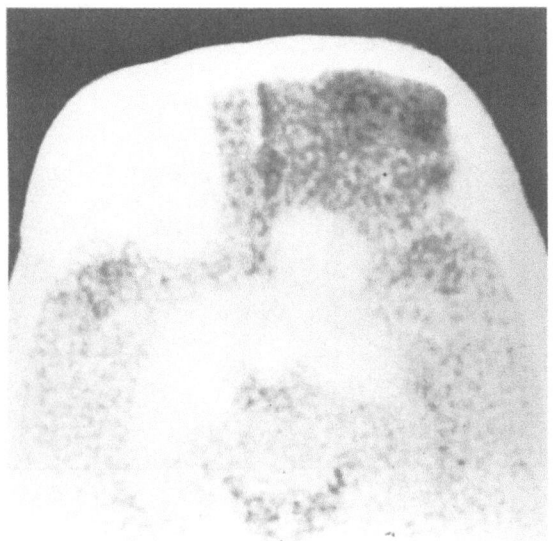

F

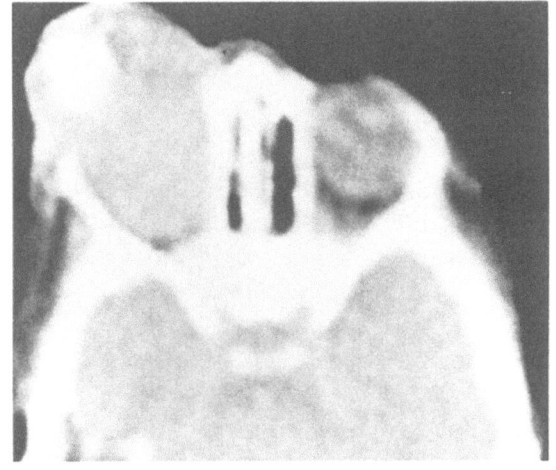

G

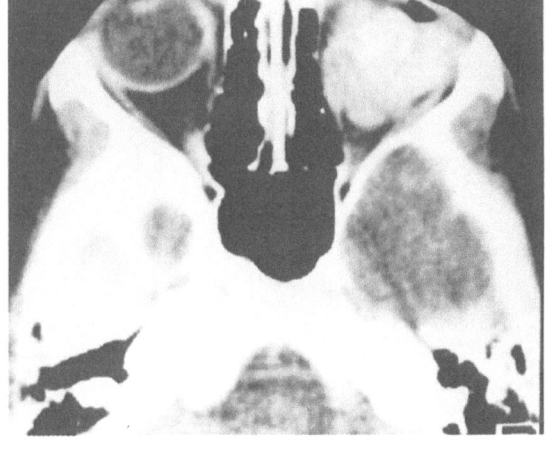

H

Fig. 11.22F. Axial CT scan showing intracranial extension of retinoblastoma into the optic chiasma and optic tracts. **G.** Retinoblastoma on an axial CT scan demonstrates extraocular extension into the orbit by a homogeneous mass lesion, with large anterior calcification due to a neglected retinoblastoma (Courtesy of I Chams, M.D., Iran). **H.** Retinoblastoma on an axial CT scan shows massive orbital involvement by recurrent tumor surrounding an Iowa implant (Courtesy of JA Shields, M.D., Wills Eye Hospital, Philadelphia, PA).

It may progress to a subretinal exudation and, possibly, to retinal detachment. Large patches of telangiectatic and aneurysmal vessels strongly suggest this disorder. The involved area of the retina frequently has a greenish-yellow sheen, and detached portions of the retina may be dark gray or black due to marked proliferation of the retinal pigment epithelium. The subretinal space usually is filled with blood, cholesterol crystals, and "ghost cells," which are lipid-laden macrophages arising from the pigment epithelium. The vascular lesions seen with Coats' disease resemble those seen in von Hipple disease (18, 32).

Malignant Melanoma

Malignant melanoma is the most common primary malignancy of the globe in adults. Most of these tumors arise from the choroid of the globe, where the melanocyte cells are extensively distributed (63). Two histologic varieties can be encoun-

tered—a relatively benign form with spindle cell predominance and a better survival rate, and a more aggressive epithelial variety with a 60% 5-year mortality (63). Melanoma is commonly associated with glaucoma, retinal destruction, and vitreous hemorrhage. Loss of visual acuity is the most common clinical presentation. Like retinoblastomas, these tumors are usually discovered on ophthalmoscopic examination (Fig. 11.23A).

On CT scans, melanoma is recognized as a homogeneous area of increased density in the posterior segment of the globe (Fig. 11.23A, 11.23B, and 11.23C) (64A). When contrast media is injected, enhancement is not usually present. Diffuse scleral thickening may be seen, and it is very useful in determining the extraocular extension of the tumor, if that is present. Intraorbital extraocular melanomas are rare and usually are metastatic deposits from distant primary tumors or direct extensions from facial or intraocular melanomas. The usual B-scan ultrasonic appearance of malignant

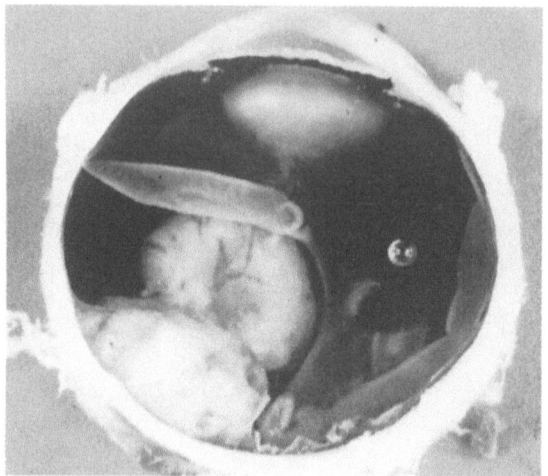

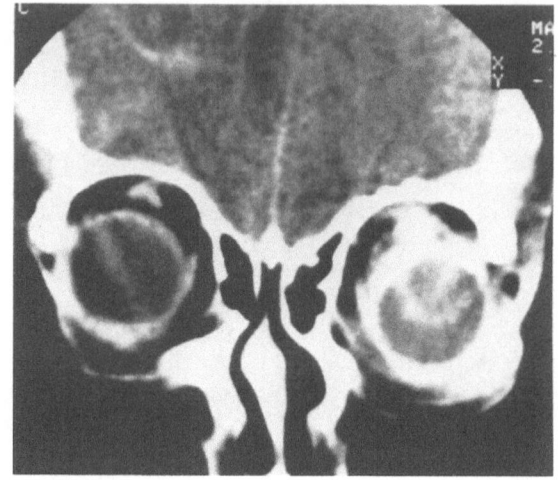

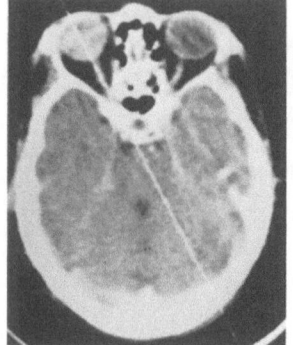

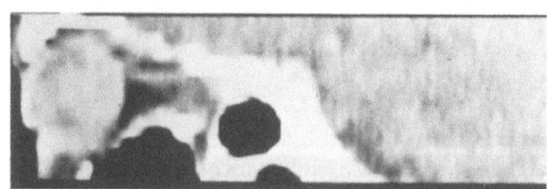

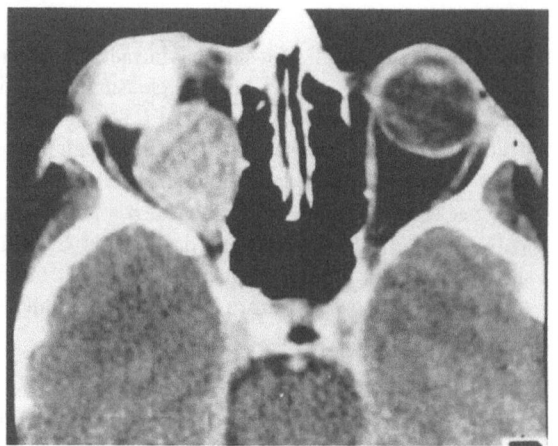

Fig. 11.23A. Choroidal melanoma, anatomic specimen. A large mass lesion is located in the posterior portions of the globe. **B.** Choroidal melanoma, coronal view. A well-defined intraocular lesion is seen attached to the posterior and superior walls of the left globe. **C, D.** Choroidal melanoma in a 61-year-old woman, with progressive loss of vision. Axial and sagittal views of the orbit show a high-density lesion filling the posterior portion of the right globe. **E.** Recurrent melanoma on an axial CT scan showing a sharply defined, homogeneous mass lesion posterior to the spherical implant. (A, B, E courtesy of JA Shields, M.D., Wills Eye Hospital, Philadelphia, PA.)

melanoma is a mass along the inner contour of the globe (Fig. 4.7). A polypoid appearance or a concave indentation of the normal globe posterior to the tumor is also indicative of melanoma. CT and MRI may help to identify the presence of unnoticed retinal detachment (5A, 64A). On MRI, melanomas exhibit shorter T1 and T2 relaxation times, and the appearance is similar to retinoblastoma. However, densely pigmented tumors may yield low signals on T2-weighted images (Fig. 8.5).

Like retinoblastoma, recurrence after enuclea-tion may develop (Fig. 11.23D). Small lesions are treated with cryosurgery, photocoagulation, and local medication. Larger lesions are treated with surgery and radiation therapy (See Chapter 17).

Metastatic Disease

Metastasis to the orbit characteristically presents with a sudden onset of pain, swelling, and diplopia (27). There is a predilection for the metastasis to

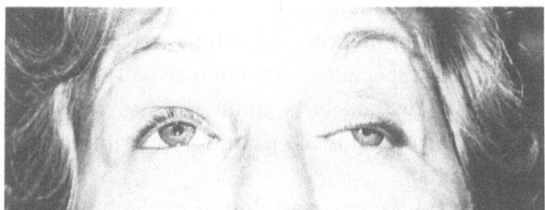

A

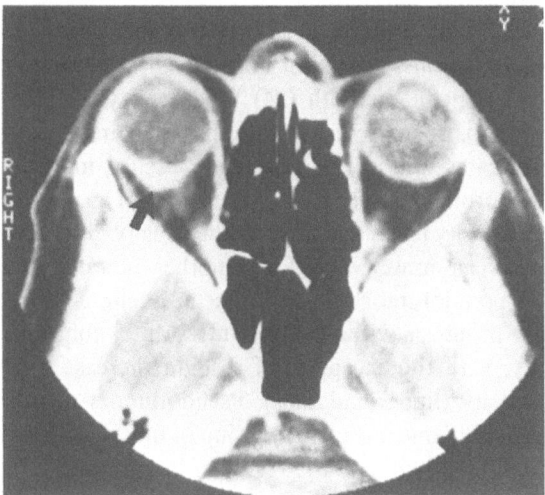

C

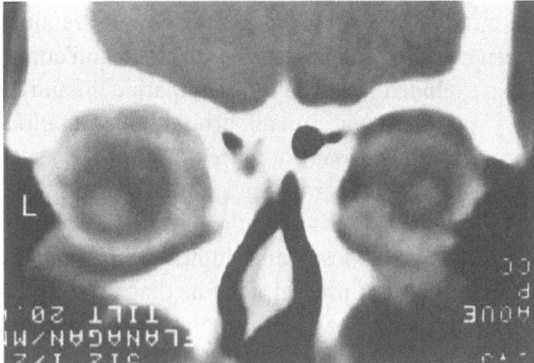

B

Fig. 11.24A. Breast carcinoma metastatic to the superior aspect of the left orbit. A 52-year-old woman presenting for evaluation of ptosis of the left upper eyelid and diplopia with a left mastectomy for a carcinoma 5 years previously. **B.** Coronal CT scan documenting a diffuse infiltrative mass in the superior medial lateral aspect of the left orbit. **C.** Choroidal metastatic melanoma in the right globe of another patient, axial view. Note the contrast-enhancing thickened area (arrow) along the posterior margin of the right globe. The patient had a primary tumor in the chest (Courtesy of Robert Peyster).

locate in the anterior superior orbit (51). This causes ptosis, hypotropia, and a palpable mass. Another common site of metastasis is the orbital apex, with the associated findings of visual loss and ophthalmoplegia. When confronted with these findings, the clinician must maintain a high index of suspicion that metastatic disease is present.

The most common sites of primary disease metastasizing to the orbit in adults are lung and breast, followed by gastrointestinal, genitourinary, and thyroid tumors. Breast carcinoma is a tumor that is commonly metastatic to the orbit (Fig. 11.24A, B and 13.26). Unlike other carcinomas previously mentioned, breast carcinoma frequently metastasizes late in its course; orbital signs may not appear until several years after the mastectomy (1, 11). In the pediatric population, neuroblastoma, Ewings sarcoma, and Wilms tumor are usually the primary tumors. Infiltration of the orbit by leukemic cells (chloroma) is also more common in the younger age group.

Often, the existence of the primary tumor is unknown at the time of ophthalmic presentation. In Henderson's (36) review of orbital metastasis from the Mayo Clinic, the primary carcinomas were undiagnosed in 30% of the patients. In a retrospective study from the Armed Forces Institute of Pathology, 17 of 28 patients presented with orbital metastasis before an underlying primary tumor was discovered (25). Metastatic orbital lesions on CT scans usually are seen as homogeneous, ill-defined, extraconal soft-tissue density masses. Bone destruction is frequently seen. Occasionally, the tumors are hyperdense and enhance slightly after injection of contrast media (Fig. 13.26). Metastasis involving the optic nerve sheath are rare and produces irregular enlargement of the nerve that has to be differentiated from meningiomas and optic gliomas. Intraocular metastases usually are very difficult to demonstrate on CT scans. The breast and lung are the most frequent primary sites of tumors metatasizing to the globe. The choroid is the most frequent site of metastasis (Fig. 11.24C) (45, 79).

Inflammations and Lymphomas

Orbital Pseudotumor

Most clinicians and pathologists agree that the term orbital pseudotumor is unsatisfactory. (7) (36) (37) (49). Orbital pseudotumor may be defined as an idiopathic inflammation of orbital structures. By definition, therefore, all orbital inflammations of a known cause are excluded, such as leaking dermoid cysts, ruptured hemangiomas, retained foreign bodies, and bacterial or parasitic infections. Also excluded from the term idiopathic inflammatory pseudotumor are all orbital inflammations secondary to regional or systemic disorders, such as sinusitis, lethal midline granuloma, ruptured mucocele, Wegener's granulomatosis, sarcoidosis, polyarteritis, nodosa, and lupus erythematosus. Pseudotumor, at present, may be diagnosed histologically on the basis of a polymorphic cellular pattern of predominance of inflammatory lymphocytes and a nonneoplastic histology.

The purpose of diagnostic imaging in the management of these patients is two-fold. First, to establish the local etiology of the orbital inflammation when one exists; and second, to define the extent of inflammation when a causative factor cannot be found. This will help the clinician to decide if a biopsy procedure is indicated; additionally, it will give the clinician an objective criteria to follow if steroid therapy or radiation therapy is considered. A CT scan, more than any other diagnostic modality, is uniquely suited to these requirements.

The clinical spectrum of idiopathic inflammatory pseudotumors is highly variable. The presentation may range from diffuse inflammation to focal inflammatory tumefaction. The onset of the symptoms usually is rapid and is characterized by marked proptosis, soft-tissue swelling, and impairment of muscle motility (Fig. 11.25A). De-

pending on which orbital structures are involved in the inflammation and which are included in the biopsy specimen, the clinical picture may be narrowly defined as a diffused mass lesion, dacryoadenitis, myositis, posterior scleritis, or lipogranuloma.

On CT scanning pseudotumor commonly presents as a poorly defined "halo" or "ring" of increased density around the globe (posterior scleritis) (Fig. 11.25B) or as a poorly defined retroocular mass lesions, with either intraconal or extraconal components, or both (24). The density of the lesions is increased, and it appears to involve the sclera as well as the retroocular tissues, including the orbital fat and the rectus muscles. The increase in density tends to obliterate the density differences between muscle and fat. Another manifestation of pseudotumor on the CT scan is characterized by proptosis without other intraorbital abnormality, with the exception of a slight increase in fat density (lipogranulomas). Pseudotumors may affect only one muscle or a group of muscles (myositis), in which case the CT scan image shows uniform muscular enlargement. In cases where this is the only finding, pseudotumor should be differentiated from thyroid ophthalmopathy (see Chapter 10).

Pseudotumor may be localited in the lacrimal gland (dacryoadenitis) and has to be differentiated from other pathology common to this area. Pseudotumors produce diffuse ultrasound findings. The retrobulbar fat pad generally is the most involved

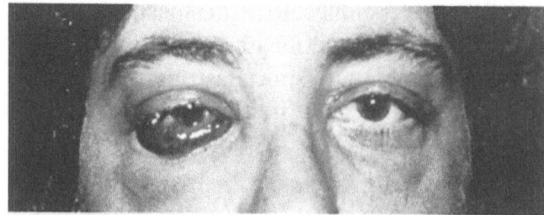

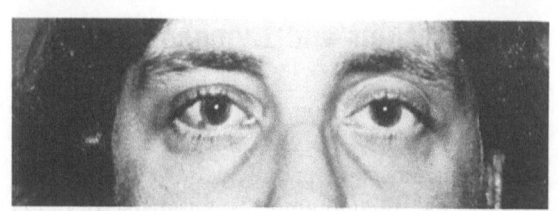

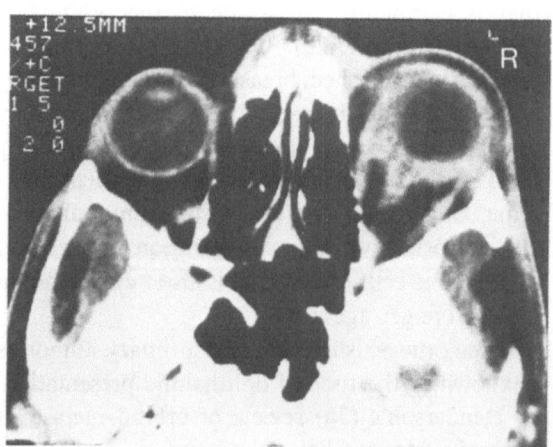

Fig. 11.25A. Pseudotumor of the right orbit. A 24-year-old man presenting with pain, redness, and swelling of the right eye. **B.** Axial CT scan after contrast injection reveals a diffuse "halo" or "ring" of increased den-

sity around the globe. **C.** Pseudotumor of the right orbit after 1 week of systemic steroid therapy shows complete resolution.

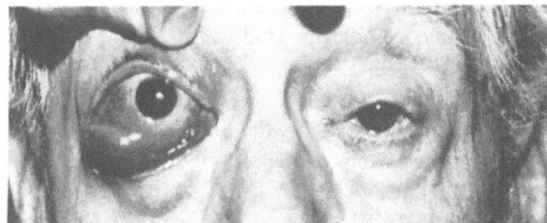

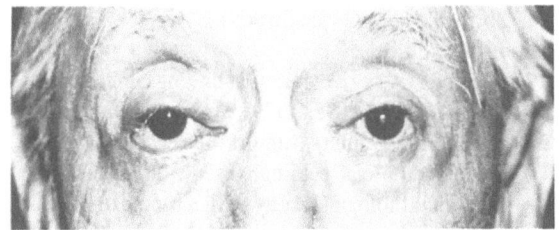

A

C

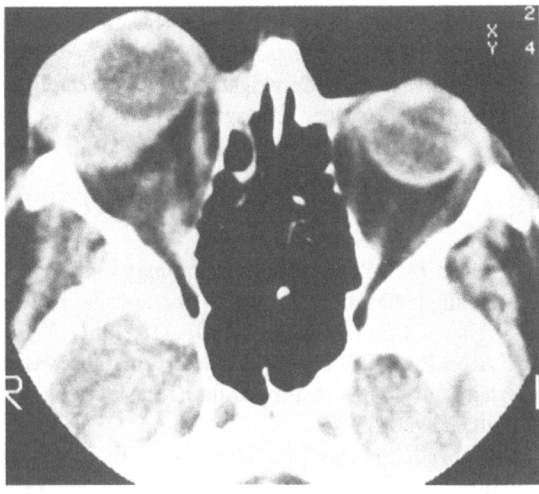

B

Fig. 11.26A. A well-differentiated lymphocytic lymphoma of the right orbit. An 83-year-old man with a 1-month history of swelling of the right eye. A salmon-colored conjunctival mass was found on examination.

B. Axial CT scan after contrast injection demonstrates a large, well-circumscribed homogeneous mass lesion around the right globe corresponding to a lymphoma. **C.** The patient after radiation therapy.

tissue, with an abnormal diffuse mottle texture identified ultrasonically. These changes probably result from the interstitial edema separating fat globules and from connective tissue abnormalities. On MRI, there is a relative decrease in signal intensity of the retrobulbar fat on both T1- and T2-weighted images (Fig. 8.9). Using coil MRI imaging, the optic nerve can be seen surrounded by inflammatory tissue (5A) (see also Chapters 13 and 15).

Lymphoma

Lymphocytic infiltrations of the orbit range from the relatively benign, reactive lymphoid hyperplasia to the frankly malignant lymphocytic lymphoma of the orbit. A pleiomorphic cellular infiltrate is correlated with the more benign biological activity. The more uniform the cellular appearance, the greater the likelihood that malignancy exists. Of all patients with orbital lymphoma, 75% have or will develop systemic lymphoma (47). Through the use of T- and B-cell marker studies, Jakobiec has defined subpopulations of lymphocytes with either monoclonal or polyclonal origins. A polyclonal origin correlates with the more benign biological activity, whereas a monoclonal origin is a sign of malignancy (53). The opinion of the pathologist in judging the biological activity of lymphocytic infiltration is of primary importance. Reactive lymphoid hyperplasia and well-dif-

ferentiated lymphocytic lymphoma have similar clinical features. They tend to occur in elderly patients as proptosis or a palpable mass, which develops insidiously over several months. The eye is usually quiet, and there is rarely pain. When the tumor presents in the subconjunctival space, it has a characteristic salmon color. An incisional biopsy procedure is indicated.

The CT scan appearance of these tumors could be similar to that of pseudotumor, or mimic any other intraorbital tumor. However, homogeneous masses of relatively high density (sometimes sharply marginated) are more often seen in the anterior portion of the orbit, the retrobulbar area, or the superior orbital compartment. In general, the lesions mold themselves to preexisting structures without eroding the bone or enlarging the orbit. Mild enhancement is present (Fig. 11.26).

Summary

When ocular and/or orbital masses suggesting tumors are noted clinically, diagnostic imaging is indicated. Routine X-ray films are of limited value. Computed tomography and ultrasound studies will yield images to help diagnose the lesion and its extent. Ultrasound is particularly useful in the evaluation of intraocular tumors, cystic lesions, and cavernous hemangiomas. In the future, MRI may be useful in studying these lesions (see Chapter 8).

Acknowledgment. Figures 11.11E, F, 11.13D, 11.24C reproduced with permission from Peyster, R.G., and Hoover, E.D.: *Computerized Tomography in Orbital Disease and Neuro-ophthalmology.* Copyright ©1984 by Year Book Medical Publishers, Inc., Chicago.

References

1. Alper MG: Management of primary optic nerve meningiomas: Current status—therapy and controversy. *J Clin Ophthalmol* 1:101–118, 1981.

2. Aron Rosa DS, Doyon DL: Malformations vasculaires orbitaires (a propos de 62 cas). *ANN Ocul* 205:667–712, 1972.

3. Barber JC, Barber LE, Guerry D, et al: Congenital orbital teratoma. *Arch Ophthalmol* 9:45–48, 1974.

4. Behrens MM: Neuro-opthalmic aspects of orbital disease, in Jones IS, Jacobiec FA (eds): *Diseases of the Orbit.* New York, Harper & Row, 1979, pp 105–122.

5. Berges O, Vignaud J, Aubin ML: Comparison of sonography and computed tomography in the study of orbital space occupying lesions. *AJNR* 5:247–251, 1984.

6. Bilaniuk LT, Vignaud T, Clay C: Venography of the orbit: An analytical report of 413 cases. *Radiology* 110:373–382, 1974.

7. Blodi FC, Gass JDM: Inflammatory pseudotumor of the orbit. *Br J Ophthalmo* 52:79, 1968.

8. Blodi FC: Vascular anomalies of the fundus, in Duane TD (ed), *Clinical Ophthalmology.* Hagerstown, MD, Harper and Row, 1980, vol 3, chap 22.

9. Brown DH: The clinicopathology of retinoblastoma *Am J Ophthalmol* 61:508, 1966.

10. Bryan N, Craig JA: The eye, in Bergeron RT, Osborn AG, Som PM (eds): *Head and Neck Radiography Excluding the Brain.* St. Louis, CV Mosby, 1983, pp 575–625.

11. Bullock JD, Yinens B: Ophthalmic manifestations of metastatic breast cancer. *Ophthalmology* 87:961, 1980.

12. Cabanis EA, Savolini U, Radallec A, et al: Computed tomography of the optic nerve: part II. Size and shape modifications in papilledema. *J Comput Assist Tomogr* 2:150–155, 1979.

13. Centeno RS, Bryan RN, Cheatham BA: Computerized tomography of intraocular neoplasia, Amercian Society of Head and Neck Radiology, presentation, May 1981, Los Angeles, CA.

14. Coleman DJ, Jack RL, Fanzen LA: High resolution B-scan ultrasonography of the orbit: Hemangiomas of the orbit. *Arch Ophthalmol* 88:368–374, 1972.

15. Conley JJ: Sinus tumors invading the orbit. *Trans Am Acad Ophthalmol Otolaryngol* 70:615–619, 1966.

16. Craig WM, Gogela LJ: Intraorbital meningiomas: A clinicopathologic study. *Am J Ophthalmol* 32:1663–1680, 1949.

17. Cromwell LD, Kerber C, Margolis MT: Selective carotid angiography in the diagnosis of orbital hemangiopericytoma: Report of two cases. *AJR* 129:730–733, 1977.

18. Daniels DL, Williams AL, Syvertsen A, et al: CT recognition of optic nerve sheath meningioma: Abnormal sheath visualization. *AJNR* 3:181–183, 1982.

19. Danziger A, Price HI: CT findings in retinoblastoma. *AJR* 133:695, 1979.

20. Davis FA: Primary tumors of the optic nerve (a phenomenon of Recklinghausen's disease): A clinical and pathological study with a report of five cases and a review of the literature. *Arch Ophthalmol* 23:735–821, 957–1022, 1940.

21. Davis KR, Hesselink JR, Dallow RL, et al: CT and ultrasound in the diagnosis of cavernous hemangioma and lymphangioma of the orbit. *Comput Tomagr* 4:98–104, 1980.

22. Dilenge D: Arteriography in angiomas of the orbit. *Radiology* 113:355–361, 1974.

23. Dunphy EB: The story of retinoblastoma: The twentieth Edward Jackson memorial lecture. *AM J Ophthalmol* 58:539, 1964.

24. Enzmann D, Donaldson SS, Marshall WH, et al: Computed tomography in orbital pseudotumor (idiopathic orbital inflammation). *Radiology* 120:597, 1976.

25. Ferry AP, Font RL: Carcinoma metastatic to the eye and orbit I: A clinical pathologic study of 227 cases. *Arch Ophthalmol* 92:276, 1974.

26. Flanagan JC: Vascular problems of the orbit. *Ophthalmology* 86:896–913, 1979.

27. Font RL, Ferry AP: Carcinoma metastatic to the eye and orbit III: A clinical pathologic study of 28 cases metastatic to the orbit. *Cancer* 38:1326–1335, 1976.

28. Font RL, Hidayat AA: Fibrous histiocytoma of the orbit. *Human Pathol* 13:199–209, 1982.

29. Fox AJ, Debrun G, Vinuela F, et al: Intrathecal metrizamide enhancement of the optic nerve sheath. *J Comput Assist Tomogr* 3:653–656, 1979.

30. Glaser JS, Hoyt WF, Corbett J: Visual morbidity with chiasmal glioma. *Arch Ophthalmol* 83:3, 1971.

31. Gyldensted C, Lester J, Fledelius H: Computed tomography of orbital lesions. A radiological study of 144 cases. *Neuroradiology* 13:141–150, 1977.

32. Harris GS: Coats' disease diagnosis and treatment. *Can J Ophthalmol* 5:311, 1970.

33. Hammerschlag SB, Hesselink JR, Weber AH; *Computed Tomography of the Eye and Orbit.* Norwalk, CT, Appleton-Century-Crofts, 1983.

34. Harris GH, Jakobiec FA: Cavernous hemangiomas of the orbit. *J Neurosurg* 51:219–228, 1979.

35. Hart WM Jr, Burde RM, Klingele TG, et al: Bilateral optic nerve sheath meningiomas. *Arch Ophthalmol* 98:149–151, 1980.

36. Henderson JW: *Orbital Tumors,* ed 2. New York, Brian C. Decker & Co, 1980.

37. Heersink B, Rodriquez MR, Flanagan JC: Inflammatory pseudotumor of the orbit. *Ann Ophthalmol* 9:17–29, 1977.

38. Hesselink JR, Davis KR, Dallow RL, et al: Computed tomography of masses in the lacrimal gland region. Radiology 131:143–147, 1979.

39. Hesselink JR, Weber AL, New PFJ, et al: Evaluation of mucoceles of the paranasal sinuses with computed tomography. *Radiology* 133:397–400, 1979.

40. Hobbs HE: Capilary and cavernous hemangiomata of the orbit. *Trans Ophthalmol Soc UK* 81:229, 1961.

41. Howard CW, Osher RH, Tomsak RL: Computed tomographic features in optic neuritis. *Am J Ophthalmol* 89:699–702, 1980.

42. Hilal SK, Trokel SL: Computerized tomography of the orbit using thin sections. *Semin Roentgenol* 12:137–147, 1977.

43. Hoyt WF, Bagdassarian SA: Optic glioma of childhood, a natural history and rationale for conservative management. *Br J Ophthalmol* 53:793–798, 1969.

44. Hoyt WF, Meshel LG, Lessell S, et al: Malignant optic glioma of adulthood. *Brain* 96:121–132, 1973.

45. Jacobs L, Weisberg LA, Kinkel WR. *Computerized Tomography of the Orbit and Sella Turcica.* New York, Raven Press, 1980.

46. Jakobiec FA, Bonanno PA, Siegleman J: Conjunctival adnexal cysts and dermoids. *Arch Ophthalmol* 96:1404–1409, 1978.

47. Jakobiec FA, Gibralter RA, Knowles DM, et al: Lymphoid tumors of the lid. *Ophthalmology* 87:1058–1064, 1980.

48. Jakobiec FA, Howard GM, Jones IS, et al: Hemangiopericytoma of the orbit. *Am J Ophthalmol* 88:816–834, 1974.

49. Jakobiec FA, Jones IS: Orbital inflammations. Vascular tumors, malformations, and degenerations, in Duane TB (ed): *Clinical Ophthalmol,* Hagerstown, MD, Harper & Row, 1980, chaps 35, 37.

50. Jakobiec FA, Jones IS: Mesenchymal and fibro-osseous tumors, in Jones IS, Jakobiec FA (eds): *Diseases of the Orbit.* Hagerstown, MD, Harper & Row, 1979, chap 20, pp 461–502.

51. Jakobiec FA, Rootman J, Jones IS: Secondary metastatic tumors of the orbit, in Duane TD (ed): *Clinical Ophthalmology.* Hagerstown, MD, Harper & Row, 1980, chap 46.

52. Jones IS, Jacobiec FA: Orbital inflammations, in Jones IS, Jacobiec FA (eds): *Diseases of the Orbit.* New York, Harper & Row, 1979, pp 187–262.

53. Knowles DM, Jakobiec FA: Orbital lymphoid neoplasms: Clinical, pathologic and immunologic characteristics, in Jakobiec FA (ed): *Ocular and Adnexal Tumors.* Birmingham, AL, Aesculapius Press, 1978, pp 806–838.

54. Lallemand DP, Brasch RC, Devron HC, et al: Orbital tumors in children. *Radiology* 151:85–88, 1984.

55. Lauten GJ, Eatherly JB, Ramirez A: Hemangioblastoma of the optic nerve: Radiologic and pathologic features. *AJNR.* 2:96–99, 1981.

56. Lloyd LA: Gliomas of the optic nerve and chiasm in childhood. *Trans Am Ophthalmol Soc* 71:488–535, 1973.

57. Manelfe C, Pasquini U, Bank WO: Metrizamide demonstration of the subarachnoid space surrounding the optic nerves. *J Comput Tomogr* 2:545–547, 1978.

58. Mark LE, Kenerdell JS, Maroon JC, et al: Microsurgical removal of primary intraorbital meningioma. *Am J Ophthalmol* 86:704–709, 1978.

59. Maurer HM: Rhabdomyosarcoma. *Pediatr Annals* 8:17–24, 1979.

60. Maurer HM et al.: The intergroup rhabdomyosarcoma study. *Cancer* 40:2015–2026, 1977.

61. McQuire WL: Current status of estrogen receptors in human breast cancer. *Cancer* 36:638–644, 1975.

62. Mohan H, Sen DK, Gupta DK: Orbital affection in nasal and paranasal neoplasms. *Acta Ophthalmol* 47:289–294, 1969.

63. Paul EV, Parnell BL, Fraker M: Prognosis of malignant melanomas of the choroid and ciliary body. *Int Ophthalmol Clin* 2:387, 1962.

64. Perugini S, Pasquini U, Menichelli F, et al: Mucoceles in the paranasal sinuses involving the orbit: CT signs in 43 cases. *Neuroradiology* 23:133–139, 1982.

65. Peyster RG, Hoover ED, Hershey BL, et al: High resolution CT of lesions of the optic nerve. *AJNR* 4:169–174, 1983.

66. Price JI, Danzinger A: The computerized tomographic findings in paediatric orbital tumors. *Clin Radiol* 30:435–440, 1979.

67. Reese AB, Ellsworth RM: The evaluation and current concept of retinoblastoma therapy. *Trans Am Acad Ophthalmol Otolaryngol* 67:164, 1963.

68. Reese AJ: *Tumors of the Orbit. Tumors of the Eye,* ed 3. Hagerstown, MD, Harper & Row, 1976.

69. Rothfus WE, Curtin HD, Slamovits TL, et al: Optic nerve/sheath enlargement. A differential approach based on high resolution CT morphology, *Radiology* 150:409–415, 1984.

70. Savoiardo M, Harwood-Nash DC, Tadmor R, et al: Glimoas of the intracranial anterior optic pathways in children. *Radiology* 138:601–610, 1981.

71. Savoiardo M, Strada L, Passerini A: Intracranial cavernous hemangiomas: Neuroradiologic review of 36 operated cases. *AJNR* 4:945–950, 1983.

72. Smith LJ, Vuksanovic MNM, Yeats BM, et al: Radiation therapy for primary optic nerve meningiomas. *J Clin Neuroophthalmol* 1:85–100, 1981.

73. Spencer WH: Primary neoplasms of the optic nerve and its sheaths: Clinical features and current concepts of pathogenetic mechanisms. *Trans Am Ophthalmol Soc* 70:490–528, 1972.

74. Stewart WB, Krohel GB, Wright JE: Lacrimal gland and fossal lesions: An approach to diagnosis and management. *Ophthalmology* 86:886–895, 1979.

75. Som PM, Sacher M, Weitzner I Jr, et al: Sarcoidosis of the optic nerve. *J Comput Assist Tomogr* 6:614–616, 1982.

76. Trobe JD, Glaser JS, Post JD, et al: Bilateral optic canal meningiomas: a case report. *Neurosurgery* 3:68–74, 1978.

77. Trokel SL, Hilal SK: Recognition and differential diagnosis of enlarged extraocular muscles in computed tomography. *Am J Ophthalmol* 87:503–512, 1979.

78. Trokel SL, Hilal SK: Submillimeter resolution CT scanning of orbital diseases. *Ophthalmology* 87:412–417, 1980.

79. Yanoff M, Fine BS: *Ocular Pathology*. Philadelphia, Harper & Row, 1975, chaps 13, 14.

80. Wende S, Aulich A, Nover A, et al: Computed tomography of orbital lesions. Cooperative study of 210 cases. *Neuroradiology* 13:123–134, 1977.

81. Wilson WB: Hemangiomas of the anterior visual system. *Surv Ophthalmol* 26:109–127, 1981.

82. Wright JE, Call NB, Liaricos J: Primary optic nerve meningioma. *Br J Ophthalmol* 64:553–558, 1980.

83. Wright JE, McDonald WI, Call NB: Management of optic nerve gliomas. *Br J Ophthalmol* 64:545–552, 1980.

84. Zimmerman RA, Bilaniuk LT, Littman P, et al: Computed tomography of pediatric craniofacial sarcoma. *Comput Tomogr* 2:113–121, 1978.

85. Zimmerman LE: Discussion at the International Symposium on Ocular Tumors. Houston, Texas, 1962, in Bonuik M (ed): *Ocular and Adnexal Tumors: New and Controversial Aspects*. St. Louis, CV Mosby, 1964.

12
Lesions Involving the Visual Pathways

CARLOS F. GONZALEZ, EDWARD W. GERNER, GARY DEFILIPP, and
MELVIN H. BECKER

Intracranial disease involving the visual pathways gives rise to visual impairment with ophthalmologic signs. These conditions are diagnosed by history and physical examination. They are demonstrated by computed tomography (CT), magnetic resonance imaging (MRI), and vascular studies. The visual pathways consist of nerve fibers arising in the retina and radiating to the visual cortex of the occipital lobe. Within the orbit, the visual pathway is formed by the retina and the anterior or orbital portion of the optic nerve. In the cranial cavity, the pathway is formed by the intracranial portion of the optic nerve, the optic chiasm, the optic tract, the lateral geniculate body, the optic radiations, and the occipital pole. Lesions involving the visual pathways are responsible for decreased vision, unilateral or bilateral blindness, and visual field defects. The clinical signs and symptoms, as well as the etiology of the lesions affecting the pathways, change from area to area. Any intracranial lesion that causes increased intracranial pressure may present ophthalmic signs, including papilledema. Only those lesions involving the visual pathways are discussed in this chapter.

The Optic Nerve

Each optic nerve has three parts. The anterior part lies within the orbit, and it has been discussed in previous chapters. the middle (intracanalicular) portion of the nerve lies within the optic canal of the sphenoid bone, and the posterior portion lies within the cranial cavity. The optic nerve passes from the apex of the orbit into the middle cranial fossa through the optic canal. The optic canal contains the optic nerve, ophthalmic artery,

and an extension of the intracranial subarachnoid space. The intracranial portion of the optic nerve is short; it extends from the intracranial opening of the optic canal to the optic chiasm. The intracanalicular portion of the optic nerve is difficult to see with CT scanning because of partial volume averaging artifacts from the adjacent bone. However, with MRI, the signal from the cortical bone is negligible, and the entire course of the nerve can be demonstrated. Using partial saturation recovery (SR) (TR 300 msec, 5-mm section thickness), Daniels, et al (11) demonstrated that the optic nerve has a comparable signal intensity to cerebral white matter. The intraorbital part has a much lower signal intensity than orbital fat. The intracranial portion, optic chiasm, and optic tracts are outlined by the lower intensity signal of the surrounding cerebrospinal fluid (CSF). The lower intensity signal from the blood in the ophthalmic artery can be identified adjacent to the intraorbital optic nerve. However, the internal carotid artery and surrounding CSF, both of which have a low-intensity signal, cannot be distinguished. Using 5-mm thickness sections with inversion recovery (IR) (TI = 100, 300, 500, and 700 msec; TR = 2,000 msec) and spin echo (SE) (TE = 25, 50, 75, and 100 msec; TR = 2,000), the optic nerves and chiasm can be seen on the axial view, although with somewhat less clarity than with SR. However, the carotid arteries are better visualized with SE (11).

Tumors and other conditions affecting the intracanalicular part of the optic nerve may cause visual deficits by compressing the nerve. The intracanalicular portion of the optic nerve, while short (6 mm), accounts for a large percentage of lesions. These are characterized by progressive loss of vision with a central scotoma or by altitudinal field defects. The nerve may be involved in the optic canal by conditions that narrow the canal, such as Paget's disease, fibrous dysplasia, osteopetrosis, and (occasionally) hyperostosis frontalis interna. (6) These conditions may be diagnosed on plain x-ray films and/or polytomography in the Rhese position, and also with CT scanning. Within the canal, the optic nerve may also be compressed by enlarged arteriosclerotic ophthalmic arteries (dolichoectatic) or by ophthalmic artery aneurysms. In these conditions—in addition to CT scanning—angiography is needed to demonstrate the abnormality. Enlargement, erosion, and hyperostosis of the bony canal in meningiomas can be demonstrated by CT scans, plain x-ray films, and polytomography. Meningiomas involving the optic canal usually represent extensions of intraorbital or intracranial meningiomas. Intracanalicular calcifications that are frequently found in meningiomas are difficult to demonstrate on CT scans due to the canal's small size and thick bony walls.

Optic nerve gliomas, which usually are extensions of intraorbital or intracranial gliomas, are the most common intrinsic tumors involving the intracanalicular portion of the optic nerve. They produce uniform enlargement of the canal that is well demonstrated on CT scans and polytomographic images. Metastatic and other malignant lesions, including multiple myeloma, also may involve the optic canal and compress the optic nerve. These lesions are usually detected by CT scans. Finally, fractures of the canal can compromise the optic nerve, as described in Chapter 16.

The Optic Chiasm and Parachiasmal Area

The optic chiasm is formed by the fusion of both optic nerves, and it lies in the chiasmal cistern. It is usually tilted 45° from the horizontal plane. It indents the anterior and superior part of the third ventricle, forming the anterior (optic) and posterior (infundibular) recess. More posteriorly, the chiasm is in close relationship to the hypothalamus. The chiasm is located above the sella turcica and the dura of the diaphragm sellae (Fig. 12.1). When the carotid arteries emerge from the cavernous sinuses, they are located beneath and lateral to the optic nerves. The vessels then travel along the lateral and inferior surfaces of the optic chiasm

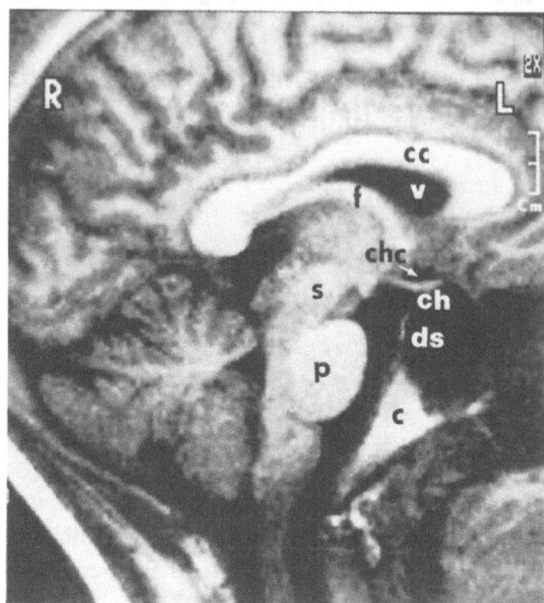

Figure 12.1. Cistern and optic chiasm. Sagittal MRI section, chiasmatic cistern (*chc*), optic chiasm (*ch*), clivus (*c*), fornix (*f*), lateral ventricles (*v*), corpus callosum (*cc*), dorsum sella (*ds*), brain stem (*s*), and pons (*p*).

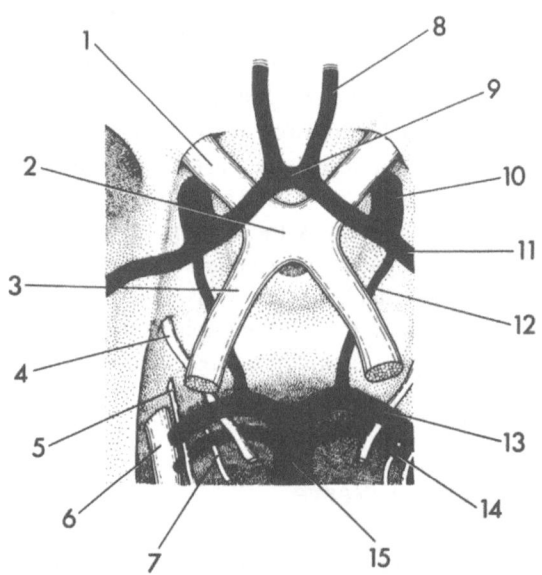

Figure 12.2. Optic chiasm anatomy. (1) Optic nerve; (2) Optic chiasm; (3) optic tract; (4) Oculomotor nerve; (5) Trochlear nerve; (6) Trigeminal nerve; (7) Abducens nerve; (8) Anterior cerebral artery; (9) Anterior communicating artery; (10) Internal carotid artery; (11) Middle cerebral artery; (12) Posterior communicating artery; (13) Posterior cerebral artery; (14) Superior cerebellar artery; (15) Basilar artery.

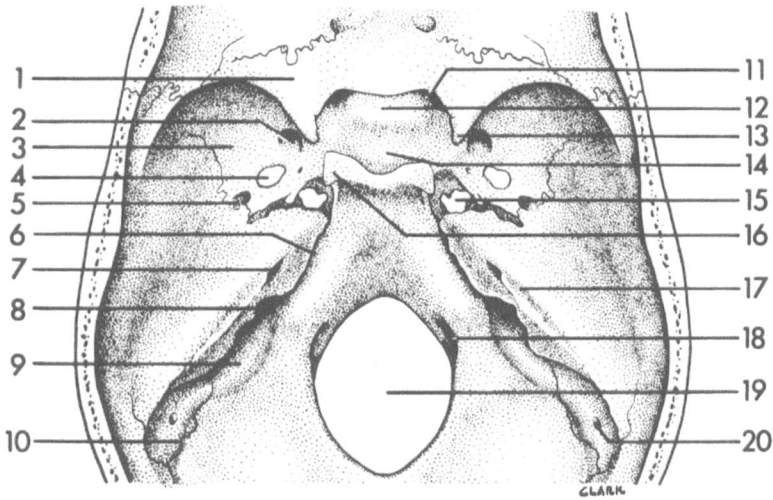

Figure 12.3. Sella turcica anatomy. (1) Sphenoid lesser wing; (2) Foramen rotundum; (3) Sphenoid greater wing; (4) Foramen ovale; (5) Foramen spinosum; (6) Petrooccipital suture; (7) Internal acoustic meatus; (8) Jugular foramen; (9) Sigmoid groove; (10) Lambdoid suture; (11) Optic foramen; (12) Tuberculum sella; (13) Anterior clinoid process; (14) Sellar floor; (15) Foramen lacerum; (16) Posterior clinoid; (17) Superior petrosal sinus (groove); (18) Hypoglossal canal; (19) Foramen magnum; (20) Mastoid foramen.

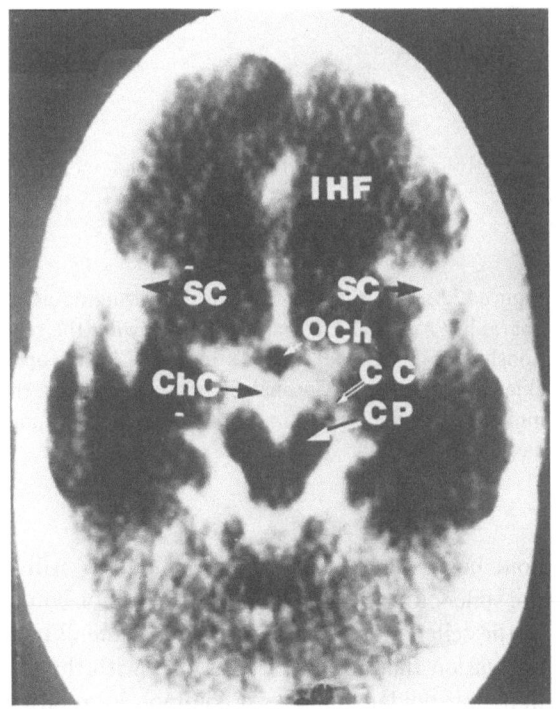

A

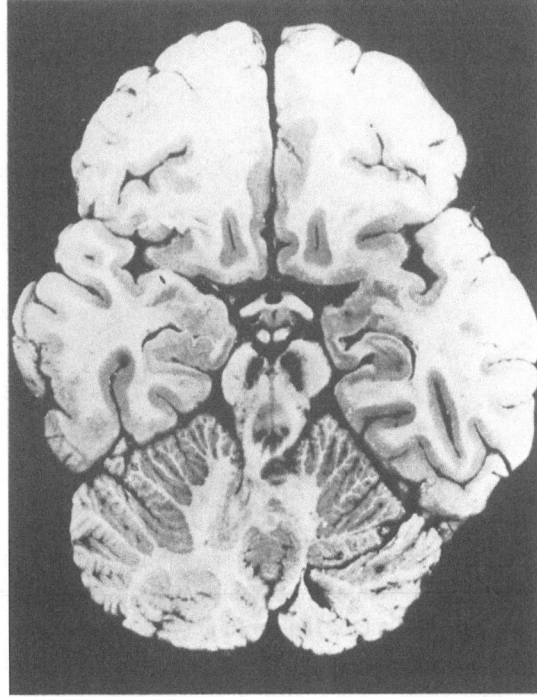

B

Figure 12.4. Chiasmal cistern anatomy. Anatomy of the chiasmatic cistern after metrizamide cisternography. **A.** A CT section at the level of the brain stem shows the interhemispheric fissure (*IHF*), optic chiasm (*OCh*), ce- rebral peduncle (*CP*), chiasm cistern (*ChC*), sylvian cistern (*SC*), and crural cistern (*CC*). **B.** Anatomic section of brain stem at the same level.

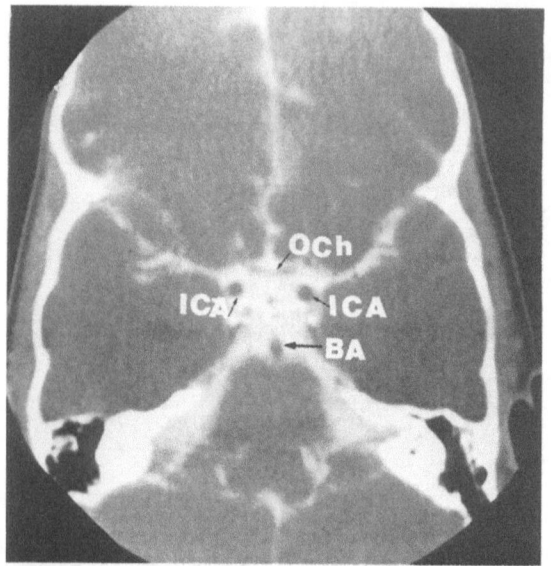

A

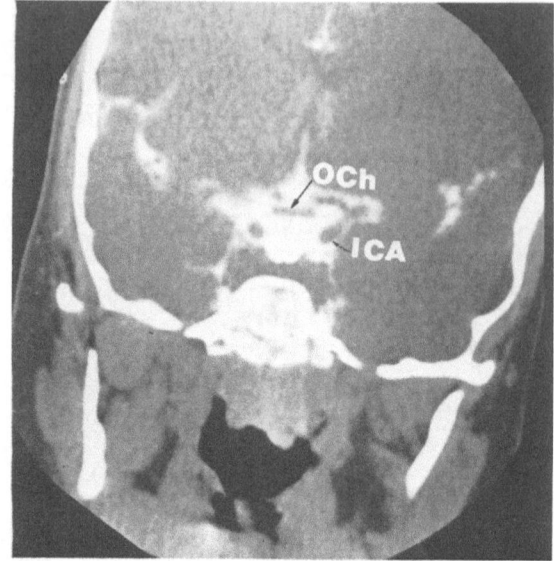

B

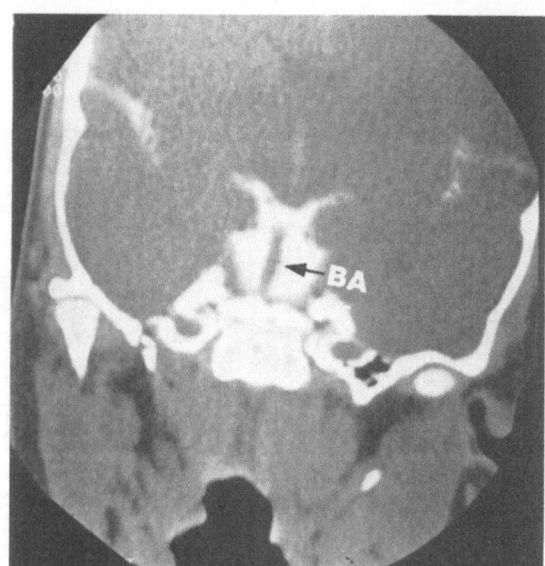

C

Figure 12.5. Cisternal metrizamide. Metrizamide cisternography. **A.** Axial CT scan section showing the relationships of the internal carotid arteries (*ICA*), and optic chiasm (*OCh*). **B, C.** Coronal CT sections showing the internal carotid artery (*ICA*), optic chiasm (*Och*), and basilar artery (*BA*).

until they branch into anterior and middle cerebral arteries. The anterior cerebral arteries cross the superior surface of the optic nerves, and they are connected in the midline by the anterior communicating artery. This anatomic relationship is important, since aneurysms often occur in this area. The posterior communicating arteries are located beneath and behind the optic tracts. Posterior to the chiasm, the infundibulum or pituitary stalk comes through the diaphragm of the sella, and it connects the hypothalamus to the pituitary gland (Fig. 12.2).

The main bony structure in the area is the sphe-

noid bone. The sella turcica is a hollow within the sphenoid bone (Fig. 12.3). The anterior border of the sella is the tuberculum sellae (a small bone protrusion that continues anteriorly with the planum sphenoidale). This is a common location for meningiomas. The shallow chiasmatic sulcus is between the tuberculum and the planum. The sella floor lies between the tuberculum sellae anteriorly and the dorsum sellae posteriorly. The dorsum sellae is a quadrangular structure that continues posteriorly with the clivus. The lateral wall of the sella consists of dural tissue that forms the cavernous sinuses. The pituitary gland lies within the

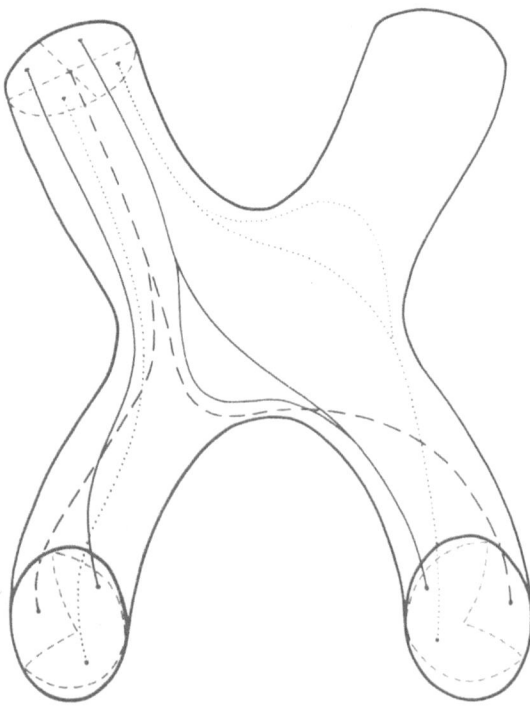

Figure 12.6. Visual pathways. Schematic representation of fibers in the chiasm. Dorsal fibers are represented by heavy continuous lines, ventral fibers by dotted lines, and macula fibers by interrupted lines (After Walsh and Ford [58]).

cistern, sellar structure, and parasellar structure is best accomplished by CT (12, 21) and MRI (Figs. 12.4 and 12.5) (11). Metrizamide cisternography, which is obtained by the intrathecal injection of metrizamide (4–6 mg, 170–190 mg I/ml), is helpful in demonstrating the chiasmatic cistern. Angiography is used to demonstrate vascular lesions, such as aneurysms or carotid-cavernous fistulae.

The visual field defect in optic chiasm lesions depends on the site of interruption (57). Approximately 60% of the fibers from each optic nerve decussate in the chiasm (Fig. 12.6). (58) The nasal retina fibers serve the temporal field. These form the crossed fibers; therefore, lesions involving the central part of the chiasm, where the fibers cross, give a bitemporal hemianopsia. In lesions impinging on the chiasm from below (i.e., pituitary adenoma), the defect starts in the superotemporal quadrants—progressing to involve the inferotemporal, then the inferonasal, and finally the superonasal quadrants. Lesions above the chiasm produce a bitemporal inferior quadrantanopsia that can progress to a bitemporal hemianopsia. Retrochiasmatic lesions usually give rise to homonymous, congruous, and hemianopic defects. Since all of the fibers behind the chiasm represent the contralateral field, the field defect is on the side opposite the lesion. The visual field defects associated with lesions of the visual system are summarized in Figure 12.7 and Table 12.1.

Suprasellar Tumors and Tumor-Like Lesions

Pituitary Adenomas

The most common tumor found in the sellar region is the pituitary adenoma (36). It occurs most commonly in the 25–55-year-old age group (25). The clinical presentation of the lesions is determined by: 1) the location of the lesion, with compression of adjacent structures; and 2) endocrine dysfunction. From a structural standpoint, clinical presentation depends on whether the tumor remains within the sella (intrasellar) or has invaded beyond the sella (extrasellar). With upward growth of the tumor, there is pressure on the diaphragma sellae; this results in headaches. Upwards of 50% of patients with pituitary adenoma complain of head-

sella turcica; therefore, pathologic processes of this structure may cause alterations of the sella. The sphenoid sinus is encompassed within the body of the sphenoid bone, and it lies below and anterior to the sella turcica.

Above the sella lies the suprasellar or chiasmatic cistern, which is an important radiologic landmark in the evaluation of lesions in this area (Fig. 12.4). The chiasmatic cistern has the shape of a hexagon. Alterations in its normal configuration are important clues to pathologic processes. From anterior to posterior, the cisterns forming the chiasmatic cistern are as follows: 1) frontal interhemisphere cistern; 2) sylvian cisterns (bilateral); 3) crural cisterns (bilateral); and 4) interpeduncular. The anatomic relationship of the optic chiasm to the pituitary gland and sella turcica varies considerably. In the majority of people, the optic chiasm is above the posterior diaphragm sella. Occasionally, the chiasm can be located anteriorly (prefix chiasm) or posteriorly (postfix chiasm) to the infundibulum.

The radiographic evaluation of the chiasmatic

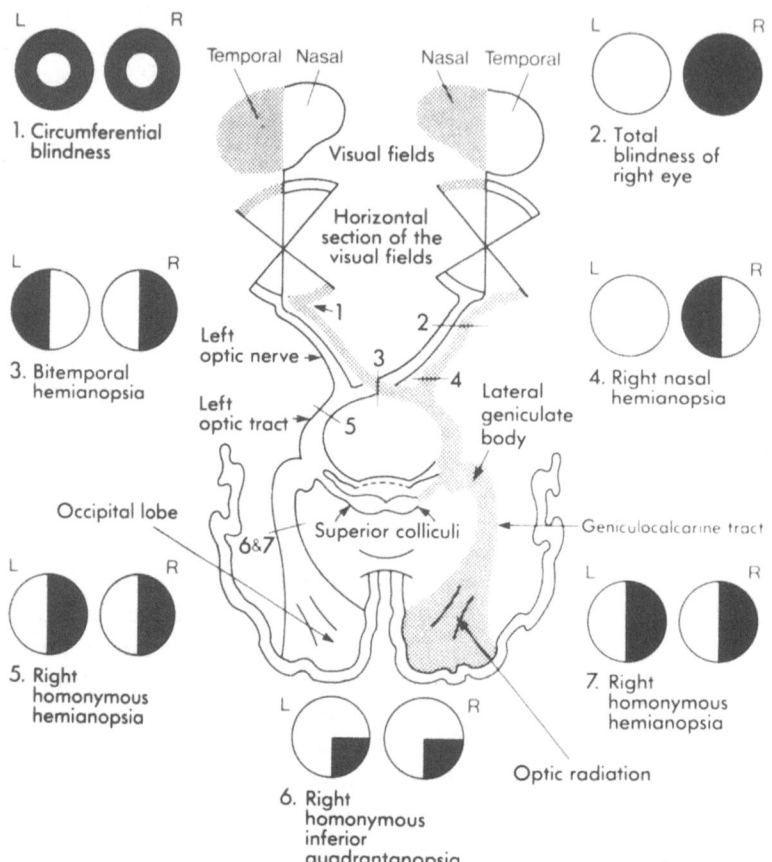

Figure 12.7. Visual field defects associated with lesions of the visual system. (1) Tubular visual field: glaucoma, optic neuritis, and hysteria; (2) Total blindness of right eye: lesion of right optic nerve, trauma, optic neuritis, tumors, and ischemia; (3) Bitemporal hemianopsia due to chiasmal lesions: pituitary tumors, craniopharyngioma, metastases, meningiomas, and others; (4) Right nasal hemianopsia due to lesions in the perichiasmal area: calcified right internal carotid artery; (5) Right homonymous hemianopsia due to lesion of the left parietal or temporal lobes with pressure in the left optic tract; (6) Right homonymous inferior quadrantanopsia due to partial involvement of the optic radiations (upper portion of left optic radiation); (7) Right homonymous hemianopsia with no pupillary change due to complete involvement of the left optic radiation.

aches. When the tumor ruptures through the diaphragma sella, the headaches subside. The patients then may have an interval free of symptoms. The next structure encountered by a pituitary adenoma growing in an upward direction is the optic chiasm. About 75% of patients have visual complaints when first examined (41). The lesion compresses the optic chiasm from below, with a resultant bilateral upper temporal field loss that may progress to a complete bitemporal hemianopsia. Optic atrophy and/or an abnormal pupillary (Marcus-Gunn) reflex may be present. Secreting adenomas produce specific endocrine syndromes, and they are classified by the hormone produced. With the advent of sensitive assays for these hormones, an earlier biochemically precise diagnosis can be made. Rapid enlargement of the tumor due to hemorrhage or necrosis is called pituitary apoplexy (7, 43, 59). The patient usually presents with violent headaches, decreased visual acuity, and ophthalmoplegia. A decreased level of consciousness and meningeal signs are also common. Pituitary adenomas occasionally become invasive, extending into the cavernous sinuses and middle fossa (56).

Pituitary adenomas are best diagnosed by using CT scanning and MRI (Figs. 12.8 and 12.9). Multiple sections of the area should be obtained, including axial, coronal, and sagittal sections, to determine the extent of these lesions. The CT appearance of these lesions is quite characteristic

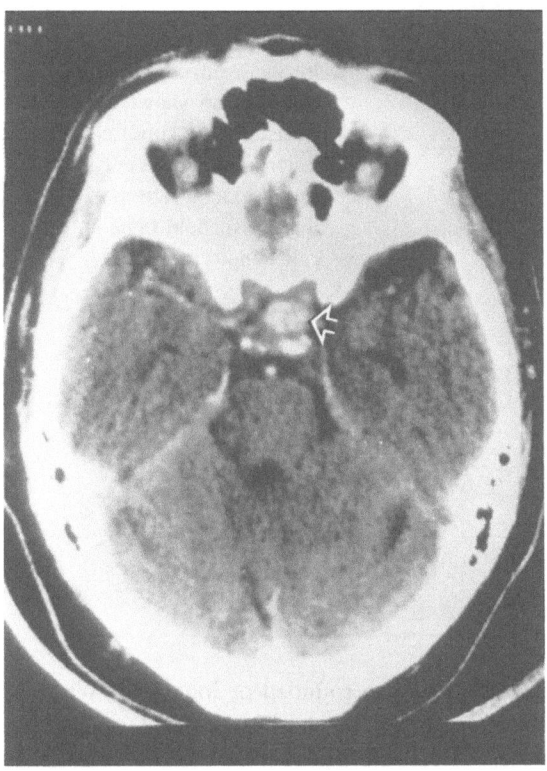

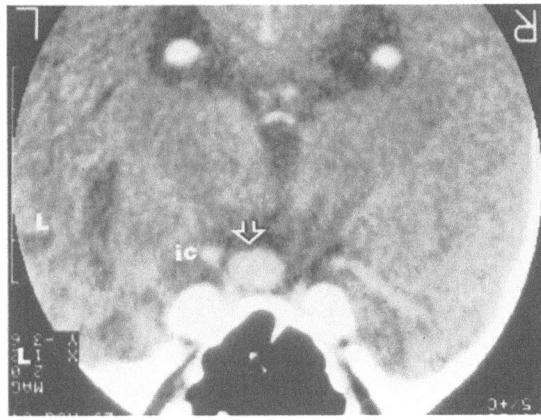

A

B

Figure 12.8. Pituitary adenoma. **A.** Axial CT scan. **B.** Coronal CT scan. Both are following contrast injection. The examination shows a round, well-defined, uniformly enhancing mass lesion (open arrow) extending into the chiasmatic cistern and compressing the left internal carotid (*IC*). It lies lateral to the mass.

Table 12.1. Common lesions affecting the optic chiasm

From below
  Pituitary adenoma
  Pituitary apoplexy
  Empty sella syndrome
  Tuberculum sella meningioma
  Sphenoid ridge meningioma
  Sphenoid mucocele
  Clivus chordoma
  Carcinoma of the sphenoid sinuses and nasopharynx
  Chondroma
  Sarcoid, tuberculosis, and other granulomas
  Metastases
  Other
From above
  Craniopharyngiomas
  Aneurysms
  Ectopic pinealomas
  Third-ventricle dilatation (hydrocephalus)
  Hypothalamic glioma
  Extension of olfactory meningiomas
  Optochiasmatic arachnoiditis
  Metastases
  Other
Lateral to the chiasm
  Parasellar meningiomas
  Carotid aneurysms
  Arteriosclerotic involvement of the carotid artery (dolichoectasia)
  Optochiasmatic arachnoiditis

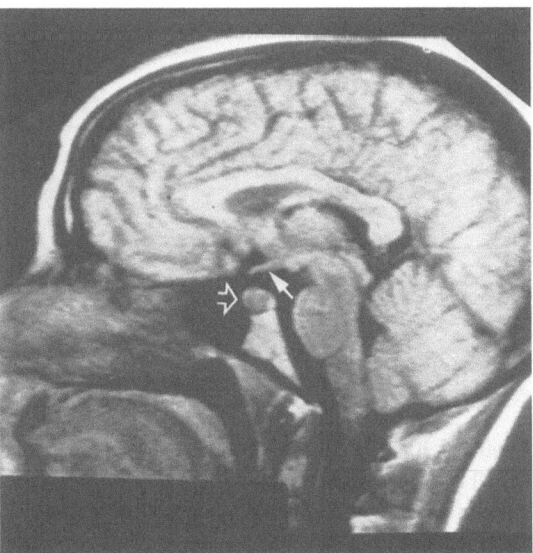

Figure 12.9. Small pituitary adenoma. Sagittal MRI scan (SE, TR 2,000 msec). Enlarged pituitary gland with a concaved upper margin and heterogeneous signal intensity (open arrow). The findings are compatible with a microadenoma. Notice that there is no compression of the optic chiasm (arrow) by the tumor.

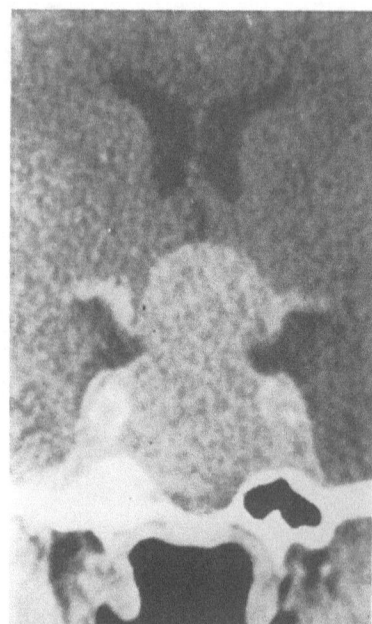
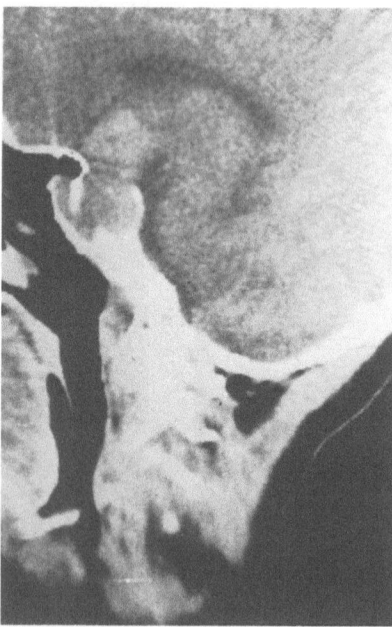

A   **B**

Figure 12.10. Large pituitary
adenoma. **A.** Coronal CT scan.
B. Direct sagital CT scan following contrast injection. The
examination shows a large intrasellar and suprasellar mass
lesion. The sella is enlarged; the
tumor extends anteriorly, eroding the spenoid bone and anterior clinoid process.

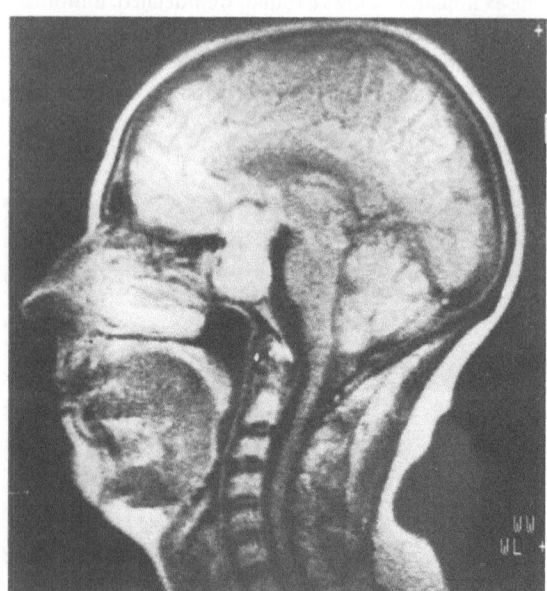

C

Figure 12.10 C. MRI sagittal section of the same patient
(SE, TE 50 msec and TR 1,000 msec). The examination
demonstrates a large mass lesion occupying the sella
and sphenoid sinus. It projects anteriorly into the chiasmatic cistern, and it appears to be involving the superior
half of the clivus as well.

(43, 52); they are rounded or lobulated. Without
contrast media, the density is equal or slightly
greater than the adjacent brain. After contrast media injection, slight homogeneous enhancement is
usually seen (22). Intrasellar lesions, with or without sellar changes (microadenomas), do not produce visual changes. These small lesions can be
detected with current imaging techniques. Large
tumors produce changes in bone (sellar enlargement or ballooning and erosion of the sella) that
are best demonstrated by CT scans and polytomography, but they may be seen on plain x-ray films.
Invasive pituitary adenomas may produce marked
destruction of the base of the skull. They have
to be differentiated from tumors such as chordomas, chondromas, nasopharyngeal carcinomas,
and metastatic lesions that may produce similar
changes (13, 23, 33). Extension of the tumor into
the suprasellar cistern and hypothalamic region,
cavernous sinuses, and sphenoid sinuses are well
demonstrated by CT scans (Fig. 12.10A, B). However, the greater anatomic detail and multiplanar
capability of MRI make this imaging modality the
procedure of choice in investigating pituitary tumors (4, 24, 38). Imaging with different pulse sequences seems to provide some information on the
specific nature of the lesions (Fig. 12.10 C–F)
(5, 60). Calcifications within the tumor are rare
and are seen on CT scans. Vascular studies usually
are performed to rule out abnormalities, such as
internal carotid aneurysms and other intrasellar

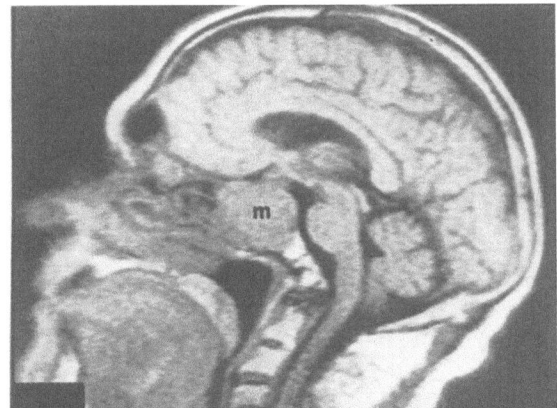

D

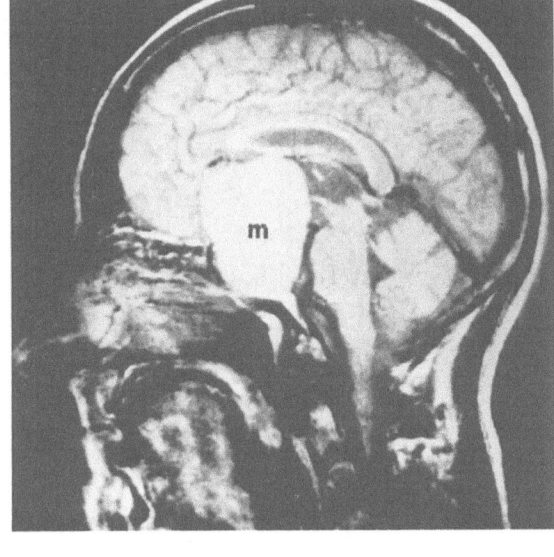

F

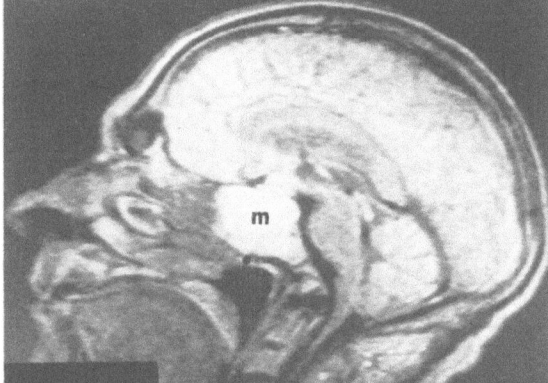

E

Figure 12.10 D, E. A second patient with a large pituitary adenoma; sagittal MRI sections. The examination shows a large pituitary tumor (*m*) extending inferiorly into the sphenoid sinus and upward into the foramen of Monro. The mass also projects anteriorly into the interhemispheric fissure and frontal lobes. **F.** Large pituitary adenoma in a third patient. Sagital MRI section shows a large pituitary tumor extending into the anterior cranial fossa and the sphenoid sinus.

or parasellar vascular tumors that may simulate pituitary adenomas.

Meningiomas

These tumors may occur in the suprasellar region; they most commonly originate in the tuberculum sellae (planum sphenoidale, anterior clinoid process), suprachiasmatic region (extension of olfactory groove meningiomas), and parasellar region (inner ridge, sphenoid wing meningiomas). Tuberculum sellae meningiomas (Fig. 12.11) and suprachiasmatic meningiomas are slow-growing and difficult to diagnose both clinically and radiographically in the early stages (45). The most common presentation is progressive visual loss, asymmetric visual field defects, and optic atrophy. Altitudinal visual field defects are seen when the intracranial optic nerve is compressed by a posterior extension of an olfactory groove meningioma. Parasellar meningiomas (Fig. 12.12), in addition to visual loss and visual field cuts, also may produce ophthalmoplegia and exophthalmos (superior orbital fissure syndrome). Meningiomas are best diagnosed by CT scans and MRI. They usually are seen on CT scans as homogeneous high-density lesions attached to the bone of the base of the skull. Significant enhancement after injection of contrast media may be seen (Fig. 12.13) (19). Sclerosis of the underlying bone and dense calcification or ossification of the associated dural structures usually are visualized on CT scans, plain x-ray films of the skull, and polytomography (Fig. 12.11). Although not enough sudies are available, high-resolution MRI (1.5 Tesla) seems to provide the best overall delineation of the tumor. Suprasellar meningiomas have to be differentiated from large pituitary adenomas and large calcified aneurysms. This is not always possible when using only CT scanning or MRI. Angiography is helpful, since it shows the vascular nature of the meningiomas, which usually are supplied from meningeal branches of the ophthalmic artery, cavernous portions of the internal carotid artery, and (rarely) branches of the external carotid artery (Fig. 12.12); it differentiates these tumors from giant aneurysms and other vascular lesions.

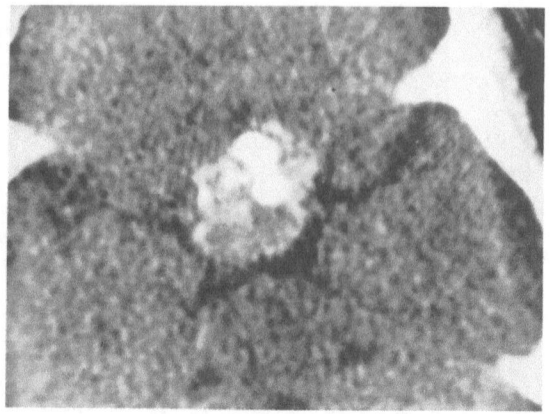

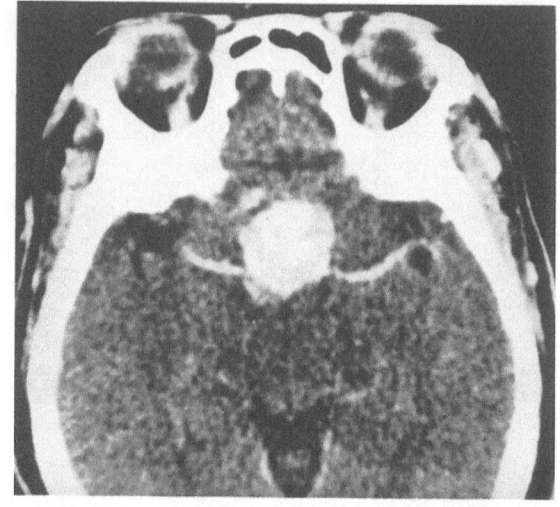

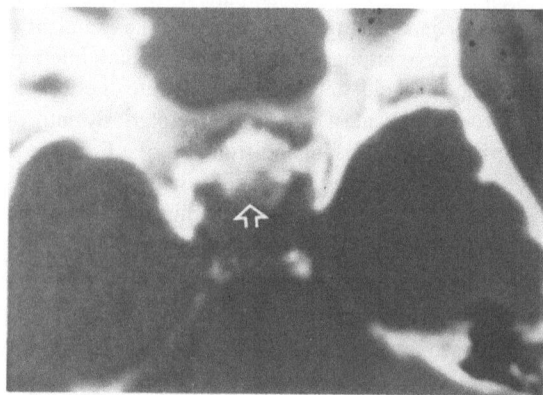

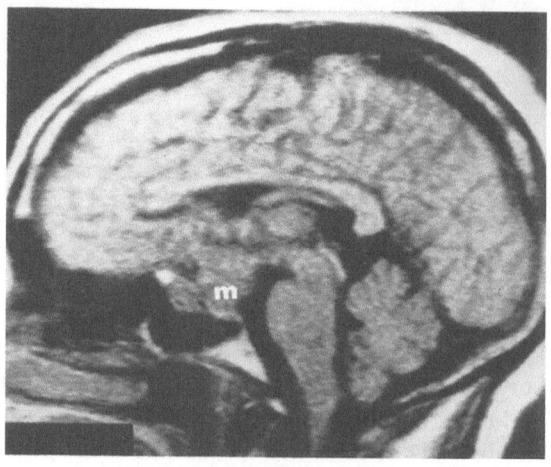

Figure 12.11. Tuberculum sella and suprasellar meningioma. **A, B, C.** Axial CT scan section. The examination prior to contrast injection (**A**) reveals a heterogeneous, high-density, calcified mass lesion occupying the suprasellar cistern. Following contrast media injection, homogeneous enhancement is seen. A section at the level of the anterior clinoid process (**C**) with bone window settings reveals irregular hyperostosis of the planum sphenoidale and tuberculum sella. **D.** Sagittal MRI section of the same patient reveals a large sellar and suprasellar lesion (*m*).

Craniopharyngioma

Craniopharyngiomas are tumors arising from the epithelial remnants of the hypophyseal stalk (Rathke's pouch). These tumors are most commonly seen in children, but they may occur at any age (8). The location is primarily suprasellar, although a small percentage is entirely or mostly intrasellar. Superior extension of the tumor into the foramen of Monro and hydrocephalus is common. Papilledema, which is due to increased intracranial pressure, is seen in children with obstructive hydrocephalus. The tumor usually compresses the dorsal and posterior surfaces of the optic chiasm, with loss of the central temporal fields. When the tumor extends posteriorly, homonymous hemianopsia, which is due to secondary involvement of the optic tract, is present. If the tumor is intrasellar, the visual changes are similar to those seen with pituitary tumors. Decreased visual acuity and optic atrophy may be present.

Craniopharyngiomas are pleiomorphic tumors with solid, cystic, and calcific elements. Both CT scans and plain x-ray films of the skull region show large, irregular calcification in the suprasellar region (Fig. 12.14) (1, 2). The appearance of the

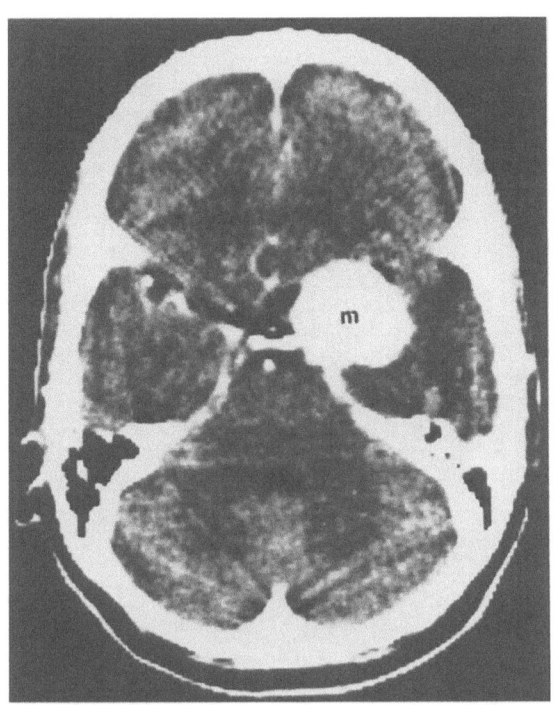

A

Figure 12.12. Large parasellar meningioma. **A.** Axial CT scan section following contrast injection. The examination reveals a large, homogeneously enhancing mass lesion (*m*) in the left parasellar region. The mass is extending into the chiasmatic cistern and anterior and middle fossa. **B, C.** Selective internal carotid arteriogram. Anteroposterior view (**B**) show marked medial displacement of right internal carotid (arrow) and elevation of the middle cerebral artery (arrowheads) produced by the tumor (**C**) Lateral view. **D, E.** Selective external carotid arteriogram. Anteroposterior (**D**) and lateral (**E**) views show a dense, homogeneous blush or stain (arrowheads) consistent with a meningioma.

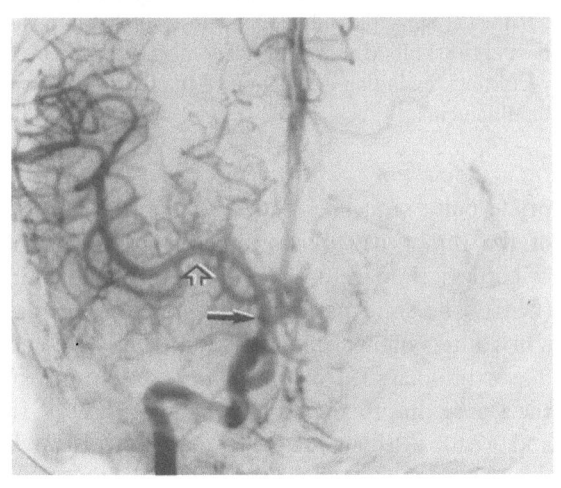

B

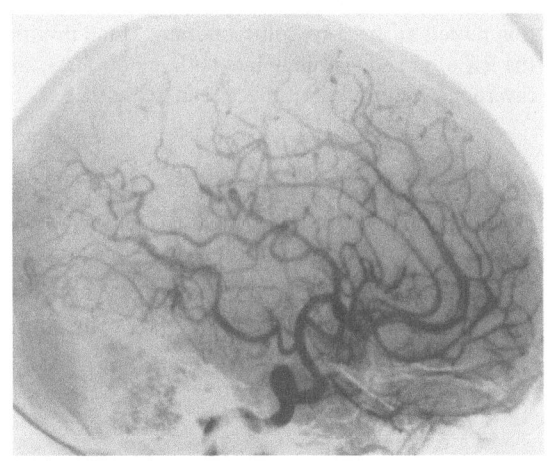

C

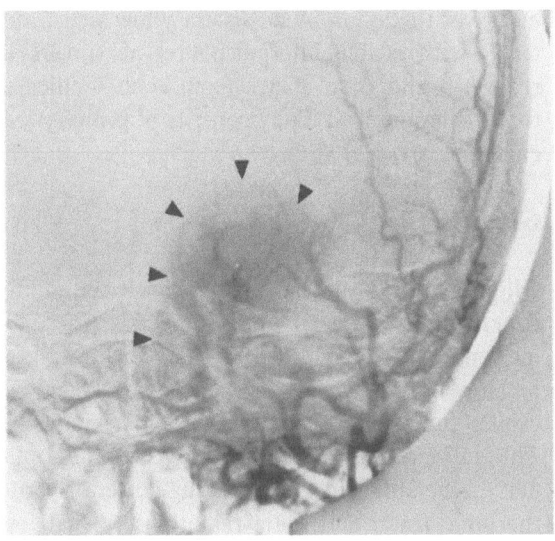

D

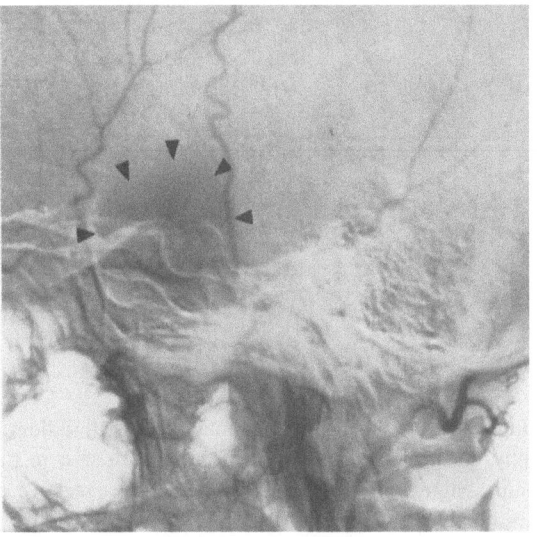

E

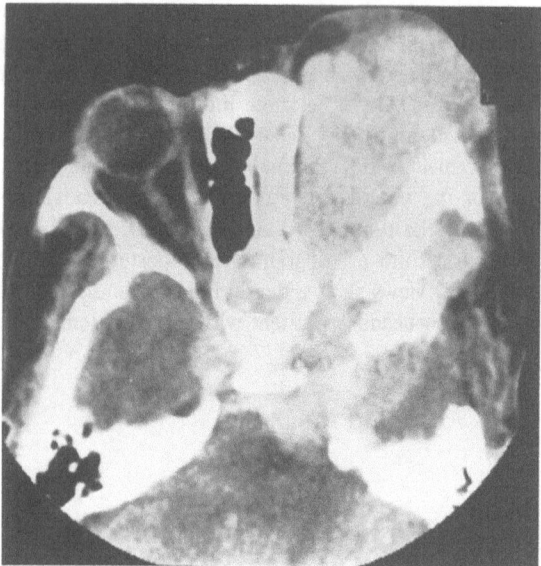

A

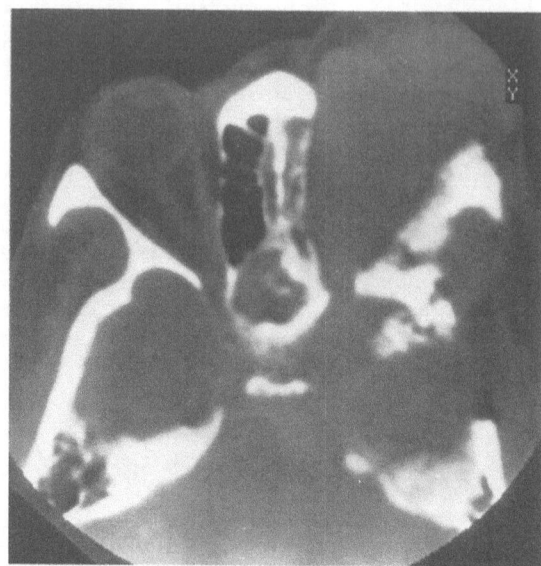

B

Figure 12.13. Recurrent orbital meningioma. **A, B.** Axial CT scan sections of the orbits and skull base performed after injection of contrast media. The examination reveals an extensive soft-tissue mass lesion invading the left orbit and extending into both middle fossas and cavernous sinuses, sella turcica, and retrosellar space, with posterior displacement of the brain stem. The tumor is a recurrent meningioma that originated in the left medial sphenoid ridge bone and extended into the base of the skull. Multiple surgical procedures have been performed, including evacuation of the left eye and orbital contents.

tumor on CT scan is very variable, ranging from cystic (sometimes multiloculated) low-density lesions to solid enhancing tumors (Figs. 12.15 and 12.16). (20). An MRI shows superior soft-tissue contrast compared to CT, provided that the appro-

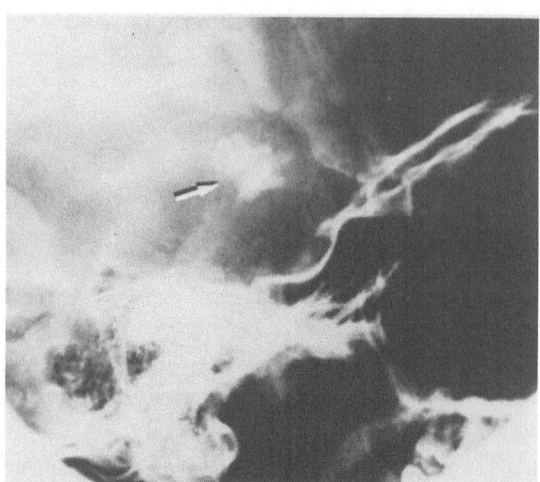

Figure 12.14. Craniopharyngioma. Plain skull radiography. Multiple suprasellar calcifications are seen in the suprasellar region. This finding is highly suggestive of craniopharyngioma (arrow).

priate pulse sequence is used. The cystic portion of the tumor usually produces a signal with a brightness similar to that of cerebrospinal fluid (CSF). The solid portion of the tumor produces a brightness higher than CSF; and if fat is present, it can be identified by the highest brightness of the signal due to the short T1 (17) (Figs. 12.15 and 12.6). Although calcifications are not well demonstrated, imaging with different pulse sequences could provide information on the specific nature of the lesion. A persistently low signal, detected with various interpulse intervals (inversion recovery) and echo delays (spin echo), indicates that the lesion most likely consists of primary calcifications (4).

Gliomas

Gliomas of the visual pathway are more commonly seen in children with neurofibromatosis. These tumors may be extracranial (in the orbit), intracranial, or contiguous between both areas. The intraorbital tumor has been described in chapter 11. The intracranial tumor can involve the optic nerves, the optic chiasm extending posteriorly into the optic tract, and optic radiations. Visual loss

Figure 12.15 **(A)** Axial CT scan section. The examination reveals a well-defined, suprasellar, homogeneous, low-density lesion with peripheral calcification. No enhancement was seen after contrast injection. **(B)** Sagittal MRI section (inversion recovery pulse sequence). The examination shows a well-defined cystic lesion of homogeneous intensity. Brightness equals that of cerebrospinal fluid on this pulse sequence. (Courtesy of Robert Steiner, M.D., Thomas Jefferson University Hospital, Philadelphia, Pennsylvania.)

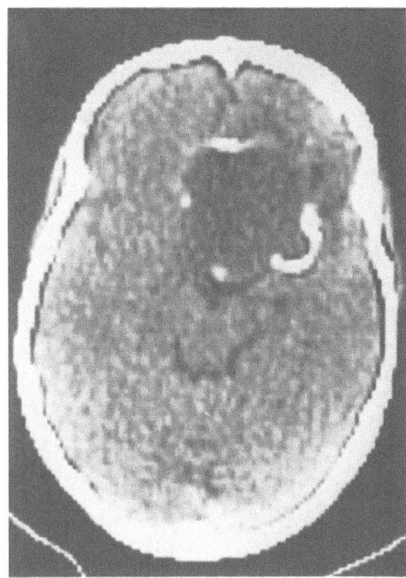
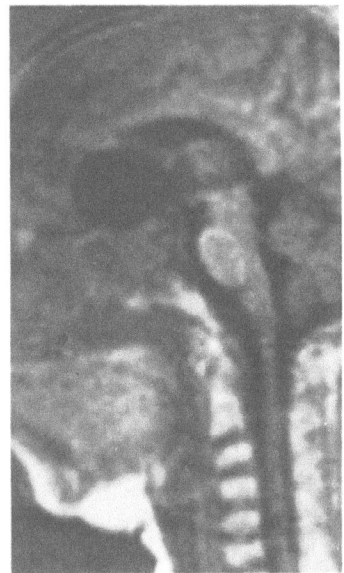

A

B

and hypothalamic dysfunction are usually present, depending on the tumor's location. A skull x-ray film may show a J-shaped deformity of the sella turcica; and if there is intraorbital extension of the tumor, the optic foramina may be enlarged. The CT scan shows a suprasellar, homogeneous, sometimes irregular mass lesion within the suprachiasmatic cistern. The density of the tumor usually is similar to the normal optic nerve density. Enhancement with intravenously given contrast media is variable. It may be intense, moderate, or

absent (16, 49). Calcifications are rare (Figs. 12.17 and 12.18).

Astrocytomas originating in the hypothalamus (hypothalamic gliomas) or septum pellucidum may produce visual changes by direct invasion or compression on the optic chiasm. These lesions occur most commonly in children who present with intracranial hypertension and diencephalic syndrome (Fig. 12.19). Other gliomas, such as oligodendrogliomas and (occasionally) ependymomas, may also grow in this area and may extend

Figure 12.16. Solid craniopharyngioma. **(A)** Direct sagittal CT scan section following intravenous injection of contrast medium. The examination shows an inhomogeneous, low-density, suprasellar lesion that enhances after injection of contrast medium. **(B)** Sagittal MRI section (inversion recovery pulse sequence) The examination reveals a poorly-defined suprasellar lesion of inhomogeneous intensity, brighter than cerebrospinal fluid on this pulse sequence. (Courtesy of Robert Steiner, M.D., Thomas Jefferson University Hospital, Philadelphia, Pennsylvania.)

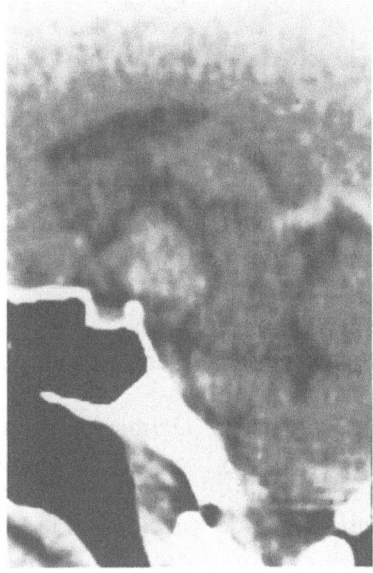
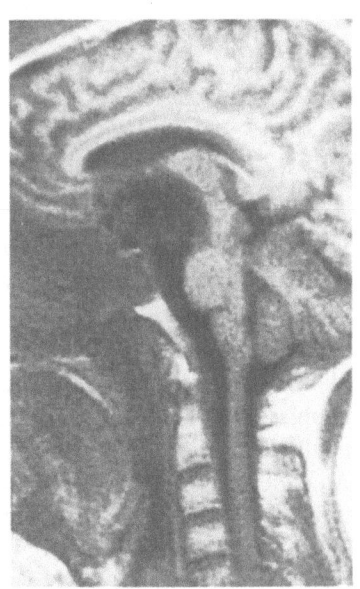

A

B

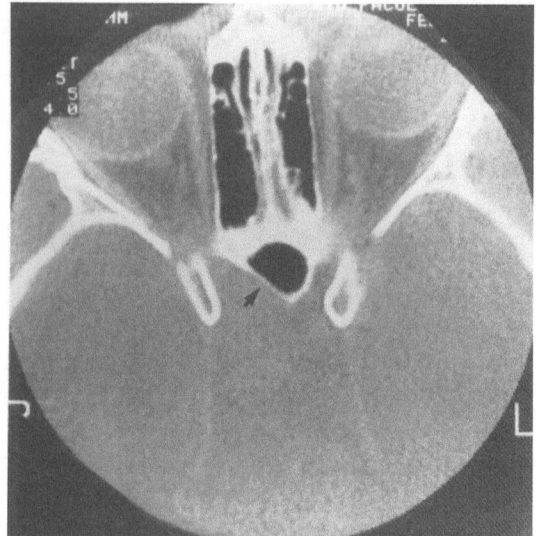

A

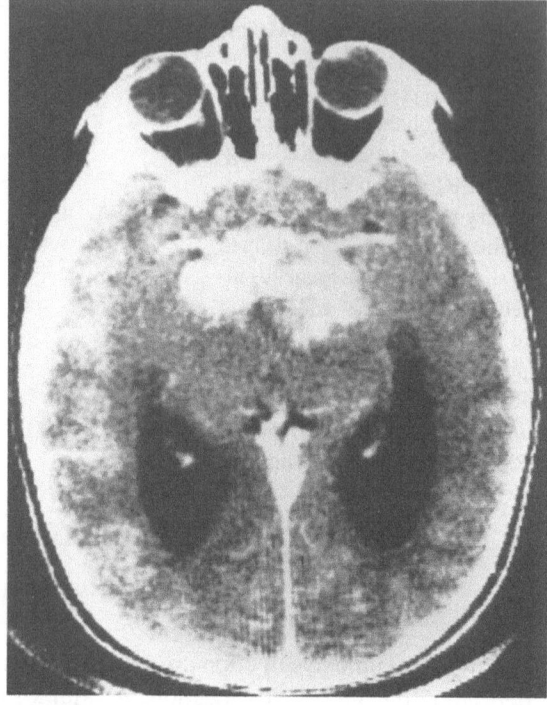

C

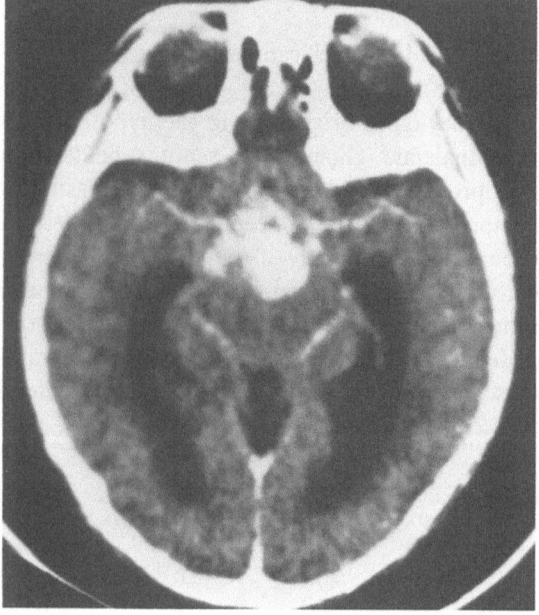

B

Figure 12.17. Optic nerve and chiasm glioma. **A.** Axial CT scan section at the level of the anterior clinoid processes. The examination reveals significant enlargement and erosion of the right optic canal due to an extension of the tumor into the canal (arrow). The intraorbital optic nerves are normal. **B, C.** Axial CT scan at the level of the chiasmatic cistern and hypothalamus performed after contrast injection. The chiasmatic cistern is occupied by an irregular, but homogeneously enhanced, mass lesion that extends upwards into the hypothalamic region.

into the chiasmatic cistern. Both CT scanning and MRI are the best imaging methods for diagnosing these lesions (39).

The other malignant gliomas—malignant optic glioma of adulthood, malignant astrocytomas, or glioblastomas—are found in early middle-aged adults, and they tend to be more rapidly fatal. A sudden onset of visual loss progressing rapidly to bilateral blindness is characteristic. Death usually occurs within 6 months of the onset of disease (29).

Other Suprasellar Tumors and Tumor-Like Lesions

Germinomas

Germinomas (atypical teratomas or ectopic pinealomas) are tumors that histologically resemble seminomas. These tumors are most commonly seen in childhood in the pineal region or the suprasellar area. Visual loss, diabetes insipidus, and pituitary

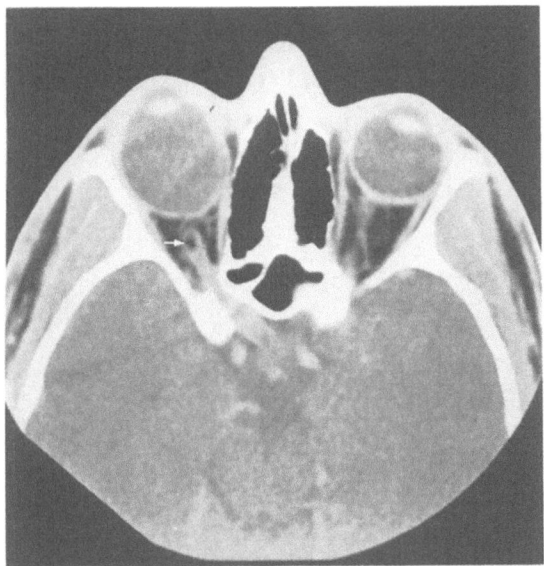

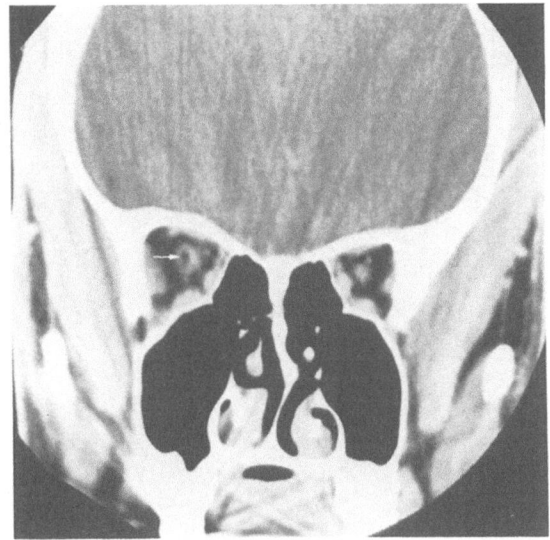

E

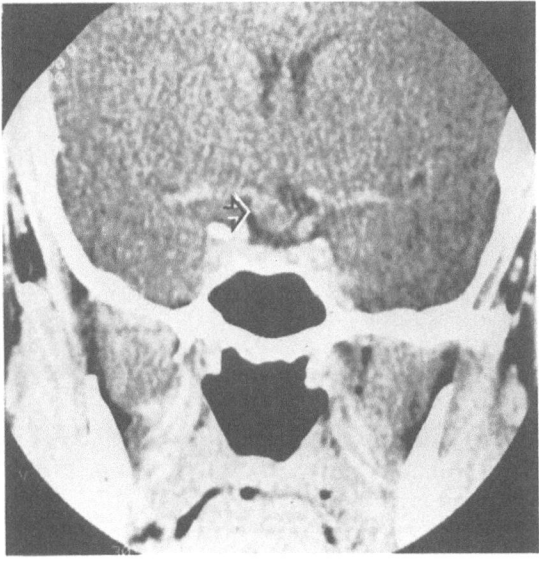

F

D

Figure 12.17. D, E, F. Another case of optic and chiasm glioma in a patient with neurofibromatosis. **D.** Axial CT scan performed after injection of contrast media. The examination shows that the right orbit is enlarged; also shown is a large right globe (buphthalmus). The right optic nerve in the orbit is thick and irregular. It has a central area of decreased density (arrow). The right optic canal is enlarged due to the extension of the tumor from the orbit into the chiasmatic cistern. **E.** Coronal CT sections at the level of the orbit and **F.** Coronal CT scan at the level of the optic chiasm revealing the enlargement of the optic nerve (arrow) and optic chiasm (open arrow) produced by the tumor.

dysfunction are characteristic. The CT scan appearance in the suprasellar region shows a nonspecific mass lesion that may mimic craniopharyngioma, hypothalamic glioma, and other suprasellar tumors (50). Calcifications are rare. Intraparenchymal extension or metastasis to the ventricular wall may occur.

Congenital or Embryonic Tumors
Suprasellar Epidermoid, Dermoid, and Teratomas

Epidermoid cysts are cystic masses lined by simple stratified squamous epithelium that occur more commonly in the third to fifth decades. Common extracranial sites for epidermoid cysts are the posterior fossa, the cerebellar-pontine angle, and the sellar and juxtasellar regions (46). In the latter location, the tumors may produce ocular symptoms (bitemporal hemianopsia and optic atrophy). Orbitofrontal epidermoids have been discussed in Chapter 11. The CT scan appearance of epidermoid tumors in the suprasellar region shows an irregular, low-density (usually CSF density) mass lesion enlarging the chiasmatic cistern (Fig. 12.20). Mixed densities, including fat or tissue with a density similar to brain tissue, have been observed occasionally within the tumor. Normally, no en-

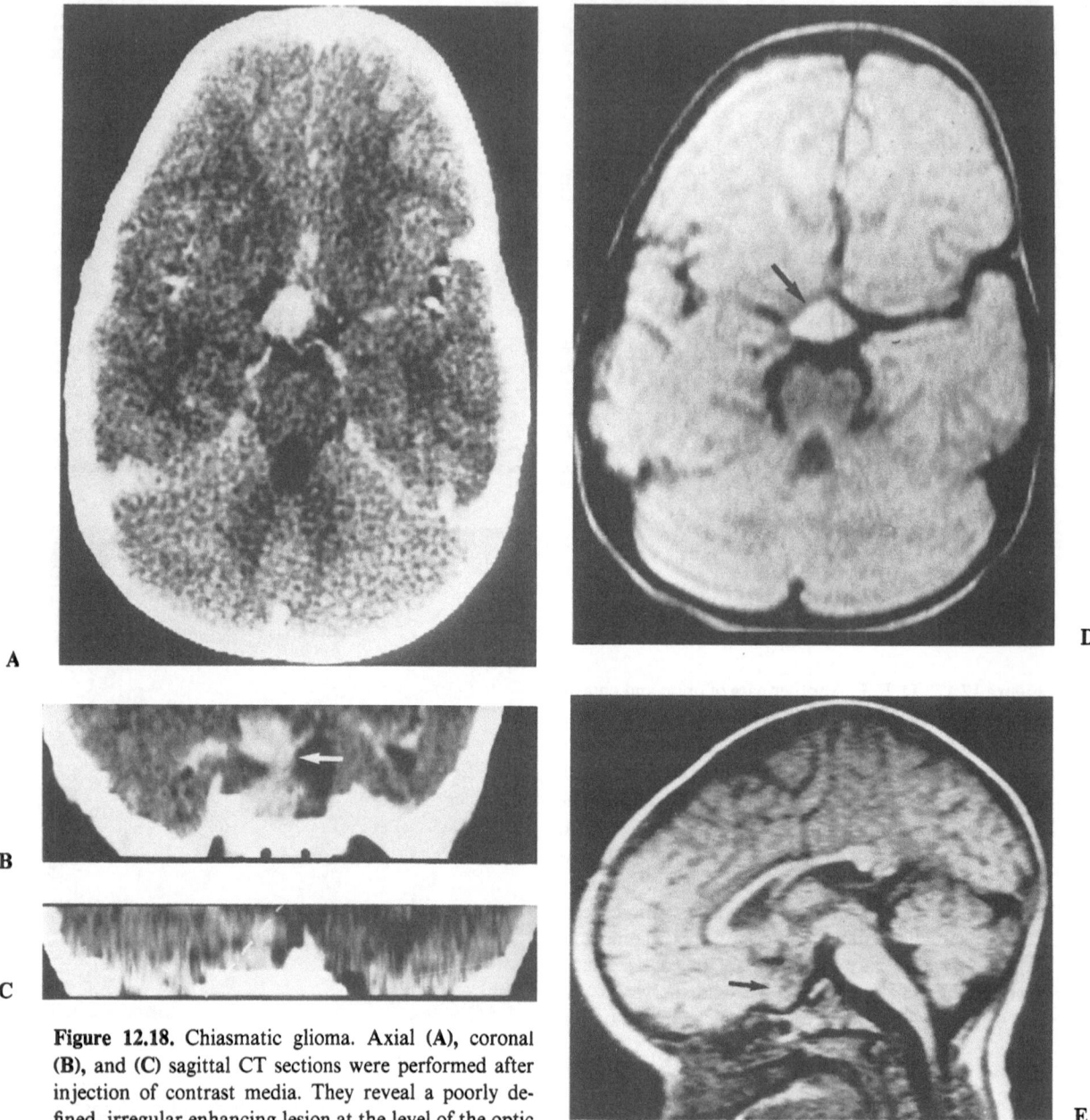

Figure 12.18. Chiasmatic glioma. Axial (**A**), coronal (**B**), and (**C**) sagittal CT sections were performed after injection of contrast media. They reveal a poorly defined, irregular enhancing lesion at the level of the optic chiasm. In the coronal reconstruction, the mass seems to extend into the hypothalamus (arrow). **D, E.** Axial and sagittal MRI sections (SE, TE 28 and 56 msec and TR 556 to 2,000 msec) at the level of the suprasellar cistern. The examination reveals a lesion in the cistern, with no evidence of intraorbital involvement or posterior extension along the optic tracts.

Figure 12.19. Hypothalamic glioma. **A.** Axial CT scan section at the level of the chiasmatic cistern in an 11-year-old boy with decreased vision and diencephalic symptoms. The examination was performed following the injection of contrast media; it reveals a large, partially enhanced mass lesion that obliterates the suprasellar cistern and extends to the anterior and both middle fossas. **B, C.** Coronal MRI sections reveals extension of the tumor up to the level of the foramen of Monro with obliteration of the third ventricle.

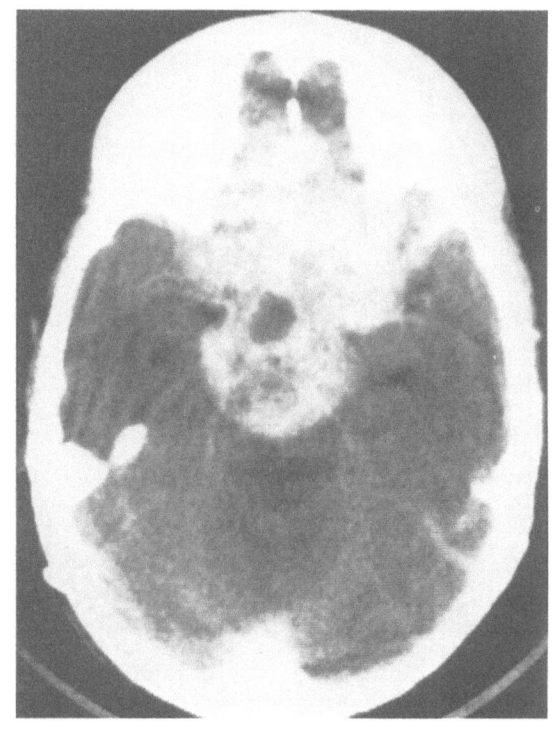

A

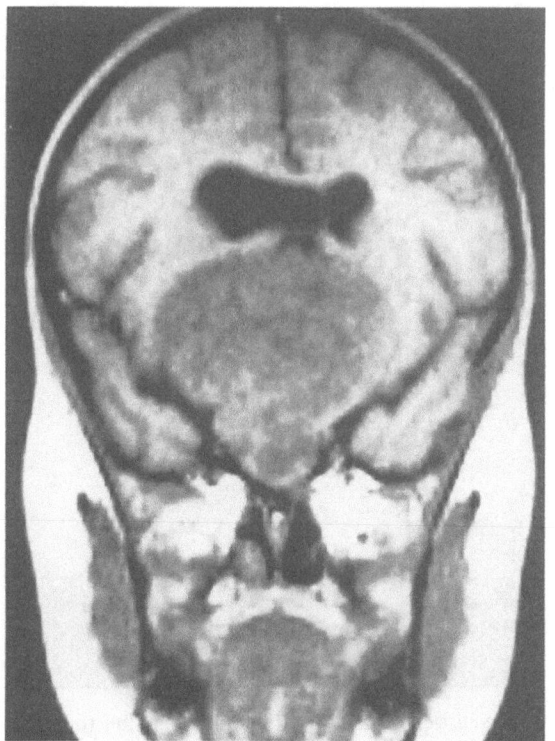

B

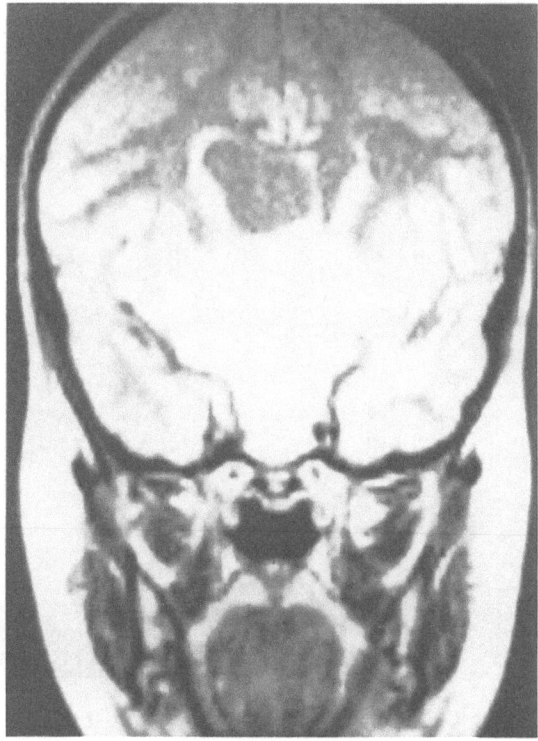

C

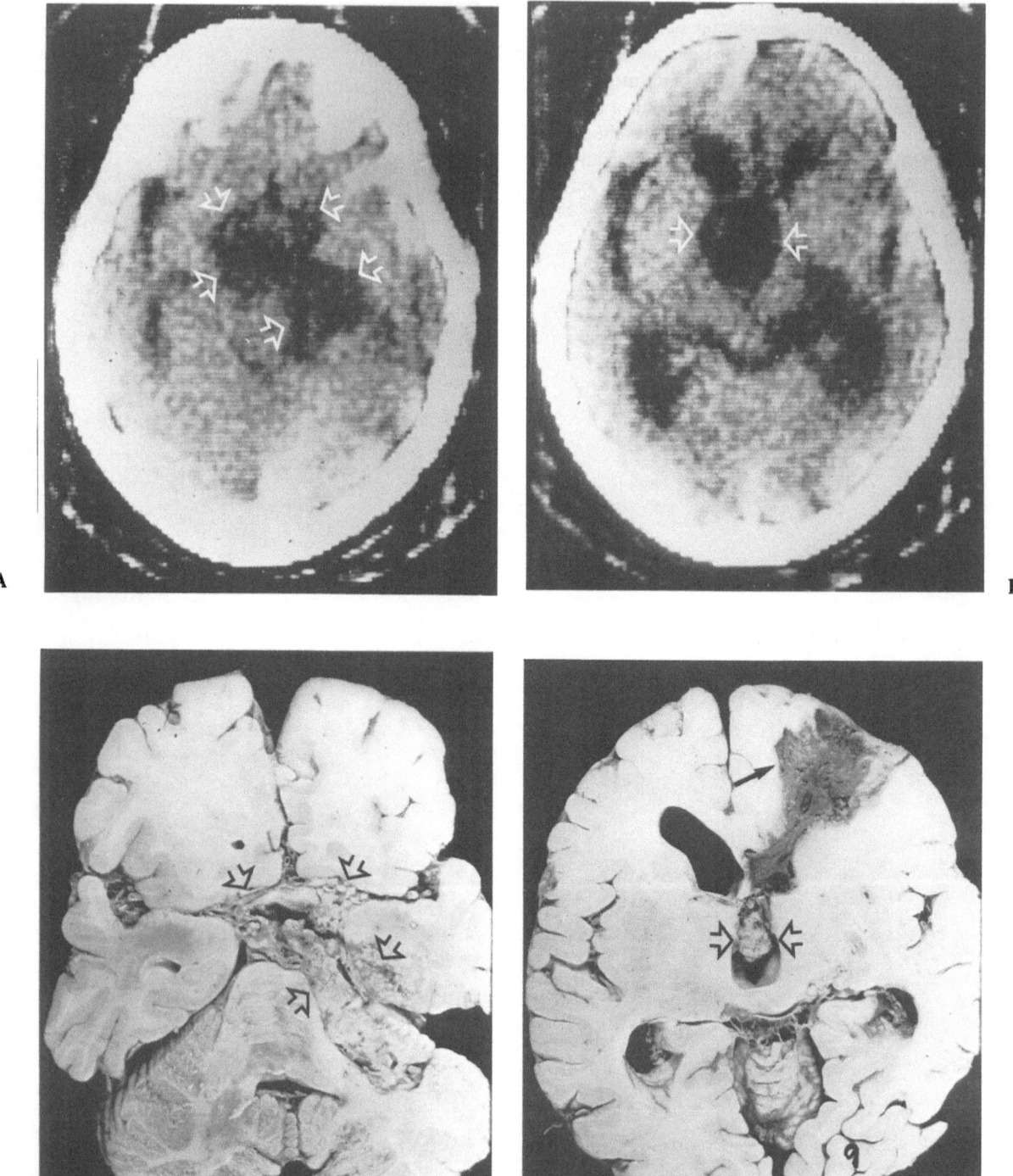

Figure 12.20. Epidermoid tumor. **A, B.** Axial CT scan sections of the brain at the level of the chiasmatic cistern and third ventricle, respectively. **A.** The examination reveals an irregularly marginated low-density mass lesion in the suprasellar region extending into the right cerebello-pontine cistern and displacing the brain stem laterally (open arrows) **B.** The mass is seen within the third ventricle as a round low-density lesion (open arrows). The lateral ventricles are enlarged. **C, D.** Brain sections of the same patient demonstrating the irregular tumor in the right cerebello-pontine cistern and the third ventricle (open arrows). Postsurgical changes are seen in the right frontal lobe (solid arrow).

hancement is seen after contrast media injection (14, 18). Epidermoid cysts are considered to be congenital lesions secondary to inclusion of the epidermoid elements during closure of the neural tube in early embryonic life. If the tumors contain (in addition to keratin sebaceous material) hair follicles and other elements of the deeper layers of the skin, the lesions are called dermoid cysts. These tumors differ from epidermoid cysts in that they occur mainly in the first decade of life and are localized in the midline of the cerebellar vermis, the fourth ventricle, the orbits, and less commonly in the suprasellar regions (46). In this location, they may cause foramen of Monro obstruction, hydrocephalus, and hypothalamic dysfunction. The CT scan appearance of the tumor shows a low-density, poorly defined cystic lesion. Fat density is more commonly seen scattered within the tumor or forming intratumoral fat fluid levels. If the cyst ruptures into the ventricular system or subarachnoid spaces, extension of fat density particles into these structures is usually found. Suprasellar teratomas are very rare (51).

Arachnoid Cysts

Arachnoid cysts are intraarachnoid collections of CSF that may act as mass lesions. The cysts usually are congenital, but they may be the result of inflammatory meningeal processes (55). Arachnoid cysts may occur in the posterior cranial fossa, middle fossa, and (occasionally) the suprasellar region. Most suprasellar cysts are large, and they may produce obstructive hydrocephalus. On CT scan, the cysts are identified as well-defined suprasellar lesions with a density similar to CSF (Figs. 12.21 and 12.22) (27, 34). The cysts usually are completely enclosed and do not communicate with the ventricular system or the subarachnoid space. The cyst wall usually is very thin and may not be seen on CT scan, in which case metrizamide CT cisternography is helpful in defining the extension of the cyst (48).

Metastatic Lesions

Metastatic lesions of the pituitary gland or hypothalamus may or may not have ophthalmologic signs or may only cause diabetes insipidus. Visual defects may occur in a small group of patients where there is compression or invasion of the optic chiasm by the tumor (9, 10). The CT and MRI appearance of metastatic tumors usually is nonspecific and may resemble any other suprasellar tumor (Fig. 12.23). Intrasellar metastatic lesions may cause bone destruction, which is best detected by CT scans or plain skull radiography. Sellar and juxtasellar metastasis are seen more frequently in patients with carcinoma of the breast (31). Enhancement after contrast media injection is seen occasionally.

Hypothalamic Hamartomas

Hypothalamic hamartomas are tumors consisting of all embryonic elements that form the central nervous system (such as neuroglial cells and myelinated fibers that are found occasionally in the hypothalamus and chiasmatic region). They usually do not produce visual symptoms, but they may cause precocious puberty in males. The tumors present on CT scans as small nodules or large solid tumors in the suprasellar cistern. The CT density is homogeneous and isodense with the rest of the brain. Calcifications are rare (Fig. 12.24) (35). Differentiation with other tumors occurring in this area (such as chiasmatic gliomas, metastatic lesions, and other chiasmatic lesions) usually is impossible. On MRI (T2-weighted spin echo images), there has been a slight increase in signal intensity compared to the normal brain. Although this finding may suggest the diagnosis of hamartoma, it also has been found in chiasmatic gliomas. Since only a few suprasellar hamartomas have been studied with MRI, there is no definitive evidence that MRI is superior to CT scanning in determining the nature of these tumors.

Granulomatous Disease

The CT and MRI changes seen in granulomatous lesions (sarcoidosis, tuberculosis, fungal disease, and histiocytosis) of the suprasellar region reflect the pathologic changes provided by these diseases—mainly granulomatous infiltration of the leptomeninges with resultant cranial nerve palsies, arteritis, and brain infarctions. Extension of chronic meningitis to the optic chiasm, hypothalamus, floor of the third ventricle, and pituitary gland account for the variable CT and MRI appearances (Fig. 12.25) (3, 15, 37, 53). Visual difficulties, diabetes insipidus, insomnia, obesity, amenorrhea, and impotence are common clinical findings. On CT scans, the lesions could resemble tumors that enhance after the injection of contrast media (Fig. 12.25), or they may be seen as diffuse enhancement of the basal cisterns. Hydrocephalus is a common complication. Angiography may show narrowing and other changes of the vessel's wall that are suggestive of arteritis.

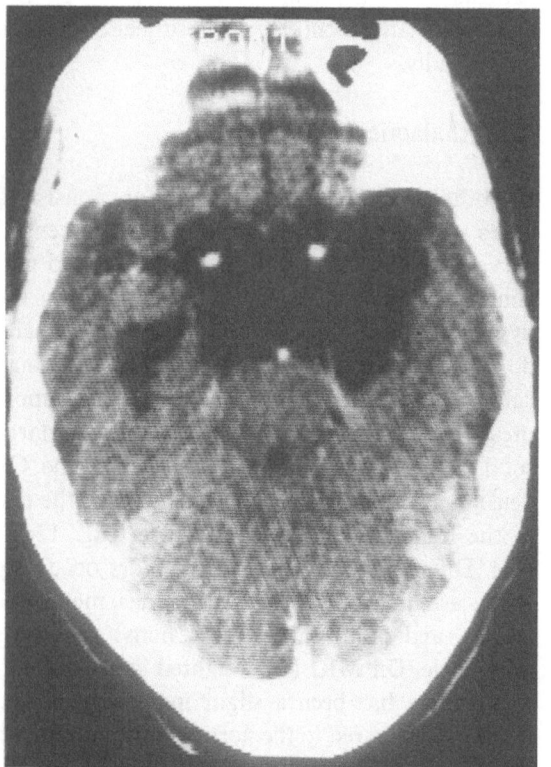

A

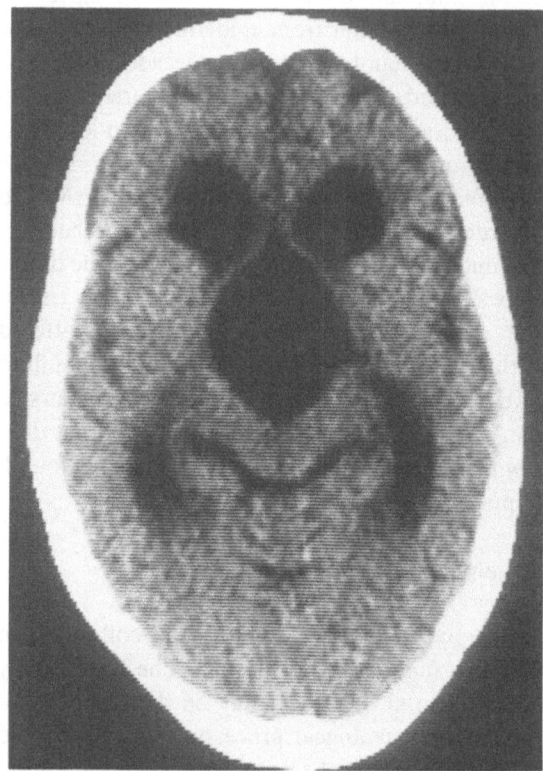

B

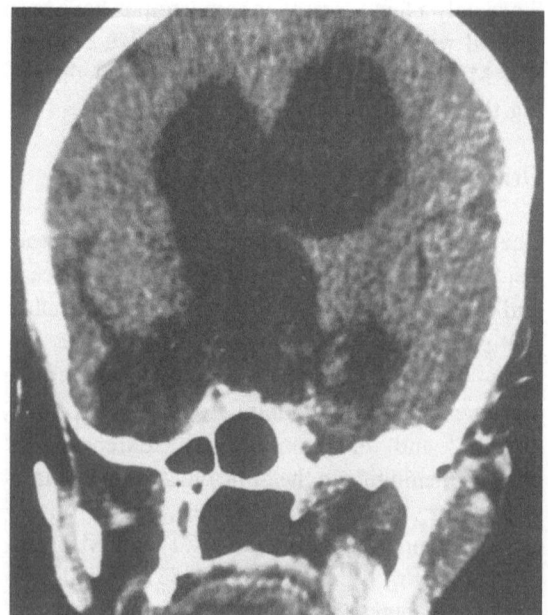

C

Figure 12.21. Suprasellar arachnoid cyst. **A, B.** Axial and **C.** reverse coronal CT scan sections at the level of the chiasmatic cistern and third ventricle. The examination reveals a large midline suprasellar cystic lesion extending into the left middle cranial fossa. The superior extension of the lesion is indistinguishable from a severe dilated third ventricle. Significant ventricular dilatation is observed. **D, E.** Axial MRI sections (SE, TE 28 msec and TR 500 and 556 msec) demonstrate the markedly enlarged lateral ventricles, as well as the midline fluid-continuing structure that represents a suprasellar cyst extending into the left middle fossa.

D 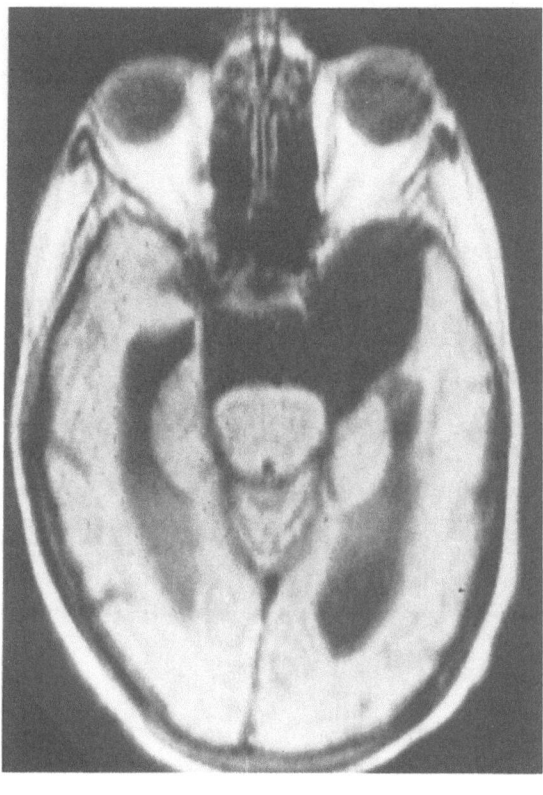   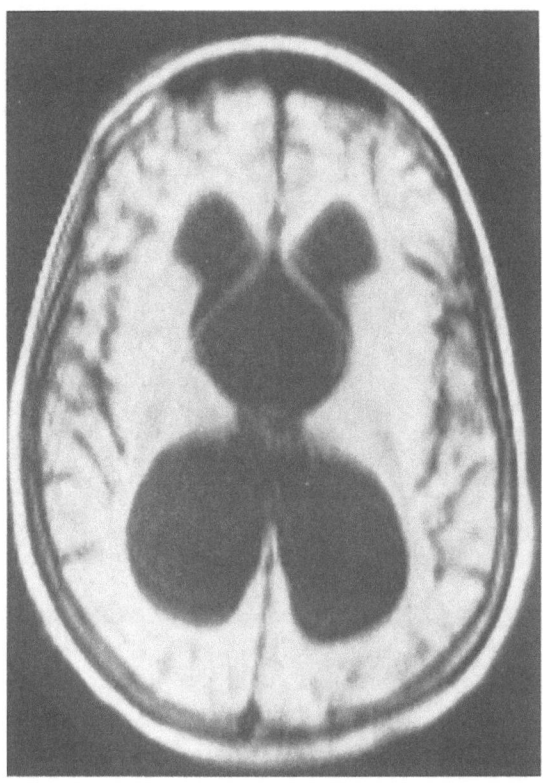 E

Empty Sella

The term empty sella generally indicates enlargement of the sella turcica, with or without signs of chiasmal involvement in the absence of a demonstrable intrasellar mass. Enlargement of the sella can result from a congenital defect of the sellar diaphragm or, secondarily, be due to spontaneous involution of pituitary adenoma. Demonstration of an empty sella can be accomplished by plain CT scanning, but metrizamide cisternography may be necessary to rule out the presence of an intrasellar arachnoid cyst (Fig. 12.26) (28).

Aneurysms and Vascular Lesions

The most common vascular abnormalities compressing the chiasm in the suprasellar region are internal carotid aneurysms arising from the suprasellar portion of the artery (Fig. 12.27). Aneurysms originating in other arteries of the Circle of Willis also may compress the chiasm or optic nerves, producing characteristic visual defects, such as

junctional scotomas and others (Figs. 12.28 and 12.29) (40). Giant aneurysms (greater than 25–30 mm in diameter) are often found in the suprasellar area (Figs. 5.3 and 12.30). Intrasellar extensions of internal carotid aneurysms are rare and can be confused with intrasellar tumors (61). Subarachnoid hemorrhage is a rare occurrence in giant aneurysms. On clinical examination, these lesions are recognized by symptoms and signs produced by compression of the adjacent structures due to their mass effect (47). Plain skull x-ray films may reveal curvilinear calcifications in the suprasellar region, which is characteristic of the lesions. On CT scanning (without use of contrast media), giant aneurysms usually manifest as irregular, loculated suprasellar or parasellar mass lesions. Calcifications seen in the thrombosed wall of the aneurysm are frequently found. Following intravenous (IV) contrast media, the nonthrombosed lumen of the aneurysm enhances (42).

Other vascular abnormalities that may effect the optic chiasm and may be responsible for focal field defects are ectatic tortuous vessels (due to arteriosclerosis involving the supraclinoid segment of the

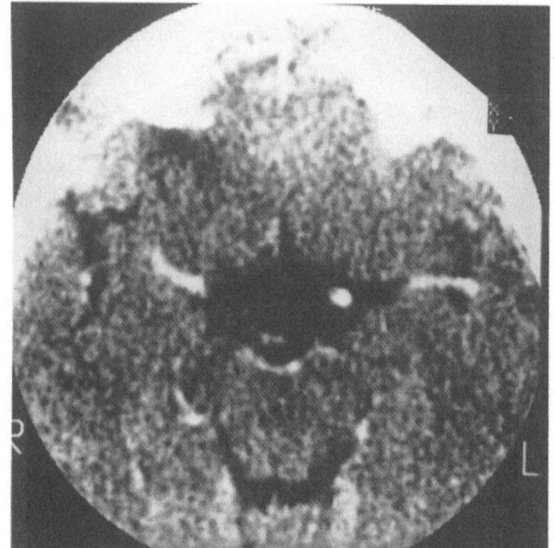

A

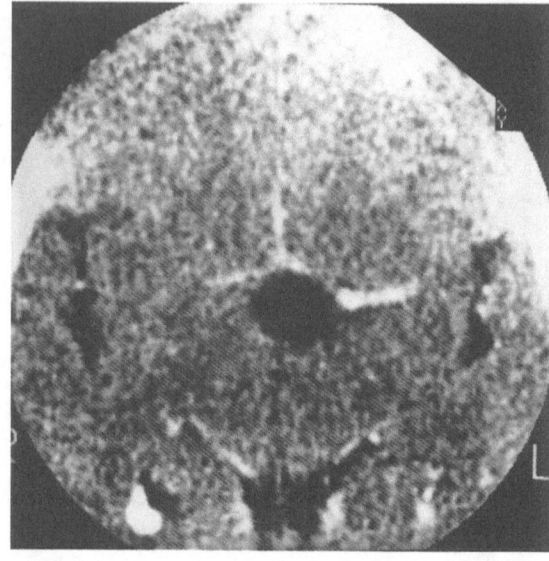

B

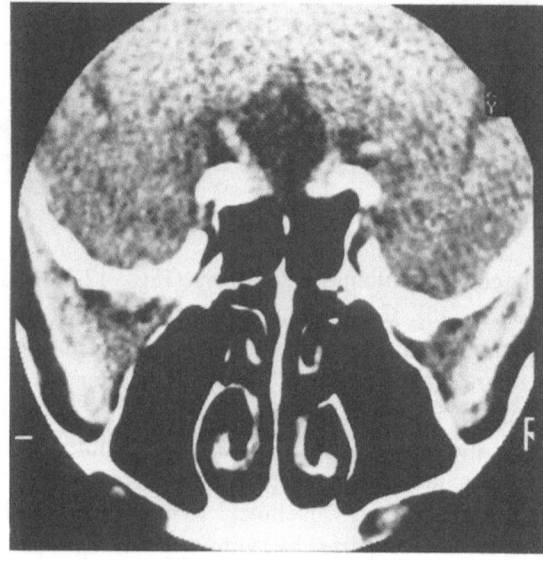

C

Figure 12.22. Intrasellar and suprasellar arachnoid cyst. **A, B.** Axial CT scan. **C.** Coronal CT scan sections. These were performed following the injection of contrast media. They show a cystic lesion in the sellar and suprasellar region that compresses the optic chiasm, producing symptoms that are indistinguishable from pituitary adenoma.

internal carotid or anterior cerebral arteries), large arteriovenous malformations of the brain extending into the suprachiasmatic cistern (Fig. 12.31), and cryptic arteriovenous malformations that may bleed into the chiasm—producing hematomas that may be visualized on CT scanning.

Parasellar and Base of the Skull Lesions

The most important structures lateral to the sella are the cavernous sinuses. They are paired venous structures lying at each side of the sphenoid bone and extending from the superior orbital fissure to the apices of both temporal bones. The cavernous sinuses are connected to each other via the intercavernous (circular) sinuses and the basilar plexus on the clivus. The superior and inferior ophthalmic veins and the sphenoparietal sinuses drain into the cavernous sinuses. The cavernous sinuses drain posteriorly into the petrosal sinus, and then into the internal jugular vein. The third, fourth, and sixth cranial nerves, the first division of the fifth cranial nerve, the internal carotid artery, and the sympathetic plexus lie within the sinuses (Fig. 12.2). The bony structures of the base of the skull in this region are the sella turcica, clivus, and sphe-

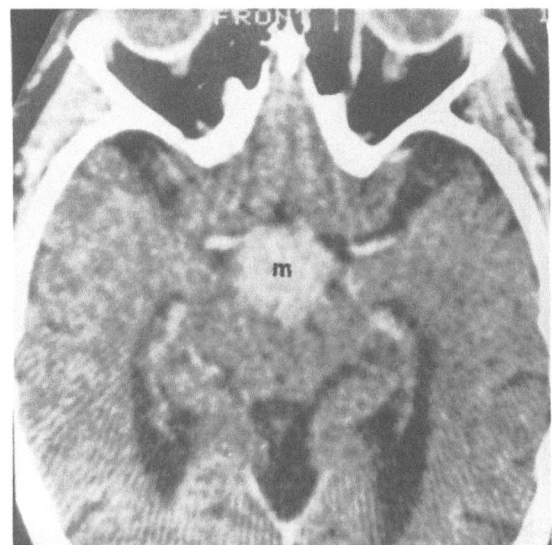

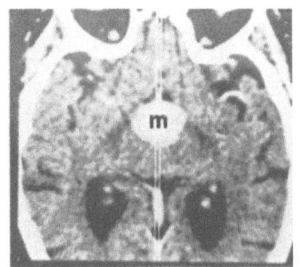

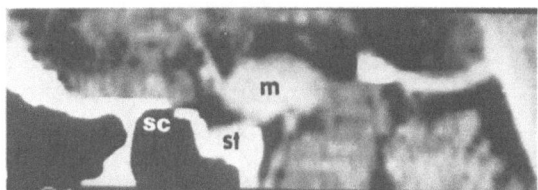

A

B

C

Figure 12.23. Metastatic lesion on the hypothalamus from breast carcinoma. **A & B.** Axial CT scan after contrast injection at the level of the chiasmatic cistern reveals a well-defined, homogeneously enhancing mass lesion (*m*) that obliterates the cistern and displaces the brain stem posteriorly. **C.** Sagittal reformation of the lesion on the midline (shown in **B**) shows that the lesion is originating in the hypothalamus, and it obliterates only the posterior portion of the suprasellar cistern. The sella turcica and pituitary gland are intact.

noid sinuses (Fig. 12.3). The anatomy of these structures can be demonstrated with CT scans and MRI; it has been described previously (32).

Tumors in the cavernous sinus are characterized by isolated unilateral dysfunction of two or more cranial nerves. Pain may be present if the ophthalmic and/or maxillary division of the trigeminal nerves are involved. Slow-growing masses, such as intracavernous meningiomas or intracavernous aneurysms, can give rise to the unusual syndrome of primary aberrant oculomotor regeneration.

Among the large number of lesions that originate or extend into the cavernous sinus, meningiomas are frequently found (Fig. 12.32) (44, 54). However, primary intracavernous meningiomas are rare lesions; more commonly, meningiomas originating in the juxtasellar region (lateral to the optic chiasm) may extend into the cavernous sinuses. These lesions usually produce asymmetric visual field defects. Large lesions can produce hyperostosis and bony erosion of the base of the skull. On noncontrast CT scanning, meningiomas can be distinguished from pituitary adenomas by their higher density on plain CT scans and their enhancement after contrast media injection. Angiography is extremely important in ruling out the presence of aneurysms (Figs. 12.12 and 12.13).

Carotid-cavernous aneurysms account for about 25% of the cavernous sinus syndromes. The CT scan appearance is similar to the suprasellar giant aneurysm. Erosion of the sella may be present (Fig. 12.33). Angiography establishes the diagnosis. Carotid-cavernous fistulae are discussed in Chapter 5 and 11 (Figs. 5.4 and 11.12).

Infiltrating pituitary adenomas are rare. The invasion is primarily downward, with extensive destruction of the bone of the sella and base of the skull (Fig. 12.10). Lateral extension into the cavernous sinus may produce ophthalmoplegia and cavernous sinus syndromes.

Neuromas of the fifth cranial nerve are uncommon lesions that usually arise from the Gasserian ganglion, erode the petrous bone, and extend into the middle fossa. Significant enhancement is seen after contrast injection. Neuromas arising from the oculomotor nerves are very rare.

Benign or malignant primary bone lesions at the base of the skull can either invade the cavernous sinuses involving one or more oculomotor nerves or destroy the sella turcica extending into the chiasmatic cistern, with or without compression of the optic chiasm. Plain x-ray films of the skull base, CT scans, and MRI are necessary to establish the diagnosis.

Chordomas are relatively rare, aggressive lesions

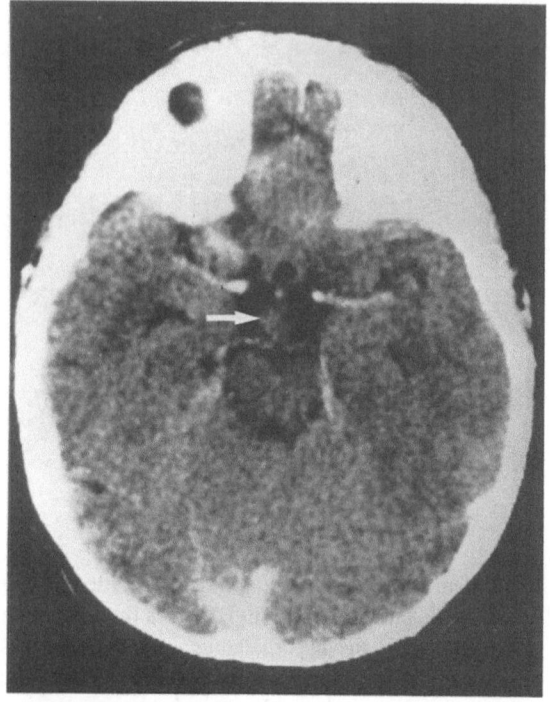

A

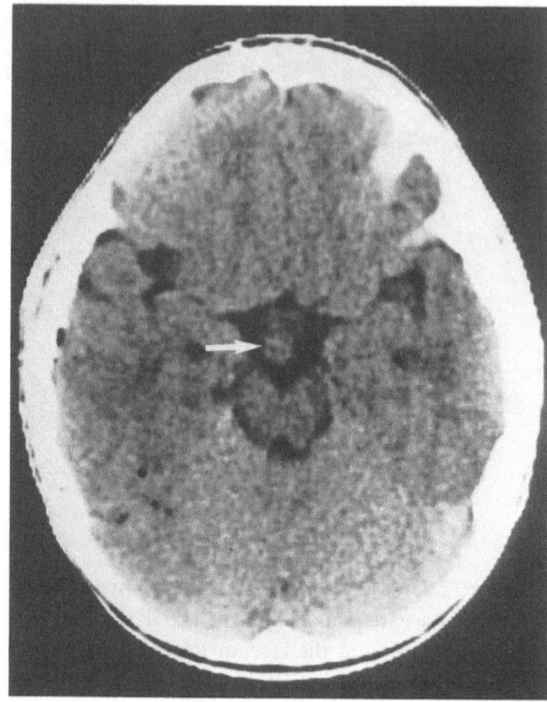

B

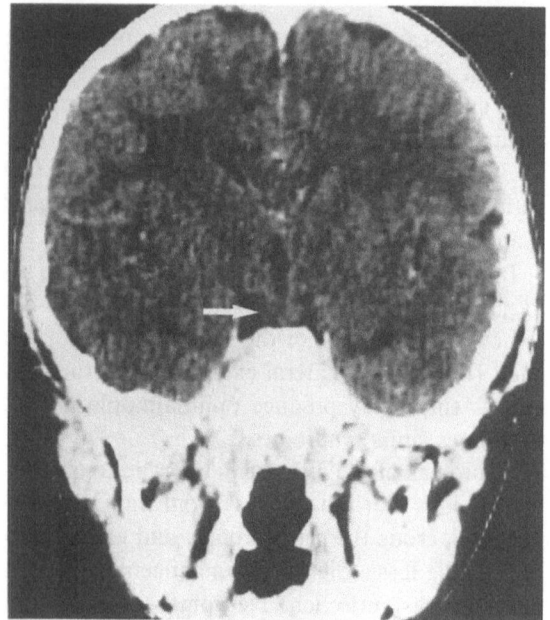

C

Figure 12.24. Hypothalamic hamartoma. **A.** Axial CT section at the level of the chiasmatic cistern. The examination reveals an isodense lesion in the suprasellar cistern (arrow). **B.** After injection of contrast media, no enhancement is seen. **C.** Coronal CT section at the level of the sella shows a sharply defined, isodense mass lesion in the chiasmatic cistern that is continuous with the hypothalamus structures (arrow).

arising from remnants of the notochord (30). Plain x-ray films of the skull and CT scans usually show destruction of the clivus and sellar structures, as well as occasional calcifications (Fig. 12.34). Chondroid tumors (chondromas, osteochondromas, and osteosarcomas) arise from contiguous tissue of the base of the skull. These tumors are characterized by bone destruction and dense, irregular calcifica-

tions characteristic of chondroid tissue. Malignant tumors of the nasopharynx (squamous cell and poorly differentiated carcinomas, reticulum cell sarcomas, and lymphoepitheliomas) and tumors of the paranasal sinuses also may invade the base of the skull and extend into the cavernous sinuses and sellar region. These tumors are recognized by extensive destruction of the bone of the base

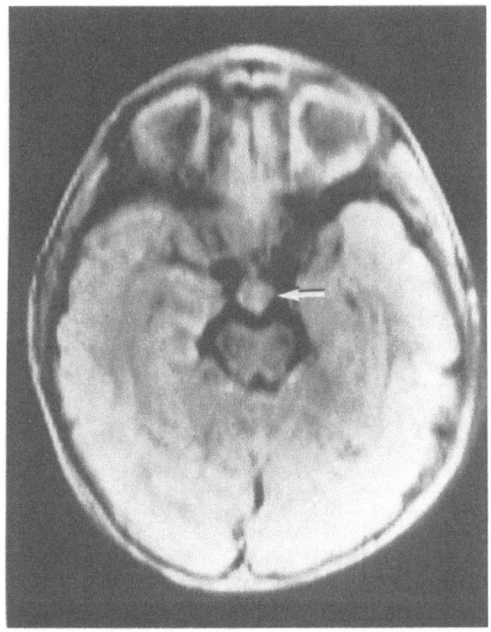

D

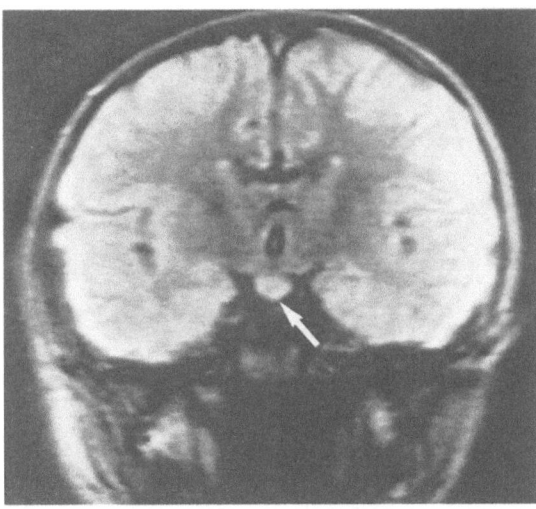

E

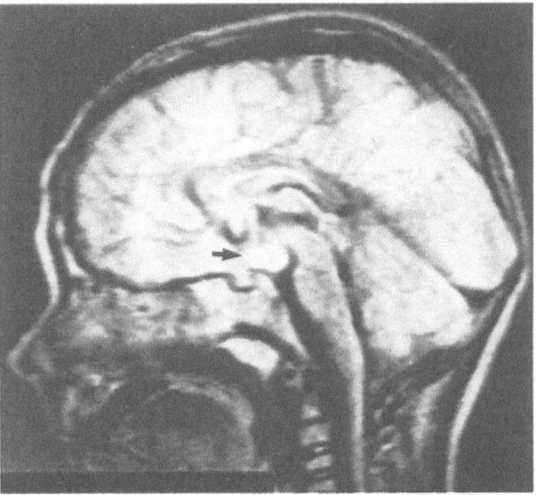

F

Figure 12.24. D, E, F. Axial, sagittal, and coronal MRI sections taken at the same level as the CT sections (SE, TE 28 msec and 56 msec and TR 556 msec and 2,000 msec). The examination demonstrates that the lesion is at the base of the brain posterior to the sella (arrow). On the T2-weighted SE image, there is a slightly increased signal intensity when compared to the normal brain stem, which suggests a slightly prolonged T2 value. These characteristics suggest a hamartoma, but a glioma related to the optic pathways cannot be totally excluded.

of the skull and a soft-tissue mass lesion that is well visualized on CT scans and MRI. Similar changes are produced by metastatic lesions in the area.

Sphenoid sinus mucoceles may expand either laterally into the cavernous sinus (producing multiple cranial nerve palsies) or superiorly into the suprasellar region (compressing the optic chiasm) (see Fig. 13.9).

Lesions of the Posterior Visual Pathways

The optic tracts encircle the cerebral peduncles and terminate in the lateral geniculate bodies. These are gray masses of cells in the lateral portions of the cerebral peduncles. Laterally, the tracts are covered by the anterior portion of the temporal lobe. The visual fibers that originate in the cells of the geniculate bodies (geniculocalcarine fibers) run superolaterally, and then turn posteriorly to end in the visual cortex on the medial surface of the occipital lobe in the region of the calcarine fissure. This thick band constitutes the optic radiation. However, some of these fibers loop forward a variable distance around the temporal horn of the lateral ventricle (Meyer's loop) before they pass backward and join the rest of the fibers on the way to the occipital cortex. Lesions that interrupt the visual pathways behind the chiasm produce homonymous hemianopsia. The visual defects may be congruous or incongruous. Defects of the fields that are similar in two eyes are called congruous. Lesions that interrupt the anterior portion of the optic radiation produce homonymous

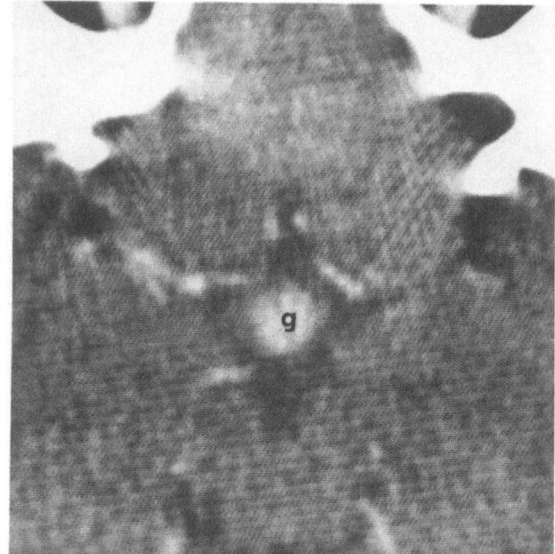

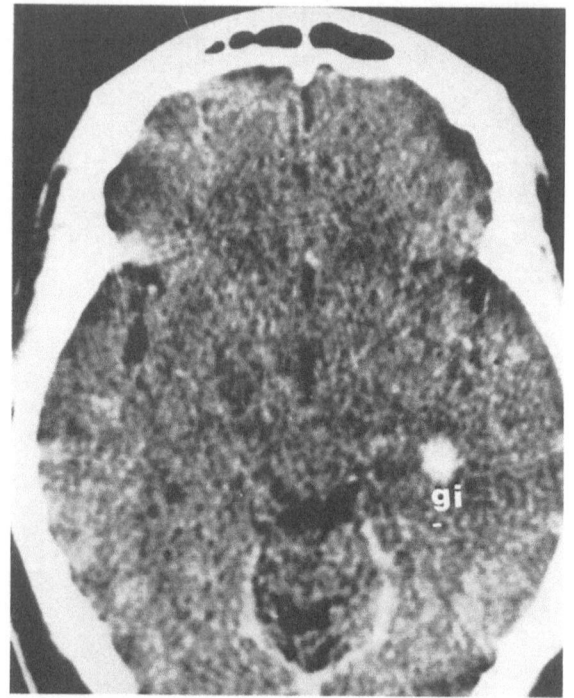

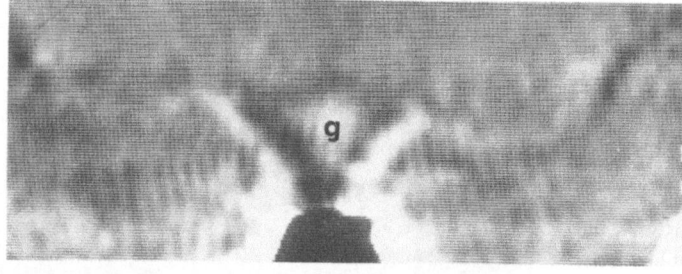

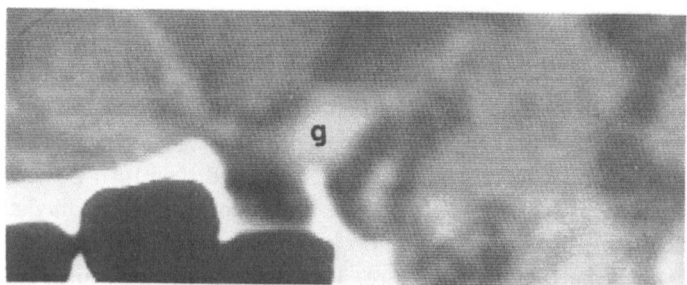

Figure 12.25. Granuloma sarcoidosis, intraparenchymal and hypothalamic chiasmatic. **A, B.** Axial CT scan sections were performed after contrast media injection. The examination reveals a well-defined, homogeneously enhancing hypothalamic chiasm lesion (*g*). A second intraparenchymal lesion is seen in the left temporal area (*gi*). **C, D.** Coronal and axial CT reformations confirmed the suprasellar location of the lesion (*g*).

Figure 12.26. Empty sella. Direct sagittal CT scan section after intrathecal injection of Metrizamide (Metrizamide cisternography). The examination shows an enlarged sella turcica filled with Metrizamide (arrow). (Courtesy of Robert Steiner, M.D., Thomas Jefferson University Hospital, Philadelphia, Pennsylvania.)

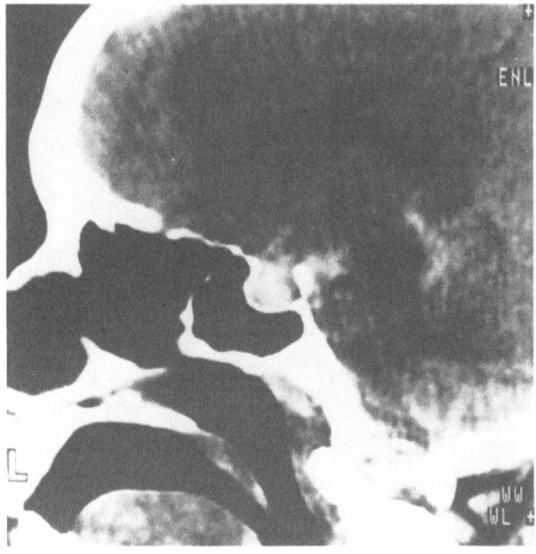

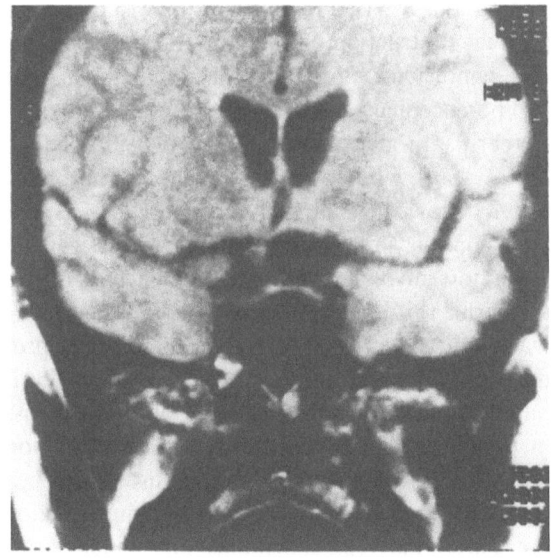

A

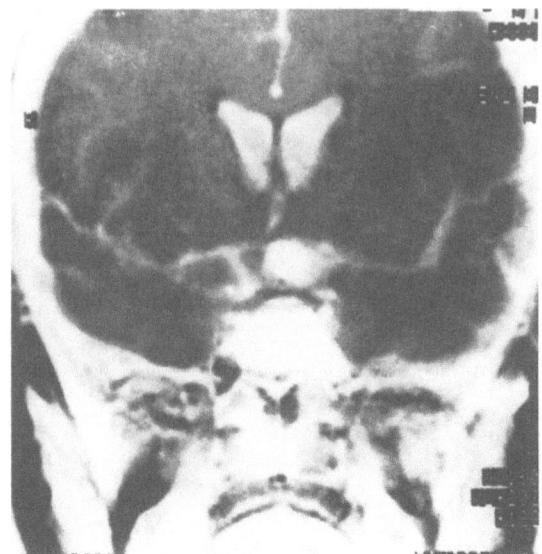

B

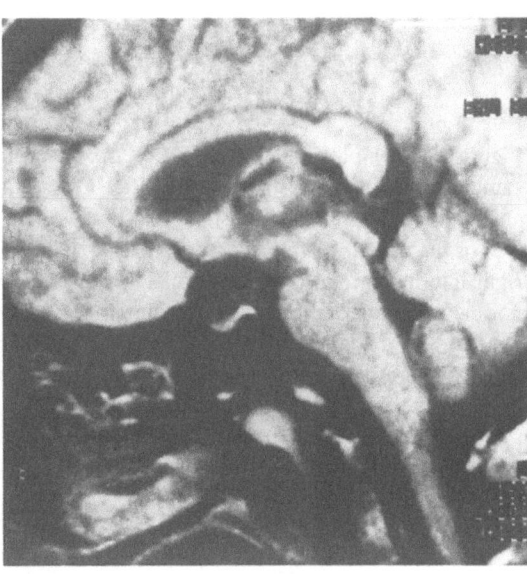

C

Figure 12.27. Internal carotid artery aneurysm. **(A, B)** Coronal and **(C)** Sagittal MRI sections. SE: a) TE = 50 msec, TR = 500 msec b) TE = 50 msec, TR = 2000 msec c) TE = 50 msec, TR = 500 msec. The examination reveals a large suprasellar aneurysm originating in the left internal carotid. The lesion is recognized in the MRI by the absence of the signal. (Courtesy of Robert Steiner, M.D., Thomas Jefferson University Hospital, Philadelphia, Pennsylvania.)

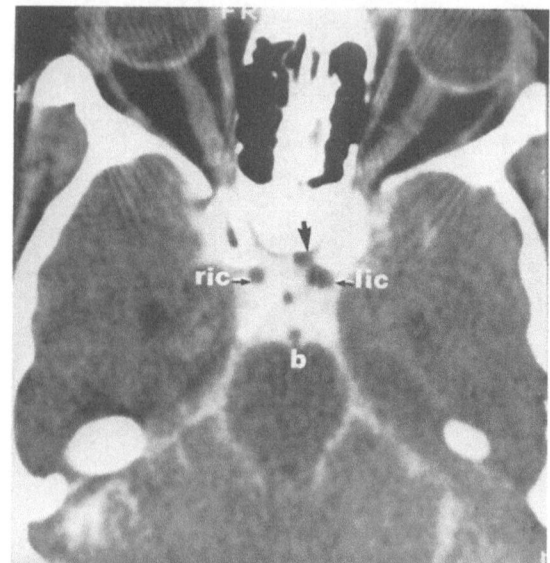

A

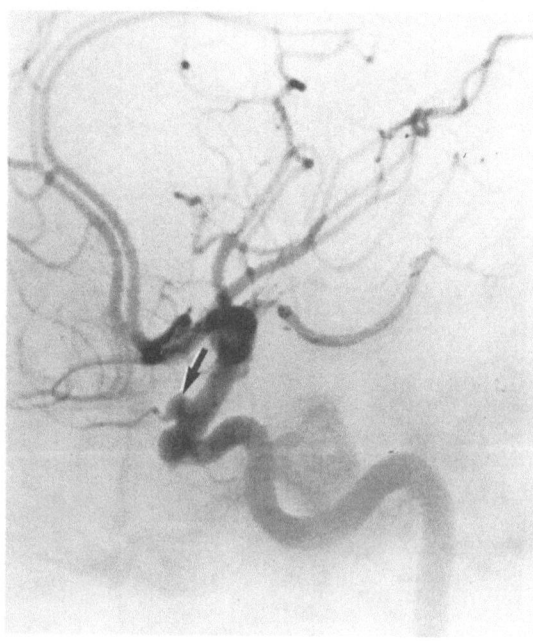

B

Figure 12.28. Ophthalmic artery aneurysm. **A.** Metrizamide cisternography showing a sagittal CT section at the level of the chiasmatic cistern. Excellent visualization of the cistern is attained with contrast media. The right internal carotid (*ric*) and basilar (*b*) arteries are normal. At the level of the left internal carotid-ophthalmic junction, (*lic*) there is an irregular filling defect (arrow) that corresponds to a small aneurysm. The patient's only clinical finding was a small junctional scotoma. **B.** Selective left internal carotid arteriogram confirmed the presence of the aneurysm at the carotid-ophthalmic junction (arrow).

defects that are slightly incongruous. Occipital pole lesions, on the contrary, produce congruous defects and have macular sparing. The reason for sparing of the macula is controversial.

Neoplasms, either primary or secondary of the brain, may interrupt the fibers of the optic radiations by direct pressure or by interference with the blood supply. These lesions are best demonstrated on CT scans (Fig. 12.35) and MRI (Figs. 12.35 and 12.36). Vascular disturbances, ranging from intracerebral hemorrhage to cerebral infarction, are also best visualized on CT scans and MRI (Fig. 12.37). The infarction usually is due to thrombosis or spasm of the middle or posterior cerebral arteries that supply the temporal and occipital lobes. The CT scan appearance of the infarct is characteristic of the territory of distribution of the arteries involved (26). Trauma may produce destruction by direct damage or by indirect contusions. Posttraumatic residual changes and porencephaly can be readily seen on CT scans. Cerebritis produces diffuse, low-density change on CT scans, while well-developed brain abscesses usually show the characteristic ring enhancement after contrast injection of contrast media.

Tumors involving the pineal and tectal region (posterior third ventricle) involve the visual pathways indirectly, but are important since they produce conjugate paralysis of vertical gaze (Parinaud's syndrome). Pupillary dilatation with loss of pupillary reflexes to light and accommodation and vertical and refractory nystagmus may be associated signs. Tumors found in the pineal region are pinealomas (pineocytomas and pineoblastomas), germinomas, teratomas, lipomas, hamartomas, meningiomas, dermoid and epidermoid tumors, metastatic lesions, and others. The CT scan appearance of these lesions are generally not specific (Fig. 12.38). However, pinealomas, meningiomas, and metastatic lesions usually enhance after contrast injection; whereas dermoid and epidermoid cysts and teratomatous lesions may reveal fat tissue density within the lesion. Calcification is seen in pinealomas. Tumors in the tectal region usually are periaqueductal gliomas and brain stem gliomas. These tumors usually are better demonstrated by MRI, since CT scanning may not show any significant change in density or compression of the neighboring structures (Figs. 12.39 and 12.40).

Finally—and to summarize this chapter—when

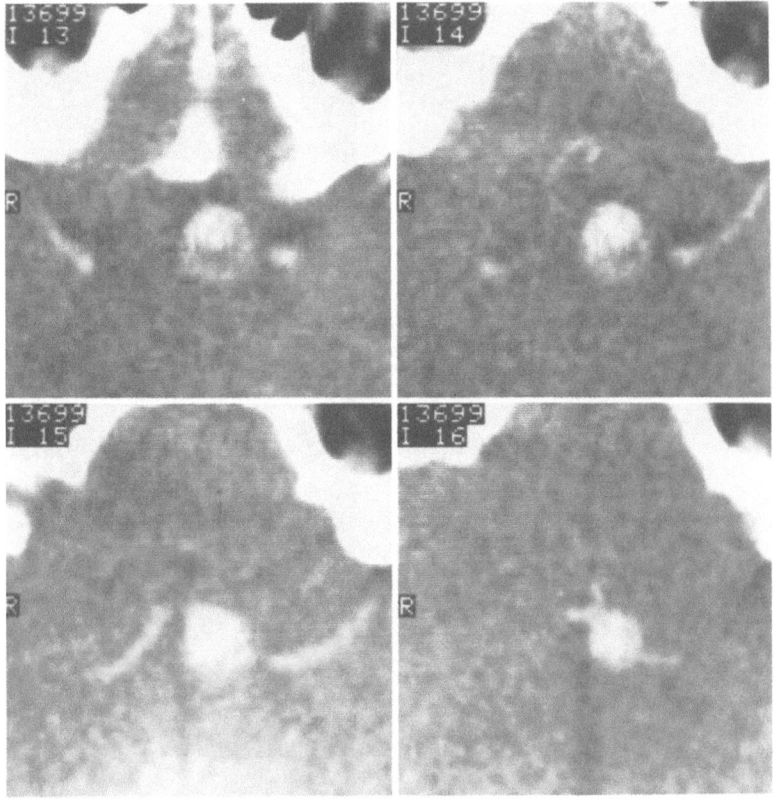

A

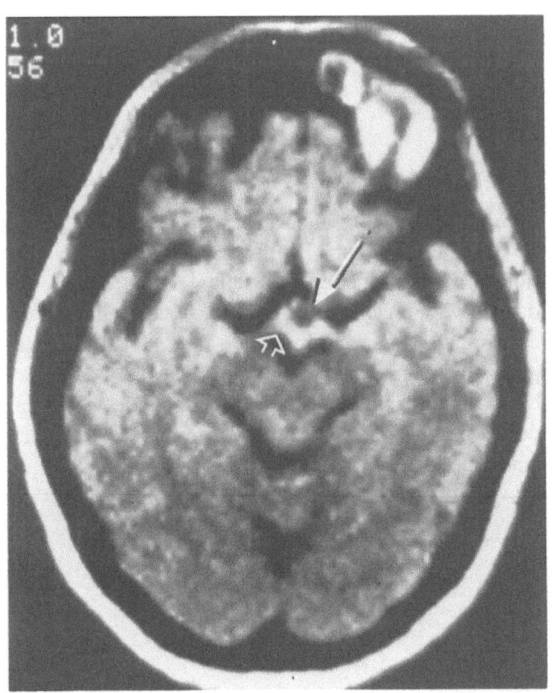

B

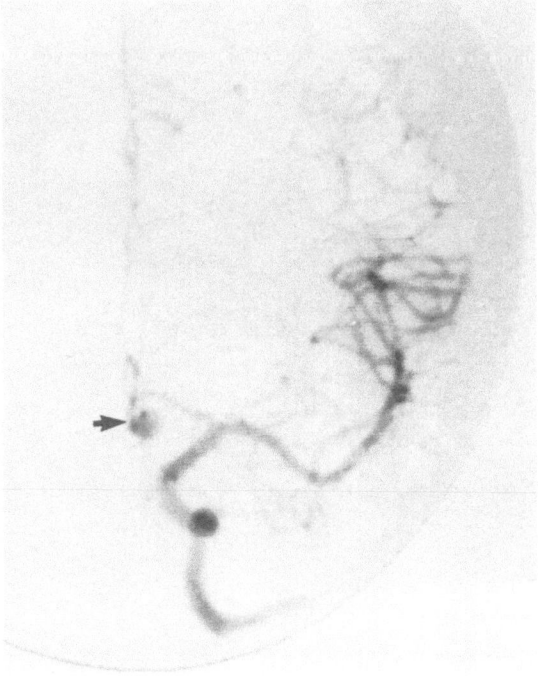

C

Figure 12.29. Anterior communicating artery aneurysm. **A.** Axial CT scan following the injection of contrast media reveals a large, irregular lobulated mass lesion in the midline, which suggests a partially clotted (low-density) anterior cerebral artery aneurysm. **B.** Axial MRI showing very clearly the location of the aneurysm (arrow) in relation to the optic chiasm (open arrow). The patient is a 56-year-old man with progressive visual loss and a junctional scotoma. **C.** Left selective internal carotid arteriogram showing the aneurysm (arrow).

267

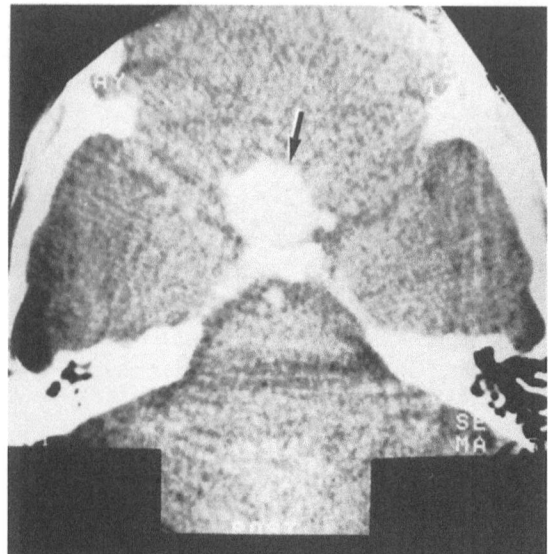

A

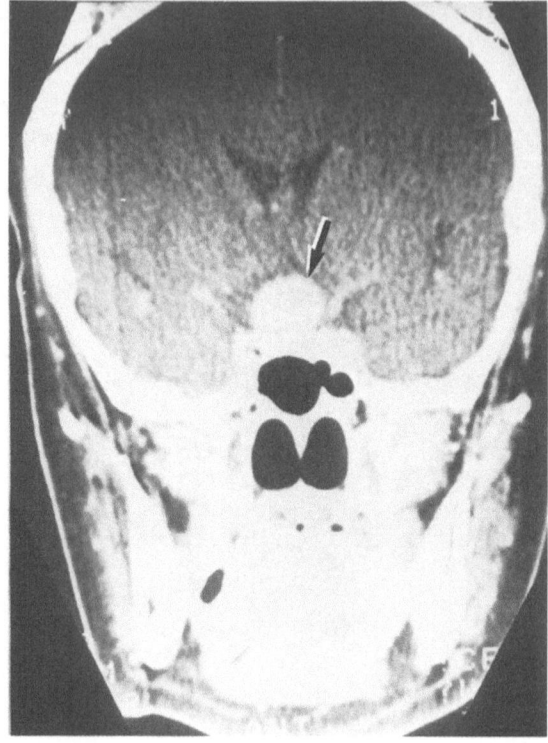

B

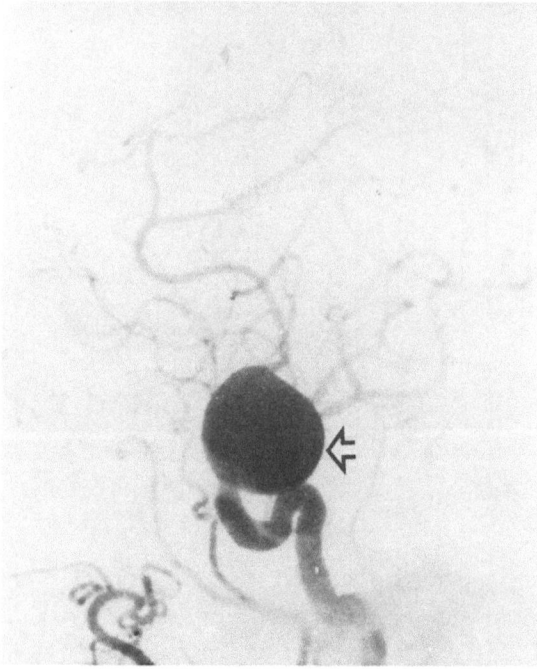

C

Figure 12.30. Suprasellar aneurysm. **A.** Axial CT scan. **B.** Coronal CT scan. These were performed after injection of contrast media. They show a suprasellar, well-defined, homogeneous enhancing lesion (arrow) that corresponds to a nonthrombosed internal carotid artery giant aneurysm. The patient, a 52-year-old woman, was blind on the right and had a hemianoptic visual field defect on the left. **C.** Carotid arteriogram revealed a giant supraclinoid aneurysm (open arrow).

a lesion of the visual pathways is suspected because of the ophthalmologic signs and symptoms, it usually can be shown with imaging techniques. Plain x-ray films and polytomography are of limited value. At present, lesions are best demonstrated by computed tomography (CT) and magnetic resonance imaging (MRI). Arteriography is helpful in the diagnosis of vascular lesions.

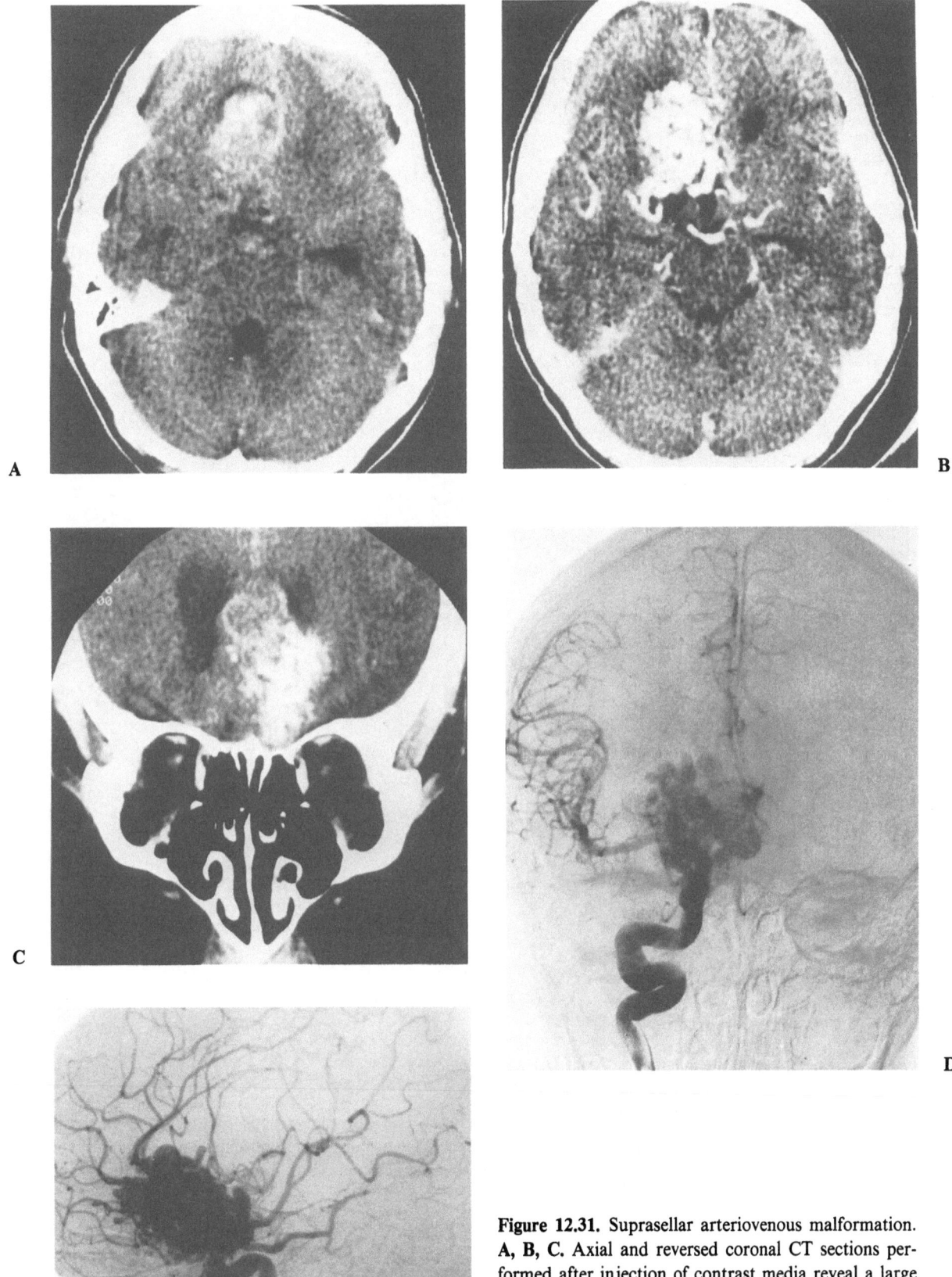

Figure 12.31. Suprasellar arteriovenous malformation. **A, B, C.** Axial and reversed coronal CT sections performed after injection of contrast media reveal a large arteriovenous malformation in the frontal and suprasellar region that extends into the hypothalamic and right ventricle regions. **D, E.** Selective right carotid arteriogram, anteroposterior and lateral views. The examination reveals marked vascularity in the area of the malformation with demonstration of large draining veins.

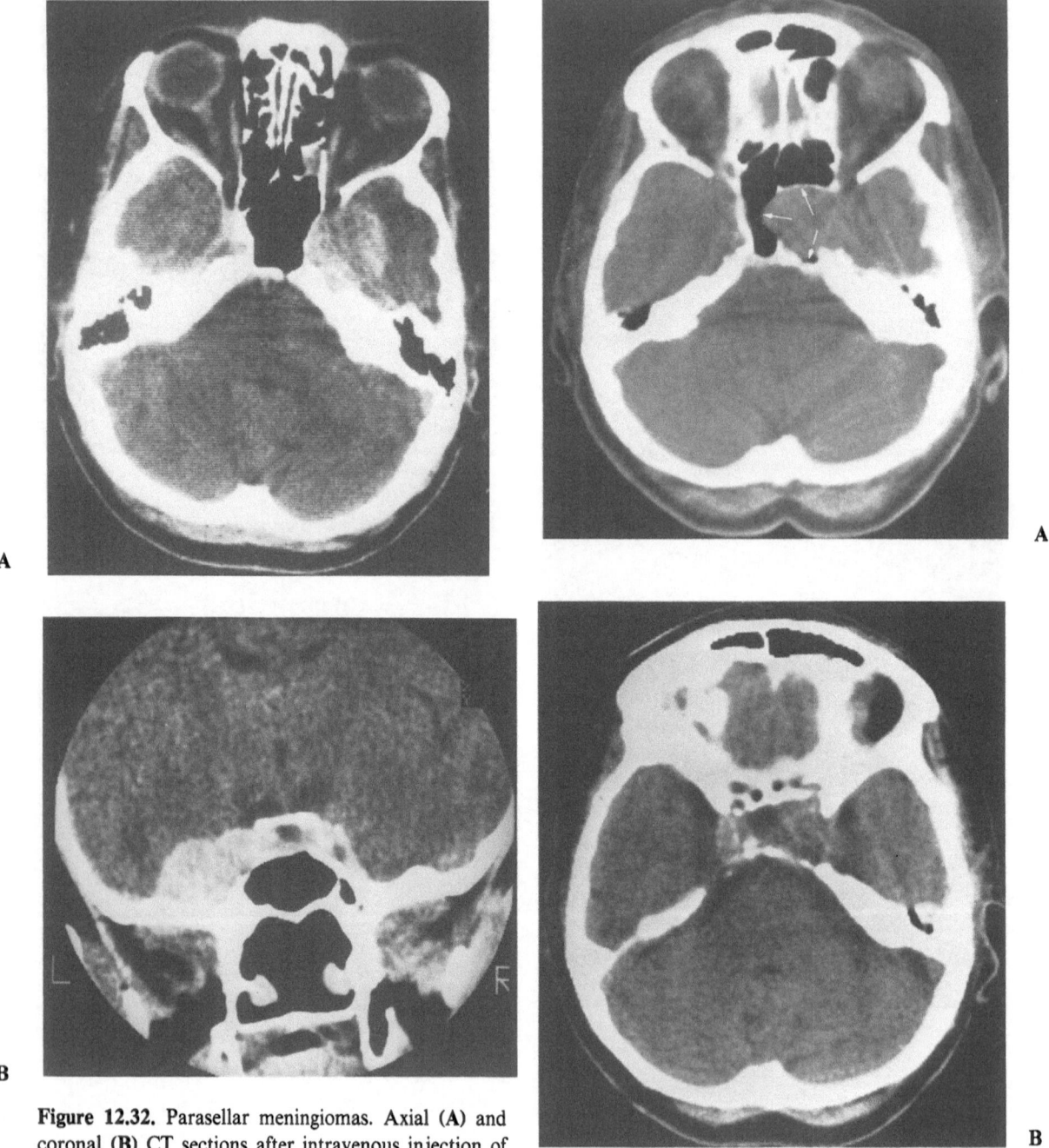

Figure 12.32. Parasellar meningiomas. Axial (**A**) and coronal (**B**) CT sections after intravenous injection of contrast media. The examination reveals a large meningioma in the left parasellar intrasellar region, involving the cavernous sinus and extending into the left middle cranial fossa.

Figure 12.33. Intracavernous aneurysm. **A, B.** Axial and CT scans showing significant bone erosion of the left cavernous sinus and sella turcica (arrows).

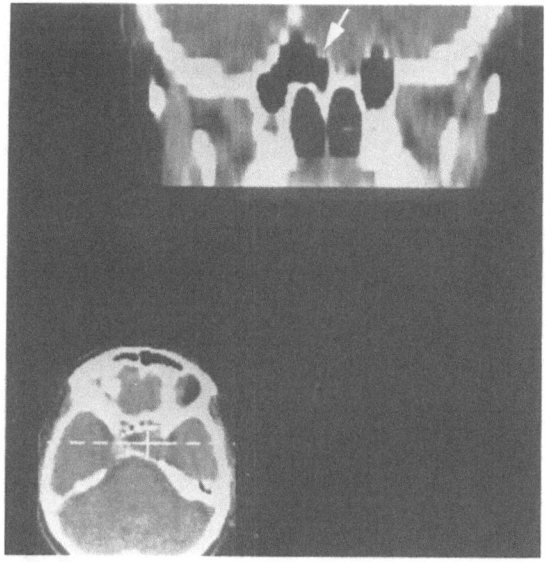

C

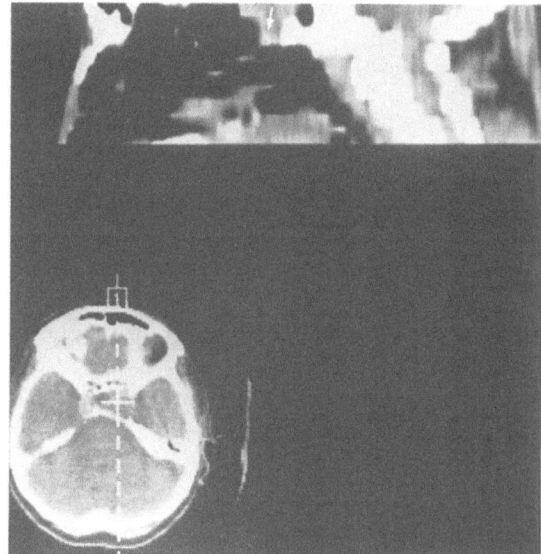

D

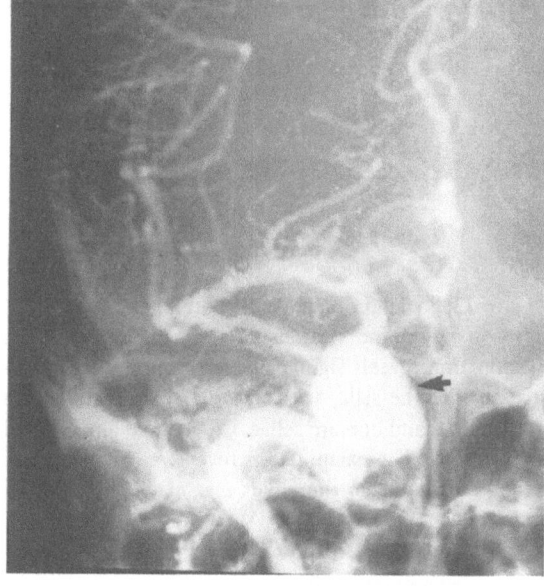

E

Figure 12.33. C, D. Coronal and sagittal CT reconstructions reveal slanting of the sellar floor and enlargement of the sella (open arrows). E. Cerebral arteriogram shows a large, round intracavernous aneurysm extending into the sella turcica (arrow).

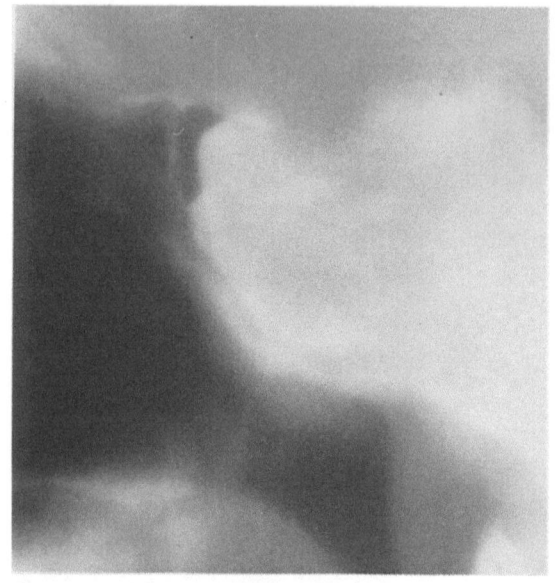

A

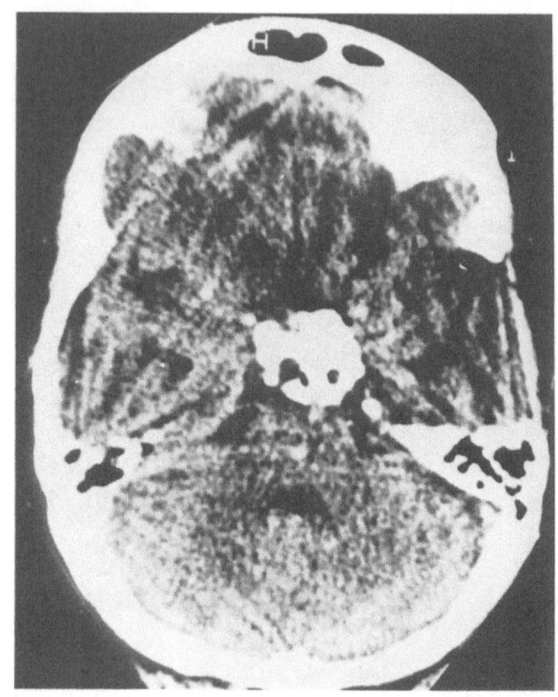

C

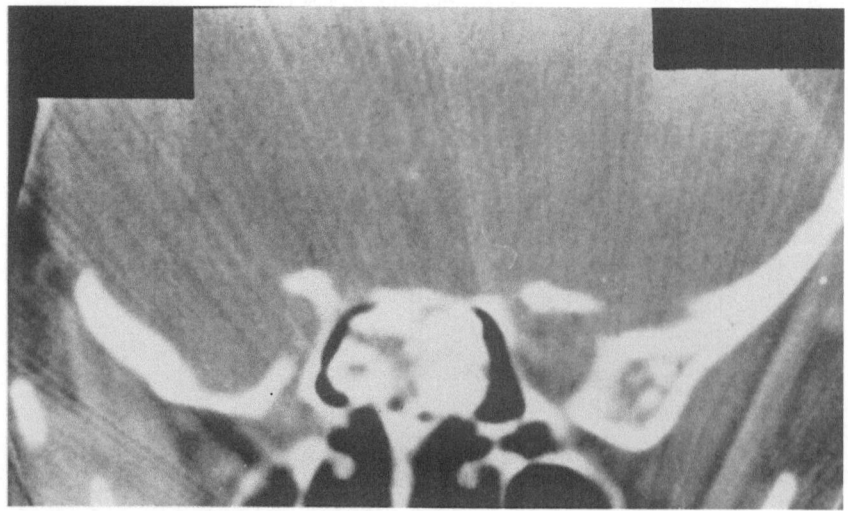

B

D

Figure 12.34. Chordoma. **A, B.** Lateral and anteroposterior tomographic sections of the sella turcica. The examination reveals significant destruction of the bony structure of the sella, with irregular calcification seen in the clivus and dorsum sellae. **C, D.** Axial and coronal CT sections. The examination reveals a calcified mass lesion originating in the clivus and extending into the suprasellar region.

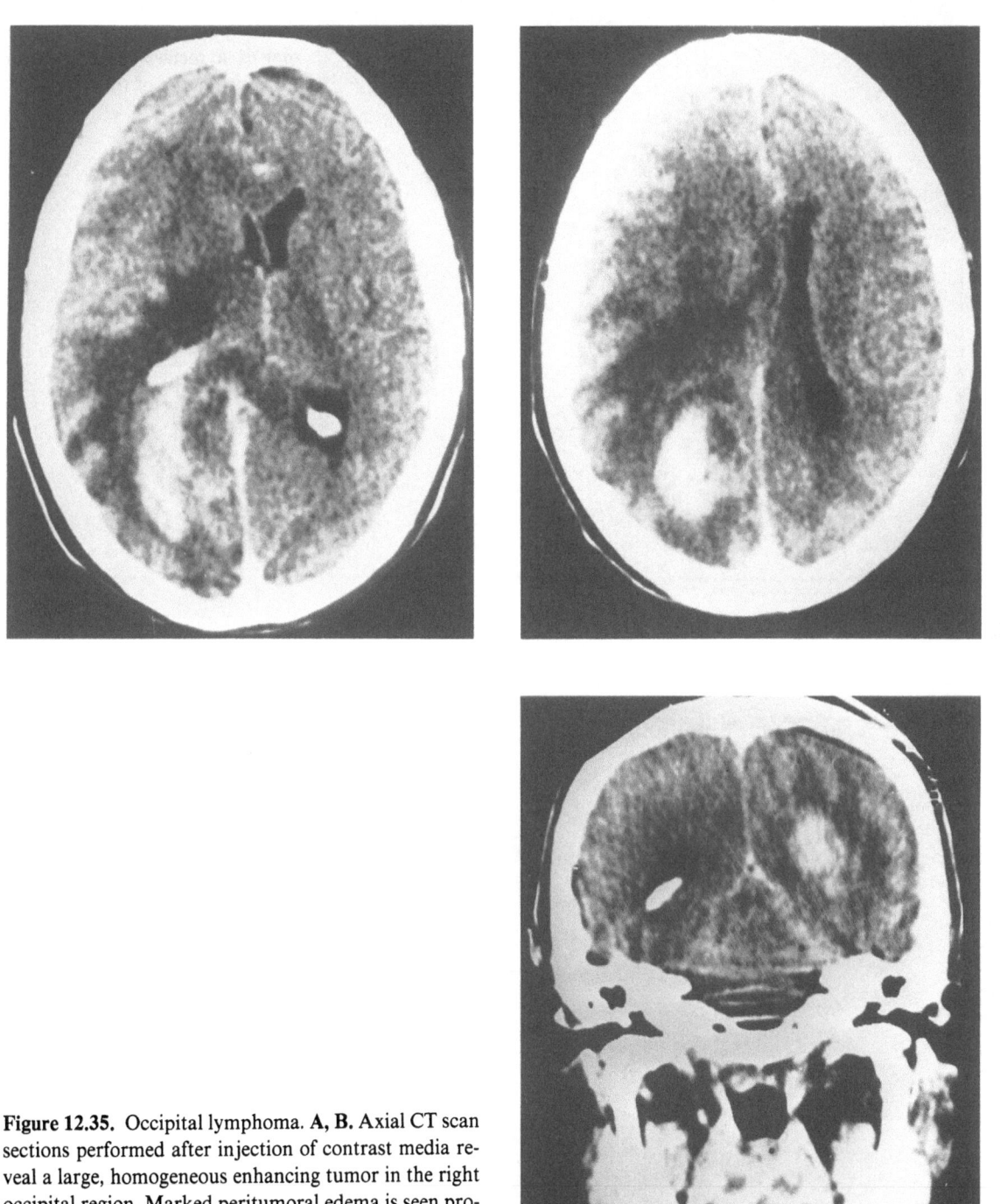

Figure 12.35. Occipital lymphoma. **A, B.** Axial CT scan sections performed after injection of contrast media reveal a large, homogeneous enhancing tumor in the right occipital region. Marked peritumoral edema is seen producing a significant mass effect and a shift of the ventricular system. **C.** Reversed coronal CT scan section showing the enhancing lesion extending posteriorly into the right occipital lobe.

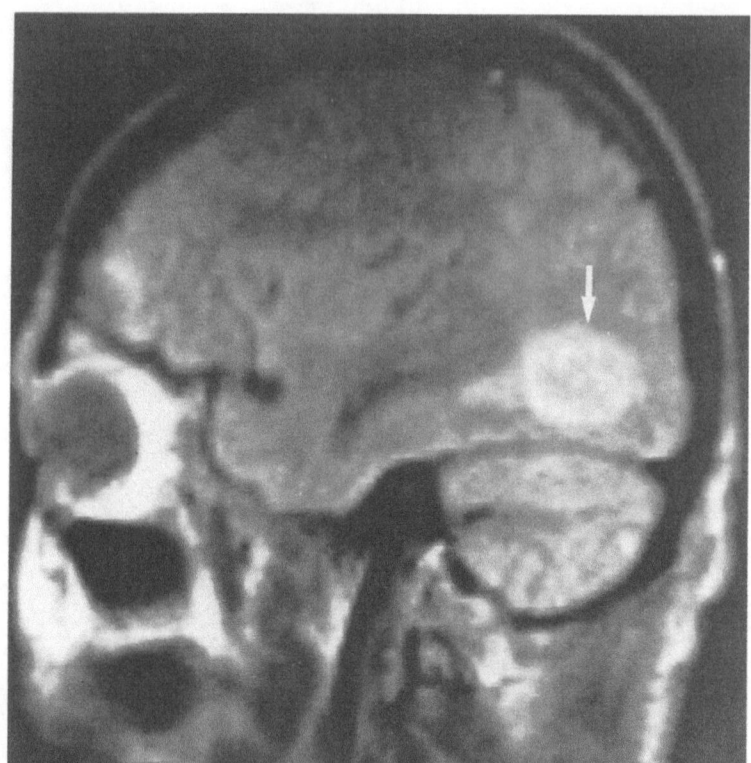

Figure 12.36. Occipital metastatic lesion. Sagittal MRI section showing a well-defined, round lesion in the occipital pole (arrow). The tumor is a metastatic brain lesion from carcinoma of the lung.

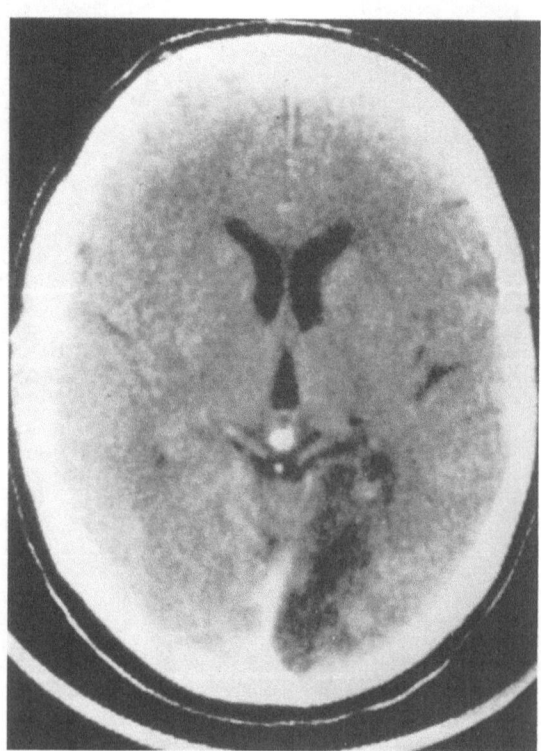

A

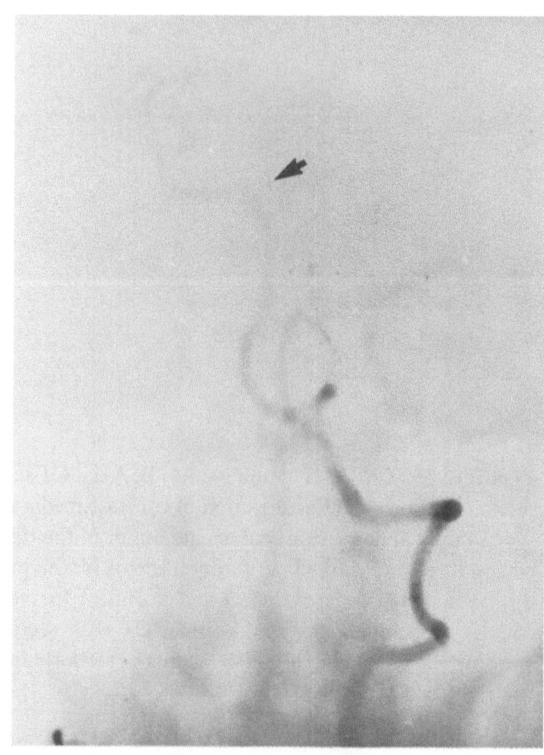

B

Figure 12.37. Occipital lobe infarction. **A.** Axial CT scan. The examination reveals an ill-defined low density in the occipital lobe corresponding to the area of distribution of the left posterior cerebral artery. **B.** Selective vertebral injection reveals a complete occlusion of the left posterior cerebral artery (arrow). The left internal carotid injection, which is not illustrated, did not show the left posterior cerebral artery coming from the left internal carotid artery.

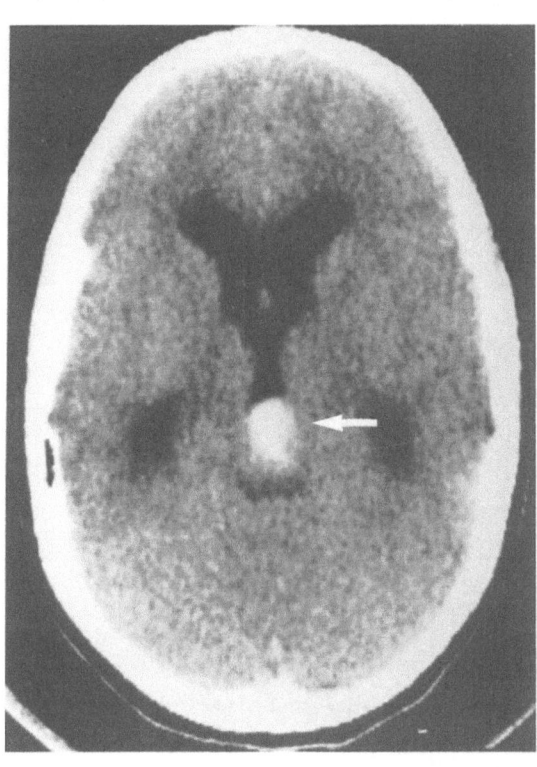
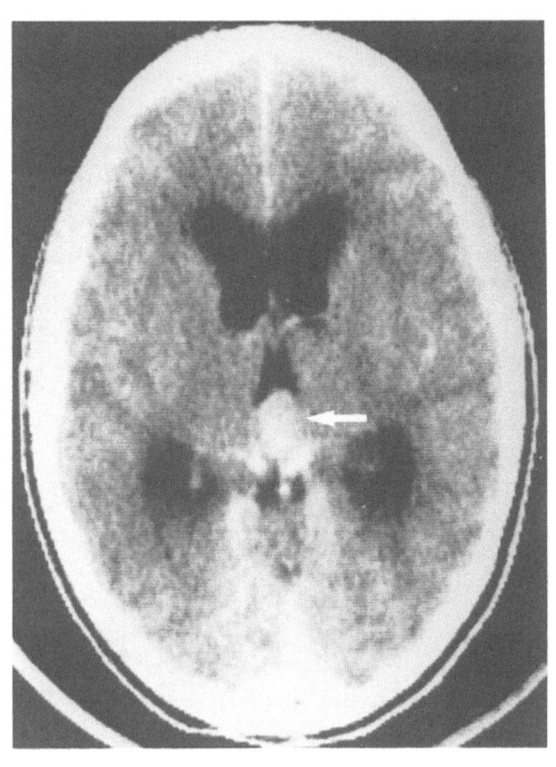

A

B

Figure 12.38. Pineoblastoma. **A.** Axial CT scan sections showing a well-defined calcified lesion at the level of the pineal gland (arrow). **B.** Axial CT scan performed after injection of the contrast media. The examination reveals homogeneous enhancement of the lesion (arrow).

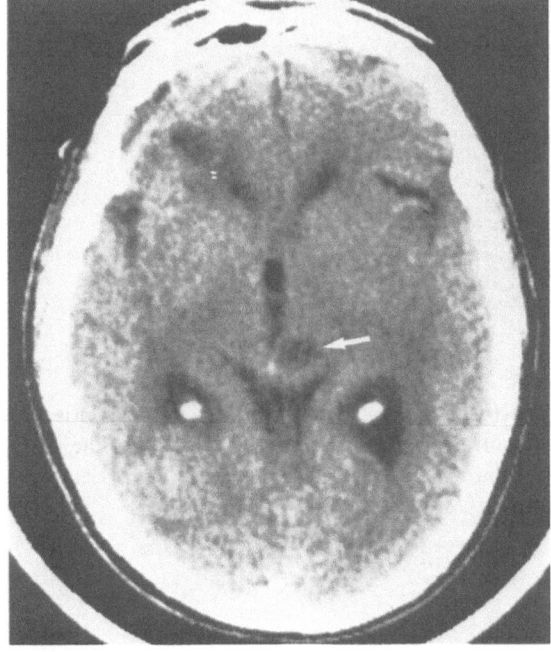
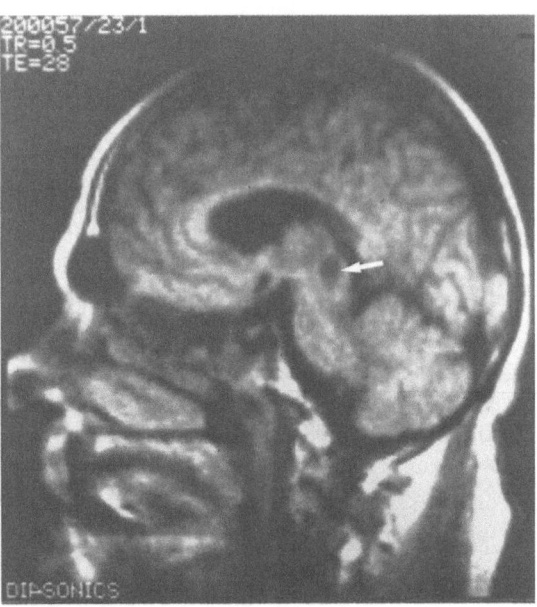

A

B

Figure 12.39. Metastatic carcinoma of the lung. **A.** Axial CT section (not enhanced). A rounded, well-defined lesion is seen in the tectal region in a 70-year-old patient with carcinoma of the lung, the CT scan was done without contrast, because the patient was allergic to the iodinated contrast media (arrow). **B.** MRI sagittal sections were performed in the same patient, and they show to greater advantage the extension of the lesion and the relationship to the normal structures (arrow).

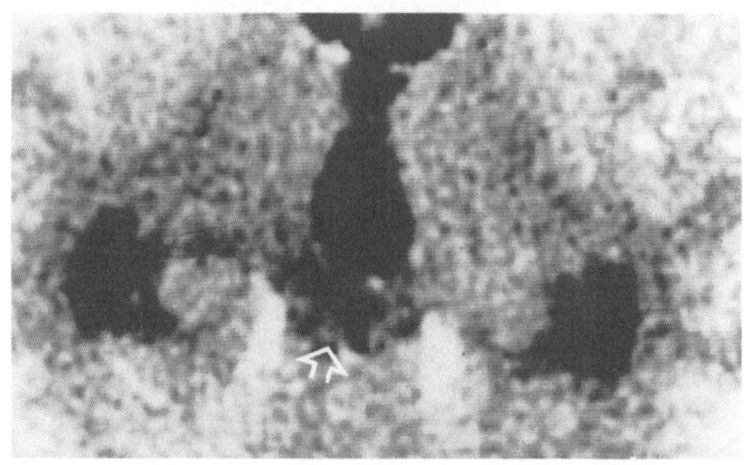

A

B

Figure 12.40. Periaqueductal glioma. **A.** Axial CT scan reveals poor visualization of the posterior portion of the third ventricle. A poorly defined small area of decreased density is shown in the posterior third ventricle area (open arrow). **B.** After intraventricular injection of contrast media, a definitive asymmetry of the posterior third ventricle produced by the lesion is seen (open arrow).

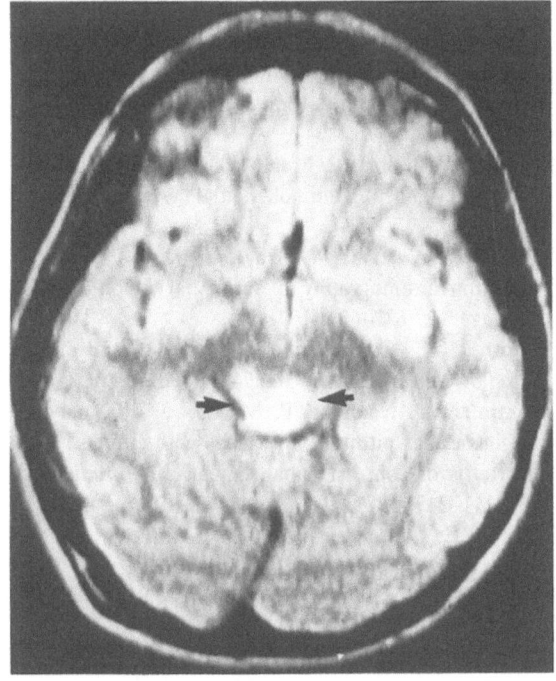

C

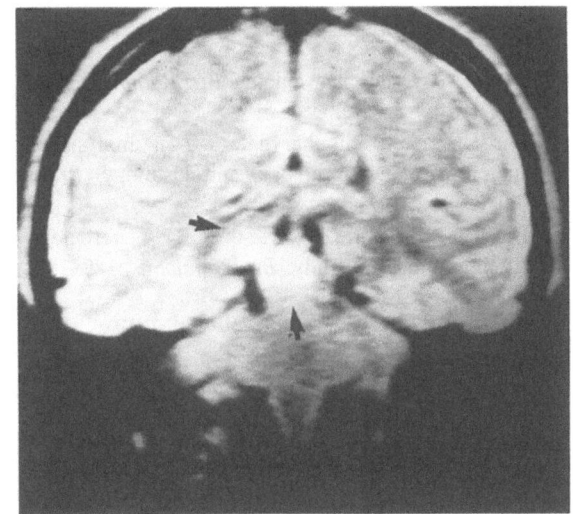

D

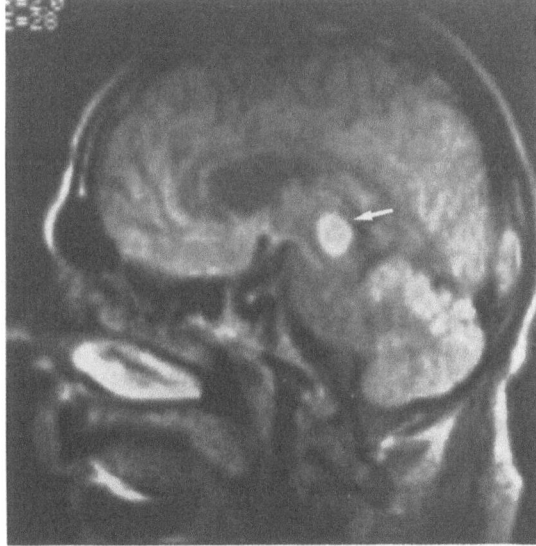

E

Figure 12.40. C, D, E. Axial coronal and sagital MRI sections reveal a well-visualized, rather large intraaxial tumor in the tectal region and upper brain stem that is poorly seen in the CT scan (arrows).

References

1. Banna M: Craniopharyngioma. *Br J Radiol* 49:206–233, 1976.
2. Bartlett JR: Craniopharyngioma—an analysis of symptomatology, radiology, and histology. *Brain* 94:725–732, 1971.
3. Bhargave S, Gupta AK, Tandon PN: Tuberculous meningitis—a CT study. *Br J Radiol* 55:189–196, 1982.
4. Bilaniuk LT, Zimmerman RA, Wehrli FW: Magnetic resonance imaging of pituitary lesions using 1.0 to 1.5 T field strength. *Radiology* 153:415–418, 1984.
5. Bilaniuk LT, Zimmerman RA, Wehrli FW, et al: Cerebral magnetic resonance: Comparison of high and low field strengths imaging. *Radiology* 153:409–414, 1984.
6. Calderon M, Brady HR. Fibrous clysplasia of bone with bilateral optic poramina involvement. *Ophthalmol* 68:513–514, 1969.
7. Citrin CM, Davis DO: Computerized tomography in the evaluation of pituitary adenomas. *Invest Radiol* 12:27–35, 1977.
8. Crane TB, Yee RD, Helper RS, et al: Clinical manifestations and radiologic findings in craniopharyngiomas in adults. *Am J Ophthalmol* 94:220–228, 1982.
9. Cohen MM, Lessell S: Chiasmal syndrome due to metastasis. *Arch Neurol* 36:565–567, 1979.
10. Cox EV III: Chiasmal compression from metastatic cancer to the pituitary gland. *Surg Neurol* 11:49–50, 1979.
11. Daniels DL, Herfkins R, Gager WE: Magnetic resonance imaging of the optic nerves and chiasm. *Radiology* 152:79–83, 1984.
12. Daniels DL, Haughton VM, Williams AL, et al: Computed tomography of the optic chiasm. *Radiology* 137:123–127, 1980.
13. Daniels DL, Williams AL, Thornton RS, et al: Differential diagnosis of intrasellar tumors by computed tomography. *Radiology* 141:697–701, 1981.
14. Davis KR, Roberson GH, Taveras JM, et al: Diagnosis of epidermoid tumor by computed tomography. *Radiology* 119:347–383, 1979.
15. Decker RE, Mardayat M, Marc J, et al: Neurosarcoidosis with computerized tomographic visualization and transsphenoidal excision of a suprasellar and intrasellar granuloma. *J Neurosurg* 50:814–816, 1979.
16. DeSouse A, Kalsbeck JE, Mealey J Jr, et al: Optic chiasmatic glioma in children. *Am J Ophthal* 87:376–381, 1979.
17. Falke THM, Ziedes des Plantes BG, Bluemm R, et al: Magnetic resonance imaging of the pituitary gland: Comparison with sagittal CT. Presented at the 70th Annual Meeting of the Radiological Society of North America (RSNA), Washington, DC, November 25–30, 1984.
18. Fawcitt RA, Isherwood I: Radiodiagnosis of intracranial pearly tumors with particular reference to the clue of computed tomography. *Neuroradiology* 11:235–242, 1976.
19. Finn JE, Mount LE: Meningiomas of the tuberculum sella and planum sphenoidale. *Arch Ophthalmol* 92:23–27, 1974.
20. Fitz CR, Wortzman G, Harwood-Nash DC, et al: Computed tomography in craniopharyngiomas. *Radiology* 127:687–691, 1978.
21. Forbes GE: Computed tomography of the orbit. *Radiol Clin North Am* 20:37–49, 1982.
22. Gardeur D, Naidich TP, Metzger J: CT analysis of intrasellar pituitary adenomas with emphasis on patterns of contrast enhancement. *Neuroradiology* 20:241–247, 1981.
23. Grote E: Characteristics of giant pituitary adenomas. *Acta Neurochir* 60:141–153, 1982.
24. Hawkes RC, Holland GN, Moore WS, et al: The application of NMR imaging to the evaluation of pituitary and juxtasellar tumors *AJNR* 4:221–222, 1983.
25. Haymaker W, Anderson E: Disorders of the hypothalamus and pituitary gland, in Baker AB, Baker LH; *Clinical Neurology.* 1984, vol III, chap 36, pp 35–36.
26. Hayman LA, Berman SA, Hinck VC: Correlation of CT cerebral vascular territories with function: II. Posterior cerebral artery. *AJNR* 137:13–19, 1981.
27. Hoffman HJ, Hendrick E, Humphreys RP, et al: Investigation and management of suprasellar arachnoid cysts. *J Neurosurg* 57:597–602, 1982.
28. Hoffman JC Jr, Tindall GT: Diagnosis of empty sella syndrome using Amipaque cisternography combined with computed tomography. *J Neurosurg* 52:99–102, 1980.
29. Hoyt, et al: Malignant optic glioma of adulthood. *Brain* 96:121, 1973. Hoyt WF, Meshel LG et al: 121–132.
30. Kendall BE, Lee BCP: Cranial chordomas. *Br J Radiol* 50:687–698, 1977.
31. Kistler M, Pibram HW: Metastatic disease of the sella turcica. *AJR* 123:13–21, 1975.
32. Kline LB, Acker JD, Post MJD: Computed tomographic evaluation of the cavernous sinus. *Ophthalmology* 89:374–385, 1982.
33. Leeds NE, Naidich TP: Computerized tomography in the diagnosis of sellar and parasellar lesions. *Semin Roentgenol* 12:121–135, 1977.
34. Leo JS, Pinto RS, Hulvat GF, et al: Computed tomography of arachnoid cysts. *Radiology* 130:675–680, 1979.
35. Lin S, Bryson MM, Gobien RP, et al: Radiologic findings of hamartomas of the tuber cinereum and hypothalamus. *Radiology* 127:697–703, 1978.

36. Merrit HH: *A Textbook of Neurology.* Philadelphia, Lea & Febiger, 1961, pp 275–277.

37. Navarro IM, Peralta VHR, Leon JAM, et al: Tuberculous optochiasmatic arachnoiditis. *Neurosurgery* 9:654–660, 1981.

38. Oot R, New PFJ, Buonanno FS: MR imaging of pituitary adenomas using a prototype resistive magnet. *AJNR* 5:131–137, 1984.

39. Pederson H, Gjerris F, Klinken L: Computed tomography of benign supratentorial astrocytomas of infancy and childhood. *Neuroradiology* 21:97–91, 1981.

40. Peiris JB, Russell RWR: Giant aneurysms of the carotid system presenting as visual field defect. *J Neurol Neurosurg Psychiatry* 43:1053–1064, 1980.

41. Peyster GR, Hoover E: *Computerized Tomography in Orbital Disease and Neuroophthalmology.* Chicago, Yearbook Medical Publishers, 1984.

42. Pinto RS, Kricheff II, Butler AR, et al: Correlation of computed tomographic, angiographic, and neuropathologic changes in giant cerebral aneurysms. *Radiology* 132:85–92, 1979.

43. Post MJD, David NJ, Glaser JS, et al: Pituitary apoplexy: Diagnosis by computed tomography. *Radiology* 134:665–670, 1980.

44. Post MJD, Glaser JS, Trobe JD: The radiographic recognition of two clinically elusive mass lesions of the cavernous sinus: meningiomas and aneurysms. *Neuroradiology* 16:499–503, 1978.

45. Pullicino P, Kendall BE, Jakubowski JL: Difficulties in diagnosis of intracranial meningiomas by computed tomography. *J Neurol Neurosurg Psychiatry* 43:1022–1029, 1980.

46. Russell DS, Rubinstein LJ: *Pathology of Tumors of the Nervous System.* Baltimore, Williams & Wilkins, 1963.

47. Sarwar M, Batnitzky S, Schechter MM: Tumorous aneurysms. *Neuroradiology* 12:79–97, 1976.

48. Spaziante R, deDivitiis E, Stella L, et al: Benign intrasellar cysts. *Surg Neurol* 15:274–282, 1981.

49. Savoiardo M, Harwood-Nash DC, Tadmor R, et al: Gliomas of the intracranial anterior optic pathways in children. *Radiology* 138:601–610, 1981.

50. Takeuchi J, Handa H, Otsuka S, et al: Neuroradiological aspects of suprasellar germinomas. *Neuroradiology* 17:153–159, 1979.

51. Takeuchi J, Mori K, Moritake K, et al: Teratomas in the suprasellar region: Report of five cases. *Surg Neurol* 3:247–255, 1975.

52. Taylor S: High resolution computed tomography of the sella. *Radiol Clin North Am* 20:207–235, 1982.

53. Tibbs PA, Chalia V, Mortara RH: Isolated histiocytosis X of the hypothalamus. *J Neurosurg* 49:929–934, 1978.

54. Trobe JD, Glaser JS, Post JD: Meningiomas and aneurysms of the cavernous sinus. *Arch Ophthalmol* 96:457–467, 1978.

55. Urich H: Malformations of the nervous system, perinatal damage and related conditions, in Blockwood W, Corsellis JAN (eds): *Greenfield's Neuropathology.* Chicago, Yearbook Medical Publishers, 1976, p. 393.

56. Virapongse C, Bhimani S, Sarwar M: Prolactin-secreting pituitary adenoma: CT appearance in diffuse invasion. *Radiology* 152:447–451, 1984.

57. Walsh TJ: *The Interpretation of Visual Fields.* Rochester, MN, American Academy of Ophthalmology, 1979.

58. Walsh TJ, Hoyt WF: *Neuro-ophthalmology,* ed 2. Baltimore, Williams & Wilkins, 1957, vol 2, p. 19.

59. Wakai S, Fukushima T, Teramoto A, et al: Pituitary apoplexy: Its incidence and clinical significance. *J Neurosurg* 55:187–193, 1981.

60. Wehrli FW, MacFall JR, Glover GH, et al: The dependence of nuclear magnetic resonance image contrast on intrinsic and pulse sequence timing parameters. *Magnet Res Imaging* 2:3–16, 1983.

61. White JC, Ballantine HT Jr: Intrasellar aneurysms simulating hypophyseal tumors. *J Neurosurg* 18:34–50, 1961.

13
Computed Tomography Assessment of Paraorbital Pathology

MAHMOOD F. MAFEE, GLEN D. DOBBEN, and GALDINO E. VALVASSORI

The orbit and its contents are often involved with diseases originating in nearby or distant organs. Computed tomography (CT) and ultrasonography frequently contribute more to the diagnosis than routine x-ray film studies (8, 18, 24, 25, 32, 34, 35, 45).

The location of a lesion is helpful in establishing a diagnosis. Hemangiomas of infancy are frequently found in the upper nasal quadrant of the orbit. Compressibility is characteristic of this lesion (20). In adults, the hemangioma is firmer. Another lesion often found in the upper nasal quadrant is the mucocele. This mass feels boggy and doughy. In the temporal quadrant, the neoplasms of the lacrimal gland and the dermoid cyst may be seen. Secondary malignant neoplasms arising from adjacent areas of the face and nose usually can be detected in either the inferior or medial orbital quadrants (20). Primary malignant lymphomas are frequently located in the more anterior portions of the orbits (20). Extraconal orbital multiple myeloma and metastasis are frequently situated in the lateral orbital compartment (see Chapter 15).

Several symptomatic sequences have diagnostic value. For example, in a child, loss of vision followed by proptosis suggests a tumor in or adjacent to the optic nerve. A blue or purple discoloration of the adnexal soft tissues aggravated by crying in an infant is characteristic of hemangioma. Lymphangiomas tend to increase in size with upper respiratory tract infections, which is a characteristic of other lymphoid structures as well. When there is a sequence in a child of ecchymosis of the eyelids, followed by proptosis (which is usually attributed to some trivial trauma), this should suggest one of the malignant orbital neoplasms of childhood (rhabdomyosarcoma, metastatic neuroblastoma). A persistent extrusion of an orbital prosthesis, implanted after enucleation of the eye, is noted in both recurrent malignant melanoma in an adult and orbital retinoblastoma in a child.

As a symptom of orbital neoplasms, moderate or severe pain is uncommon; if mentioned, it may indicate a less common orbital problem. When pain is associated with sudden proptosis and orbital swelling in an adult, an inflammatory orbital process (a well defined abscess) is more likely than a neoplasm. Any patient, whether an adult or a child, with sudden onset of proptosis and soft-tissue swelling accompanied by fever, malaise, and upper respiratory infection more likely has an inflammatory orbital disease than a neoplasm. Changes in the texture and color of the soft tissues of the eyelid occasionally may be helpful in differential diagnosis. Swelling, edema, and redness of these tissues are infrequent in the neoplasm-cyst group of disorders, although there are four common exceptions to this dictum (20). First, with malignant epithelial tumors of the lacrimal gland, early slight edema of the adjacent soft tissues of the eyelid is the rule. Second, boggy edema of the nasal portion of the upper eyelid often is associated with mucoceles that push downward into the superior nasal quadrant of the orbit from the frontal sinus. Third, some puffiness of the lower eyelid accompanies malignant lymphoma growing in the inferior quadrants of the orbit. In all of these instances, the tumors are located well forward; and, tissue swelling represents passive edema due to pressure of the tumor and interference with the lymphatic drainage. Fourth, and more puzzling, boggy edema (greater in the lower than upper eyelid) is sometimes associated with meningioma that either has been partially removed or has existed undetected in the back of the orbit for several years (20). In none of these four exceptions is the redness of the overlying skin as intense as it would appear with an inflammatory disorder.

Anatomic Consideration

The orbital cavity is pyramidal, its base is the orbital opening, and its long axis is directed posteriorly and medially. Each orbit has a roof, floor, medial and lateral walls, a base or orbital opening, and an apex. Once the sinuses are fully developed, over half the circumference of the orbit consists of thin plates of bone shared with a sinus cavity.

1) A portion of the orbit's roof is the floor of the frontal sinus; 2) a portion of its floor is the roof of the maxillary sinus; and 3) a great part of its medial wall is the lamina papyracea of the ethmoid sinus, which is very thin and is easily traversed by infection. The ethmoid and maxillary sinuses are present at birth and are of clinical significance in the young child (19, 48). The frontal sinuses, which develop later, may be detected radiographically after 5 or 6 years of age (19); but they may be present earlier and usually achieve clinical significance only at 10–12 years of age (5). The sphenoid sinuses also develop late and reach adult size in adolescence (19). Infection may spread from a sinus to the orbit by direct extension, or it may spread by way of numerous, valveless

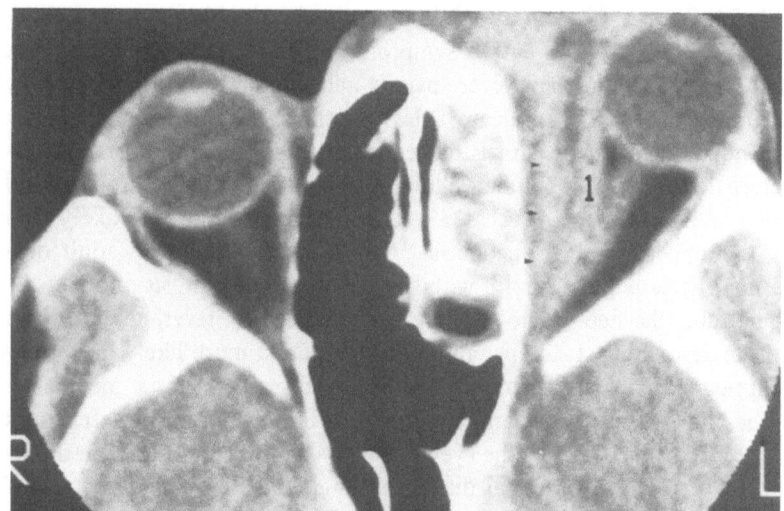

A

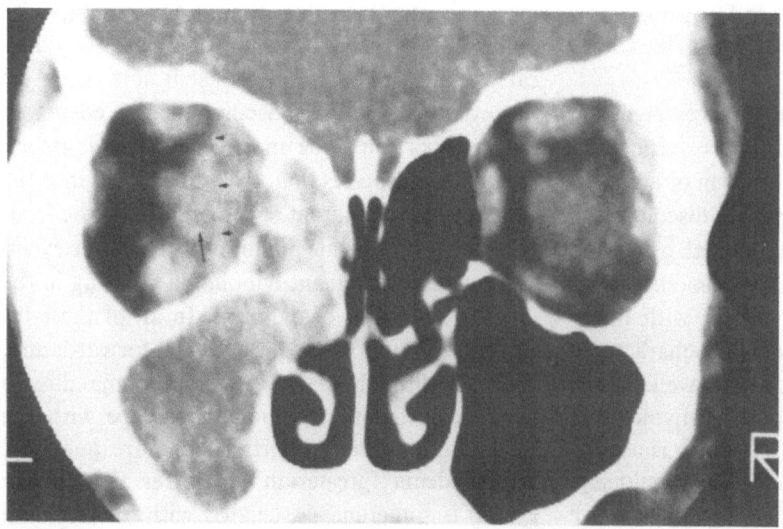

B

Figure 13.1. Subperiosteal phlegmon of the orbit. **A.** Axial CT scan showing mucoperiosteal thickening of the left ethmoid sinus, with soft-tissue density (induration) in the medial compartment of the left orbit (arrowheads) between the thickened lamina papyracea and displaced medial rectus (1). **B.** Coronal CT scan showing mucoperiosteal thickening of the left ethmoid, with soft-tissue induration in the periorbita (subperiosteal space). Note displaced orbital fascia (arrowheads) and the displaced swollen left medial rectus (arrow). The left inferior rectus is also swollen. Notice that the coronal view is reversed.

communicating veins between the sinuses and the orbit (19).

Orbital Complications of Sinus Diseases

Even though antibiotics have cut down on the incidence of complicated sinusitis with orbital involvement, it still occurs and may be the first sign of sinus infection in children (19). Orbital involvement from sinusitis has been described by many authors (5, 19, 26, 28, 36, 49). The five categories or stages of orbital involvement from sinusitis are: 1) inflammatory edema; 2) orbital periostitis; 3) subperiosteal abscess; 4) orbital cellulitis; and 5) orbital abscess (5, 19, 26, 28, 49). Limiting a particular inflammatory lesion to one of these categories is difficult, because they tend to overlap (19). Edema of the eyelid is the first stage; it often is misdiagnosed as orbital or periorbital cellulitis. The infection in this early stage actually is still confined to the sinus (19). A CT scan at this stage will demonstrate the edema of the eyelids and conjunctivae and inflammatory changes of the infected sinus or sinuses. As the reaction of the orbital periosteum begins and gradually advances, the edema of the eyelids and conjunctivae becomes more generalized and the eye begins to protrude. Inflammatory tissue collects beneath the periosteum to form a subperiosteal phlegmon (Fig. 13.1); subsequently, pus may form to represent a subperiosteal abscess (Fig. 13.2) (19, 36). As the disease progresses, the bacteria may infiltrate the periorbital and retroorbital fat to give rise to a true orbital cellulitis (Fig. 13.3). These two conditions frequently coexist (19). At this stage, extraocular mobility is progressively impaired. With severe involvement, visual disturbances can result from optic neuritis and/or ischemia. Abscess formation in the orbit may result from extension of a subperiosteal abscess through the periosteum or from localization of an orbital cellulitis (Fig. 13.3) (19). Usually, the ethmoid sinus infection is the one that is frequently responsible for orbital swelling, subperiosteal abscess, and orbital cellulitis, which extends from the ethmoid through the lamina papyracea (19). A CT scan is an excellent radiologic method for evaluating an ethmoiditis (Fig. 13.1, 13.2, 13.3). The information obtained by the CT scan, together with clinical findings (proptosis, limitation of extraocular muscular movements, and decreased visual acuity), may be the best guidelines for treatment.

Not all orbital bacterial inflammations are a complication of paranasal sinusitis. Figure 13.4 demonstrates an abscess formation in the left temporal fossa, with a fistula tract into the orbit, in a patient with Crouzon's disease who had multiple surgical procedures for repair of hypertelorism. In this case, CT scanning was the only radiographic method that provided the diagnostic information leading to the presurgical diagnosis of the abscess.

Another important and more complicated orbital inflammatory process is extension of mycotic infection of both nasal and paranasal sinuses into the orbit. Mycotic infection of the nasal and para-

Figure 13.2. Subperiosteal abscess of the orbit. Axial CT scan showing mucosal thickening of the ethmoid air cells, with a surgically proven subperiosteal abscess in the medial compartment of the left orbit. Note the air bubbles within the abscess (arrows). The left medial rectus is swollen and displaced laterally (arrowheads).

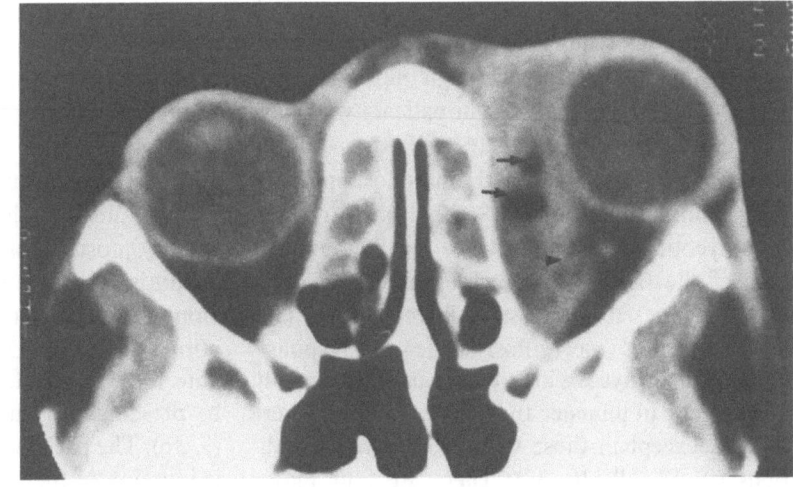

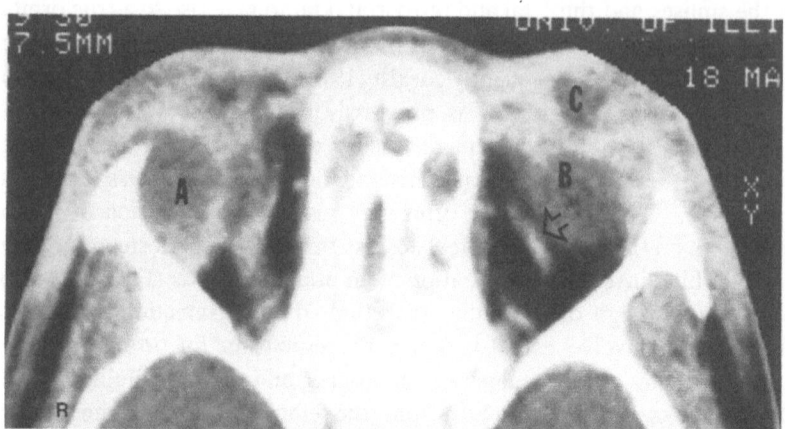

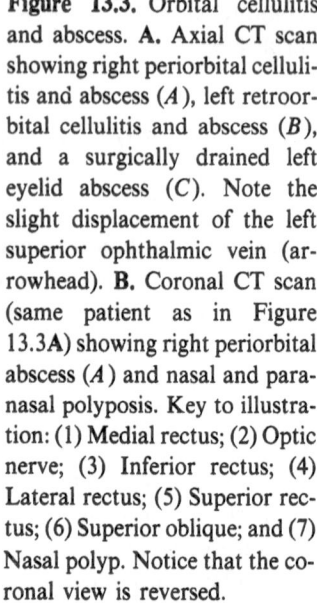

Figure 13.3. Orbital cellulitis and abscess. **A.** Axial CT scan showing right periorbital cellulitis and abscess (*A*), left retroorbital cellulitis and abscess (*B*), and a surgically drained left eyelid abscess (*C*). Note the slight displacement of the left superior ophthalmic vein (arrowhead). **B.** Coronal CT scan (same patient as in Figure 13.3A) showing right periorbital abscess (*A*) and nasal and paranasal polyposis. Key to illustration: (1) Medial rectus; (2) Optic nerve; (3) Inferior rectus; (4) Lateral rectus; (5) Superior rectus; (6) Superior oblique; and (7) Nasal polyp. Notice that the coronal view is reversed.

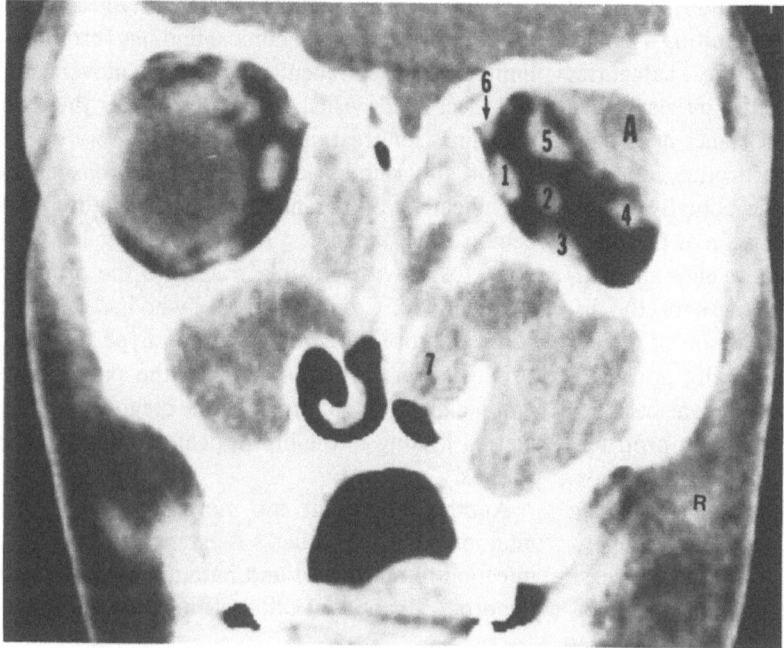

nasal sinuses and craniofacial structures is a serious disease that requires prompt surgery and medical therapy to decrease its high morbidity rate (9, 30). This usually is seen in patients who have debilitating diseases, diabetes mellitus, or who have undergone therapy with immunosuppressive drugs and antimetabolites (9, 30, 38). Rhinocerebral mycotic infection may be caused by the members of the family *Mucoraceae* (mucormycosis), which belongs to the class of Phycomycetes (12) and Aspergillus (aspergillosis). The fungi responsible for mucormycosis are ubiquitous and normally saprophytic in humans; they rarely produce severe disease, except in those with predisposing conditions (9, 12, 30, 36, 38). There are four major

types of mucormycosis: rhinocerebral, pulmonary, gastrointestinal, and disseminated (9). The most common form is the rhinocerebral form. The infection usually begins in the nose and spreads to the paranasal sinuses; then it extends into the orbit and cavernous sinus (9, 30, 36). Orbital involvement results in such orbital signs as ophthalmoplegia, proptosis, ptosis, loss of vision, and orbital cellulitis. The inflammatory process soon extends along the infraorbital fissure and into the infratemporal fossa (Fig. 13.5). Black necrosis of a turbinate is a diagnostic clinical sign, but it may not be present until late in the course of the disease (9, 36). The pathologic landmark of mucormycosis is invasion of the walls of the vessels, particularly

Figure 13.4. Temporal fossa abscess. Axial CT scan showing an image of low attenuation values (abscess) involving the left temporal fossa (arrows). Note the air bubbles and a fistula tract extending from the abscess into the left orbit in this patient with Crouzon disease who had several orbital surgeries for repair of hypertelorism.

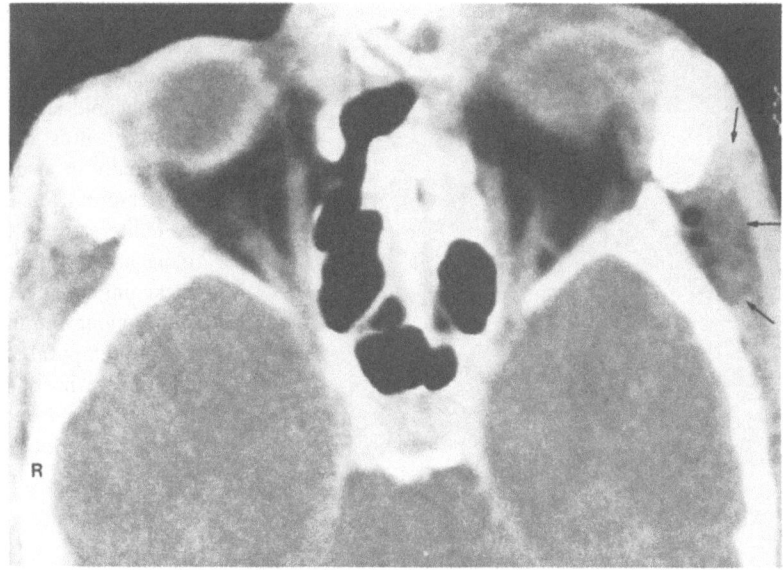

the arteries (12). The organism presumably enters the nasal cavity and paranasal sinuses in inhaled dust particles (26). It sporulates in tissues that have lost their internal resistance to the fungus. Hyphae are produced and blood vessels are invaded (30). The organism proliferates within the muscular walls of arteries and (to a lesser extent) veins and lymphatics, thus producing purulent arteritis, thrombosis, and consequent infarction (6, 41). The nasal and sinus walls are invaded via these vessels, with subsequent invasion of the meninges, brain, cavernous sinus, cranial nerves, and carotid arteries. Fungal arteritis may result in an aneurysm, pseudoaneurysm, thrombosis, or cerebral infarction (30, 43).

The radiographic findings of mucormycosis of the sinuses were first described by Green, et al, (16) who noted three signs: nodular mucosal thickening, absence of fluid levels, and a spotty destruction of bony walls. None of these signs can be considered typical for the diagnosis of fungal sinusitis; however, a CT scan can be very helpful and sometimes (13, 14, 36) characteristic for the diagnosis of mucormycosis. The main contribution of CT scanning to the diagnosis of mucormycosis is its clear demostration of the relationship between nasal, sinus and orbital disease, a relationship so typical of mucormycosis that this diagnosis should be considered whenever combined nasal, sinus, and orbital diseases are encountered (Fig. 13.5). Invasion of the medial orbit by the infecting organism results in phlegmon of the periorbita and,

therefore, elevation of the medial rectus, which later on becomes involved via direct invasion by hyphae (9). Bone destruction of the sinus walls—and in particular, periosteal irregularity and thickening—indicative of periostitis and osteitis is common. It usually helps to differentiate the overall picture from that of the malignant process, which usually results in large areas of bone destruction.

Aspergillosis is a ubiquitous mould found primarily in agricultural dust. It may produce rhinocerebral disease and orbital involvement similar to mucormycosis, although hematogenous spread from the lungs to the brain is more common (9). This fungus also has a well-known propensity for invading blood vessels, including the internal carotid artery (27, 46). The combination of orbital and sinus involvement is not pathognomonic of rhinocerebral mucormycosis or aspergillosis; however, awareness of its possibility, particularly when any of the predisposing factors are present, would help in making an early diagnosis and treatment of this aggressive and fatal disease. Mortality now has been reduced to approximately 50% (9). In our practice, CT scanning has been the most effective radiologic imaging modality for making the correct diagnosis in two clinically unsuspected cases of mucormycosis of the nose and paranasal sinuses—one diabetic patient and one renal transplant patient. The diabetic patient presented with complete left ophthalmoplegia of unknown etiology. The diagnosis of mucormycosis was made by CT scanning (Fig. 13.5); it was confirmed on

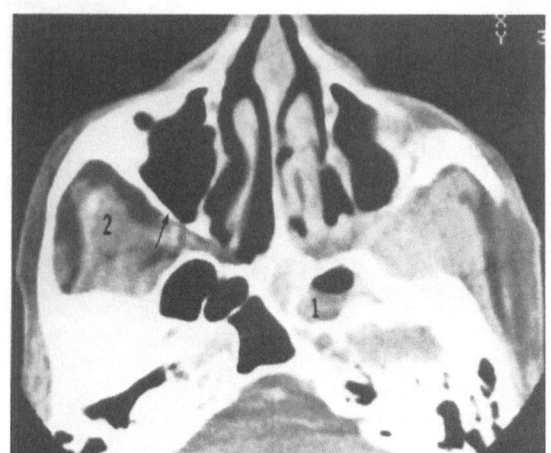

A

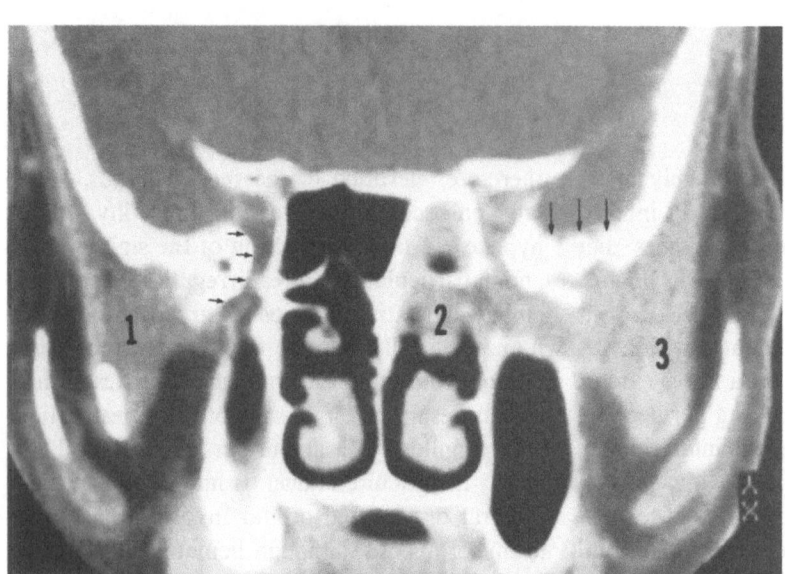

B

Figure 13.5. Mucormycosis: **A.** Axial CT scan showing soft-tissue induration in the left nasal cavity and left infratemporal fossa. Note the mucosal thickening of the left sphenoid sinus (1). The posterior wall of the left maxillary sinus, compared with the right side (arrow), is partially eroded. The fascial fat planes of the left infratemporal fossa, compared with the right side (2), are obliterated. **B.** Semicoronal CT scan showing soft-tissue induration in the left nasal cavity (2) and mucosal thickening in the left sphenoid. Note the soft-tissue infiltration along the inferior orbital fissure extending into the infratemporal fossa (3). Note the irregularity of the left greater wing of the sphenoid (vertical arrows), which is indicative of osteomyelitis. Note the normal fat along the right superior and inferior orbital fissure (horizontal arrows) and the normal appearance of the right infratemporal fossa (1). Note that the coronal view is reversed. **C.** Axial CT scan showing soft-tissue involvement of the left posterior ethmoid air cells and left sphenoid sinus (*E*), with obliteration of the left orbital apical fat by soft-tissue infiltration and with extension and involvement of the left cavernous sinus (arrows) in this diabetic patient who presented with complete ophthalmoplegia of unknown etiology. A diagnosis of mucormycosis was made on the basis of CT scans and proved by nasal biopsy.

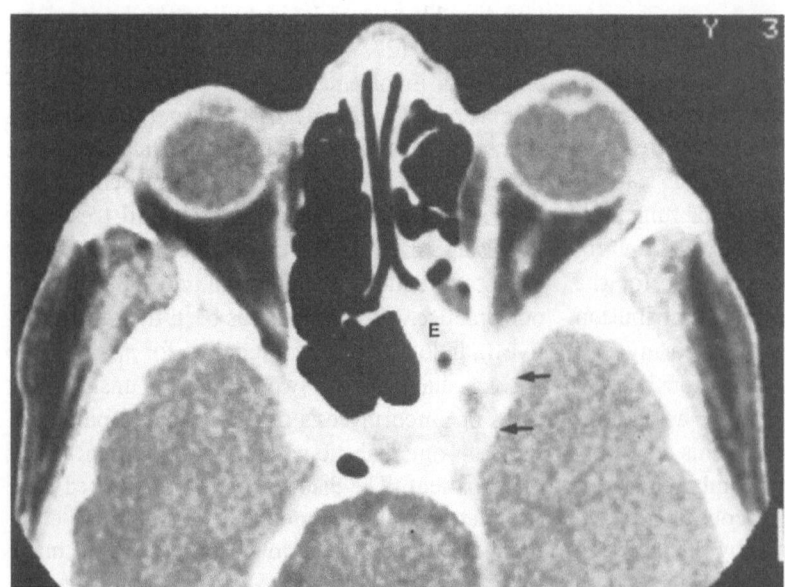

C

a nasal biopsy specimen. It is important to include the nasal cavity, nasopharynx, and base of the skull when performing CT scans in a patient with a potential diagnosis of mucormycosis or aspergillosis.

Mucoceles

The otolaryngologist and ophthalmologist should be constantly on the lookout for orbital complications of sinus disease. Most of these complications are readily apparent from their clinical manifestations. Others, however, such as mucocele and inflammatory polyps, have a slow insidious onset, which makes the diagnosis quite difficult (20). The slow and silent expansion of a mucocele may be unsuspected until bone is eroded and the cyst impinges on some other structures (20).

The etiology of a mucocele is debatable. Most otorhinolaryngologists believe that mucoceles are secondary to obstruction of the ostium of the sinus. This obstruction may be the result of inflammation, trauma, osteoma, fibrous dysplasia, or repeated surgery in and around the nasal cavity (3, 20, 55). A minority of investigators believe that mucoceles arise as small cysts within the mucous membrane, which by continued growth finally obstruct the ostium of the sinus. Similarly, inflammation, trauma, and surgery may contribute to initial cyst or it may arise de novo (20). All of these theories differ only as to whether the cyst is the primary cause or the effect of obstruction. It is likely that both circumstances prevail, and arguments about etiology are academic. For all practical purposes and whatever the pathogenesis and cause of obstruction, the mucoceles are the cyst-like lesions that most commonly produce bone destruction within the paranasal sinuses (55). They are expanding cystic lesions, covered by mucous membrane, that result from the continued accumulation of secretion and desquamation within an obstructed sinus cavity (3, 55). The degree of inflammatory changes that either initiate or accompany the mucocele determines the amount of chronic inflammatory reaction in the covering wall of the mucous membrane (20). Their secretion is usually clear, thick (mucoid), and tenacious unless the mucocele has been converted to a pyocele by the invasion of bacteria (3). In pyoceles, the cyst then contains a green or yellow thick, viscid material (20). Mucoceles are frequently discussed from

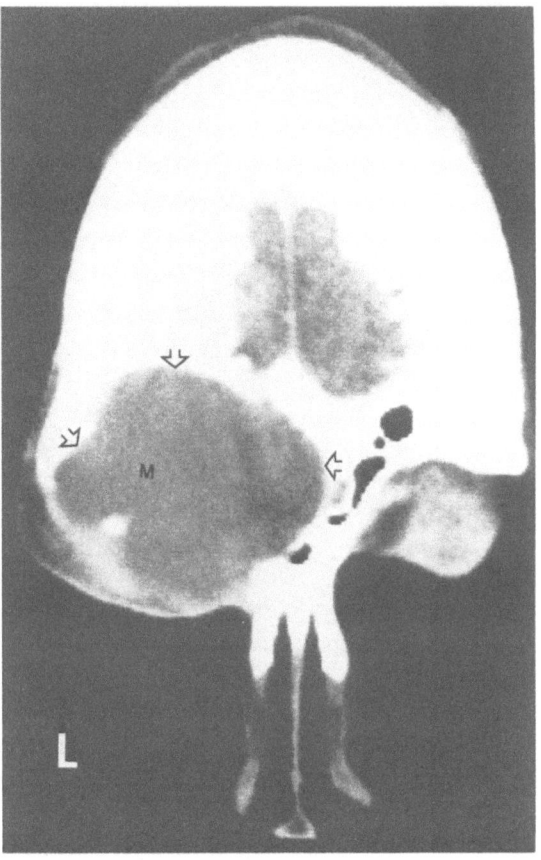

Figure 13.6. Frontal sinus mucocele. Large mucocele of the left frontal sinus. Coronal CT scan showing a large, expansile soft-tissue mass (M) of low density, with associated bone erosion of the medial, superior, and lateral orbital rims (arrows). At surgery, a large mucocele was found arising from the left frontal sinus, with extensive bone destruction of the floor and anterior wall of the left frontal sinus.

the standpoint of the sinus of origin. There is a definite predilection for the frontal and ethmoidal sinuses, presumably because of the dependent position of their ostia (55). Approximately two thirds of all mucoceles involve the frontal sinus (Fig. 13.6); the majority of the remainder involve the ethmoidal labyrinth (Figs. 13.7 and 13.8). Maxillary and sphenoidal mucoceles (Fig. 13.9) are rare (3, 55). The sinus of origin, of course, is most important for treatment planning. The persistent expansion of the mucocele causes erosion of surrounding bone, with frequent exit into the adjacent orbit (Fig. 13.8). If the cyst continues to expand within the orbital cavity, the mass may mimic the behavior of many benign growths. In these circum-

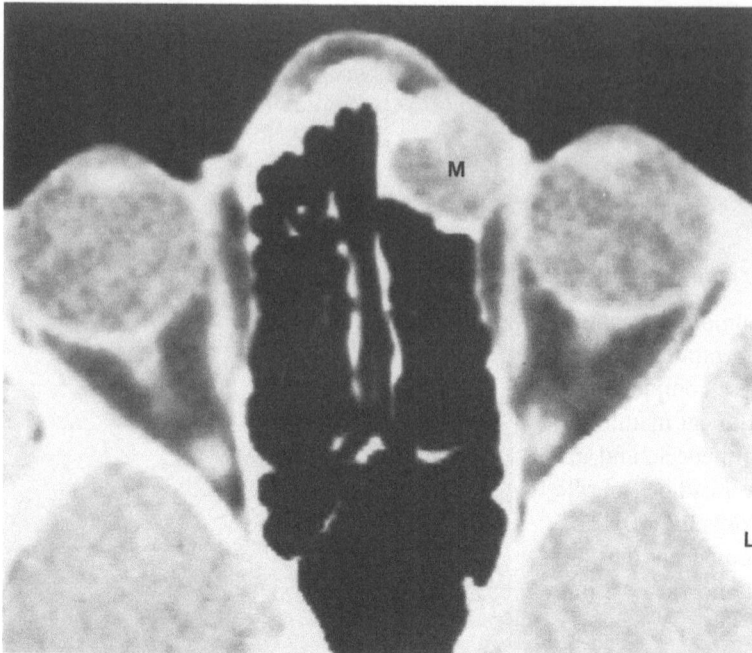

Figure 13.7. Ethmoid mucocele. Axial CT scan showing an expansile soft-tissue mass (*M*) localized to the left anterior ethmoidal air cells. Note the erosion of the nasal process of the left maxilla and anterior portion of the left lamina papyracea.

stances, the tumor is of concern to ophthalmologists because displacement of the eye may be the initial symptom of an otherwise insidious lesion. Proptosis or displacement of the eye, puffiness of the upper eyelid, a mild ophthalmoplegia, some degree of visual disturbance, and a palpable mass are clinical features encountered with an orbital mucocele (3, 20). When the mucocele enters the more anterior portion of the orbital cavity (usually from the frontal and ethmoid sinuses), it usually

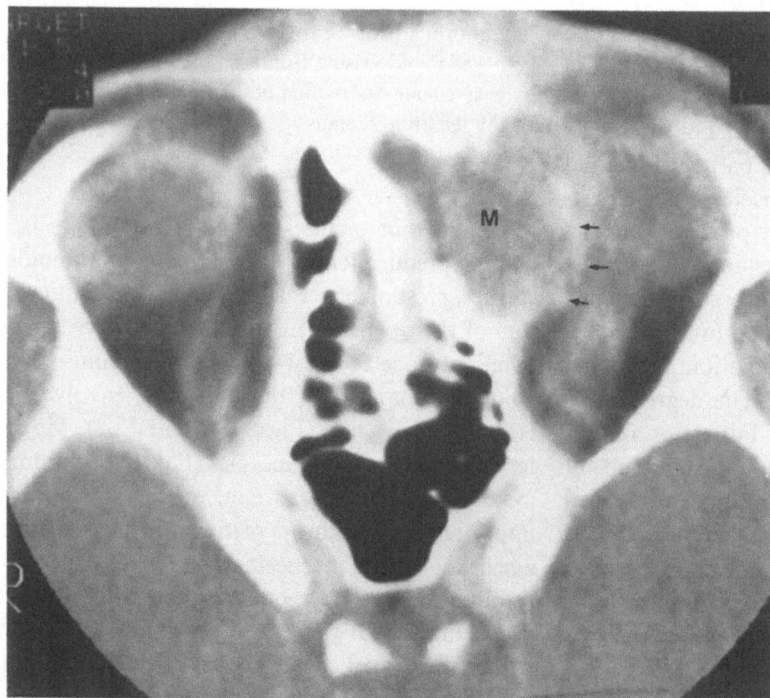

Figure 13.8. Ethmoid mucocele. Axial CT scan showing an expansile soft-tissue mass (*M*) involving the left ethmoid sinus, with erosion of the left lamina papyracea and extension into the left orbit. Note a faint rim of calcification (arrows) along the lateral aspect of the capsule of the mucocele.

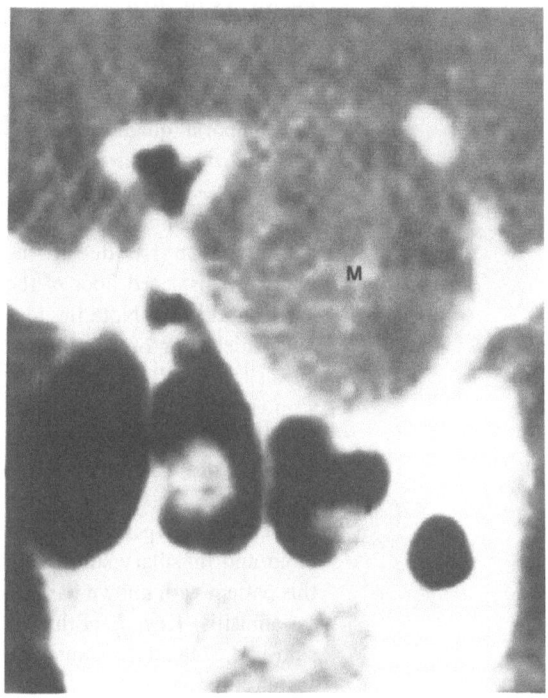

Figure 13.9. Sphenoid mucocele. Coronal CT scan showing an expansile destructive soft-tissue mass (*M*) of low attenuation values involving almost the entire sphenoid sinuses.

will do so in the upper nasal quadrant (Fig. 13.8); this results in a peculiar droopy appearance, and the puffy soft tissue of the upper eyelid and a mass will be palpable beneath and slightly behind the superior orbital rim. In a large frontal sinus mucocele, if bone erosion occurs along the orbital roof, it may imitate signs of other tumors of the posterior orbit and sphenoid (20). The sphenoidal mucocele may cause serious neurologic symptoms by intracranial extension (36, 55). There may be destruction of the floor of the sella and encroachment on the pituitary gland. An orbital apex syndrome with loss of vision or constriction of the visual fields may occur (Fig. 13.9) (33). A mucocele of the maxillary sinus, although infrequent, may result in upward displacement of the orbital contents and enophthalmos caused by a loss of the roof of the antrum. A CT scan should be considered the diagnostic method of choice for the diagnosis and management of the mucocele (36).

The radiographic characteristics of mucoceles have been well described (8, 21, 22, 36, 44, 47, 55). A large mucocele produces a classic roentgenographic appearance of an enlarged, distorted si-

nus with a large bony defect representing a breakthrough into the adjacent structures (Fig. 13.8). Not all mucoceles are so classic, and there are many with subtle bone erosion. Those cases having minimal bone defects pose the greatest difficulty in diagnosis (Fig. 13.7). The gradual pressure atrophy and erosion of the bone by the enlarging soft-tissue mass of the mucocele, the expansile appearance on CT scanning (Fig. 13.7, 13.8, 13.9) with no enhancement after contrast infusion (except around the inflamed capsule and peripheral induration), and occasional peripheral calcification (Fig. 13.8) all make the CT diagnosis of mucocele almost certain. The location, the intraorbital and intracranial extensions, and the surrounding inflammatory changes of a mucocele and the extent of bone erosion (using high-resolution CT with extended bone CT range technique) can be best evaluated by combined axial and coronal CT scans. Occasionally, a large frontal sinus inflammatory polyp, if bone erosion occurs along the orbital roof, may imitate the CT scan appearance of a mucocele (Fig. 13.10) or other tumors of the orbit.

Orbital Trauma

Conventional plain x-ray film examination and selective complex motion tomography remain the basis for radiologic diagnosis of the isolated maxilloorbital facial fracture (36, 37). These modalities are clinically accessible and acceptable, cost-effective, and diagnostically functional. In complex maxillofacial trauma, CT scanning now provides a very effective imaging modality (17, 36, 37, 54). Current-CT scanners with extended bone range imaging possibility provides excellent bone detail (37). The orbital findings in trauma are well documented (8, 17, 36, 37, 53, 54). The fracture fragments and foreign bodies projecting into the orbit and fat, and muscle herniation into the ethmoid or maxillary sinuses, are readily identified—together with any hematoma and/or pneumoorbit (Figs. 13.11, 13.12, 13.13). The CT scan is helpful in evaluating the position of the silastic implant for the repair of the orbital floor fracture. The intraorbital and intracranial extension of the complex maxilloorbital facial fractures, shattering craniofacial fractures, splayed ethmoid fractures, and medial and lateral orbital wall and apex fractures can now be imaged in a manner not previously possible (37) (see Chapter 16).

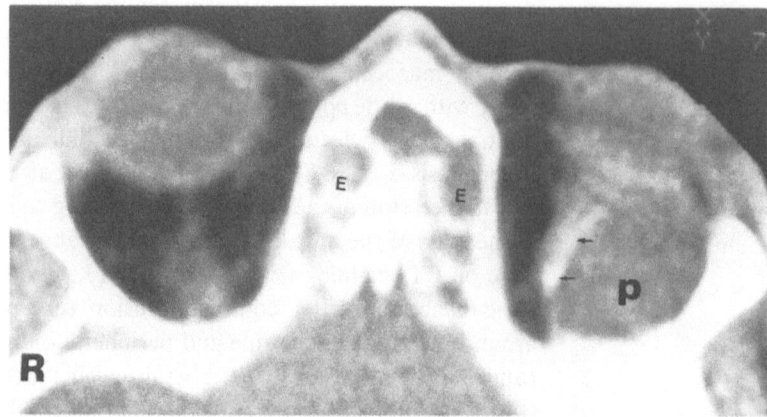

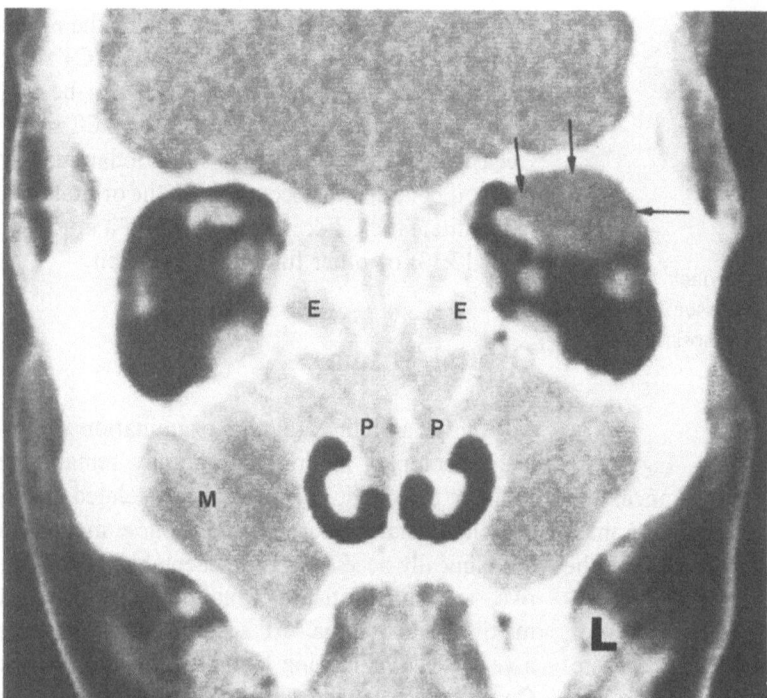

Figure 13.10. Extension of a frontal sinus polyp into the orbit. **A.** Axial CT scan showing a soft-tissue mass (*P*) in the superotemporal quadrant of the left orbit due to extension of a frontal sinus polyp into the orbit. The curvilinear increased density (arrows) is due to the inferiorly displaced floor of the left frontal sinus. Note the mucosal thickening of the ethmoid air cells (*E*). **B.** Coronal CT scan showing a soft-tissue mass (arrows) in the superior compartment of the left orbit (same patient as in Fig. 13.10A). Note the chronic hyperplastic ethmoid and maxillary sinusitis in this patient with known paranasal sinusitis. Key: *E,* Ethmoid sinus; *M,* Maxillary sinus; and *P,* Nasal polyp.

Subperiosteal Orbital Hematomas of the Orbit and Hematic Cysts

Subperiosteal orbital hematomas are rare; but they are a serious complication of trauma, usually occurring soon after blunt head trauma—although they may be delayed for months or years (42, 52). They may develop so insidiously as to defy explanation, and with no definite history of injury (20, 50). The hematomas develop between the bone and separated periosteum (42). This usually occurs as a result of the direct rupture of the subperiosteal

blood vessels (42). The orbital roof is the most common place; subperiosteal hematomas of the orbital roof occur almost exclusively in children and young adults, since the orbital periosteum is not firmly adhered to the bone (42). They are less likely to occur later, since the periosteal bony connection may grow firmer with age (42). Most orbital hematomas are due to trauma, although a spontaneous hemorrhage may occur as complications of systemic disease, such as leukemia, thrombocytopenia, and hemophilia (20). Most of the orbital hematomas, like other localized collections of blood, disappear within days (20). Seldom do

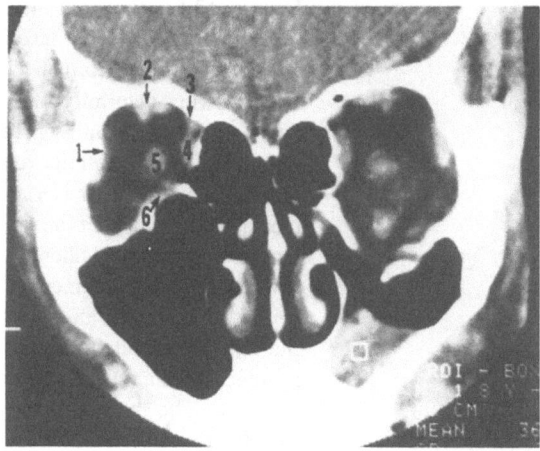

A

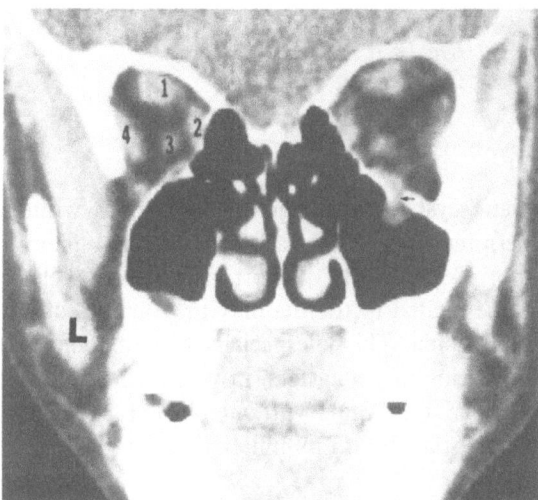

B

Figure 13.11. Blow-out fracture of the orbital floor. **A.** Coronal CT scan showing a fracture of the floor of the right orbit, with inferior displacement of the periorbital fat. The right inferior rectus is enlarged and round in appearance (compared with the left side). This is due to an intramuscular hematoma. This CT scan appearance of the inferior rectus is frequently observed in a blow-out fracture. Note fluid with a high attenuation value within the right maxillary sinus due to hemorrhage. Key to illustration: (1) Lateral rectus; (2) Superior rectus–Levator palpebra complex; (3) Superior oblique; (4) Medial rectus; (5) Optic nerve; and (6) Inferior rectus. **B.** Blow-out fracture of the orbital floor with inferior rectus muscle entrapment. Axial CT scan showing a fracture of the floor of the right orbit (arrow), with inferior displacement of the inferior rectus (arrow). Key to illustration: (1) Superior rectus–Levator palpebra complex; (2) Medial rectus; (3) Optic nerve; and (4) Medial rectus.

we think of hematoma, in reference to the orbit, as a deeply placed cystic structure that may remain unchanged and unidentified for long periods. For this type of hemorrhagic condition, hematic cyst seems the preferable term (20). Hematic cysts may develop as a complication of head trauma or from prolonged retention of an orbital foreign body. They may also develop because orbital hemorrhage is too great to be quickly absorbed, and it silently remains as a cystic accumulation of hematogenous debris surrounded by a wall of fibrous tissue (20). An epithelial covering or lining is not present. A history of trauma may be remote or even absent in such cases (20, 42, 52). The cyst may be several centimeters in size (Fig. 13.14) (20). Consistency and color of the contents vary according to the duration of the cyst. All degrees and stages of organization are encountered: cholesterol clefts, hemosiderin deposition, foreign body cells, pigment-collecting macrophages, and foam cells containing liquid (20). The CT scan is extremely useful for evaluating orbital hematomas (Fig. 13.13). Orbital CT scanning permits a precise delineation of the size and extent of this hematoma (42). An orbital subperiosteal hematoma appears as a sharply delineated soft-tissue image of high CT attenuation values (blood density), with a broad base abutting the superior orbital wall (42). The differential diagnoses include neoplasms and inflammation; however, when the clinical history is combined with the CT findings, a diagnosis should be easily established. Confusion occurs in a case of blood cyst (Fig. 13.14), while a history of trauma may be remote or even absent—and also hemorrhagic systemic disease, which might otherwise furnish a clue in differential diagnosis, may be absent. In such situations, the following CT signs would help to establish the diagnosis: 1) the cyst appears as a well-defined extraconal mass in the superolateral portion of the orbit, which may be homogeneous or nonhomogeneous in appearance (Fig. 13.14); (It should be noted that hematic cysts are seldom reported along the floor of the orbit, (20) and we have not seen cyst formation as a major complication of blow-out fractures and associated traumatic orbital floor hematomas, which are frequently observed.) 2) the cyst-like mass or its cystic component—despite its lucent appearance (Fig. 13.14)—demonstrates high CT attenuation values, which are most likely related to the hemosiderin deposition; 3) bone expansion of the orbit, which indicates chronicity of the lesion (Fig.

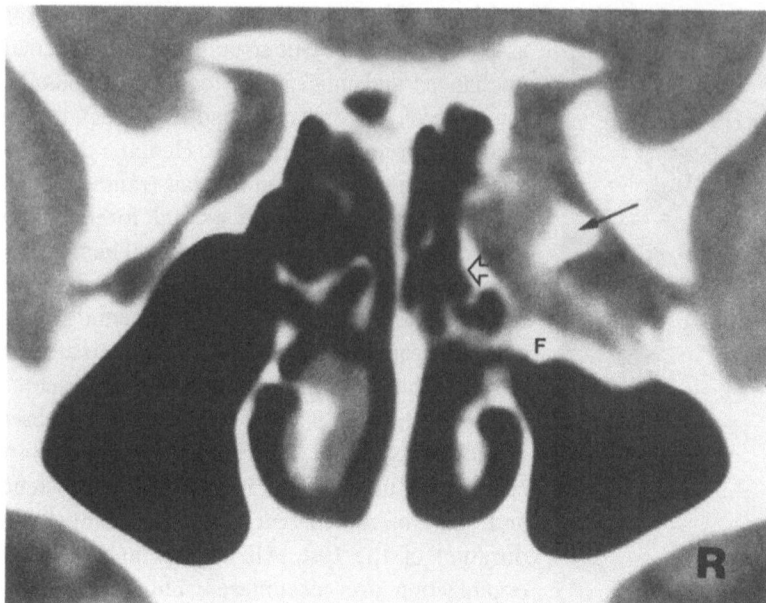

Figure 13.12. Blow-out fractures of the floor and medial wall of the orbit. Coronal CT scan showing deformity of the floor and medial wall of the right orbit. Note inferior displacement of the floor (*F*) and medial displacement of the right lamina papyracea (hollow arrow). Note a bone fragment (arrow) and increased density of the right retroorbital fat, which is indicative of a retroorbital hematoma. The bone fragment was due to a fracture of the orbital apex.

13.14); 4) occasional flecks of calcium may be present in the wall of the lesion (42), and 5) there will be no enhancement following administration of contrast material. These cysts are infrequent, but they occasionally pose a challenge in the differential diagnosis of unilateral proptosis. The location, CT scan appearance, and bone expansion (cavity formation) should raise the question of hematic cyst, hemorrhagic extravasations within a dermoid cyst, and/or a benign lacrimal gland tumor. Some of the hemorrhagic masses believed to be related to trauma may be examples of lymphangioma. This is especially true of some cases appearing in youngsters, in whom sudden orbital hemorrhage occurs without obvious explanation or associated with minimal trauma (20).

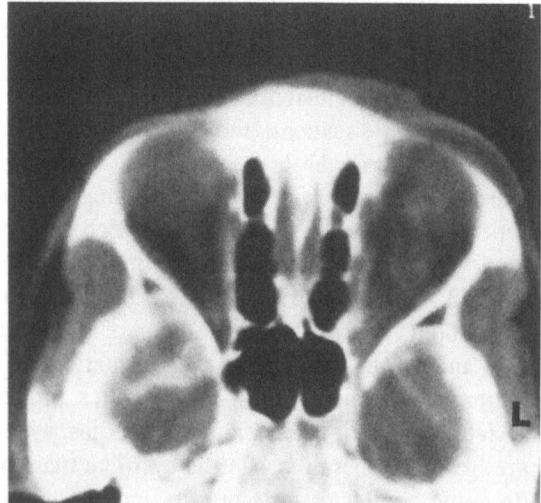

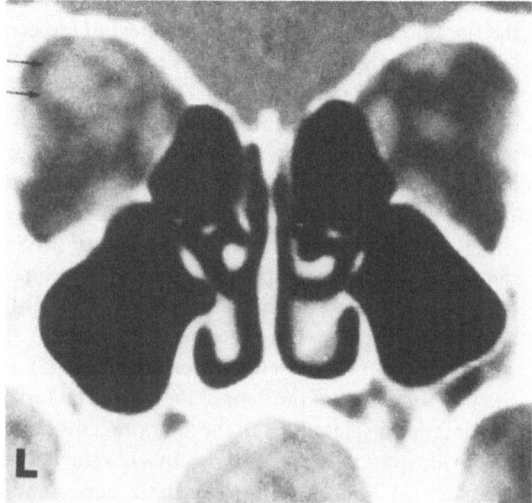

Figure 13.13. Orbital hematoma. **A.** Axial CT scan showing an image of high attenuation values (hollow arrow) in the superior compartment of the left orbit due to a retroorbital hematoma. **B.** Coronal CT scan (same patient as in **A**) showing an image of high attenuation values (arrows) in the superotemporal compartment of the left orbit due to an intraconal hematoma.

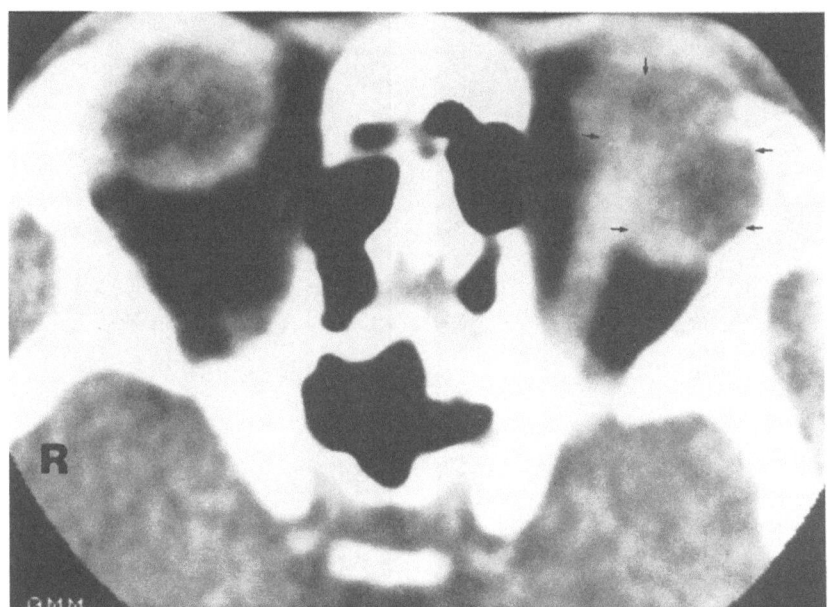

A

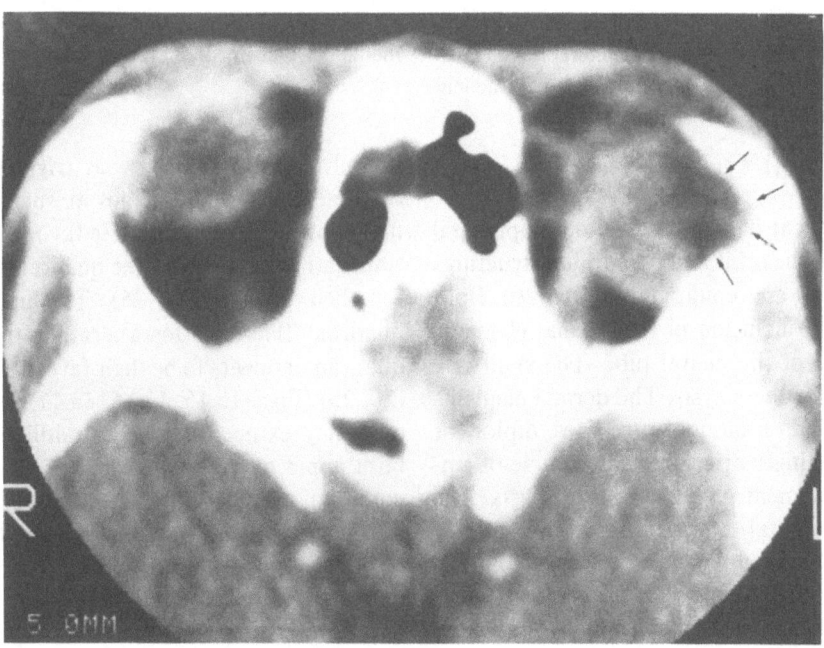

B

Figure 13.14. Orbital hematic cyst. **A.** Axial CT scan showing a well-defined nonhomogeneous mass in the superolateral portion of the left orbit (arrows). The left globe is displaced inferiorly; therefore, it is not included in the plane of section. The lucent component of the mass showed high attenuation values due to hemosiderin deposition. Note bone expansion of the orbit in the lacri- mal fossa, which indicates compression atrophy of the bone and the chronic nature of the lesion. **B.** This CT scan is taken 5 mm above the CT scan in Figure 13.14A. The cavity formation (arrows) in the left lacrimal gland fossa is better demonstrated in this scan. The patient has multiple previous head traumas. At surgery, a large hematic cyst was found in this patient.

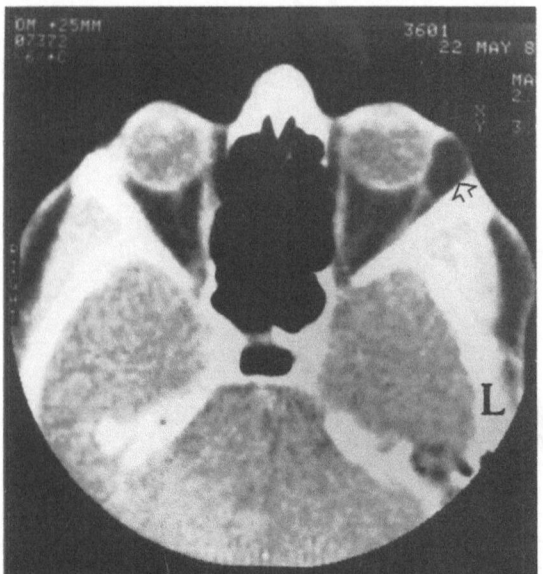

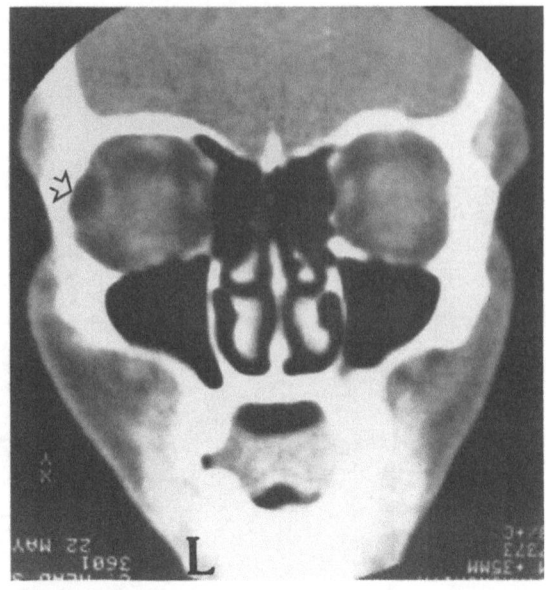

Figure 13.15. Dermoid cyst of the left orbit. **A.** Axial CT scan showing an extraconal mass of fat density (arrow) within the anterolateral aspect of the left orbit, displacing the anterior portion of the lateral rectus muscle medially. **B.** Coronal CT scan showing an extraconal image of fat density (arrow) within the superolateral aspect of the left orbit. Note that the lesion is in the vicinity of the frontozygomatic suture. Also note the medial displacement of the left lateral rectus muscle.

Developmental Orbital Cysts

The most frequent of the so-called developmental cysts involving the orbit and paraorbital structures are the dermoid and epidermoid cysts (20). Both result from the inclusion of ectodermal elements during closure of the neural tube. The skull is a common site for these cysts. The dermal elements that are pinched off along suture lines, diploe, or within the meninges or scalp in the course of embryonic development give rise to these cysts. The orbit and paraorbital structures may house almost 50% of those tumors involving the head (20). Both have a fibrous capsule of varying degree of thickness and toughness. The epidermoid has a lining of epithelial cells, which are usually stratified and capable of producing keratin (20). The dermoid contains sebaceous secretions and desquamated epithelium and elements of normal skin, including hair. These cysts occur almost equally in males and females. Although they may appear at any age from 2–50 years, the peak age for onset seems to be from 3–10 years, and again in the third and fourth decades (20). They usually grow slowly. In children and young adults, the cyst may enlarge for several months and then remain dormant for an interval. In adults, the cyst may have a long period of latency. Just what triggers the growth of these embryonic anlages at such a late age is not known (20). These cysts favor the upper portion, rather than the lower quadrants, of the orbit for their growth (20, 25). The upper temporal quadrant (lacrimal fossa), rather than the nasal quadrant, appears to be their favorite area of origin (20, 25) (Figs. 13.15, 13.16, 13.17). An occasional cyst may extend across the midline and occupy both upper quadrants. Although the cysts are not common, they have always been easily recognized by their classic radiolucent defects that are seen on x-ray films. The bone defect varies in size, but it usually is relatively large in proportion to the overall size of the orbit and has a well-corticated margin. On CT scans, the lesion is seen as a low-density image with smooth margins, with a sharp interface visible against the retrobulbar fat (25) (Figs. 13.15, 13.16, 13.17). Occasionally, these lesions have a density equivalent to surrounding muscle (25). There will be no enhancement following intravenous (IV) administration of contrast material (Fig. 13.15). If the cyst involves the paraorbital structures, such as eyelids and eyebrows, the epidermoid or dermoid cyst may be entirely confined to adnexal tissue. Figure 13.16 shows a dermoid of the left upper eyelid, anterior to the

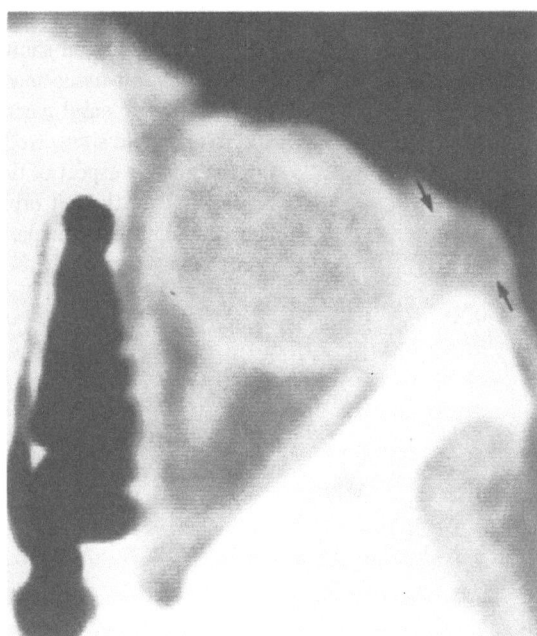

Figure 13.16. Dermoid cyst. Axial CT scan showing a round image of low attenuation values in the lateral orbital angle (arrows) confined to the lateral portion of the upper eyelid.

orbital septum. In some instances, the surgeon may find that the orbital septum is eroded by the enlarging cyst and that the tumor seems to straddle the border between eyelids and orbits; the question arises as to whether the cyst originated in a bony crevice within the orbit, with subsequent anterior expansion through the orbital septum (20). Figure 13.17 shows a dermoid cyst in the vicinity of the left frontal zygomatic suture along the lateral side of the left orbit. Although there is no evidence for intraorbital extension of the cyst, both its location adjacent to the frontozygomatic suture and the associated deformity and flattening of the lateral wall of the orbit would tend to imply that the anlage of the tumor originally was situated along the suture—with subsequent lateral and posterior expansion along the temporal fossa (Fig. 13.17).

Paraorbital Tumors

Extraconal neoplasms may arise extraorbitally; i.e., from the nasal cavity, paranasal sinuses, facial skin, parotid gland, and from the anterior and middle cranial fossae or temporal fossa. They may invade the orbit secondarily or arise in the extraconal component—but still within the orbital cavity, such as the lacrimal gland, lacrimal sac, and lacrimal caruncle.

Neoplasms from the nasal cavity (Fig. 13.18) and the maxillary (Fig. 13.19 and 13.20), ethmoid (Fig. 13.21), and sphenoid sinuses can invade the orbit and produce an extraconal tumor. Extension of the tumor to involve the orbital muscles and intraconal area, and the relationship of the tumor to the optic nerve, is an important feature for patient management. It should be noted and described in every examination (25). Ophthalmoplegia due to fixation of the eye in the orbit by neoplastic invasion of extraocular muscles appears late in the course of disease (Fig. 13.22).

Lacrimal gland tumors may be of mixed types, with both epithelial and mesenchymal components; or they may be carcinomas, usually of the adenocystic variety (8, 20). Adenoid cystic or adenocystic carcinoma is generally infiltrative. After identification and initial removal of the tumor, the course usually is one of slow relentless spread. There may be extensive local involvement (Fig. 13.23). Tumors arising from the lacrimal sac and nasolacrimal canal can invade the intraorbital and paraorbital structures (Fig. 13.24). The CT scan

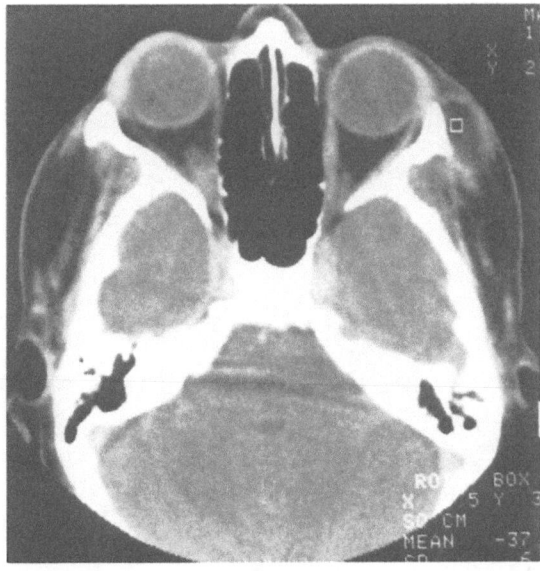

Figure 13.17. Dermoid cyst. Axial CT scan showing an image of low attenuation values in the vicinity of the left frontozygomatic suture along the lateral side of the left orbit. Note flattening of the lateral wall of the orbit adjacent to the mass.

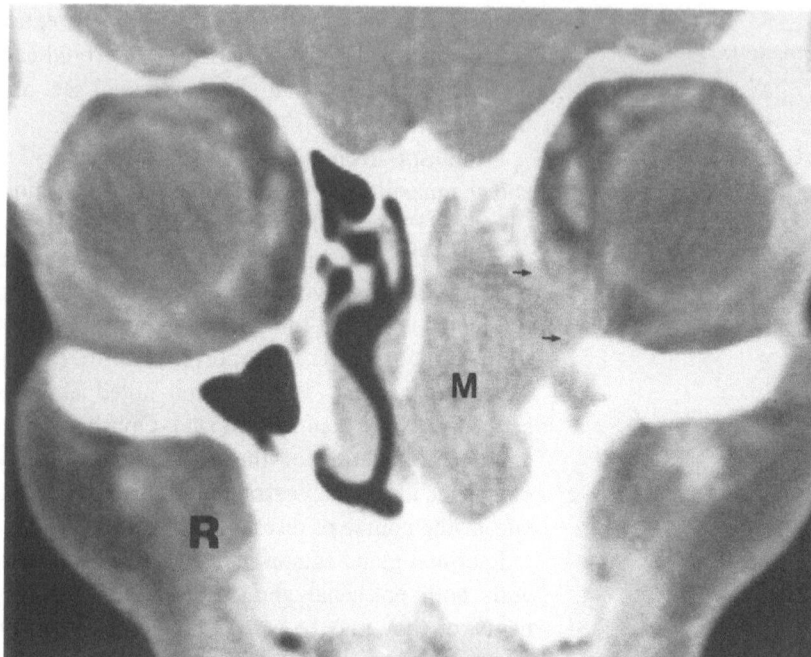

Figure 13.18. Extension of nasal carcinoma into the orbit. Coronal CT scan showing a large soft-tissue mass (*M*) in the left nasal cavity and left ethmoid sinus, eroding the inferior aspect of the medial wall of the left orbit and extending into the periorbital space (arrows).

is a very good method for showing the orbital spread from squamous cell carcinoma of the eyelid, the skin of the face, and the skin of the temple (Fig. 13.25). This is usually seen in patients with squamous cell carcinoma of the skin and with several previous excisions and skin grafts.

Orbital Metastasis

Metastases to the orbit are found in the choroid, retrobulbar soft tissues, and bony orbits. Metastatic disease to the eye and orbit is not rare; it accounted for 3% of patients with unilateral ex-

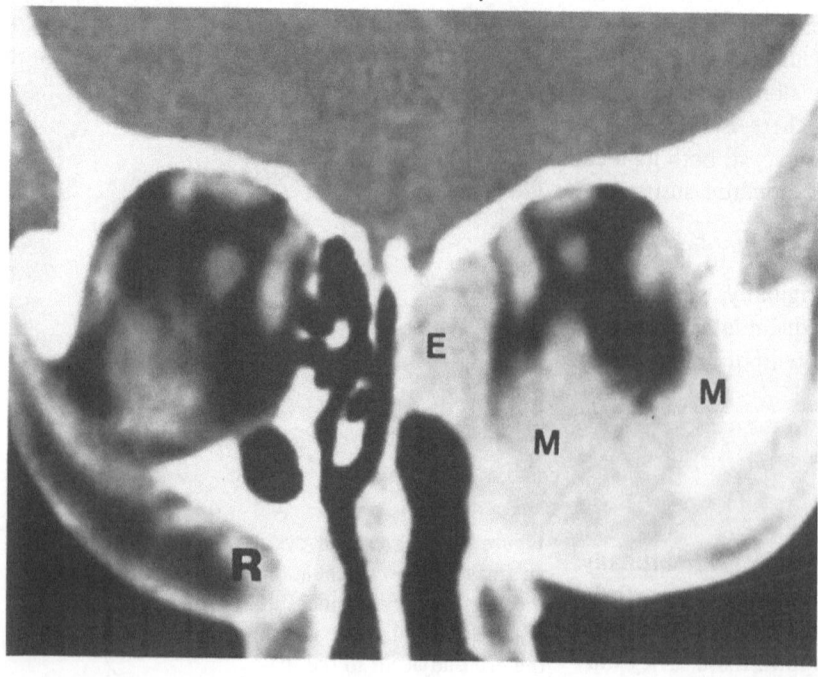

Figure 13.19. Extension of maxillary sinus carcinoma into the orbit. Coronal CT scan showing irregular soft-tissue mass (*M*) within the left orbit due to extension of a recurrent left maxillary sinus carcinoma into the orbit. Also note tumor involvement of the left ethmoid (*E*).

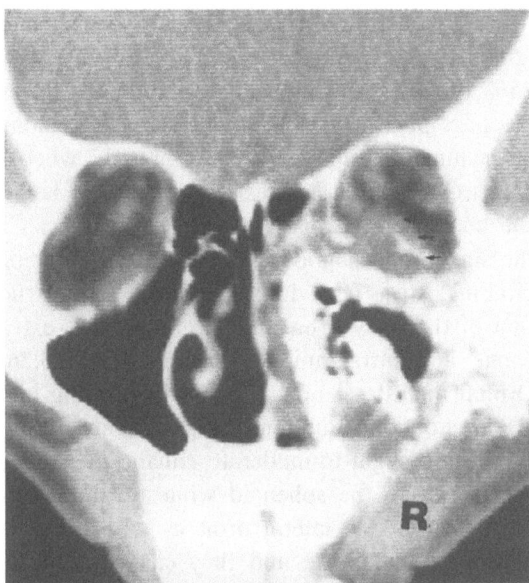

Figure 13.20. Osteosarcoma of the right maxillary sinus. Coronal CT scan showing a destructive mass (M), with islands of new bone formation involving the right maxillary sinus and extending into both the nasal cavity and the inferior compartment of the orbit (arrows).

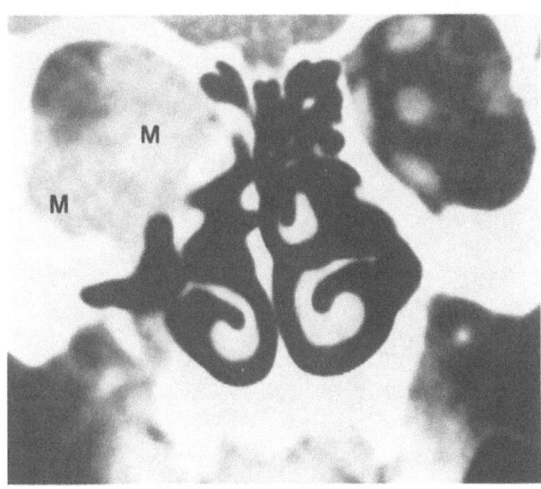

Figure 13.22. Extension of a maxillary sinus carcinoma into the orbit. Coronal CT scan showing a large soft-tissue mass (M) within the intraconal and extraconal spaces of the right orbit due to extension of a recurrent carcinoma of the right maxillary antrum.

ophthalmos at the Columbia Eye Institute (40) and 7% of 465 orbital tumors at the Mayo Clinic (20). Retrobulbar metastasis can involve both extraconal and intraconal spaces (23). Metastasis to the bone and retrobulbar soft tissues causes exophthalmos. The greater wing of the sphenoid is the most common site of bone metastasis (Fig. 13.26) (23). These lesions often have soft-tissue components in both the lateral extraconal space of the orbit and the middle cranial fossa (Fig. 13.26) (23). The most common primary sources

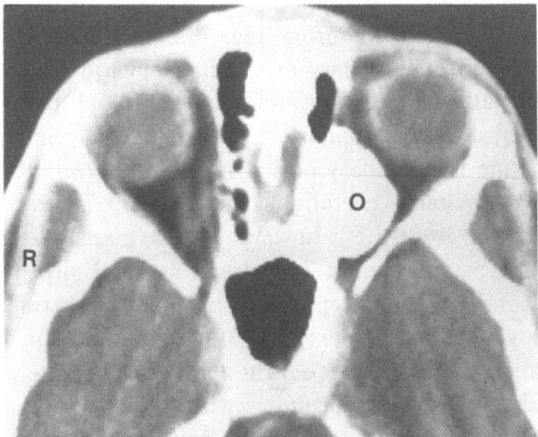

Figure 13.21. Osteoma. Axial CT scan showing a large osteoma (O) of the left ethmoid encroaching on the left orbit and abutting the optic nerve.

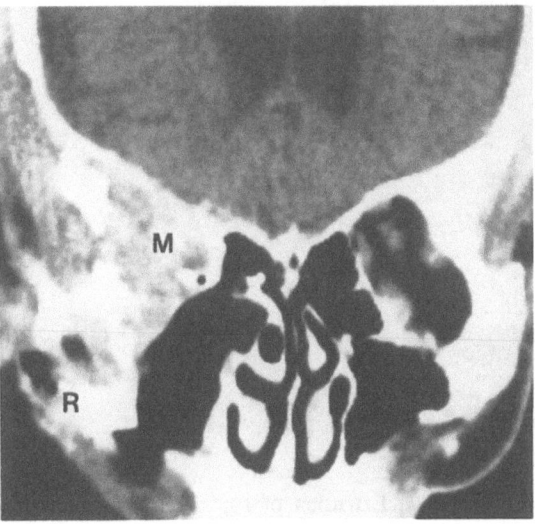

Figure 13.23. Extensive local involvement of adenocystic carcinoma of the lacrimal gland. Coronal CT scan showing destruction of the superior and lateral wall of the right bony orbit, with an enhanced tumor mass (M) filling the entire posterior orbital space.

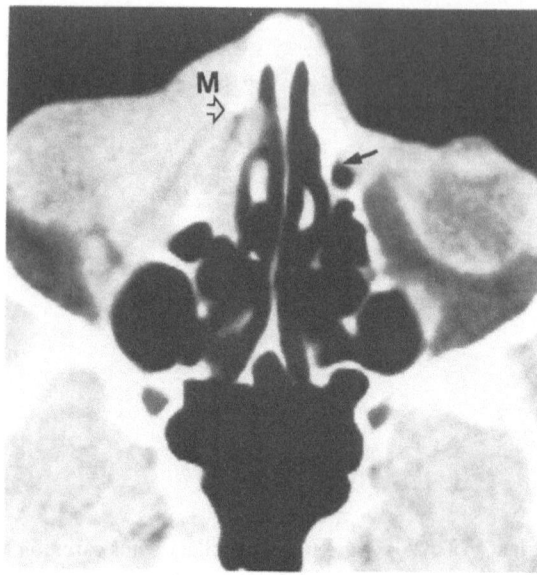

Figure 13.24. Carcinoma of the lacrimal sac. Axial CT scan showing a large soft-tissue mass (*M*) in the right nasoorbital angle extending into both the nasal cavity and medial portion of the right orbit. Note erosion of the nasal process of the right maxilla (hollow arrow); and posterior to that, destruction of the lacrimal bone and nasolacrimal canal. Note the normal left nasolacrimal canal (arrow).

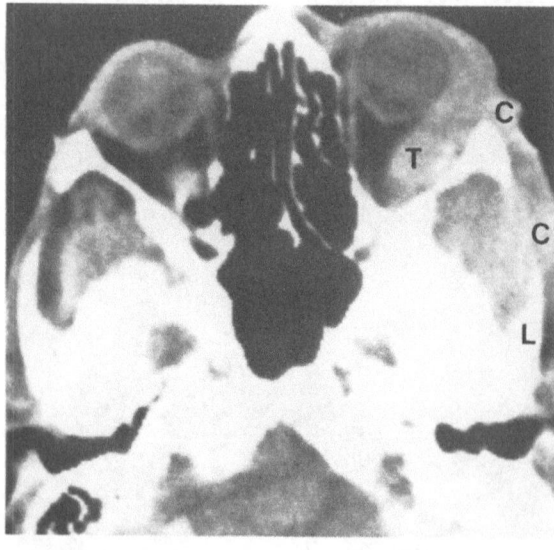

Figure 13.25. Extension of squamous cell carcinoma of the skin of the temple into the orbit. Axial CT scan showing an irregular soft-tissue tumor in the left (*L*) temporal fossa, just above the zygomatic arch, due to recurrent squamous cell carcinoma of the skin (*C*). Note the extensive tumor involvement along the lateral wall of the left orbit (*T*).

of orbital metastases are the breast and lung, followed by gastrointestinal and genitourinary sites (20, 23, 40). Orbital metastases are bilateral in 25% of cases, and associated pulmonary metastases are present in 80–85% (23, 40). Carcinoma of the lung metastasizes to the orbit early, whereas breast carcinoma metastasizes to the orbit late in the course of the disease (15). The CT scan is the single-best diagnostic test for extraocular orbital metastasis (Fig. 13.26), showing the destruction of the bony orbit and the intraconal, extraconal, and intracranial extensions (Fig. 13.26). Orbital metastases appear as masses having high CT attenuation values and irregular margins, and they show slight-to-moderate enhancement (23). Metastases to the sphenoid wing are often seen as a mass in the lateral orbit as well as in the middle cranial fossa, and they can be confused with meningiomas; however, meningiomas show greater enhancement, and angiographic demonstration of a middle meningeal arterial supply to the mass favors meningioma (23). In the differential diagnosis of orbital metastases, orbital myeloma always should be a consideration. The diagnosis of orbital myeloma in the presence of generalized multiple myeloma does not usually create a problem. Myeloma presenting only with proptosis usually is only diagnosed on a biopsy specimen (Fig. 13.27) (39). Multiple myeloma can affect the eye in many ways. Involvement of the conjunctiva (4), cornea (1), ciliary body (2), sclera, choroid, and iris (2, 7) have all been described. Clark (10) had divided orbital myeloma into two categories: 1) primary orbital myeloma, in which the patient has ocular features suggestive of an orbital tumor and the lesion arises from the walls or contents of the orbit (Fig. 13.27) (1, 2, 7, 10, 39); and 2) secondary orbital myeloma, in which the patient has paraorbital myeloma (nasal, paranasal sinuses, nasopharynx, and cranial bones), resulting in secondary orbital invasion (1, 2, 7, 10, 39). Myeloma generally occurs in the 40–70-year-old age group (39); however we have seen it in three patients under 34 years of age and also in several published reports on myeloma occurring in young patients (11, 31, 39). Paraorbital myeloma on CT scan appears as a mild to moderately enhanced soft-tissue tumor, with frequent tumor extension into the temporal fossa (Fig. 13.27). At times, myeloma may be only presenting as an intraconal or both intra- and extraconal mass with no extraorbital component.

Figure 13.26. Orbital metastasis. Axial CT scan showing extensive bone destruction of the posterior lateral wall of the right (*R*) orbit, with a marked soft-tissue mass (*M*) involving the right periorbital and retroorbital spaces in this patient with metastatic lung carcinoma.

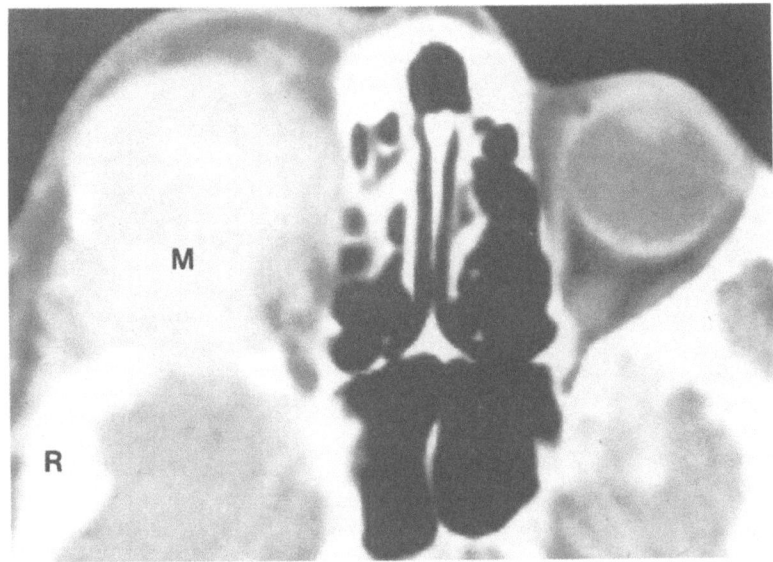

Meningioma

The most common tumor invading the orbit from outside the muscle cone is meningioma (25). Meningioma arising from the sphenoid wings, cavernous sinus, and parasellar region may extend into the orbit (Fig. 13.28) (20, 25, 29). Both intracranial and orbital soft-tissue components usually are enhanced with contrast media injection (Figs. 13.28 and 13.29). The tumor also frequently extends into the extracranial temporal fossa (Fig. 13.29). Hyperostotic changes of the adjacent bony structures often can be recognized on the CT scan (Fig.

13.28). A tumor originating from the sphenoid ridge and the vicinity of the cavernous sinus shows a tendency to spread along the surface of the meninges (51). This spread produces what has been called a meningioma en-plaque (Figs. 13.30 and 13.31) (51). A meningioma arising from the greater wing of the sphenoid typically displaces the lateral rectus muscle (Fig. 13.30 (25). An en-plaque meningioma tends to pass along the nerves that leave the cranium, especially in the superior orbital fissure and the optic foramina (51). It penetrates the dura early to involve the adjacent bone and usually produces a significant thickening (Figs.

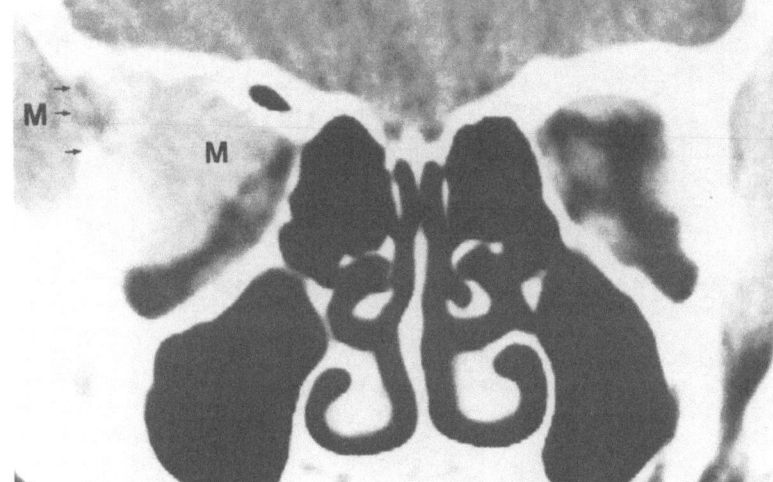

Figure 13.27. Orbital myeloma. Coronal CT scan showing bone destruction of the superolateral portion of the right orbit (arrows), with a large extra- and intraorbital soft-tissue mass (*M*) in this patient who presented initially with proptosis.

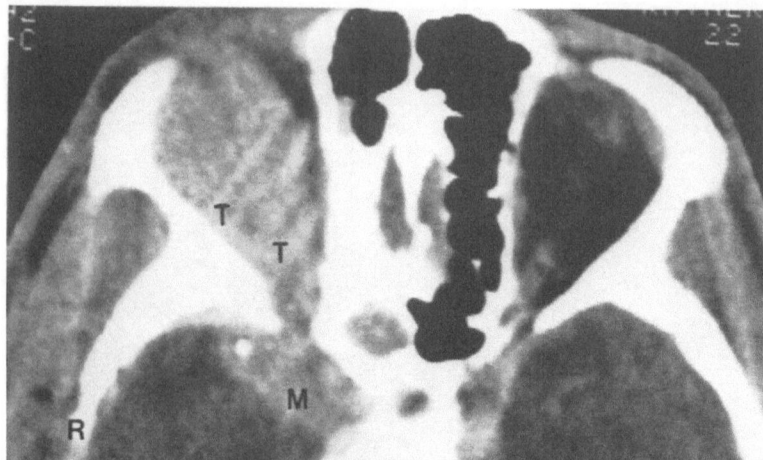

Figure 13.28. Meningioma. Axial CT scan showing recurrence (*M*) and extension of the right (*R*) middle cranial fossa meningioma (*M*) into the orbit (*T*). Note the hyperostotic changes of the adjacent greater wing of the sphenoid.

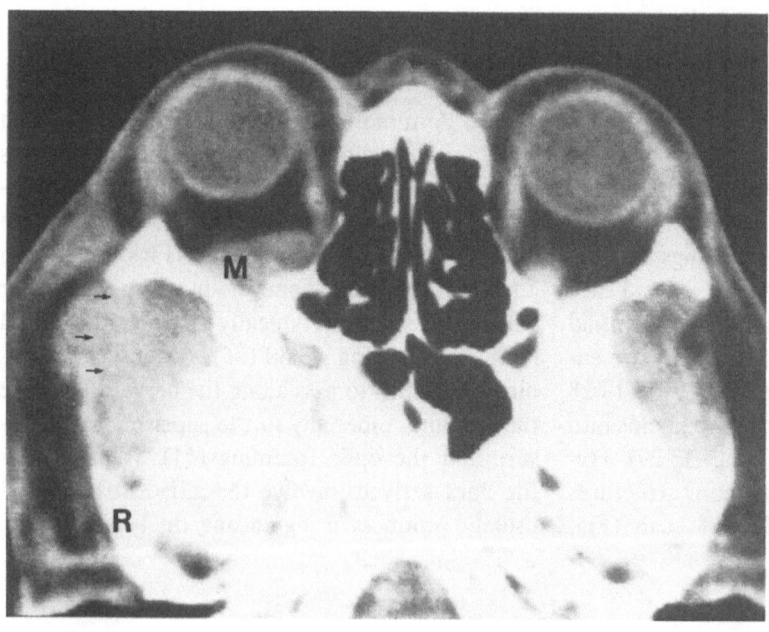

Figure 13.29. Meningioma. Axial CT scan showing extension of a right middle cranial fossa meningioma into both the right orbit (*M*) and the right infratemporal fossa (arrows). This patient presented with a nasopharyngeal mass, which revealed a meningioma in the biopsy specimen. The intracranial component of the tumor was barely recognized on the CT scan along the medial aspect of the right middle cranial fossa.

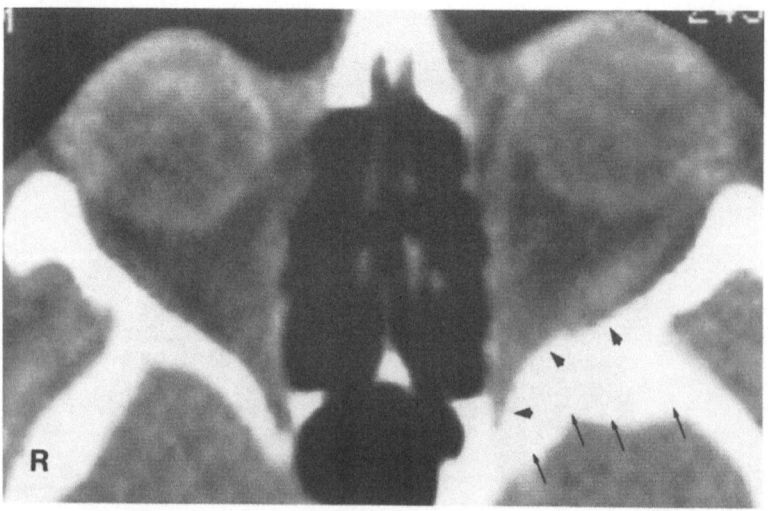

Figure 13.30. En-plaque meningioma. Axial CT scan showing marked hyperostotic changes of the greater wing of the left sphenoid along its intracranial (arrows) and intraorbital (arrow heads) portions. Note elevation of the thickened left lateral rectus. Despite marked hyperostotic changes, note that the intradural mass (soft-tissue component) is not recognized in this postinfusion CT scan.

Figure 13.31. En-plaque meningioma. Axial CT scan showing postsurgical changes of a left lateral orbitotomy and hyperostotic changes of the left greater wing of the sphenoid (arrows) and along the apex of the orbit (1). Note the recurrent soft-tissue mass (2) along the posterior aspect of the left eye.

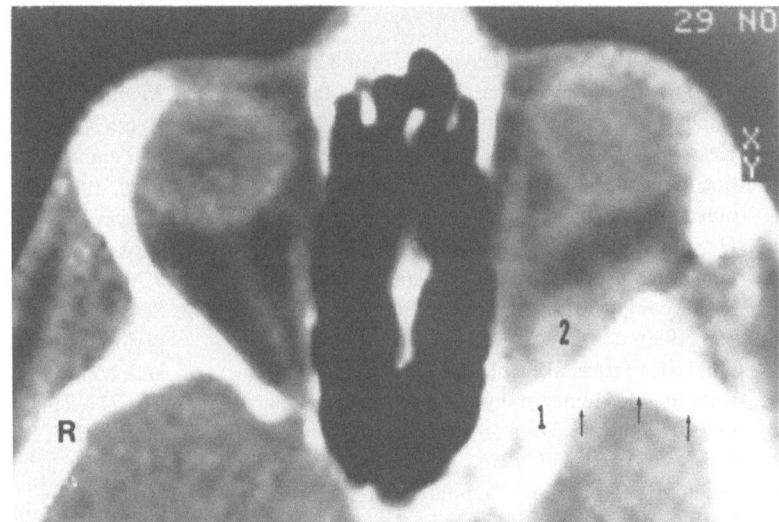

13.30 and 13.31). At times, the tumor cells may be widely disseminated through the adjacent bone, even though the intradural mass is no thicker than a few cell layers (Fig. 13.30) (51). A meningioma of the orbit may be en-plaque or globoid. One that originates primarily in the meninges around the optic nerve seldom invades the cranium, but it may involve the bony orbit (51). Extraconal meningioma may also arise from the orbital roof and, more rarely, from its floor (25). The importance of CT scans in meningiomas of the orbital wall is to determine the extent of the intra- and extraorbital components. Most important is the delineation of its medial boundary, so as to establish how close it is to the optic nerve and optic canal (25).

References

1. Aronson SB, Shaw R: Corneal crystalis in multiple myeloma. *Arch Ophthalmol* 61:541–546, 1979.
2. Ashton N: Ocular changes in multiple myelomatosis. *Arch Ophthalmol* 73:487–497, 1965.
3. Ballenger JJ: *Diseases of the Nose, Throat and Ear,* ed 11. Philadelphia, Lea & Febiger, 1969.
4. Benjamin F, Taylor H, Spindler J: Orbital and conjunctival involvement in multiple myeloma. *Am J Clin Pathol* 63:811–817, 1975.
5. Bernstein L: Pediatric sinus problems. *Otolaryngol Clin North Am* 4:127, 1971.
6. Bergstrom L, Hemenway WJ, Barnhart RA: Rhinocerebral and otologic mucormycosis. *Ann Otol* 79:70–81, 1970.

7. Bronstein M: Ocular involvement in multiple myeloma. *Arch Ophthalmol* 55:188–192, 1956.
8. Carter BL: Computer tomography, Part III, in Valvassori GE, Potter GD, Hanafee WN, et al (eds): *Radiology of the Ear, Nose and Throat.* Stuttgart, Georg Thieme Verlag, 1982, pp 212–240.
9. Centeno RS, Bentson RJ, Mancuso AA: CT scanning in rhinocerebral mucormucosis and aspergillosis. *Radiology* 140:383–389, 1981.
10. Clark F: Plasma cell myeloma of the orbit. *Br J Ophthalmol* 37:543–554, 1953.
11. Clough V, Delamore IW, Whittaker JA: Multiple myeloma in a young woman. *Ann Intern Med* 86:117–118, 1977.
12. Courey WR, New PFJ, Price DL: Angiographic manifestations of craniofacial phycomycosis. Report of three cases. *Radiology* 103:329–334, 1972.
13. De Weese DD, Schleuning AJ II, Robinson LB: Mucormycosis of the nose and paranasal sinuses. *Laryngoscope* 75:1298–1407, 1965.
14. Eisenberg L, Wood T, Boles R: Mucormycosis. *Laryngoscope* 87:347–356, March 1977.
15. Ferry AP, Front RL: Carcinoma metastatic to the eye and orbit. 1—A clinical pathologic study of 227 cases. *Arch Ophthalmol* 92:276–286, 1974.
16. Green WH, Goldberg HI, Wohl GT: Mucormycosis infection of the craniofacial structures. *Am J Roentgenol* 101:802–806, 1967.
17. Grove AS Jr: Orbital trauma evaluation by computed tomography. *Comput Tomogr* 3:267–278, 1979.
18. Hassani SN, Bard RL: Real-time ophthalmic ultrasonography. *Radiology* 127:213–219, 1978.
19. Hawkins DD, Clark RW: Orbital involvement in acute sinusitis. *Clinical Pediatrics* 16(5):464–471, 1977.

20. Henderson JW: *Orbital Tumors*. Philadelphia, WB Saunders, 1973.
21. Hesselink JR, New PH, Davis KR, et al: Computer tomography of the paranasal sinuses and face. Part I and II. *J Comput Assist Tomog* 2:559–576, 1978.
22. Hesselink JR, Weber AL, New PFJ, et al: Evaluation of mucoceles of the paranasal sinuses with computed tomography. *Radiology* 133:397, 1979.
23. Hesselink JR, Davis KR, Weber AL, et al: Radiological evaluation of orbital metastasis, with emphasis on computed tomography. *Radiology* 137:363–366, 1980.
24. Hilal SK, Trokel SL, Coleman DJ: High resolution computerized tomography and B-scan ultrasonography of the orbits. *Trans Am Acad Ophthalmol Otolaryngol* 81:607–617, 1976.
25. Hilal SK, Trokel SL: Computerized tomography of the orbit using thin sections. *Senin Roentgenol* 12:137–147, 1977.
26. Hubert L: Orbital infection due to nasal sinusitis. *NYS J Med* 37:1559, 1937.
27. Khoo TK, Sujai K, Leong TK: Disseminated aspergillosis. Case report and review of the world literature. *Am J Clin Pathol* 45:697–704, June 1966.
28. Kronschnabel EF: Orbital apex syndrome due to sinus infection. *Laryngoscope* 84:353, 1974.
29. Lampert VL, Zelch JV, Cohen DM: Computed tomography of the orbits. *Radiology* 113:351–354, 1974.
30. Lazo A, Wilner HI, Metes JJ: Craniofacial mucormycosis: Computed tomography and angiographic findings in two cases. *Radiology* 139:623–626, 1981.
31. Levin SR, Spaulding AG, Wirman JA: Multiple myeloma orbital involvement in a youth. *Arch Ophthalmol* 95:642–644, 1977.
32. Lloyd GA: The impact of CT scanning and ultrasonography on orbital diagnosis. *Clin Radiol* 28:583–593, 1977.
33. Lundgreen A, Olin T: Muco-pyocele of sphenoidal sinus or posterior ethmoidal cells with special reference to the apex orbital syndrome. *Acta Otolaryngol* 53:61, 1961.
34. Mafee MF, Valvassori GE: Radiology of the craniofacial anomalies. *Otolaryngol Clin North Am* 14(4):939–988, 1981.
35. Mafee MF, Goldberg MF, Valvassori GE, et al: Computed tomography in the diagnosis of persistent hyperplastic primary vitreous (PHPV). *Radiology* 145:713–717, 1982.
36. Mafee MF: Computerized tomography (CT) and its application to otolaryngology, in Ballenger JJ (ed): *Diseases of the Nose, Throat and Ear, ed 13*. Philadelphia, Lea & Febiger, 1985, pp. 810–85.
37. Noyek AM, Kassel EE, Wortzman G, et al: Sophisticated CT and complex maxillofacial trauma. *Laryngoscope* 92(6, Suppl 27):1–17, 1982.
38. Pillsbury HC, Fischer ND: Rhinocerebral mucor-

mycosis. *Arch Otolaryngol* 103:600–604, 1977.
39. Price HI, Danziger A, Wainwright HC, et al: CT of orbital multiple myeloma. *American Journal of Neuroradiology* 1:573–575, 1980.
40. Reese AB: Metastatic tumors of the eye and adnexa, in *Tumors of the Eye*, ed 3, New York, Harper & Row, 1976, chap 16, pp 423–431.
41. Reeves DL, Dickson DR, Benjamin EL: Phycomycosis (mucormycosis) of the central nervous system. *J Neurosurg* 23:82–84, 1965.
42. Seigel RS, Williams AG, Hutchison JW, et al: Subperiosteal hematomas of the orbit. Angiographic and computed tomographic diagnosis. *Radiology* 143:711–714, 1982.
43. Smith HW, Yanagisawa E: Rhinomucormycosis: Report of a fatal case. *N Engl J Med* 260:1007–1012, 1959.
44. Som PM, Shugar JMA: The classification of ethmoid mucoceles. *J Comput Assist Tomogr* 4:199–203, 1980.
45. Tadmor R, New PF: Computed tomography of the orbit with special emphasis on coronal sections; Part I and II normal and pathological anatomy. *J Comput Assist Tomogr* 2:24–44, 1978.
46. Tveten L: Cerebral mycosis. A clinical-pathological report of four cases. *Acta Neurol Scand* 41:19–33, 1965.
47. Valvassori GE, Putterman AM: Ophthalmologic and roentgenographic findings in sphenoidal mucoceles. *Trans Am Acad Ophthalmol Otolaryngol* November-December 1973, 77:703–713.
48. Warwick R and Williams PL: *Gray's Anatomy*, British ed, 35. Philadelphia, WB Saunders, 1973.
49. Welsh LW, Welsh JJ: Orbital complications of sinus disease. *Laryngoscope* 84:848, 1974.
50. Whitwell J: Spontaneous hematoma of the orbit. *Br J Ophthalmol* 40:250–251, 1956.
51. Wilson CB, Moossy J, Boldrey EB, et al: Pathology of intraorbital tumors, in Newton TH, Potts DG (eds): *Radiology of the Skull and Brain. Anatomy and Pathology*. St Louis, CV Mosby, 1976, chap 93, pp 3016–3048.
52. Wolter JR: Superiosteal hematomas of the orbit in young males: A serious complication of trauma or surgery in the eye region. *Trans Am Ophthalmol Soc* 77:104–120, 1979.
53. Zilkha A: Computed tomography of blow-out fracture of the medial orbital wall. *American Journal of Neuroradiology* 2:427–429, September–October 1981.
54. Gilbard SM, Mafee MF, Lagouros PA, Langer BG. The prognostic significance of computed tomography of orbital blow-out fractures (in press) Ophthalmology.
55. Zizmor J, Noyek AM: Cysts, benign tumors, and malignant tumors of the paranasal sinuses. *Otolaryngol Clin North Am* 6:(2):487–507, 1973.

14
Computed Tomography in Evaluation of the Orbits in Patients with Basal and Squamous-Cell Tumors of the Face

Hossein Firooznia and Cornelia Golimbu

The computed tomographic (CT) evaluation of the orbit is helpful in assessing the spread of cutaneous basal cell and squamous cell carcinomas. The CT examination shows areas of involvement that are not seen by other methods. This information is valuable for planning treatment.

Basal cell carcinoma is the most common carcinoma involving the scalp and face. It usually begins as a discrete, small, pearly papule that slowly enlarges; over several months to years, it may ultimately undergo central necrosis leading to ulceration. Most basal cell carcinomas are slow-growing. They remain relatively small (under 1 cm.) and do not invade underlying tissues, even when present for years. A significant number of larger (greater than 2 cm.) basal cell carcinomas also do not invade beyond the subcutaneous fat. However, there is a subgroup of primary basal cell carcinomas that are significantly more aggressive in growth and invasiveness. These lesions may grow relatively rapidly and may invade the underlying tissues extensively. At present, there is no clinical or microscopic way to identify this subgroup (2, 3, 8, 9, 11).

Squamous cell carcinomas of the head and neck are widely variable in biological aggressiveness. Some of these lesions may invade the underlying tissues very extensively. Squamous cell carcinomas are potentially dangerous lesions; they not only have the ability to metastasize via the lymphatic system and blood vessels, but also regionally along the nerve sheaths. Peripheral portions of the fifth and seventh cranial nerves seem to be most commonly involved. This is extremely important, because these neural extensions of the tumor can invade the brain.

Both basal and squamous cell tumors may arise on the bridge of the nose, eyelids, and inner canthus. For basal cell tumors of the head and neck, these areas are the most common sites of involvement. These tumors may invade the nasal cavity, orbits, and ethmoidal sinuses—and through these, the brain. The management of these lesions is particularly difficult, because clinical presurgical assessment of the precise extent of these lesions is practically impossible. Prior to the CT era, tomography, bone scanning, and angiography had to be performed to detect bone erosion and extension of these tumors into the orbits and/or cranium. At present, in the vast majority of patients, a tailored high-resolution CT examination of the orbits will detect erosion of bone and invasion of the orbits, ethmoid cells, and nasal cavities (1, 4–7, 10, 12).

Technique

Basal and squamous cell tumors of the orbital region usually infiltrate along the walls, floor, and roof of the orbit; they may extend into the brain, ethmoidal cells, and maxillary sinuses. For these reasons, axial slices are needed for evaluation of the medial and lateral wall, and coronal slices are needed for the floor and roof of the orbit. The study has to be monitored by a physician while it is being performed. If the lesion is noted to extend beyond the orbit (e.g., inferiorly into the maxillary sinus), appropriate slices must be obtained to include all of the involved periorbital tissues. The patient's head must remain absolutely motionless during the examination. Computed tomographic studies with very high spatial resolution are needed for detection of minute changes along

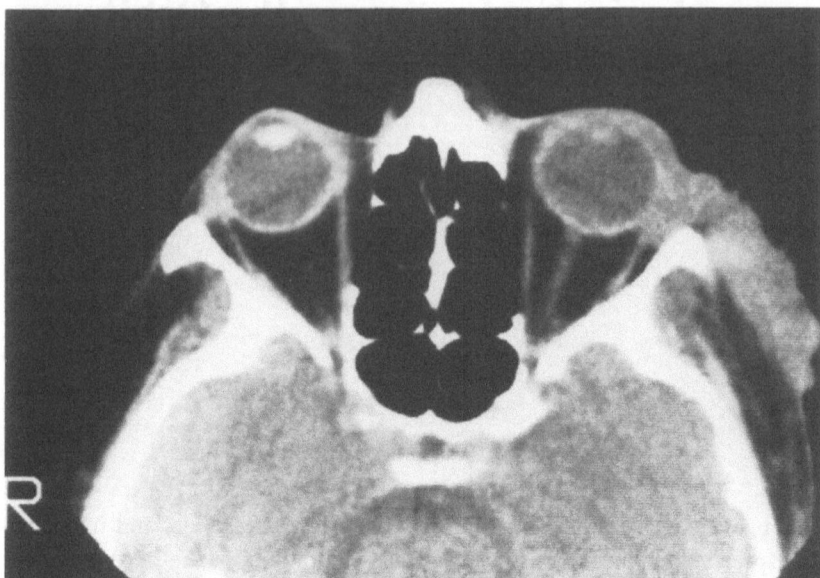

Figure 14.1. A soft-tissue mass is shown extending onto the surface of the face into the left orbit on its lateral side, along the lateral orbital wall, and over the surface of the globe. The tumor was attached to the surface of the globe and the lateral rectus muscle.

the walls of the orbit and for an assessment of the integrity of the ethmoidal cells and retroorbital structures. If the lesion is fairly large (i.e., several centimeters or more), consecutive 5-mm slices are obtained. In smaller lesions, 1.5-mm or thinner slices (if possible) are desirable. Although it is possible to obtain axial images and then to produce coronal images with reformatting, we believe that to obtain both more information and a more accurate and precise localization of these lesions, both axial and coronal images should be obtained directly. For the axial images, the patient is supine.

A lateral scout view of the orbits is obtained. Then, axial images are obtained with the gantry tilted, so as to obtain images parallel to the axis of the orbit. The axial images must start at least a few millimeters above the roof and extend for a few millimeters below the floor of the orbit. The coronal images are obtained with the patient prone and the patient's head extended 60–65°. A lateral scout view is obtained. The coronal images are best obtained in a plane perpendicular to the axis of the orbits to lessen distortion of the image, although the gantry must be tilted so as to avoid

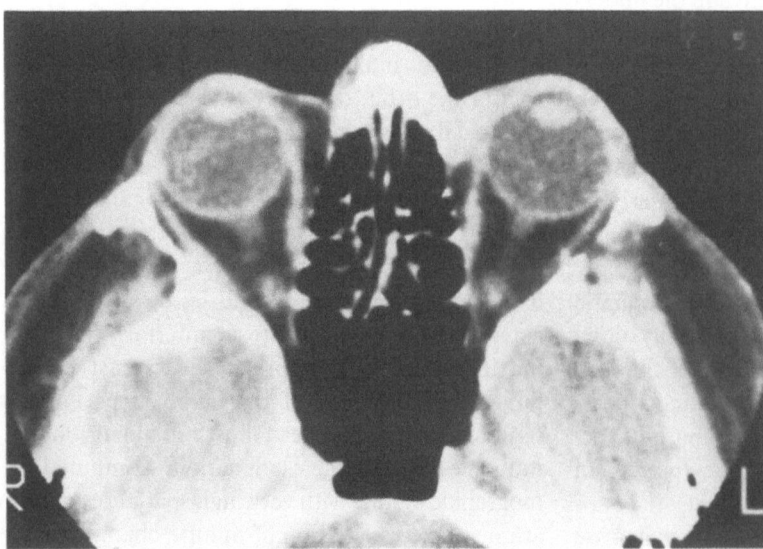

Figure 14.2. A soft-tissue mass is shown in the inner canthus of the left eye extending into the orbit and along the medial wall of the orbit. The mass lesion is attached to the globe and to the internal rectus muscle.

including metallic dental (molar) fillings in the images. For further evaluation, images in sagittal, off-axis sagittal, and other desired planes may be reformatted as needed (4–6). Intravenous (IV) contrast enhancement may be useful in these patients.

CT Findings

We have examined 42 patients with basal cell and squamous cell tumors of the face with a GE 8800 CT/T unit. Involvement of the orbit was found in 11 patients (Fig. 14.1). We found that the size of the tumor mass or ulceration on the skin surface usually was a fair indication of the extent of invasion of the underlying soft tissues; the smaller tumors essentially were limited to the skin with no (or only minimal) invasion of the underlying tissues. However, this was not always true. There were two patients with tumors measuring 7 mm

or less who had invasion of the underlying tissues beyond the confines of the base of the tumor (Fig. 14.2). This information was not available prior to CT examination. There were six patients with extensive involvement of the orbit, which consisted of infiltration by the mass along the medial wall and the floor of the orbit and invasion of the bone and extension of the tumor into the ethmoidal cells, through the medial wall, and into the maxillary sinuses through the floor of the orbit. There were two patients with erosion of the bony structures of the apex of the orbit, with the tumor extending into the cranium (Fig. 14.3). In one patient, the tumor had caused diffuse infiltration of the orbit. Nineteen patients were examined following surgery. Recurrence of the lesion was noted in five of these patients.

A CT-scan diagnosis of involvement of the orbit by basal cell carcinoma ordinarily is simple and based on demonstration of a mass lesion invading

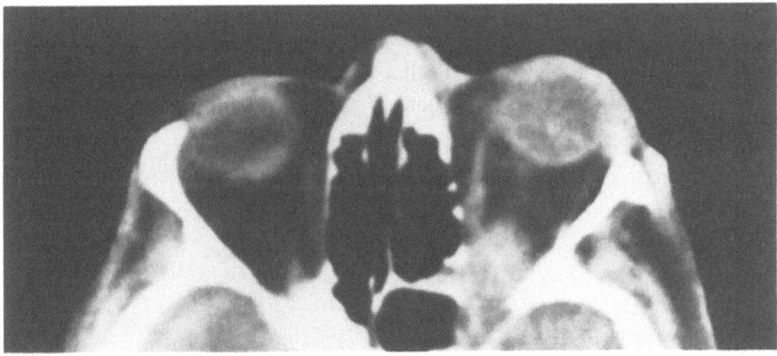

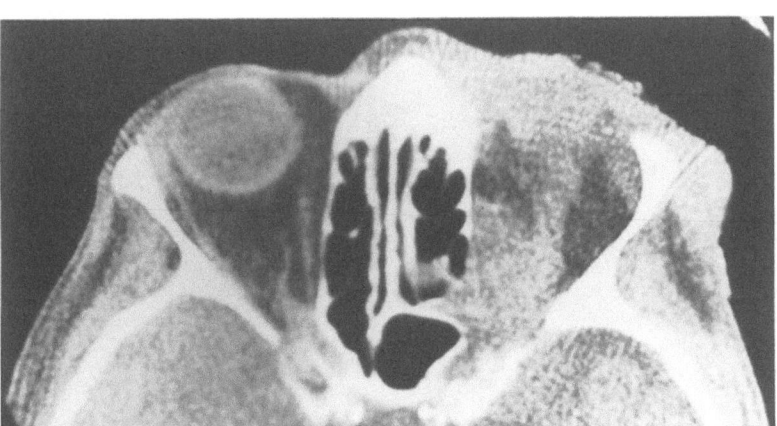

Figure 14.3. A soft-tissue mass is noted extending into the left orbit, along its lateral wall, and extending over the surface of the globe. A soft-tissue mass is noted at the apex of the left orbit, with destruction of bones of the apex of the orbit and with extension beyond this point. There is also destruction of the bones of the medial wall of the orbit posteriorly, with extension of the mass into the ethmoidal cells.

the orbit. In specific instances where an advanced basal cell carcinoma has caused extensive involvement of the orbit, the lesion has to be distinguished from infection, lymphoma, and pseudotumor of the orbit. Correlation with clinical and laboratory findings usually will establish the correct diagnosis.

In our experience, CT scanning is indispensable in presurgical assessment of the size and precise extent of invasion of the adjacent bone and soft tissues by these tumors. This information is critical for assessment of operability and for the planning of a proper course of treatment. Follow-up CT examinations will reveal thoroughness of tumor ablation, detect evidence of recurrence, and reveal extension of the lesion into new anatomic compartments.

References

1. Bilaniuk LT, Zimmerman RA: Computed tomography in evaluation of paranasal sinuses. *Rad Clin North Am* 20(1):50, 1982.
2. Conley JJ: Malignant tumors of the scalp. *Plast Reconstr Surg* 33:1, 1964.
3. Firooznia H, Kricheff I, Young R, et al: Basal cell carcinoma of head and neck: Radiologic evaluation and value of angiography. *NYS J Med* 71(4):429, 1971.
4. Forbes GS, Sheedy PF II, Waller RR: Orbital tumors evaluated by computed tomography. *Radiology* 136:101, 1980.
5. Forbes G: Computed tomography of the orbit. *Rad Clin North Am* 20(1):37, 1981.
6. Hesselink JR, Davis KR, Weber AL, et al: Radiological evaluation of orbital metastases, with emphasis on computed tomography. *Radiology* 137:363, 1980.
7. Leo JS, Halpern J, Sackler JP: Computed tomography in the evaluation of orbital infections. *Comput Tomogr* 4:133, 1980.
8. Lund HZ: How often does squamous-cell carcinoma of the skin metastasize? *Arch Dermatol* 92:635, 1965.
9. MacKenzie I, Tucker HH: Extensive malignant lesions of the scalp. *Can J Surg* (7:64, 1964.
10. Nugent RA, Routman J, Robertson WD, et al: Acute orbital pseudotumors: Classification and CT features. *American Journal of Roentgenology* 137:957, 1982.
11. Pollack SV: Moh's chemosurgery for skin cancer. *Progr Dermatol* 14:1, 1980.
12. Zimmerman RA, Bilaniuk LT: CT of orbital infection and its cerebral complications. *American Journal of Roentgenology* 134:45, 1980.

15
Infection of the Orbit

K. Jack Momose

Orbital infections often are local, self-limited lesions arising in different areas. They can potentially progress to damage the eye, produce blindness, or develop life-threatening intracranial complications (27). In addition to other laboratory examinations, imaging studies can help in the diagnosis and management of these infections by demonstrating the local lesion and its extent (if any) into surrounding anatomic structures (i.e., paranasal sinuses and intracranial spaces). All imaging methods may be employed in studying these infections. Ultrasonography, computed tomography (CT), and Magnetic Resonance Imaging (MRI) are especially helpful in showing soft tissues (12, 27). This information can indicate which lesions should be treated with antibiotics alone and which will require surgical drainage as well. High resolution CT scans and magnetic resonance image with surface coil can show changes of the intraocular structures which was previously not possible except by ultrasonography.

The bacteria most commonly involved in ophthalmologic infections are staphylococcus, streptococcus, pneumococcus, pseudomonas, neisseriaceae, hemophilus, and mycobacteria. Staphylococcus and streptococcus are causal agents of diseases of the eyelids, conjunctiva, and cornea. Pneumococcus is a common etiologic factor in infectious corneal ulcers. Pseudomonas is a cause of corneal ulcers, endophthalmitis, meibomanitis, and blepharoconjunctivitis. Neisseriaceae infection results in a purulent conjunctivitis. Hemophilus may be responsible for acute bacterial conjunctivitis, orbital cellulitis, episcleritis, and a distinct form of preseptal cellulitis in children between 6–

36 months of age (19). Mycobacterium tuberculosis can affect nearly all ocular tissues, often starting as a form of lupus vulgaris that may spread to produce ulceration, scarring, ectropion, and keratitis. Tuberculosis also may involve the uveal tract.

Herpes simplex and Herpes zoster are the major virus infections of the orbit. They may mimic orbital cellulitis, or a true cellulitis may develop from secondary infection. Herpes simplex often causes ocular disease, corneal dendritic scarring, blepharoconjunctivitis in the newborn, and (rarely) a diffuse chorioretinitis associated with encephalitis. Herpes simplex infection often begins as a keratoconjunctivitis. Herpes zoster infection usually involves the ophthalmic division of the trigeminal nerve but any division may be involved. The skin lesions of Herpes zoster may involve the eyelids or lid margins and can lead to permanent scarring of these areas. Late complications may develop in almost any segment of the eye due to zoster involvement.

The number of fungal infections seen by the ophthalmologist has increased in the past 25 years secondary to the use of immunosuppressive drugs, the increased longevity of debilitated patients, and the long-standing use of intravenous (IV) hyperalimentation (4). Candida albicans is frequently implicated in endogenous fungal endophthalmitis. Aspergillus fumigatus, coccidioides immitis, blastomyces dermatidis, cryptococcus neoformans, and other phycomycetes may be involved in ophthalmic infections. Actinomyces may cause a canaliculitis and may form fungus balls in the tear sac.

In severely immune-suppressed patients (11)

and in the acidotic diabetic patient, mucormycosis (Absidian rhizopus and Mucor infection) may develop with a severe nasosinoorbital involvement (see Chapter 13).

Eyelid

A knowledge of the anatomy of the eyelid is needed to understand infections involving it. This anatomy is illustrated in Figure 15.1. Infection of the skin of the eyelid with streptococci and staphylococci may lead to folliculitis, with multiple pustules surrounding individual hairs around pilosebaceous orifices. Furuncles are in deeper position in the eyelid, and they vary in size. External hordeolum (sty) essentially is a staphylococcal abscess of the eyelash follicle and gland of Zeis. An internal hordeolum (acute chalazion) is acute staphylococcal infection of a meibomian gland. It occurs on the conjunctival side of the eyelid. Chalazion is a chronic granuloma of a meibomian gland char-

acterized by swelling due to retention of meibomian secretions and by formation of granulation tissue. It may remain contained in the tarsus or it may break through anteriorly beneath the skin (dumbbell chalazion); or it may break through on the conjunctival side to produce a fistula through which granulation tissue protrudes (1). Acute infection of the eyelid is a very common condition. The patient presents with pain in the lid margin. There is generalized periorbital edema due to inflammation in the preseptal or postseptal spaces. Pus may be discharged from the infected eyelid. The CT scan generally shows periorbital swelling, with distention of the preseptal space.

Conjunctiva

The conjunctiva forming the inner lining of the eyelid is contiguous with the lining of the lacrimal apparatus, is reflected over the globe, and is continuous with the limbus of the cornea. Inflammation

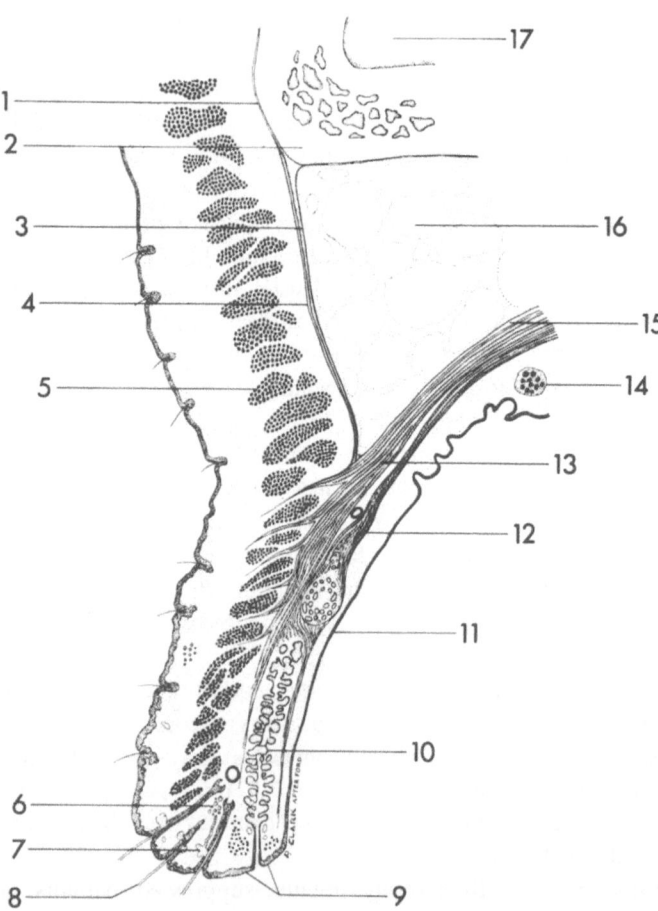

Figure 15.1. Diagram of the eyelid: (1) Periosteum; (2) Bone; (3) Orbital septum; (4) Preseptal space; (5) Orbicularis oculi; (6) Gland of Moll; (7) Gland of Zeis; (8) Eyelash; (9) Tarsal plate; (10) Meibomian gland; (11) Conjunctiva; (12) Muller muscle; (13) Fibers of levator muscle; (14) Gland of Krause; (15) Postseptal space; (16) Fat; (17) Frontal sinus.

of the cornea results in photophobia, tearing, itchiness, and an irritating sensation. Conjunctivitis can be noninflammatory (allergy, drug reaction) or inflammatory (11). Discharge from conjunctivitis may be watery, sanguinous, or purulent. Swelling (chemosis) of the conjunctiva or eyelid may be caused by edema or cellular infiltration. Such cases generally show generalized periorbital edema on CT scans.

Sclera

The sclera is the outer coat of the eye that supports the eye and protects the inner structure. It is fibrous and is nearly devoid of blood vessels. Inflammation of the loose connective tissue over the sclera is called episcleritis. It is often localized over one quadrant of the globe. The area is tender to touch, and it may be a forerunner of iritis or iridocyclitis. Scleritis is a rare disease that is often associated with rheumatoid arthritis. Scleritis may take a malignant form and develop localized necrosis, ulceration, and eventual perforation (scleromalacia perforans).

Uveal Tract

The uvea includes the iris, ciliary body, and choroid. Inflammation of the iris and the ciliary body is known as anterior uveitis. Lesions behind the iris and ciliary body are referred to as posterior uveitis. Inflammation of the choroid may exist as single or multiple focal inflammatory spots of choroiditis. Acute choroiditis is the most resistant form of uveitis. It is manifested by a huge elevated abscess involving practically the entire superior or inferior quadrant. Chronic uveitis commonly involves either the posterior pole or portions of the entire uveal tract. This usually is a devastating progressive disease that frequently causes blindness unless the disease process is interrupted (14).

Cornea

The cornea is the transparent structure that forms the anterior part of the fibrous tunic of the eye. It consists of five layers: 1) the anterior corneal epithelium continuous with that of the conjunctiva; 2) the basement membrane of the epithelium; 3) the stroma; 4) Descemet's membrane; and 5)

the endothelium. The cornea is well protected by its own tough structure, as well as by the eyelid. The corneal surface also is protected by tearing and by the blink reflex. Most diseases affecting the cornea can be identified on the basis of clinical appearance alone. Bacteria-produced ulcerations of the cornea usually are pyogenic in variety and occur as a result of a break in the corneal epithelium through trauma, edema, or drying. A typical bacterial ulcer usually is situated centrally or paracentrally in the cornea. The bacteria that produce corneal ulcers are staphylococcus aureus and epidermitis, diplococcus pneumoniae, streptococcus hemolyticus, pseudomonas aerogenosa, and Friedlander's bacillus, and others.

Lacrimal System

For normal functioning of the eye, an adequate supply of fluid is required to cover its surface. The maintenance of the fluid covering the eye is dependent on the secretory and excretory mechanisms. The secretory component includes the lacrimal gland, the accessory lacrimal gland, the sebaceous glands of the eyelids, and mucin-secreting cells of the conjunctiva (15). The elimination of the lacrimal secretion is dependent on the lacrimal drainage system. The drainage system (see Fig. 6.1) consists of the lacrimal puncta, canaliculi, nasolacrimal sac, and nasolacrimal duct. Dacryocystitis can result from intermittent or constant obstruction anywhere along the course of the lacrimal drainage system (15). The retained normal secretions of the eye provide a favorable media for bacterial growth. Obstruction in the nasolacrimal system can be congenital in origin or secondary to trauma or inflammation spreading from the sinuses or other adjacent structures of the nasolacrimal system. Acute dacryocystitis is usually caused by pneumococci, streptococci, and staphylococci. Chronic dacryocystitis can be due to pneumococci, streptococci, staphylococci, hemophilus, pseudomonas, and Escherichia coli. In mycotic canaliculitis, the concretions most commonly formed by actinomyces israeli can present an almost diagnostic appearance on x-ray films. The canaliculi are dilated, there are filling defects resulting from the concretions lying in the canaliculi or the sac, the system usually irrigates through to the nose, and there may be diverticuli or fistulas originating from the canaliculi or the sac. Periorbital cellulitis is seen with acute dacryocystitis, with or without occlusion of the nasolacrimal sac. Dacryocystography is required to demonstrate the point of obstruction (Figs. 15.2 and 15.3) (see Chapter 6).

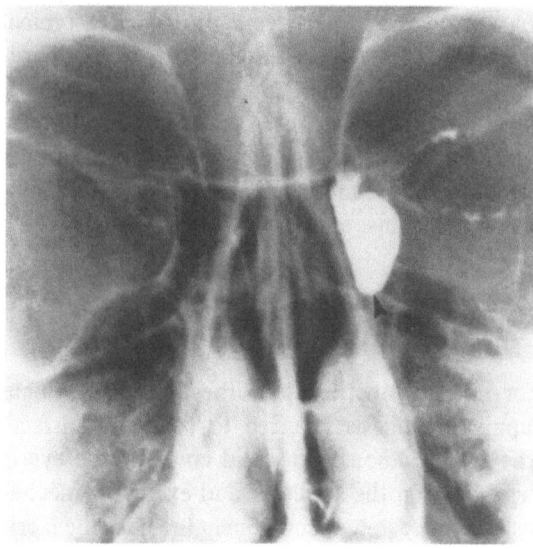

Figure 15.2. A 62-year-old woman complaining of unilateral overflow tearing. The dacryocystogram shows dilation of the nasolacrimal sac due to a complete block at the junction (arrow) between it and the nasolacrimal duct, thus demonstrating changes due to dacryocystitis.

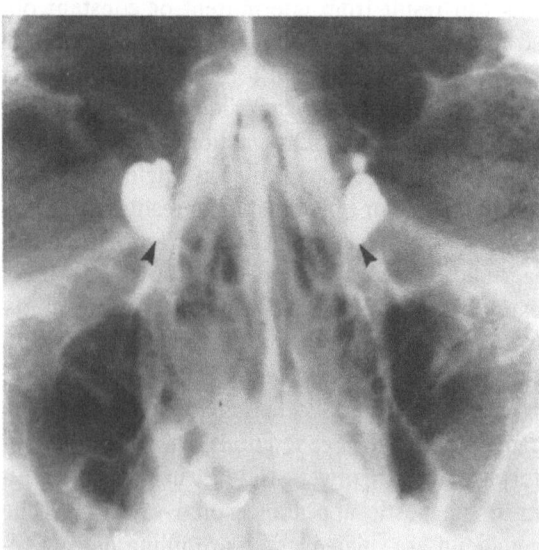

Figure 15.3. A 60-year-old man with bilateral overflow tearing. Blocks are shown at the junction (arrows) of the sac with the nasolacrimal duct, indicating bilateral dacryocystitis.

Paranasal Sinuses

Direct extension of purulent sinusitis (23) is the most common cause of orbital cellulitis, especially in young patients (18). It is estimated that 60% of orbital cellulitis results from sinus etiology (24, 26). In children, ethmoid or sphenoid sinusitis is the most likely source of infection. The anatomic factors that make orbital cellulitis a common condition is the intimate relationship between the orbit and the sinuses. The "paper plate" of the ethmoid sinus separates the content of the bony orbit from the ethmoid sinuses (6), and it may have preexisting foramina or congenital dehiscence. The lack of lymphatic drainage of the orbit and the lack of valves in the ophthalmic venous system also allow easy bacterial invasion of the orbit. Orbital cellulitis and abscess affecting the fibrofatty tissue results from the interference of the venous drainage of the orbital content and the infection of the ethmoid sinus (16). With the addition of a bacterial phlebitis and direct entry of bacteria into perivascular structures, orbital inflammatory and infective changes are likely to result.

Clinically, the patient will develop swelling of the eyelid, proptosis, limitation of movement of the eye, and loss of vision. During the stage of thrombophlebitis, there is proptosis due to edema; but there is a lack of pus macroscopically in the extravascular tissue, even though there are clots and pus in the veins (8). When the suppuration establishes itself in the tissues, rapid spread is the rule. A CT scan of the orbit will show orbital edema, subperiosteal abscess, and/or orbital abscess (see also Chapter 13).

Direction of Spread and Clinical Correlation

The pus from skin and paranasal sinus infections usually spreads anteriorly, perforating the skin of the eyelid or conjunctival fornix (16). Discharge of pus from the conjunctiva indicates that its site is within the orbital tissue. Nonspecific periorbital swelling is seen at this phase in CT scans; orbital edema cannot be distinguished from inflammation unless clinical information is obtained (Fig. 15.4). Alternately, if the pus spreads posteriorly, it may extend to the orbital apex through the sphenoidal fissure or optic canal and may produce necrosis about the surrounding tissue. Encapsulation of the

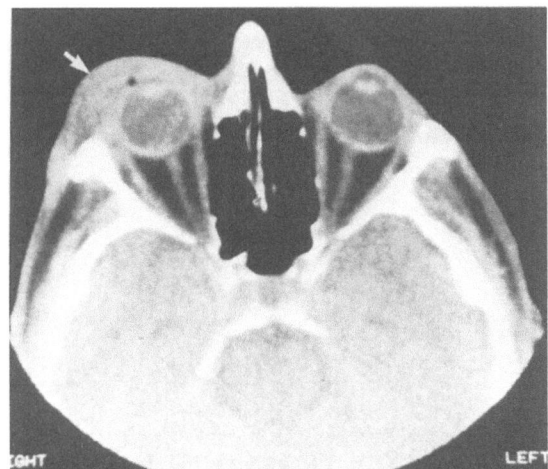

Figure 15.4. Axial CT scan showing severe preseptal space distention (arrow) and a slightly enlarged lateral rectus. These are the changes of periorbital cellulitis.

abscess rarely occurs, although this may be suggested in the CT scan and may not be found at surgery. The periosteum of the bony wall usually prevents inflammation from entering the orbital space. When a subperiosteal abscess develops, it appears as an elliptical mass with lucent tissue contiguous with the wall of the sinus, with a lateral curvilinear rim of variable thickness represented by a displaced periosteum. In time, the subperiosteal abscess may rupture spontaneously into the orbit. This can be prevented by surgical drainage.

Anterior Abscess-Producing Fistula in the Upper Eyelid

Frontal sinusitis may develop complications, such as orbital cellulitis, frontal bone osteomyelitis, meningitis, subdural empyema, and intracerebral abscess. If the infection extends into the diploic spaces from the frontal sinus, osteomyelitis can spread to any portion of the calvarium. In frontal sinusitis, subperiosteal abscess occurs most frequently in the superior temporal quadrant of the orbit. An abscess in the anterior portion of the orbit can produce osteoperiostitis. If untreated, the loculated pus may form a fistula. The most common site of the fistula in adults is under the upper margin of the eye near the center. It is near the inner margin in children when the frontal sinus is at fault.

Fistula in the Lower Eyelid

A special type of periostitis with orbital cellulitis can be seen during infancy. This is due to staphylococcal osteomyelitis of the maxillary sinus that results from an infection of the tooth bud, particularly the upper deciduous unerupted molar. Cavanaugh (5) collected 24 cases of this type. The child develops swelling of the lower lid and then both lids, with proptosis due to subperiosteal abscess in the floor of the orbit. The entire cheek swells; the abscess can point at the inner or outer canthus. An external fistula eventually develops, usually in the median part of the lower lid in the region of the lacrimal sac. Nasal discharge is often found on the affected side. Swelling and fistula may occur in the palate and alveolar process. Eventually, the entire maxillary bone may be involved unless the process is treated. The source of infection is often obscure. Some investigators maintain that the lacrimal sac is first affected, rather than the tooth bud; others believe that the maxillary sinus is the original site (5).

Orbital Cellulitis

With the use of CT scanning, the anatomic changes of the six different stages of orbital cellulitis (6) can be demonstrated in the axial and coronal views.

Preseptal Edema and Cellulitis

Superficial infection of the eyelids and bacterial facial cellulitis are confined initially to the preseptal portion of the eyelid. The orbital septum, which arises from the anterior bony orbit margin, inserts on the tarsal plates of the eyelid and acts as a barrier to the spread of infection into the orbit (Figs. 15.5 and 15.6). Eyelid edema is the first manifestation of preseptal orbital cellulitis. These changes are seen as periorbital swelling. The swelling is nonspecific, and simple edema cannot be distinguished from cellulitis on CT scanning. The position of the preseptal and postseptal spaces are well demonstrated in the axial views (Fig. 15.7). The other spaces to which the infection may spread can be shown in the axial and coronal views, including the intraconal space (central surgical space), extraconal space (peripheral surgical space), and subperiosteal space.

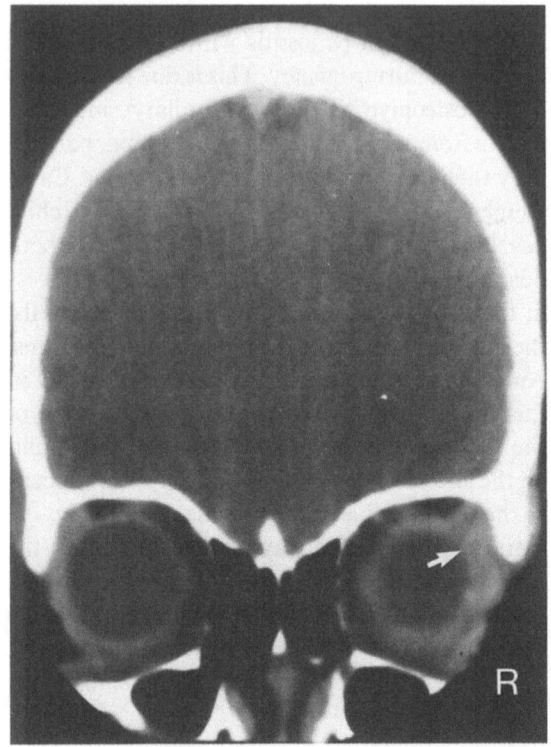

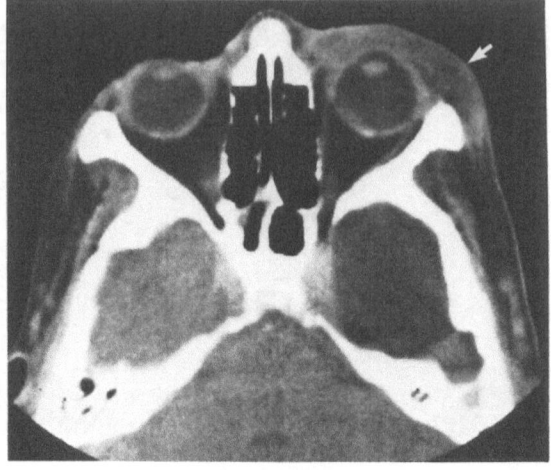

Figure 15.6. Periorbital cellulitis. A 47-year-old woman with erysipelas that had spread and developed swelling about the left eye. The axial CT scan shows changes of periorbital cellulitis involving the preseptal space. Note the considerable swelling in the preseptal space (arrow). This space was lanced, but no pus was shown except for serosanguinous fluid.

A

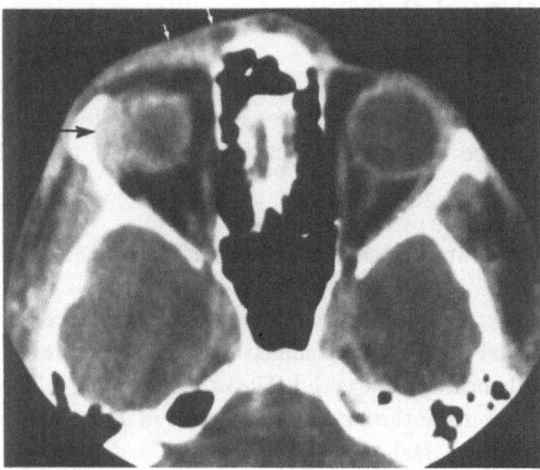

B

Figure 15.5. A 29-year-old man studied with CT scanning because of recent onset of periorbital edema on the right. **A.** Soft-tissue thickening in the lacrimal fossa and areas of the orbital rim (white arrow) seen on the coronal view. **B.** Periorbital swelling (white arrows) and thickening of the lacrimal gland (arrow) seen on the axial view indicating dacryoadenitis and adjacent periorbital cellulitis.

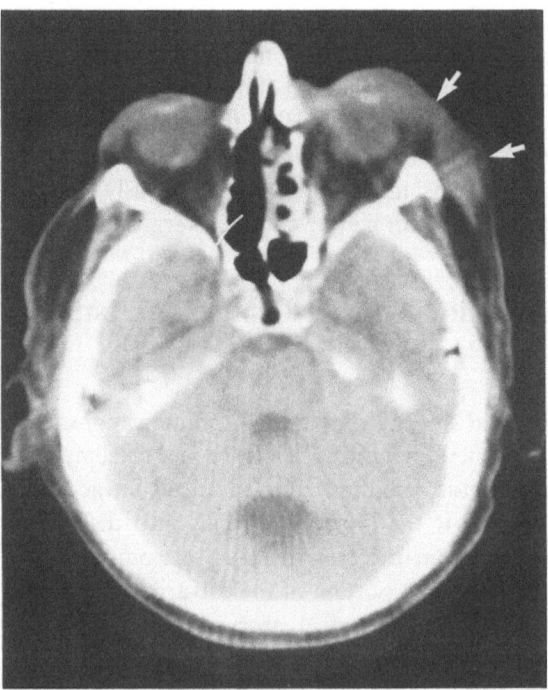

Figure 15.7. Axial CT scan showing distention of the preseptal space with extension to the lateral aspect of the orbit (arrows). Left ethmoiditis is present.

Intraconal Cellulitis

Inflammation of the intraconal space is shown on CT scanning by obliteration of the normal soft-tissue and fat planes between the optic nerve, retroorbital fat, and muscles. Rarely, infection within the intraconal space pushes the eye forward (Fig. 15.8)

Periostitis of Orbital Wall

The bony walls of the orbit formed by the frontal, ethmoid, and maxillary sinuses may show changed density in relation to the contiguous orbital tissue involved by cellulitis. These changes are suggested in the "paper plate" of the ethmoid sinus, when the contiguous medial rectus muscle and the periosteum are thickened (Figs. 15.9 and 15.10).

Subperiosteal Abscess

Progression of periostitis leads to subperiosteal abscess, which arises between the bony orbital wall and the periosteum. The periosteal abscess appears as an elliptical mass formed by the displaced periosteum, which forms its lateral border (Figs. 15.10, 15.11, and 15.12). The collected pus lies

medial to the dense periosteum and appears to be of low tissue density. The deformed periosteum, which encloses the pus, often enhances with IV contrast media. There may be gas within the abscess from gas-producing bacillus or from air in the communicating sinus. When ethmoiditis is the cause of the orbital cellulitis, the subperiosteal abscess acts as a mass, displacing the medial rectus muscle and the globe laterally. When the subperiosteal abscess develops from frontal sinusitis and occupies the superior aspect of the orbit, the globe is displaced anteriorly and downward.

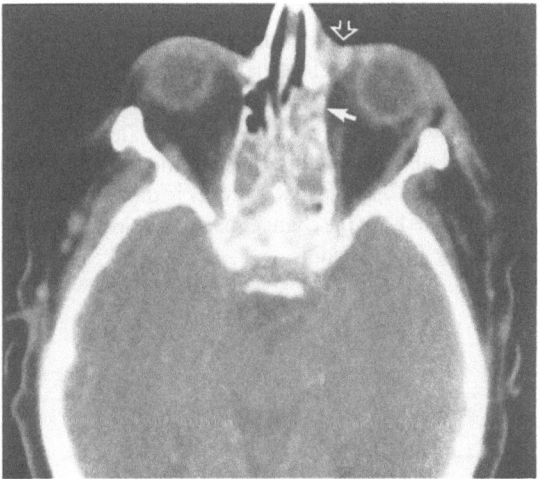

A

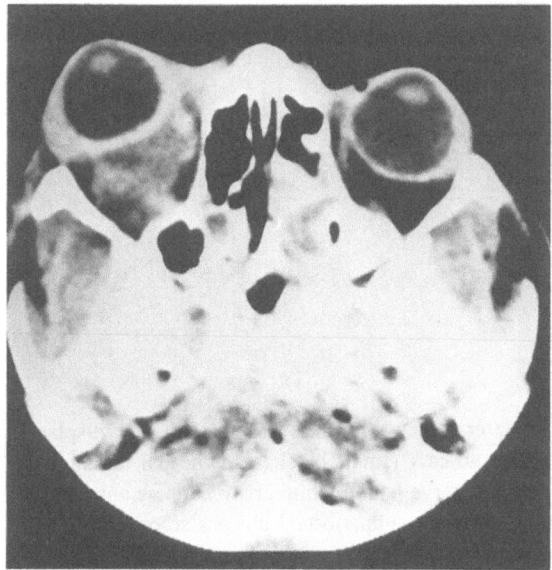

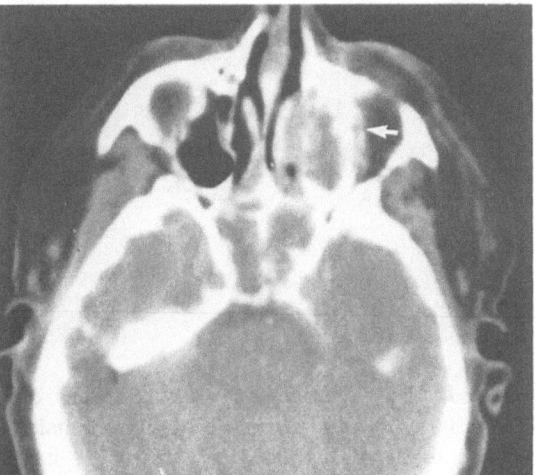

B

Figure 15.8. Orbital cellulitis. Axial CT scan shows obliteration of the normal soft-tissue and fat planes between the optic nerve and the muscles by inflammatory infiltrate on the left.

Figure 15.9. A 72-year-old woman seen with a complaint of headache, proptosis, and otorrhea. A. Ethmoid sinusitis (arrow) and periorbital edema (open arrowhead) are shown on the axial CT scan. B. The axial CT scan reveals a change of maxillary and sphenoid sinusitis with periostitis (arrow).

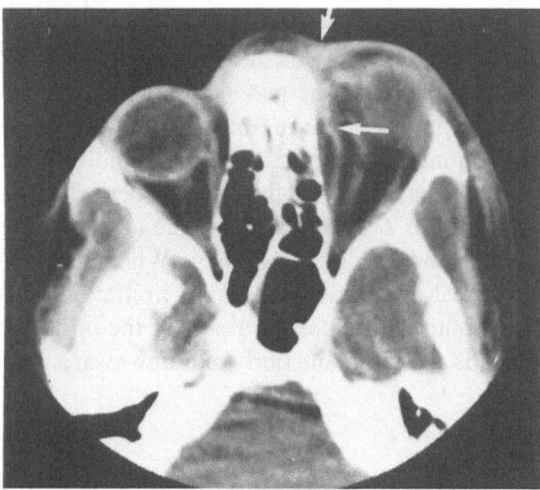

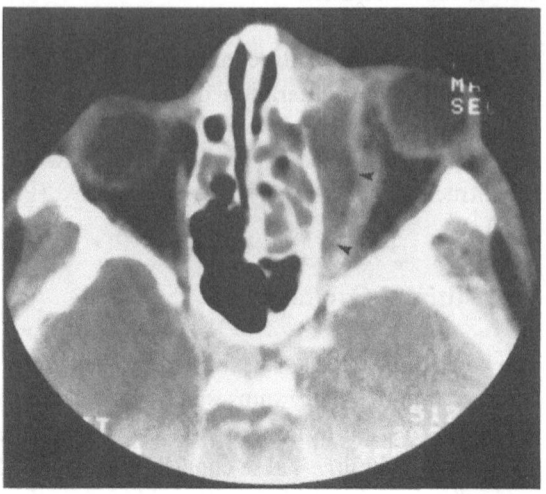

Figure 15.10. Patient with headaches and swelling about the left eye. The axial CT scan shows changes of preseptal (vertical arrow) and postseptal cellulitis in the medial canthal area of the left orbit (horizontal arrow) and also ethmoiditis. The left medial orbital wall periosteum is displaced laterally, as is the medial rectus muscle. These are the changes of a subperiosteal abscess secondary to ethmoiditis.

Figure 15.12. The axial CT scan demonstrates opacification of the left ethmoid sinus and marked lateral displacement of the periosteum of the medial orbital wall (arrowheads), which is adjacent to a displaced medial rectus muscle. The eyeball is displaced anterolaterally. This is a case of ethmoiditis with a large subperiosteal abscess.

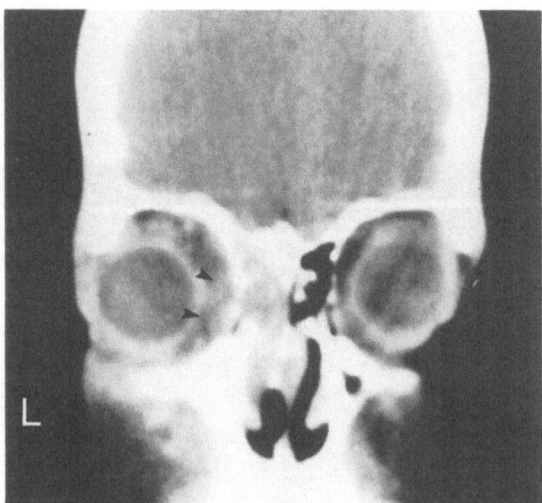

A

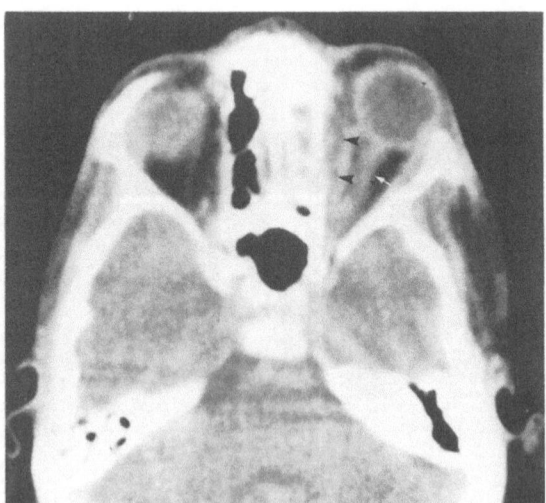

B

Figure 15.11. A. Patient seen with complaint of a "runny nose," headaches, and fever. Left ethmoiditis with periostitis and increased periosteal space lateral to the paper plate of the ethmoid (arrowheads), as seen on the coronal CT scan. **B.** In the axial view, the medial and lateral rectus muscles are swollen and displaced by the abscess (small black arrowheads), along with the optic nerve (small white arrow). These changes are indicative of a subperiosteal abscess secondary to ethmoiditis.

Orbital Abscess

Orbital abscess may develop within the preseptal space or retrobulbar space (20). It may be identified as an area of increased tissue density (Fig. 15.13) and/or by the presence of gas within the areas of soft-tissue changes in the preseptal, intraconal, or extraconal spaces. Epidural, subdural, and intracerebral abscesses are readily identified by their enhancing rims on CT scans (Fig. 15.14). Cerebritis is shown as an area of decreased density (without enhancement) with IV contrast media.

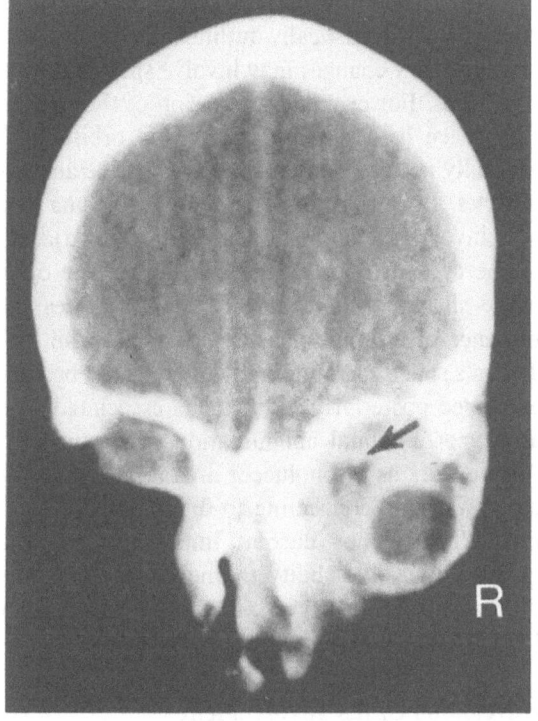

A

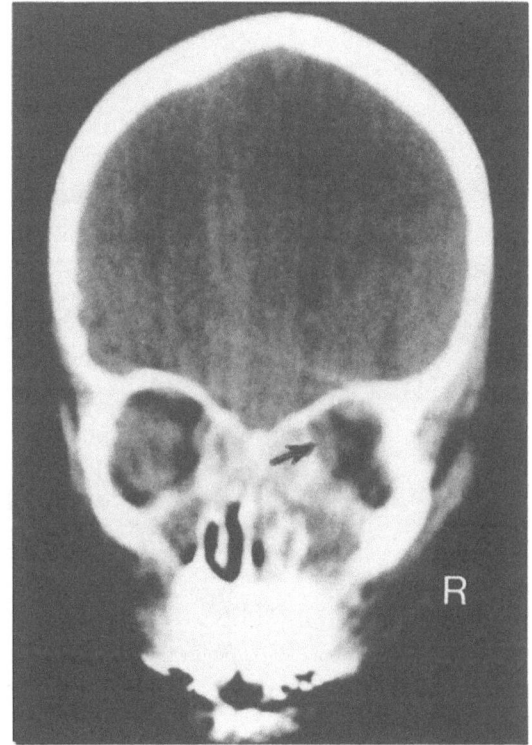

B

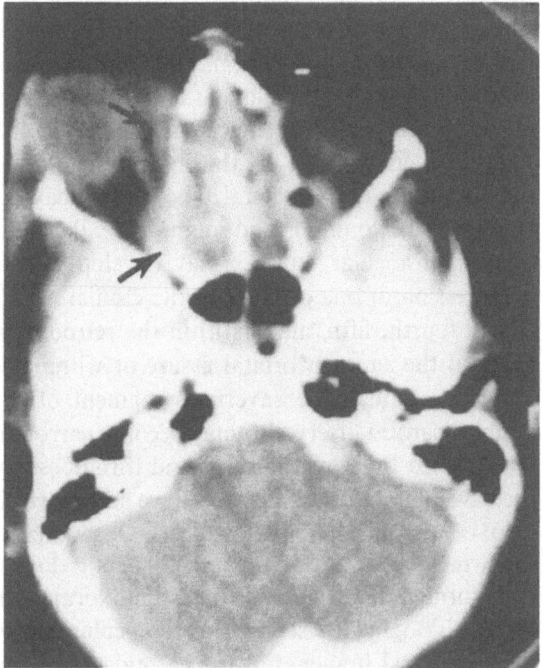

C

Figure 15.13. A. Anterior coronal CT scan showing a diffuse increase in density of the periocular fat, with gas seen in the medial superior area (arrow). The eyeball is displaced downward and laterally. **B.** Posterior coronal section behind the eye revealing a subperiosteal abscess lateral to the paper plate of the ethmoid (arrow). An increased density in the ethmoid and antra sinuses suggest a pansinusitis. **C.** A low-axial section shows the periorbital and retrobulbar cellulitis (arrows) and the forward displacement of the eyeball on the right. All of these changes suggest a medial orbital abscess secondary to pansinusitis.

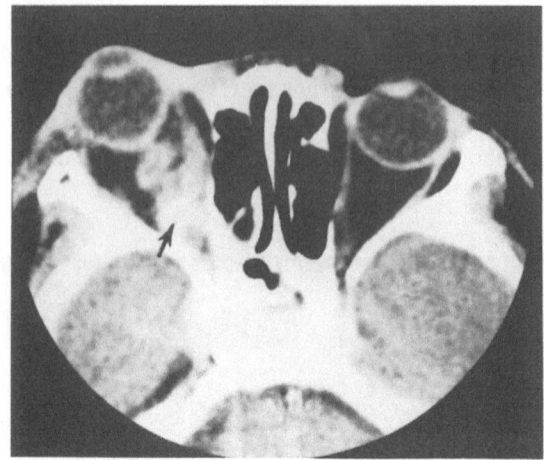

A

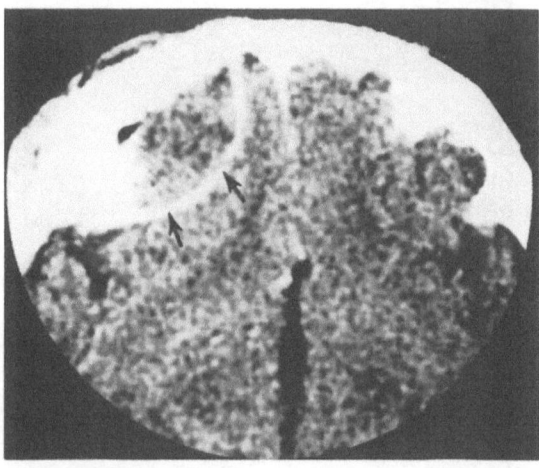

B

Figure 15.14. Following treatment of a penetrating wound through the right orbit into the brain, this patient developed an apical orbital abscess. After this was evacuated, an extradural empyema was found. **A.** Axial CT scan, obtained subsequent to the evacuation of the apical abscess, shows thickening of the medial rectus muscle and the optic nerve (arrow). The eyeball is displaced anteriorly. **B.** Axial view of right frontal lobe shows an epidural mass with an enhancing rim (arrows). These changes are consistent with an epidural empyema.

Abscess formation can be diagnosed by ultrasonography (Fig. 15.15) (13). However, ultrasonography may not delineate an abscess located in either the orbital apex or the posterolateral roof of the orbit.

B-Scan Ultrasonography in Orbital Cellulitis

Coleman (7) classifies inflammatory changes of the orbit as being diffuse or localized to a particular area or tissue in the orbit, depending on the specific inflammatory process. A generalized, abnormal mottling of the orbital fat pad is indicative of diffuse orbital inflammation, such as cellulitis. In this instance, echoes within the fat are more widely spaced than normal and are of high amplitude, giving the fat pad a more heterogeneous appearance without circumscribed borders. Some cases of orbital cellulitis may have discrete cavities, which can be acoustically outlined. Other localized inflammatory changes may involve specific orbital structures. For example, expansion of the sonolucent space between the fat pad and orbital wall generally indicates enlargement of the extraocular muscles. Localized inflammation and edema also may involve the optic nerve or the space adjacent to the eye posteriorly. Accentuation of the optic nerve sheath without enlargement indicates the presence of an optic neuritis or edema. The sub-Tenon's space surrounding the globe may become expanded posteriorly from edema associated with any type of orbital inflammation. Ultrasonically, this appears as a sonolucent area adjacent to the globe wall and connecting to the optic nerve outline. With the most current, improved ultrasonographic units, the ability to analyze the anatomy of orbital cellulitis has also improved considerably (21).

Cavernous Sinus Involvement

In untreated orbital cellulitis, the infection may spread to the orbital apex and produce septic cavernous sinus thrombosis (27). Ophthalmic symptoms usually start with pain of the eye and increasing exophthalmos. This may be associated with signs of meningismus. In the majority of cases, the exophthalmos is bilateral. The patient may develop nausea, vomiting, and somnolence. Paralysis of the extraocular muscles may develop due to compression of one or more of the cranial nerves (third, fourth, fifth, and sixth) in the retroorbital space at the superior orbital fissure or within the cavernous sinus. The cavernous segment of the internal carotid artery also may become narrowed or occluded by septic phlebitis and thrombosis of the cavernous sinus; some cases have added arteritis of the carotid siphon at that level. Occasionally, the arteritis may become the site of septic thrombus formation or pseudoaneurysm formation. With dislodging of septic emboli, occlusions of the peripheral branches of the carotid artery can

Figure 15.15. B-scan ultrasonogram of a large orbital abscess. **A.** The axial section shows a large sonolucent area compressing the orbital fat and flattening the posterior surface of the eye. Sketch shows anatomy.

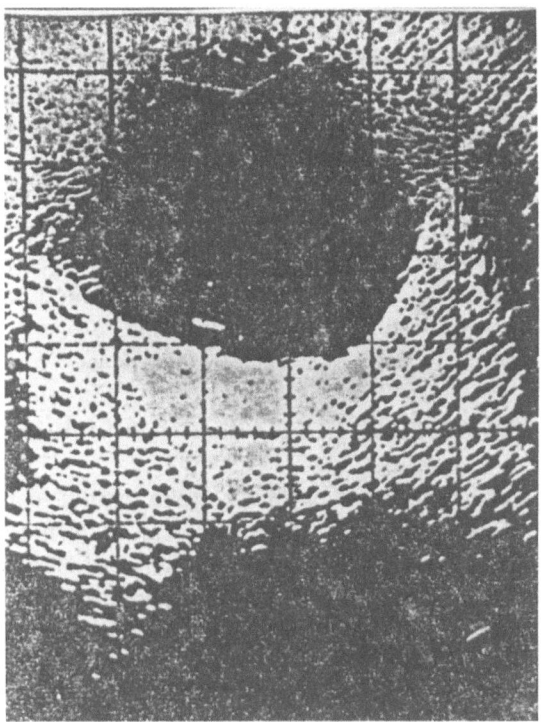

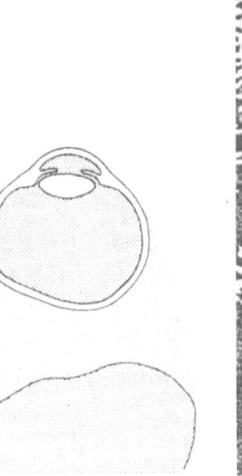

lat.

ABSCESS →

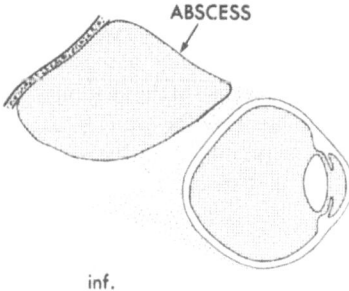

ABSCESS

inf.

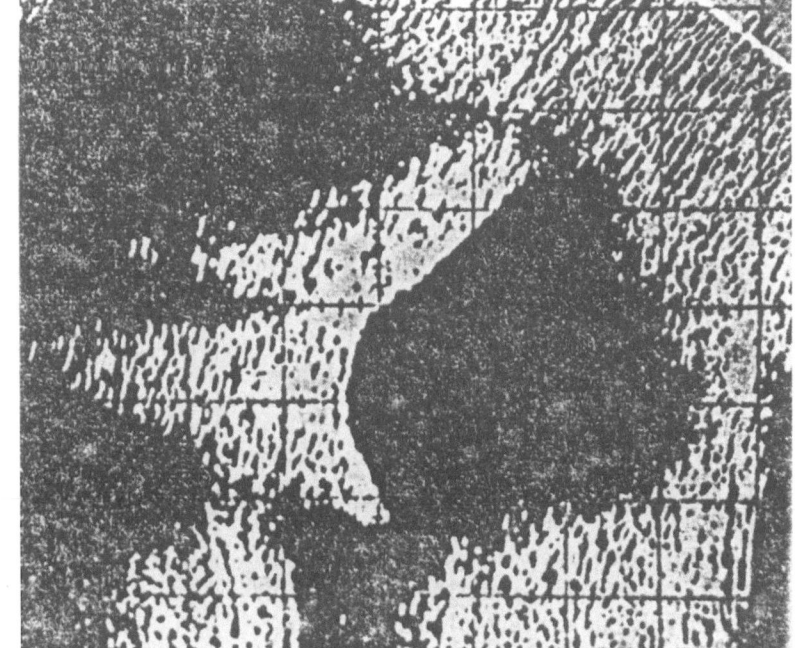

B. Sagittal section shows a large sonolucent area superior and above the optic nerve, with compression and deformity of the superior posterior portion of the eye. Sketch shows anatomy.

result in cerebral infarctions (29). As the infected clot travels into the intracranial tissue by arterial or venous routes, the patient can develop meningitis, subdural empyema, or intracranial abscess secondary to orbital cellulitis. The vascular changes usually are shown by angiography; cavernous sinus thrombosis can be shown by orbital venography or dynamic CT scanning of this region. Cerebral abscess, infarction, and subdural or epidural abscess are well shown by CT scanning.

Postsurgical Infection of the Orbit

Postsurgical infection of the eyelid, cornea, conjunctiva, or uveal tract may occur. It is not a common complication, but it is seen after surgical procedures on the orbit or globe. Postsurgical cellulitis is most likely to be due to staphylococcus aureus.

Orbital Pseudotumor

The diagnosis of orbital pseudotumor is a well-accepted, but controversial, entity in ophthalmology (3, 10). It can mimic orbital cellulitis or orbital tumor. The histologic pattern seen with this condition can be subdivided into three categories (12, 22).

1. Known cause (virus, bacteria, foreign body, and so on)
2. Some stage of certain systemic disease (endocrinopathy, Wegener's granulomatosis, Sjogren's disease, lupus erythematosus, Boeck's sarcoid, and benign lymphoepithelioma)
3. No recognizable cause (idiopathic origin) (1, 2)

However, some investigators use the term pseudotumor only in the cases with idiopathic origin (see Chapter 11).

To make a diagnosis of idiopathic orbital pseudotumor, the histologic pattern should be carefully studied to rule out any causes listed in categories 1 and 2. The cases diagnosed as idiopathic pseudotumor should be followed for at least 1 to 5 years, since some of these cases may develop later into a local orbital or systemic lymphoma; some will develop a systemic disease, such as a collagen disease or Wegener's granulomatosis. Acute inflammatory orbital pseudotumors have a rapid onset,

and they frequently produce proptosis, eyelid swelling, chemosis, limited extraocular movement, and pain. Papilledema and optic neuropathy may also occur.

A CT study of orbital pseudotumors (23) showed that this lesion may occur in five specific anatomic locations: anterior, posterior, diffuse, in the lacrimal gland, and in muscle. The most com-

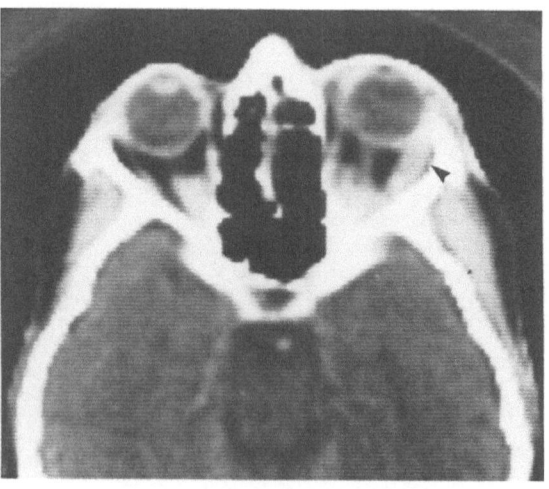

Figure 15.16. This 31-year-old man developed periorbital edema and a retrobulbar mass without associated pansinusitis. The tissue biopsy specimen of the abnormal area was diagnosed as pseudotumor of the orbit. A CT scan showed enlarged lateral rectus muscle (arrowhead), with crowding of the orbital apex tissue.

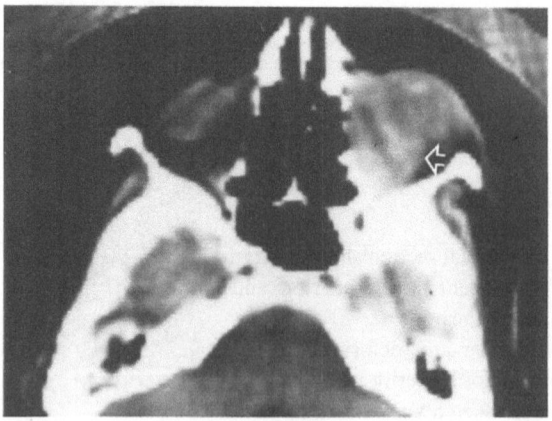

Figure 15.17. This patient was seen with a history of rapid onset of proptosis. An axial CT scan reveals a diffuse retrobulbar lesion (open arrow) with a lack of sharp delineation between the globe and the mass. This is one of the signs of pseudotumor, which was shown on a biopsy specimen.

mon site for this lesion was the lacrimal gland (dacryadenitis), in which the lateral aspect of the globe may be obscured. A pseudotumor may show the lesion being intimately related to the posterior aspect of the globe and producing a thickening of the posterior sclera and/or choroid (9), which obscures the junction of the optic nerve with the globe (Fig. 15.16). In addition, a pseudotumor may extend a variable distance posteriorly along the optic nerve. A diffuse pseudotumor involves the entire globe, with a soft-tissue mass extending from the orbital apex to the posterior margin of the globe (Fig. 15.17). The pseudotumors located in an extraocular muscle have a relatively diffuse enlargement of the muscle (Fig. 15.18), including the muscle tendon (myositis) (see Chapter 12).

Extraorbital Infections

Patients with nasal polyposis with pansinusitis are prone to cellulitis, which may progress to involve the orbit (see Chapter 13).

Mucocele is an expanding lesion of the paranasal sinuses that develops after the occlusion of a part or an entire compartment of a sinus outlet. The blockage of the sinus outlet may be due to chronic infection, polyp, tumor, or scar formation after fracture or injury to soft-tissue contiguous to sinus outlets. Frontal and ethmoid mucoceles develop most commonly in people with nasal polyposis. The mucoceles from both of these areas often grow into the orbital space to displace the orbital contents (23). Mucopyoceles develop when the fluid content in the mucocele becomes infected. Many of these cases often have accompanying periorbital cellulitis and abscesses. The CT scans and radiographs (17) show a characteristic expansile lesion

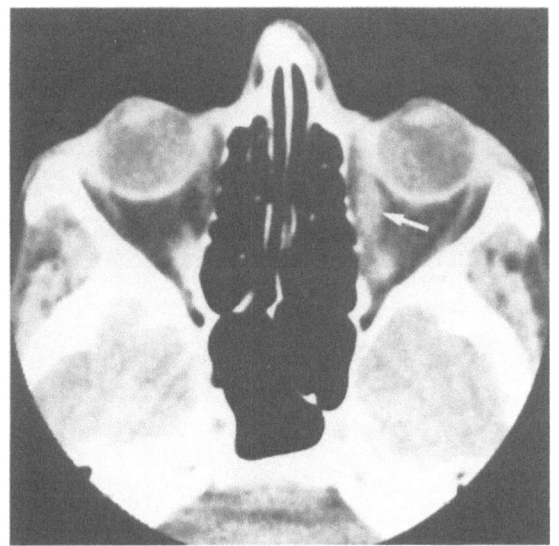

A

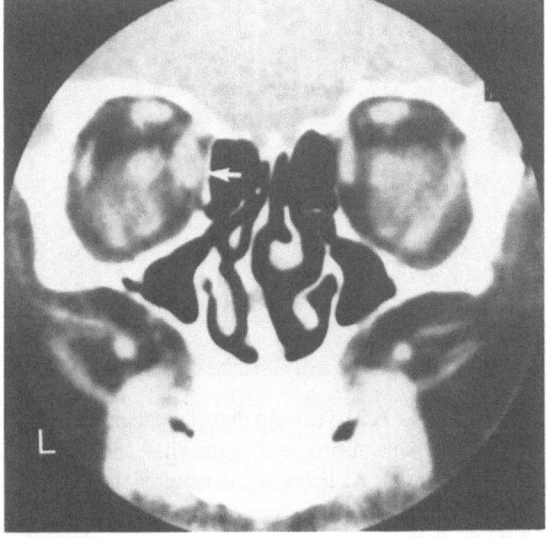

B

Figure 15.18. This patient developed sudden swelling of the left orbital area, with proptosis and difficulty in moving the eye. The (**A**) axial and (**B**) coronal CT scans show the enlarged medial rectus muscle (arrow). The patient improved with steroid treatment.

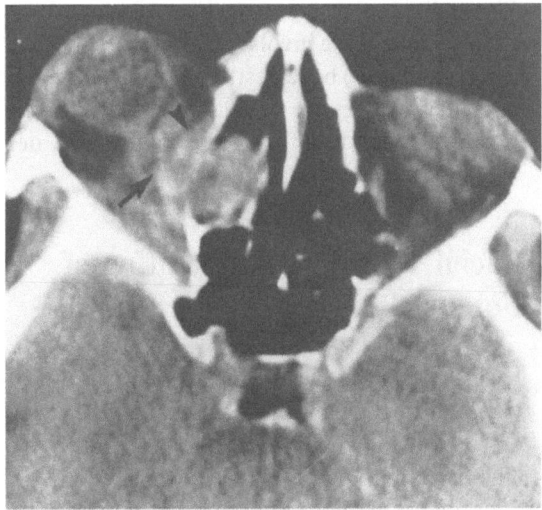

Figure 15.19. Mucopyocele arising in the midethmoid labyrinth, bulging into the medial aspect of the retrobulbar space, displacing the medial rectus muscle (arrow), and crowding the tissues in the orbital apex.

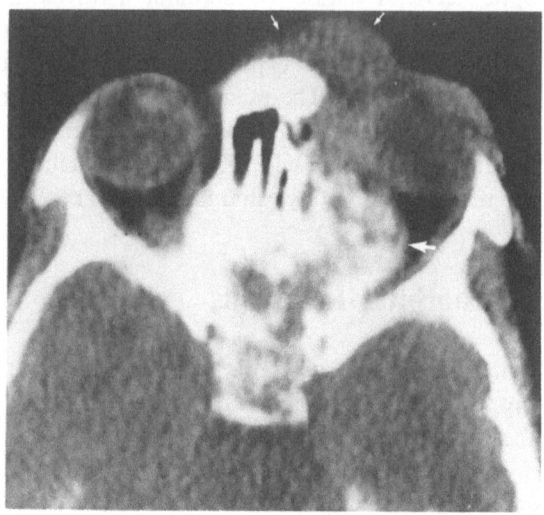

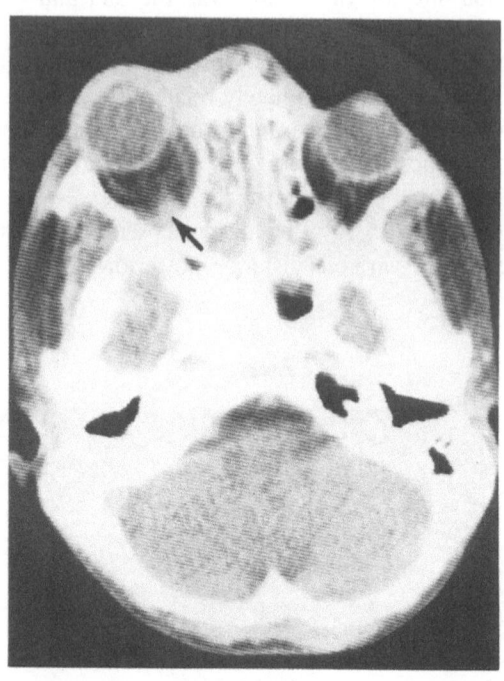

A

Figure 15.20. Axial CT scan shows periorbital edema and a chronic infection in which the preseptal space is distended (small arrows). The ethmoid-sphenoid mucoceles in the medial retrobulbar space compress the orbital apical structures (large arrow).

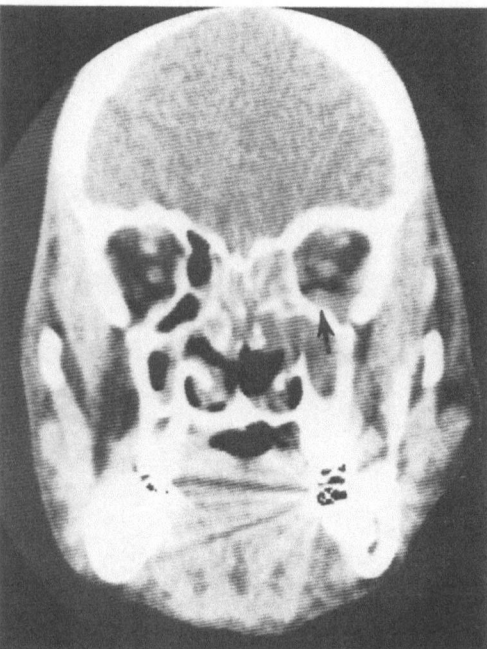

B

in the frontal or ethmoid sinus, with or without destruction of the surrounding bone (Fig. 15.19). Periorbital cellulitis and displacement of the orbital content by mucocele is well visualized with CT scanning (Fig. 15.20).

Mucormycosis frequently is a fulminating infection, with marked involvement of the paranasal sinuses leading to a facial cellulitis and gangrene. The radiographic findings (Fig. 15.21 and 13.5) are clouding of the involved paranasal sinuses and (soon thereafter) bone destruction. Then the infection may progress to orbital and brain infection. If this infection is not treated expeditiously, death will soon occur (see Chapter 13).

Facial Trauma and Retention of Foreign Body

Fractures of the facial bone and transections of any wall of the paranasal sinuses may be complicated by orbital cellulitis with abscess formation. The retention of a foreign body, infection of the overlying skin, and poor drainage of the nose and sinuses all contribute to the development of orbital cellulitis (Figs. 15.22 and 15.23) (see Chapter 14). Proper management with antibiotics and surgery may prevent orbital cellulitis.

Figure 15.21. A 21-year-old diabetic patient in acidosis developed pansinusitis and periorbital edema (due to mucormycosis). **A.** Increased density of the ethnoid sinuses, with edema of the preseptal space and soft-tissue density at the orbital apex due to enlargement of the inferior rectus muscle (arrow), as shown in the axial CT scan. **B.** The upper half of the nasal fossa and the ethmoid and maxillary sinuses on the left show soft-tissue thickening; the inferior rectus (arrow) and lateral rectus muscles are enlarged on the coronal CT.

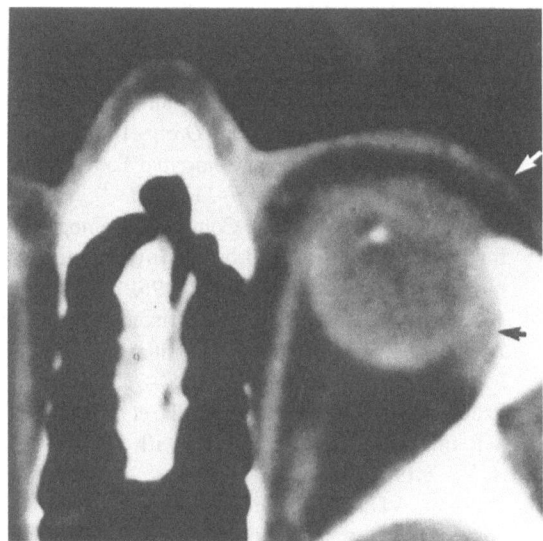

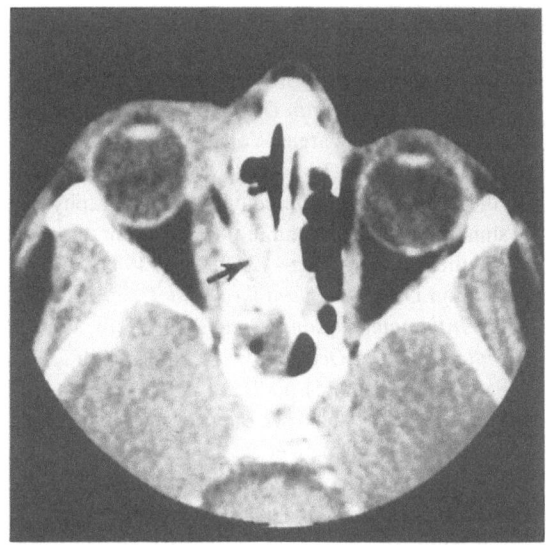

Figure 15.22. Orbital Cellulitis with metallic foreign body. A metallic foreign body is in the anterior nasal portion of the eye; there is considerable secondary periorbital edema (white arrow) and increased soft-tissue density in the anterotemporal portion of the eye (black arrow), as seen in the axial CT scan.

Figure 15.23. A twig (arrow) penetrating the medial portion of the eye, with its distal portion entering in the ethmoid labyrinth; there is considerable inflammation surrounding the foreign body with formation of preseptal edema.

Summary

The available radiological modalities in the investigation of orbital infections are routine x-ray films, polytomograms, ultrasonograms, CT scanning, and magnetic resonance imaging. Of these, CT scanning has become the single most useful method of investigating orbital infection. It allows for quick localization of the different stages of cellulitis and abscess formation in relationship to the intraocular, retrobulbar, paranasal sinus, and intracranial spaces. More recently, the use of surface coil in magnetic resonance imaging promises to give details superior (25) to ultrasonography and high resolution CT scanning in the study of inflammatory changes of the intraocular structures such as the uveal tract, lens, choroid, retina and the sclera.

References

1. Beard C: in Gordon DM (ed): *Diseases of the Lids in Medical Management of Ocular Disease.* Philadelphia, WB Saunders, 1964, (10) pp 122–171.

2. Blodi FC, Gass JDM: Inflammatory pseudotumor of the orbit. *Trans Am Acad Ophthalmol Otolaryngol* 71:17–29, 1967.

3. Blodi FC: Orbital inflammations. *Orbit* 1:1–19, 1982.

4. Clarkson JG, Green WR: Endogenous fungal endophthalmitis, in Duan TD (ed): *Clinical Ophthalmology.* Vol 3, Philadelphia, Harper & Row, 1981. pp 1–44.

5. Cavanagh F: Osteomyelitis of the superior maxilla in infants. *Br Med J* 1:468–472, 1960.

6. Chandler J, Langenbrunner D, Stevens E: The pathogenesis of orbital complications in acute sinusitis. *Laryngoscope* 80:1414–1428, 1970.

7. Coleman DJ, Lizzi FL, Jack RL: *Orbital Inflammation in Ultrasonography of the Eye and Orbit.* Philadelphia, Lea & Febiger, 1977.

8. Duke-Elder S: Inflammations of the orbit, in *System of ophthalmology,* London, Henry Kimpton, 1974. Vol 13, Part 2 (13), pp 866–884.

9. Enzmann D, Donaldson SS, Marshall WH, et al: Computed tomography in orbital pseudotumor (idiopathic orbital inflammation). *Radiology* 120: 597–601, 1976.

10. Eshaghian J, Anderson RL: Sinus involvement in inflammatory orbital pseudotumor. *Arch Ophthalmol* 99:627–630, 1981.

11. Friedlander MH: *Allergy and Immunology of the Eye.* Philadelphia, Harper & Row, 1979, pp 107–138.

12. Garner A: Pathology of pseudotumors of the orbit, in *Modern Problems in Ophthalmology: Orbital Disorders,* Basel, S Karger, Vol 14, 1975, pp 349–354.

13. Goodwin WJ Jr, Weinshall M, Chandler JR: The role of high resolution computed tomography and standardized ultrasound in the evaluation of orbital cellulitis. *Laryngoscope* 92:728–731, 1982.

14. Gordon DM: *Diseases of the Uveal Tract, Intraocular Inflammations and Optic Neuritis in Medical Management of Ocular Disease.* Philadelphia, WB Saunders, 1964, (15) pp 245–271.

15. Gullotta U, Denffer HV: *Dacryocystography.* Stuttgart, Georg Thieme Verlag, 1980.

16. Hawkins D, Clark R: Orbital involvement in acute sinusitis. *Clin Radiol* 29:501–511, 1978.

17. Hesselink JR, Weber AL, New PFJ, et al: Evaluation of mucoceles of the paranasal sinuses with computed tomography. *Radiology* 133:397–400, 1979.

18. Jakobiec F, Jones IS: Orbital inflammations, in Duane TD (ed): *Clinical Ophthalmology.* Philadelphia, Harper & Row, 1981, vol 2 (35), pp 1–75.

19. Jones DB: Microbial preseptal and orbital cellulitis, in Duane TD (ed): *Clinical Ophthalmology.* Philadelphia, Harper & Row, 1981, vol 4 (25), pp 1–19.

20. Krohel GB, Krauss HR, Winnick J: Orbital abscess: Presentation, diagnosis, therapy and sequelae. *Ophthalmology* 89:492–498, 1982.

21. Lou P: Personal communication on the use of B-Scan ultrasonography in orbital infection.

22. Momose KJ, Grove A Jr, Silberman N, et al: *Diagnosis of Pseudotumor of the Orbit.* International Symposium and Course on Computed Tomography, Las Vegas, Nevada, April 7–11, 1980.

23. Momose KJ, Grove A Jr: Computed Tomography for Evaluation of Sinus Disorders Invading the Orbit. *Internat Ophthalmol* 22:181–196, 1982.

24. Nugent RA, Rootman J, Robertson WB, et al: Acute orbital pseudotumor: Classification and CT features. *Am J Roentgenol* 137:957–962, 1981.

25. Schenck JF, Hart HR Jr, Foster TH, et al: Improved MR imaging of the orbit at 1st with Surface Coil *AJNR* 6:193–196, 1985.

26. Schramm VL Jr, Myers EN, Kennerdell JS: Orbital complications of acute sinusitis: Evaluation, management and outcome. *Trans Am Acad Ophthalmol Otolaryngol* 96:221–230, 1981.

27. Schramm VL Jr, Curtin HD, Kennerdell JS: Evaluation of orbital cellulitis and results of treatment. *Laryngoscope* 92:732–738, 1982.

28. Yanoff M, Fine BS: *Ocular Pathology,* ed 2. Philadelphia, Harper & Row, 1982.

29. Zimmerman R, Bilaniuk L: Computed tomography of orbital infection and its cerebral complications. *Am J Roentgenol* 134:45–50, 1980.

16
Orbital Trauma

Joseph A. Mauriello, Jr., Carlos F. Gonzalez, Charles B. Grossman, and Joseph C. Flanagan

The bony orbit is a four-walled (superior, inferior, medial and lateral) pyramidal structure whose main function is to support and protect the eye (19). The superior and lateral margins are particularly strong, and they shield the globe from direct trauma. The medial and inferior rims of the orbit are not as strong. The thin inferior and medial walls are prone to fracture or "blow-out," thus protecting the globe from blunt, nonpenetrating trauma. The interorbital space is the area between the orbits and beneath the floor of the anterior cranial fossa. This space contains the right and left ethmoid sinuses. The floor of the anterior cranial fossa is composed of the cribriform plate medially and the roof of each ethmoid sinus laterally.

With high-acceleration vehicular accidents and violent crimes, the variety of possible orbital and facial fractures is limitless. However, certain fractures occur with sufficient regularity to allow classification of orbital fractures into five basic types: 1) floor fractures; 2) medial wall fractures; 3) roof fractures; 4) lateral wall fractures; and 5) combined fractures including tripod, nasoorbital, and LeFort (types I–III). This classification has practical value, in that a particular mechanism tends to produce each type of fracture and that the clinical presentation and management are also peculiar to each type of fracture. Another classification defines orbital fractures as either internal or external fractures. Internal fractures spare the orbital rim, while external fractures involve the rim (19). For the purposes of this chapter, the former system will be employed.

In the investigation of trauma, standard plain x-ray film views of the orbit usually include: 1) Caldwell (modified posterior-anterior); 2) Waters; 3) optic canal; 4) lateral; and 5) basal (submentovertex). However, our routine is to obtain Waters, Caldwell, and lateral views with a horizontal beam. Computed tomography (CT) is used for further work-up, if necessary. The standard orbital CT scan views include axial and direct coronal projections. The latter view is very helpful in evaluating orbital floor and roof fractures. Since the orbital CT scan demonstrates both orbital soft tissues and bones, it is valuable in virtually all patients with orbital trauma. Sagittal and coronal reformation generally is of limited value due to lack of detail and accuracy of the method. If the injured patient cannot be scanned in the hyperextended position for direct coronal scanning, then conventional anteroposterior tomograms are obtained. High-resolution, thin-section, target technique axial and direct coronal scans demonstrate even optic canal fractures with great clarity. However, for optic canal studies, complex-motion tomography may be necessary if satisfactory CT scans cannot be obtained. Computed tomography, ultrasound, or possibly Magnetic Resonante Imaging (MRI) may be important in managing patients in whom an intraocular or orbital nonradiopaque foreign body (e.g., wood or glass) is suspected (10) (see Chapters 4 and 7).

Orbital (Blow-Out) Fractures

The blow-out fracture generally results from trauma to the globe by a relatively large, somewhat rounded object, such as a ball or a fist. The force is transmitted to the globe and surrounding orbital soft tissues; some of the force is cushioned by the surrounding orbital margin. If the intraorbital pressure is raised sufficiently, the osseous orbital confines give way at the weakest points. These points are the medial wall of the orbit in the region of the lamina papyracea (18).

Classically, a "pure" blow-out fracture involves the inferior wall; most commonly, the posterior part of the medial floor (7). The orbital rim is not fractured. In an "impure" blow-out fracture (8), there is an accompanying orbital rim fracture. In this type of fracture, the fractured orbital rim and the orbital contents are both pushed posteriorly. Posterior displacement of the orbital rim and the attached orbital septum results in a vertical shortening of the lower eyelid with scleral show. This vertical shortening may occur with or without an associated blow-out fracture. It is important to remember that an "impure" blow-out fracture accompanies an orbital rim fracture if: 1) the object causing the fracture is of greater dimension than that of the bony orbital entrance; and 2) the force is sufficient to push both the orbital rim and the orbital contents posteriorly.

Because the mechanism of medial wall fractures is the same as that of orbital floor blow-out fractures, a medial wall fracture due to blunt trauma is considered to be a form of blow-out fracture (5, 6). In one series of 20 orbital floor fractures, eight of the patients had an associated medial wall fracture (2). In none of the cases was an isolated medial wall fracture present (20).

The clinical signs of orbital floor fracture most commonly include traumatic ptosis, hypesthesia in the distribution of the second division of the fifth cranial nerve, subconjunctival and eyelid hemorrhage, vertical diplopia due to difficulty in elevation or depression, and exophthalmos or enophthalmos. Initially, extravasated blood may cause exophthalmos and may make evaluation of motility difficult. For this reason, surgery usually is not considered until approximately 1 week after the injury.

Three main factors contribute to posttraumatic enophthalmos. The first factor that causes early enophthalmos is the result of the initial volume expansion of the orbit from both the downward displacement of the orbital floor into the maxillary antrum and escape of orbital fat through the ruptured periorbita. A second possible cause of enophthalmos is entrapment of tissues within the fracture site, which may fix the globe in a posterior position. Late enophthalmos is due to the latter factors, but it is also caused by a third factor: the gradual atrophy of the incarcerated tissue,

mostly fat. Enophthalmos usually causes a deep supratarsal fold, and it may occur with or without entrapment and diplopia.

The pathophysiology of motility disturbance due to true entrapment is as follows. The orbital fat contains a network of fibrovascular septae that have intimate associations with the extraocular muscles. At the time of injury, the orbital fat prolapses through the fracture site into the maxillary sinus and entraps the fat and septae, thus limiting ocular motility. The entire globe rarely prolapses into the maxillary sinus (13).

A very helpful clinical sign in the determination of entrapment of orbital tissues into a fracture is the forced duction test. A positive forced duction test indicates that the ophthalmologist is unable to move the globe in a given direction by applying traction with forceps at the anesthetized corneoscleral limbus. A positive test suggests that there is evidence of entrapment of orbital tissues into the fracture site that is responsible for the motility disturbance. However, a positive forced duction test within the first few days posttrauma may be due to orbital hemorrhage and edema, and it may convert to a negative test as the blood resorbs

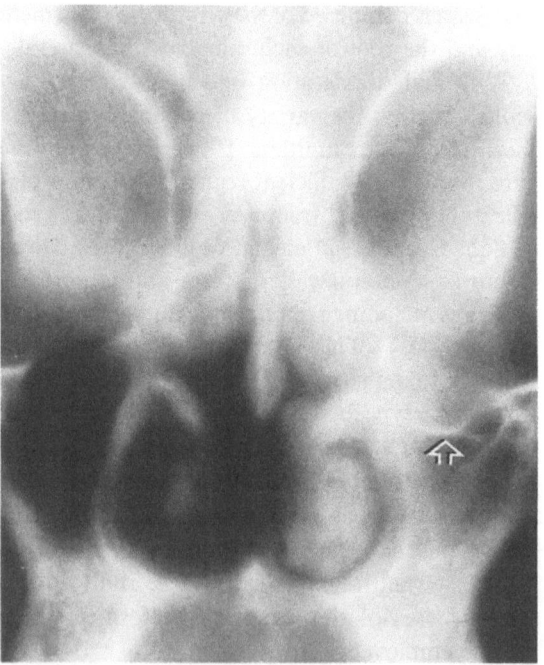

Figure 16.1. Blow-out fractures of the orbital floor. **A.** Water's view shows a blow-out fracture with depression of the bone fragments (open arrow) and diffuse opacification of the left maxillary antrum.

Figure 16.1B. Coronal CT scan showing the fracture (arrow) and diffuse opacification of right maxillary antrum.

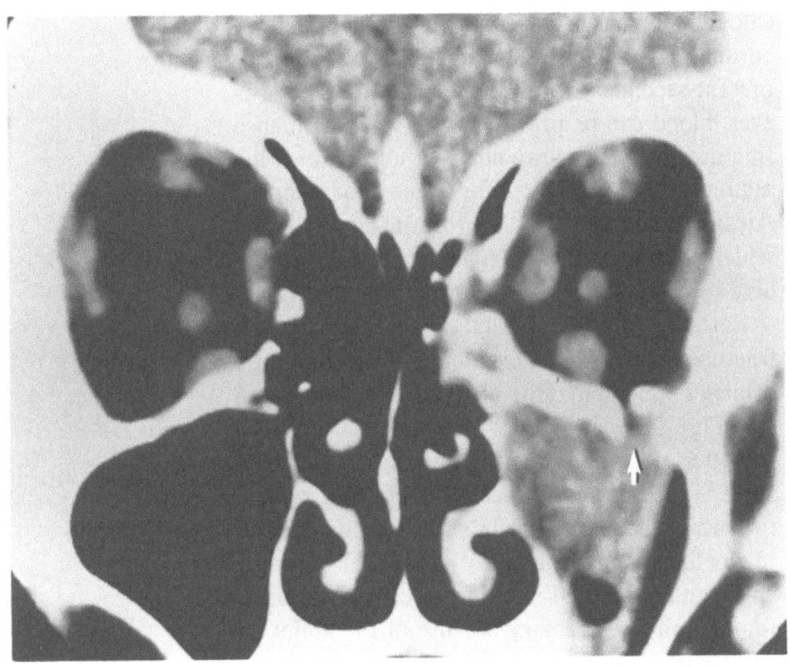

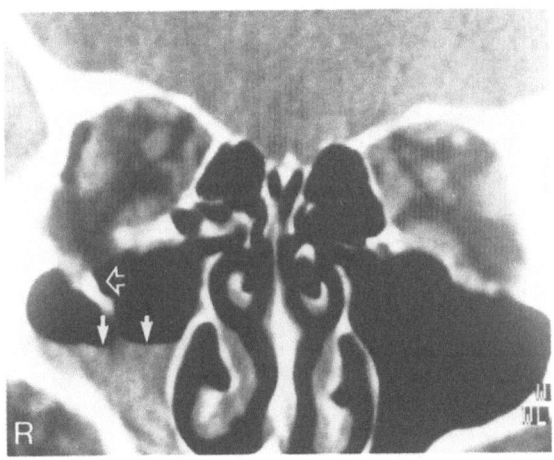

Figure 16.1C. Coronal CT scan showing the air-fluid density interface (arrows) and fracture of the orbital floor and displacement of the fragment into the right maxillary antrum (open arrow).

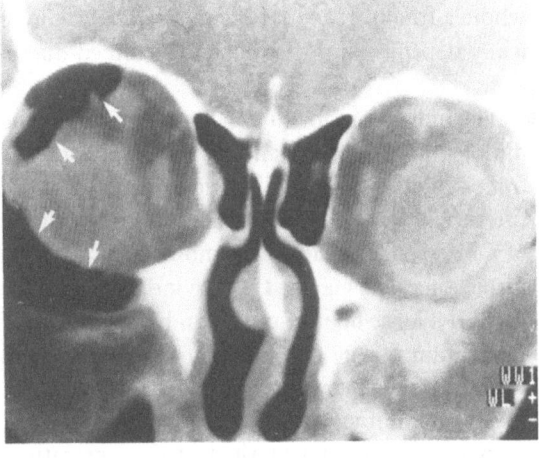

Figure 16.1D. Coronal CT scan (same patient as in Fig. 16.1C) showing orbital emphysema (arrows).

and the edema subsides. A negative forced duction test indicates that the motility disturbance is not caused by entrapment of orbital tissues into the fracture site. Causes of a motility disturbance with a negative forced duction test include traumatic neuropathy or hemorrhage into the extraocular muscle.

Routine plain facial views, CT scans, and complex-motion tomograms are the most commonly used imaging modalities for confirming the diagno-

sis. In general, plain x-ray films are not as definitive as orbital CT scans or complex-motion tomograms in diagnosing orbital floor fractures. Plain x-ray films or complex-motion tomography in the Waters projection provide the optimum view of the orbital floor, and they usually are sufficient to demonstrate the fracture, depression of the bone fragments, or prolapse of the orbital soft tissues into the maxillary sinus (Fig. 16.1A and 16.1B). Total opacification of the maxillary sinus usually indicates hemorrhage. On erect plain x-ray films or coronal CT scanning, an air-fluid level may be present secondary to bleeding (Fig. 16.1C). However, blood can be present in the sinus without a fracture. On plain x-ray films, a subperiosteal hematoma may be mistaken for a true floor fracture. Air in the orbital soft tissues (orbital emphysema), which is characteristic of blow-out fractures, is best seen on orbital CT scanning (Fig. 16.1D).

Entrapment of the orbital soft tissues into the fracture site can be adequately demonstrated by orbital tomography (Fig. 16.2) and CT scanning (see Figs. 3.16, 3.17, 3.18, and 3.19).

A trap-door blow-out fracture is one in which there is little bony displacement. For this reason, the orbital floor fracture in such cases is difficult to document on plain x-ray films (21). Coronal and sagital orbital CT scanning or complex-motion tomography is necessary because of the ability of these studies to demonstrate soft-tissue displacement (Fig. 16.3) (see Fig. 3.19). Ultimately, the decision to intervene surgically on patients in whom a fracture cannot be demonstrated radiologically depends on the results of the forced duction test.

The indications for surgical intervention include diplopia in an important field of gaze, positive forced ductions, and radiologic evidence of a floor fracture. In patients without radiologic evidence of a blow-out fracture, poor motility with positive forced ductions may be the sole indication for surgery. If a large floor fracture can be demonstrated, prevention of late enophthalmos is an indication for surgical exploration and insertion of an alloplastic floor implant. In some cases, orbital CT scan is the optimum method of demonstrating a large orbital floor defect. As previously indicated, these fractures need not be repaired within a few days of injury; optimally, they are repaired 7–10 days after injury following remission of edema and before fibrosis begins. Floor defects can be repaired months or even years later, but are best repaired as soon as demonstrated. Patients that show improvement in motility do not require surgery and usually are only observed. A traumatic ptosis may take 6 months to 1 year to resolve. Blindness due to compression of the optic nerve circulation is a well-known, although rare, complication of orbital floor exploration with or without insertion of an alloplastic implant.

We have observed two patients who developed late proptosis, 10 and 16 years, respectively, after

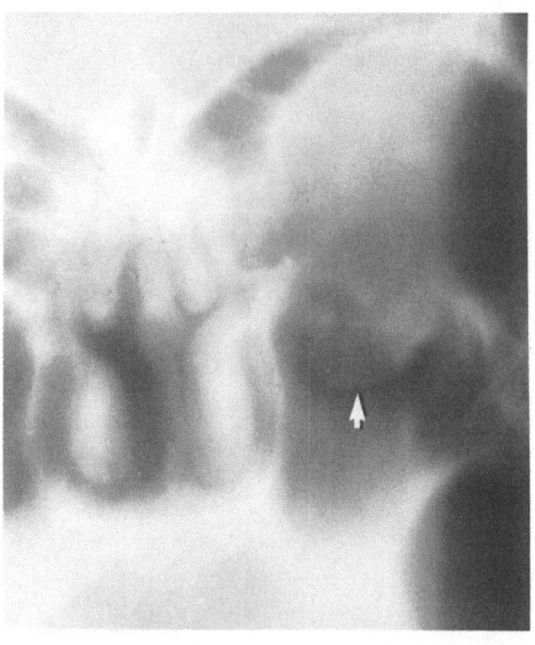

A

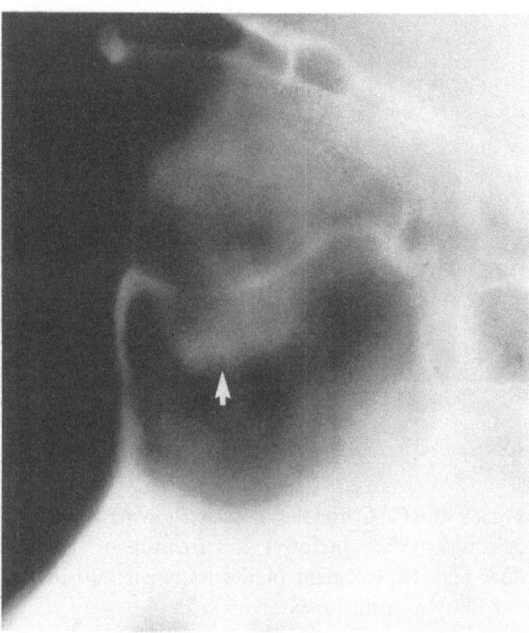

B

Figure 16.2. Blow-out fracture of the orbital floor. **(A)** Anteroposterior and **(B)** lateral tomogram of the left orbit and antrum, showing herniation of the orbital soft tissues into the left maxillary antrum (arrow).

repair of an orbital floor fracture with a teflon implant. In both cases, hemorrhage into the fibrous capsule that surrounded the implant produced a cyst-like structure, which was observed on the CT scan and was documented pathologically (15). Suc-

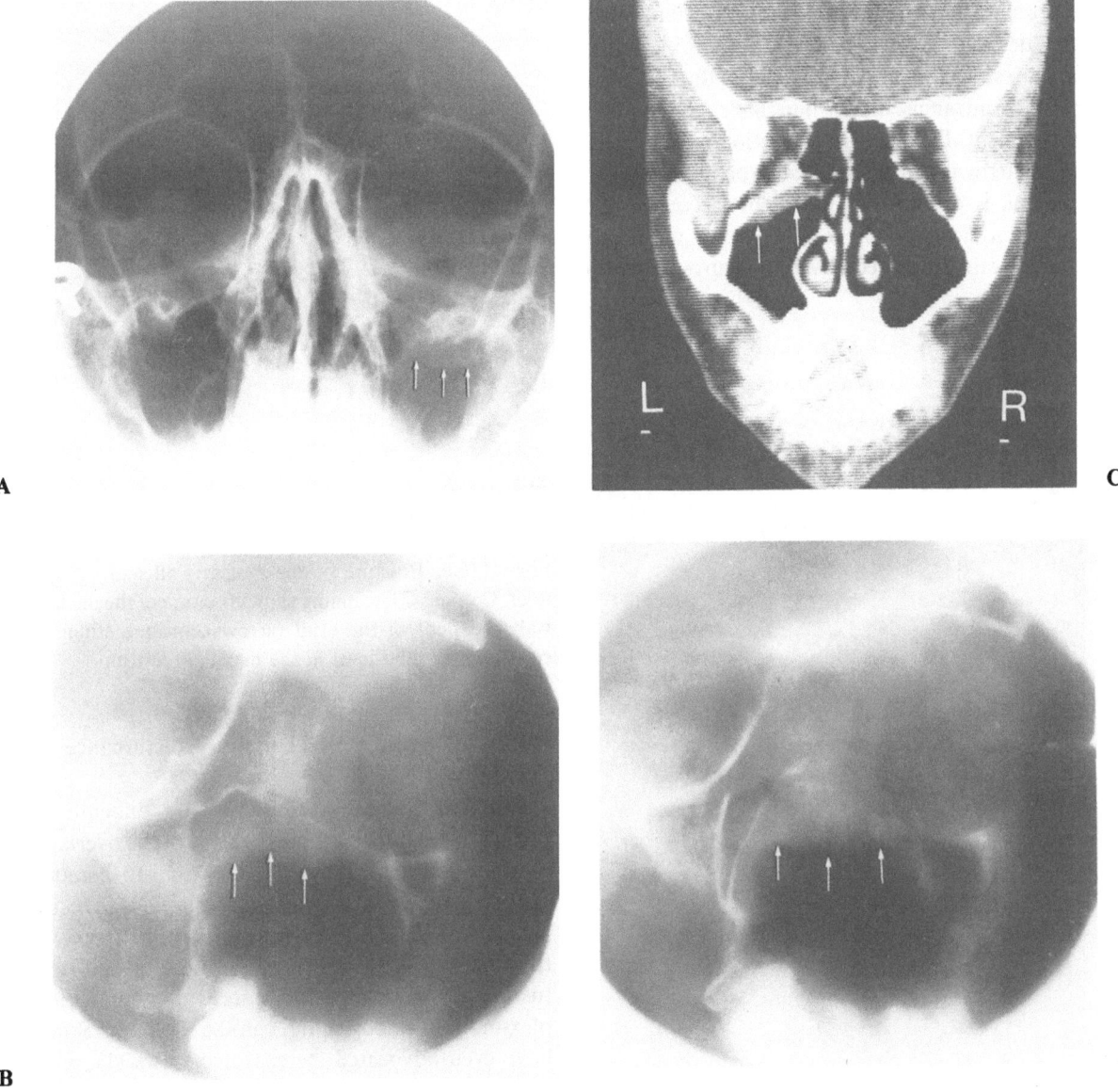

Figure 16.3. Blow-out fracture of the orbit. **A.** Water's view reveals no evidence of a fracture, but a faintly visualized herniation of orbital soft tissue into the right maxillary antrum (arrows) is shown. **B, D.** Lateral tomo-gram reveals no obvious fracture, and it localizes the entrapment of soft tissue to the superior posterior portion of the maxillary antrum (arrows). **C.** The coronal CT scan demonstrates the same changes (arrows).

cessful treatment required partial removal of the fibrous capsule and decompression of the "cyst."

Medial Wall Fracture

Medial wall fractures are more commonly due to nonpenetrating (than penetrating) injury. The pathophysiology of medial wall fractures caused by a nonpenetrating orbital injury is identical to that of an orbital floor blow-out fracture. The signs of a medial wall fracture include orbital emphysema with crepitus under the skin and/or conjunctiva. Crepitus is extremely common in medial wall fractures, but it occurs whenever there is a fracture of the common bony wall between the orbit and an adjacent sinus (1). Epistaxis is often present. As with any orbital floor fracture, significant eyelid, subconjunctival, and orbital hemorrhage and edema may cause transient exophthalmos. Motility disturbances are rare with medial wall fracture; if present, they may resolve with resorbing blood and decreasing chemosis. As with orbital floor fractures, traumatic muscle palsy due to nerve palsy or intramuscular hemorrhage may simulate entrapment. Difficulty in adduction or abduction, with narrowing of the lid fissure on attempted abduction, is due to entrapment of the orbital soft tissues adjacent to the medial rectus within the fracture site (16). Medial wall fractures should be

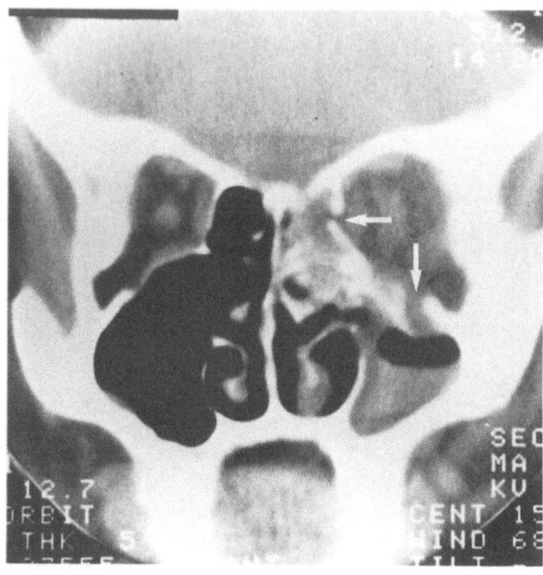

Figure 16.5. Fracture of the medial wall and orbital floor. Coronal CT scanning shows fracture of the medial wall and floor of the orbit (arrows), opaque ethmoid cells, and air-fluid level in the maxillary antrum.

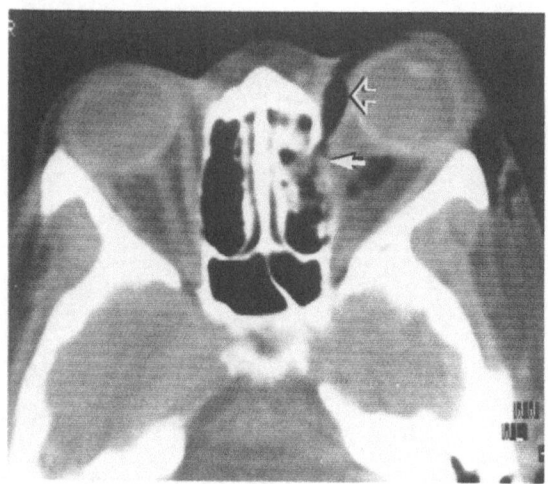

A

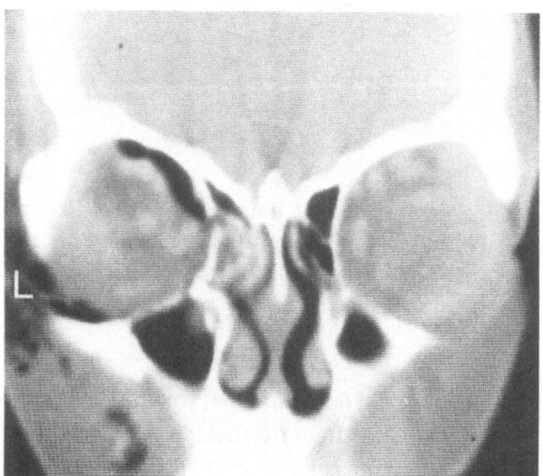

B

Figure 16.4. Fracture of the medial wall. (**A**) Axial and (**B**) coronal CT scans of the orbits reveal multiple fractures of lamina papyracea of the ethmoid bone (arrow), with opacification of the left ethmoid sinus due to hemorrhage. Orbital emphysema (open arrow), exophthalmos, and retrobulbar increased density secondary to bleeding are also seen.

suspected if any vertical motility disturbance is present.

Ethmoid fractures are sometimes difficult to identify on plain x-ray films because of the overlapping shadows. Ethmoid clouding due to hemorrhage may be the only definite clue (11). Documenting an ethmoid fracture is only necessary if there is evidence of entrapment of the medial rectus muscles with a positive forced duction. Complex-motion tomography can be helpful. Some have even advocated stereoscopic views (1). The orbital CT scan has greatly facilitated diagnosis of medial wall fractures (Fig. 16.4). Blow-out fractures of the medial orbital wall may occur alone or in association with blow-out fractures of the orbital floor (Fig. 16.5). When surgical release of the entrapped tissues is warranted, an incision is made above the lacrimal sac and the periosteum is freed from the underlying bony orbit until the incarcerated tissues are identified.

Penetrating trauma may result in a medial wall fracture and a fracture of the adjacent cribriform plate. Possible cerebrospinal fluid (CSF) rhinorrhea and pneumocephalus require neurosurgical evaluation. Nonionic intrathecal contrast media introduced via lumbar puncture is helpful in demonstrating the site of the dural tear on coronal CT scanning.

Figure 16.6. Fractures of the orbital roof. **A.** Water's view on plain skull x-ray film. Depressed, comminuted fracture of the medial orbital roof (arrows). The frontal sinus is opacified.

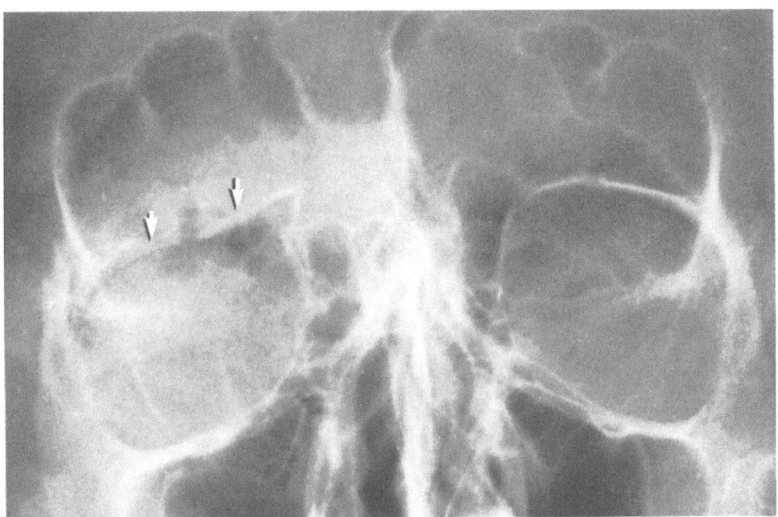

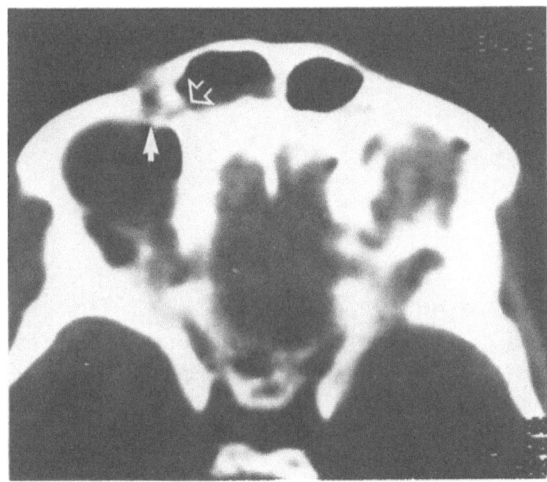

B. Axial CT scan shows the fracture of the medial orbital roof (arrow), with extension into the right frontal sinus (open arrow).

Orbital Roof Fractures

Fractures of the orbital roof account for only about 5% of facial fractures (9). The superior orbital rim is broad and well supported; it is fractured only by severe blunt trauma (i.e., from the impact of a dashboard or steering column in an automobile accident). However, the roof itself is rather thin and susceptible to penetrating injury (14). Unilateral forehead anesthesia due to supraorbital nerve damage and decreased frontalis muscle function are clinical signs unique to a frontal sinus fracture (4, 17).

The clinical signs of roof fractures vary, depending on which portion of the roof is fractured. Fractures that occur in the medial aspect of the orbital roof often cause comminuted and depressed fractures of the frontal sinus (Fig. 16.6). The comminuted fractures also may be elevated (Fig. 16.7). Theoretically, fractures in this area may sever the trochlea of the superior oblique muscle or may rupture the medial horn of the levator, causing motility imbalance and ptosis, respectively. Fractures of the lateral roof may disrupt the lateral horn of the levator as it attaches between the palpebral and orbital lobes of the lacrimal gland (Fig. 16.8). Enophthalmos with entrapment of orbital tissues may cause motility disturbances (usually limitation of upgaze). Pseudoptosis may result from depression of the globe. A true ptosis may occur from traumatic neuropathy or hemorrhage into the levator muscle, or its aponeurosis. Entrapment of the levator, causing lagophthalmos or eyelid retraction, has not been reported (4).

Since any orbital roof fracture may be associated with a frontal or ethmoid sinus and cribriform plate fracture (Fig. 16.9), the possibility of a dural tear CSF leak and pneumocephalus must always be considered. A CSF leak may lead to meningitis, with headache, neck rigidity, and changes in the level of consciousness; anosmia may be present (Fig. 16.10). Meningitis may lead to frontal lobe abscess formation. Rarely, a traumatic meningoencephalocele may occur if a large bony defect is present.

The axial and coronal CT scans are of tremendous value in diagnosing orbital roof fractures.

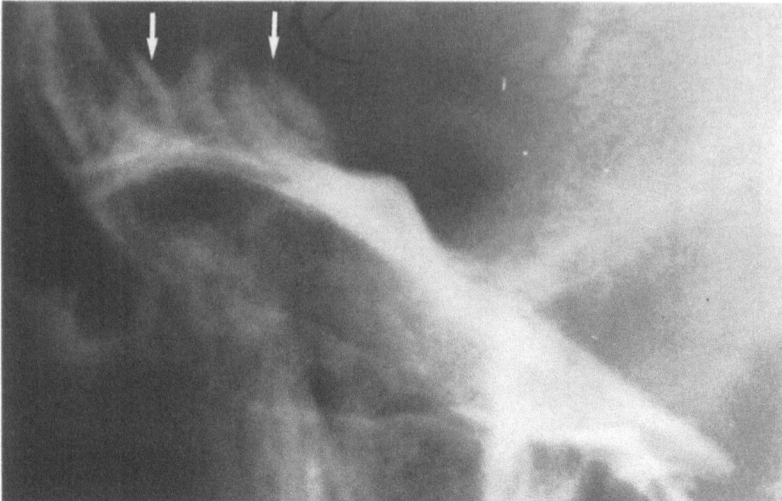

Figure 16.7. Fracture of the orbital roof. Lateral plain x-ray film of the orbit shows upward displacement of the bone fragments (arrows).

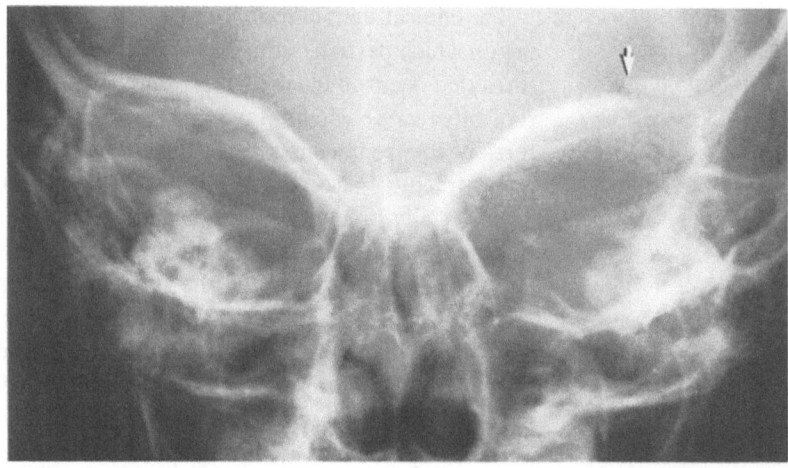

Figure 16.8. Fracture of the orbital roof. Depressed fracture of the left lateral superior orbital rim (arrow).

Moreover, CT scans can demonstrate concomitant pathologies of the orbital and cerebral soft tissues, such as orbital or cerebral hematoma, infection, or abscess formation. On the plain x-ray film views, fractures of the frontal sinus are best demonstrated in the posteroanterior and Waters views. The lateral view may be helpful. Conventional complex-tomographic studies are always recommended. On plain x-ray films, posterior wall fractures of the frontal sinus are difficult to demonstrate, and pneumocephalus may be the only evidence of such a fracture (16).

Fractures of the Lateral Wall

The lateral wall of the orbit is unique in that it is the only wall of the orbit that is not at least partially bounded by a sinus. Also, unlike with the other three walls, entrapment of extraocular muscles has not been reported in association with lateral wall fractures. The bones of the lateral wall are thick and strong. For this reason, fractures that involve only the lateral orbital rim are rare. It appears that to generate a sufficient force to disrupt the lateral wall, an adjacent structure is also injured. The most common combined fractures that involve the lateral orbital wall affect the zygomaticofrontal suture; they include tripod fractures and LeFort III fractures.

Combined Fractures

The combinations of orbital fractures that can result from trauma is limitless. The types of combined fractures that commonly involve the orbit

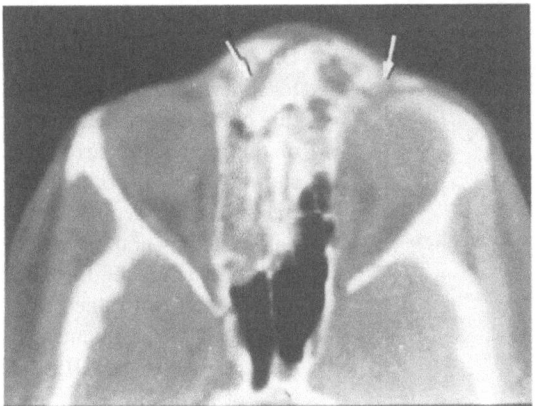

A

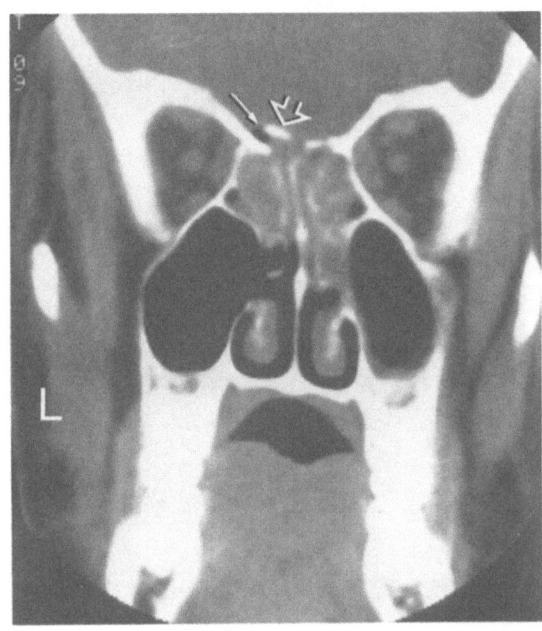

B

Figure 16.9. Fracture of the orbital roof and cribriform plate. **A.** Axial CT scan shows a comminuted fracture of the nasal bones extending into the left superior orbital rim (arrows). Also shown is opacification of both ethmoid sinuses secondary to bleeding. **B.** Coronal CT scan reveals posterior extension of a cribriform fracture (open arrow), with superior displacement of the fragment and pneumocephalus (long arrow). A CSF fluid leak was demonstrated by metrizamide cisternography.

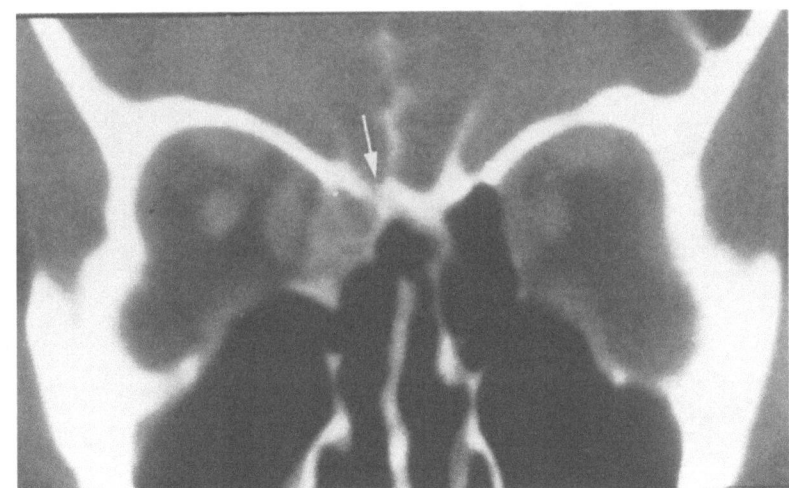

Figure 16.10. Fracture of cribriform plate with CSF. Metrizamide cisternogram. A coronal CT scan at the midorbital level shows a CSF leak (arrow) due to traumatic fracture of the cribriform plate.

and/or midfacial structures are considered below as separate entities.

Tripod or Tripartite Fractures

The tripod fracture is caused by direct trauma to the cheek. The three components of the fracture include separation of: 1) the zygomaticofrontal suture, superiorly; 2) the zygomatic arch, laterally; and 3) the zygomatic maxillary suture, medially. The zygoma usually is displaced either backward or downward (17). The backward-displaced zygoma usually results in complete detachment of the zygoma, with a step deformity of the inferior orbital rim, a depressed malar eminence, and an elevated zygomatic arch. The fractures that cause downward displacement of the zygoma usually result in incomplete displacement of the zygoma. If the zygoma remains hinged at the zygomaticofrontal suture, but is detached at the maxillary attachment, the orbital septum will be pulled down and there will be increased scleral show at the

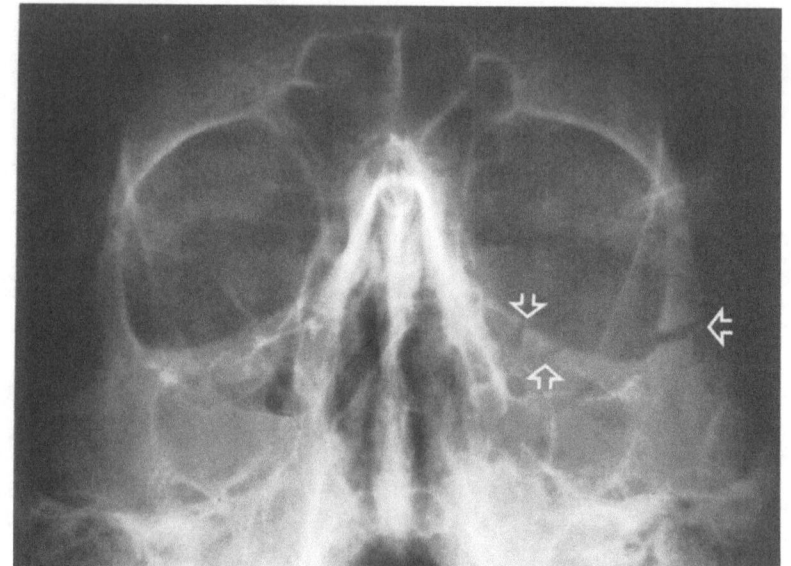

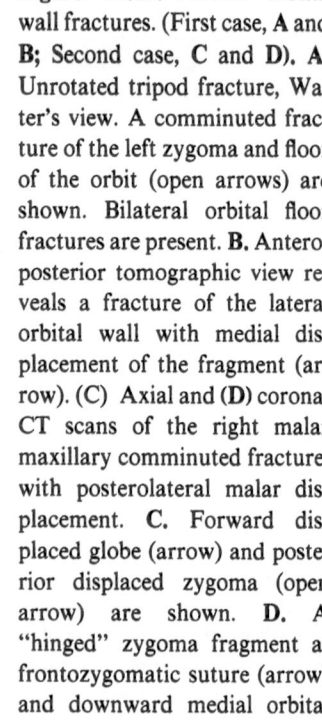

Figure 16.11. Lateral orbital wall fractures. (First case, **A** and **B**; Second case, **C** and **D**). **A.** Unrotated tripod fracture, Water's view. A comminuted fracture of the left zygoma and floor of the orbit (open arrows) are shown. Bilateral orbital floor fractures are present. **B.** Anteroposterior tomographic view reveals a fracture of the lateral orbital wall with medial displacement of the fragment (arrow). (**C**) Axial and (**D**) coronal CT scans of the right malar maxillary comminuted fracture, with posterolateral malar displacement. **C.** Forward displaced globe (arrow) and posterior displaced zygoma (open arrow) are shown. **D.** A "hinged" zygoma fragment at frontozygomatic suture (arrow) and downward medial orbital floor fragment (open arrow) are shown.

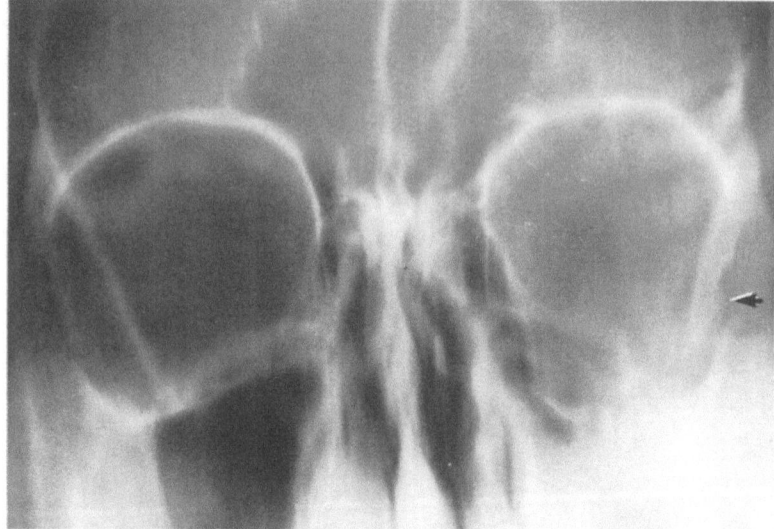

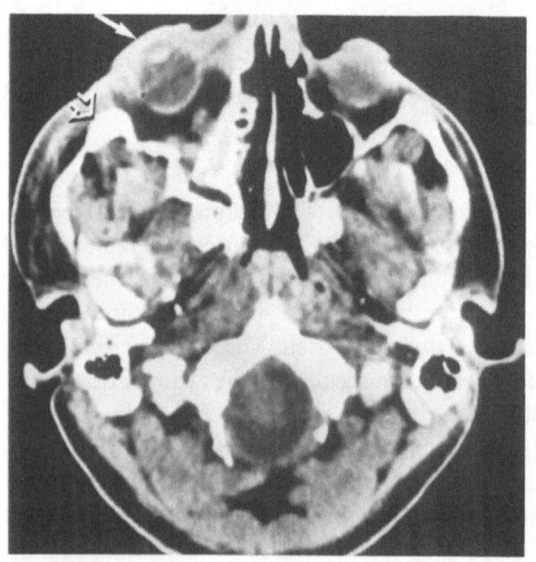

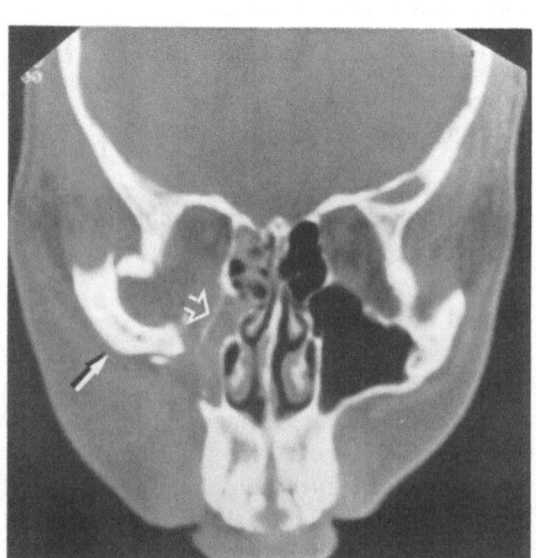

lateral aspect of the lower eyelid. The lateral canthal tendon, which inserts at the orbital tubercule 10 mm inferior to the zygomaticofrontal suture, will remain intact. If the zygoma remains hinged at the zygomatic maxillary suture, but is detached at the zygomaticofrontal suture, the lateral canthal tendon and the globe will be displaced downward. There will be no increased scleral show.

Most patients with tripod fractures have hypesthesia in the distribution of the second division of the fifth nerve. Malocclusion often develops due to the fracture of the zygomatic arch. Extraocular muscle palsies are rare.

On plain x-ray films of the skull, the basal and Waters views are most helpful in demonstrating fracture of the zygomatic bone and arch. The CT scan has no significant advantage over plain x-ray films in the diagnosis and management of simple tripod fractures (Fig. 16.11A and 16.11B). An exaggerated Townes view and a base view of the skull will be helpful. Also, CT scanning plays a significant role in more severe injuries due to the ability of CT to image the bone as well as the globe and other soft tissues (Fig. 16.11C and 16.11D).

Nasoorbital Fractures

The most frequent cause of nasoorbital fracture is the "dashboard" automobile injury, where the patient's face strikes the dashboard or steering column. Due to the anterior-to-posterior direction of the traumatic force, the narrow and thick nasal bones supported by the nasal spine of the frontal bone and the frontal process of the maxilla push the weaker posterior bones of the medial orbital wall posteriorly. A comminuted fracture of these

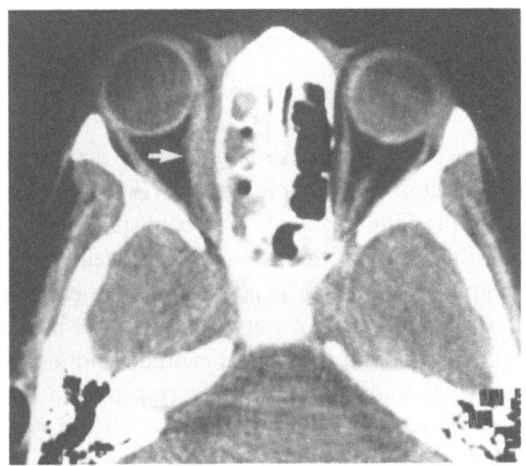

A

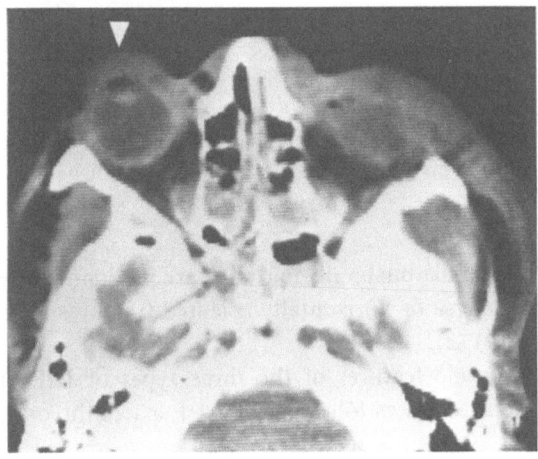

Figure 16.12. Fracture of ethmoid bones. An axial CT scan reveals multiple fractures of the ethmoid bones with increased density, secondary to bleeding, and lamina papyracea fracture. Contusion and emphysema of the facial soft tissue and right eyelid (arrowhead) are shown.

B

Figure 16.13. Fracture of the ethmoid, frontal, and maxillary bones. (A) axial and (B) coronal CT scans. Comminuted fractures of the face, involving the right frontal sinus, right ethmoid sinus, medial wall of the orbit, and right maxillary sinus are shown. Notice the apparent thickening and displacement of the right medial rectus muscle due to possible hemorrhage (arrow). The coronal scan demonstrates nasal turbinate swelling and frontal, ethmoidal and maxillary sinus opacity.

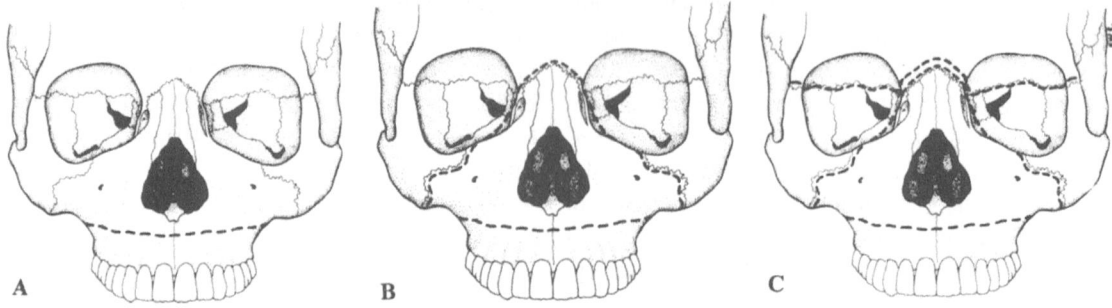

Figure 16.14. LeFort fractures. Schematic demonstration of the LeFort fractures. **A.** LeFort I. **B.** LeFort II. **C.** LeFort III.

thinner bones (the lacrimal bone and the lamina papyracea of the ethmoid) results (Fig. 16.12 and 16.13) (4). The fragments may be displaced along the orbital side of the medial orbital wall or, less commonly, they may penetrate into the ethmoid sinus and produce an out-fracture of the medial wall. In addition, the medial canthal tendon may be severed and the lacrimal sac relationship may be distorted. Clinically, the patient has a depression over the upper portion of the bridge of the nose, telecanthus, tearing, and epistaxis.

Severe trauma may cause a depressed fracture of the frontal bone and a fracture of the cribriform plate and roof of the ethmoid. In patients with roof fractures, neurologic evaluation for CSF fluid rhinorrhea and pneumocephalus may be indicated. An orbital CT scan is most helpful in evaluating comminuted nasoorbital fractures. Associated orbital injury (including orbital hemorrhage or optic canal fracture), intracranial injury (including subdural hematoma or pneumocephalus), and hemorrhage into a sinus, all may be seen on the orbital CT scan. Dacryocystography may be helpful in demonstrating a lacrimal drainage abnormality (4).

LeFort Fractures

Although LeFort fractures are not primarily orbital fractures, they may involve the orbit. The LeFort fractures (types I, II, and III) all involve

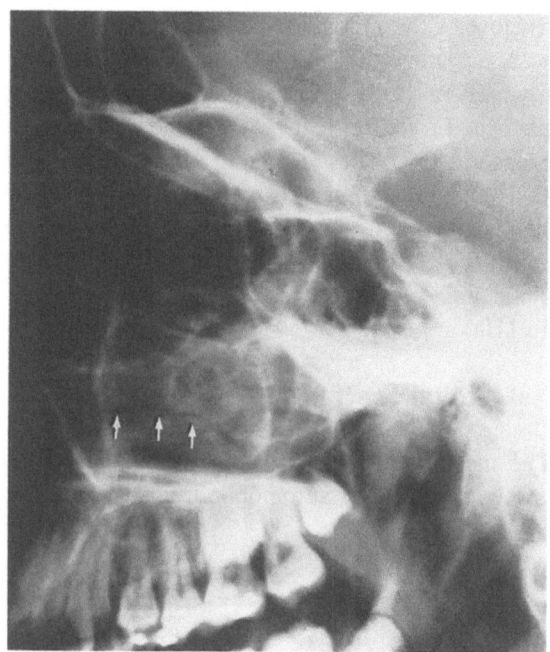

Figure 16.15. LeFort I. A plain lateral x-ray film. A transverse maxillary fracture that separates the palate from the body of the maxilla (arrows) is shown.

the maxilla bilaterally and they are predominantly transverse or horizontally oriented fractures (Fig. 16.14) (3).

Specific features of the three types of LeFort fractures are as follows. LeFort I spares the orbit

Figure 16.16. LeFort II. The first case (**A-C**) shows plain x-ray and complex motion tomograms. The second case (**D and E**) shows axial and direct coronal CT scans. **A.** Tomography of the face in the anteroposterior projection. **B.** Plain x-ray film Water's view. **C.** Lateral tomogram. Multiple bilateral fractures of the maxillary antrum and medial wall of the orbits (arrows) are shown. Also seen are extension of the fractures to the pterygoid plates (open arrows). **D.** Axial CT scan. **E.** Coronal CT scan. Shown are bilateral multiple antral fractures and pterygoid plate fractures (open arrows).

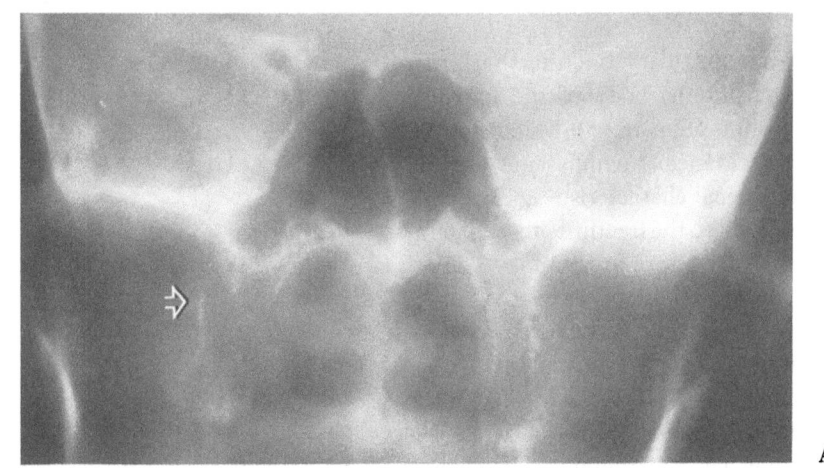

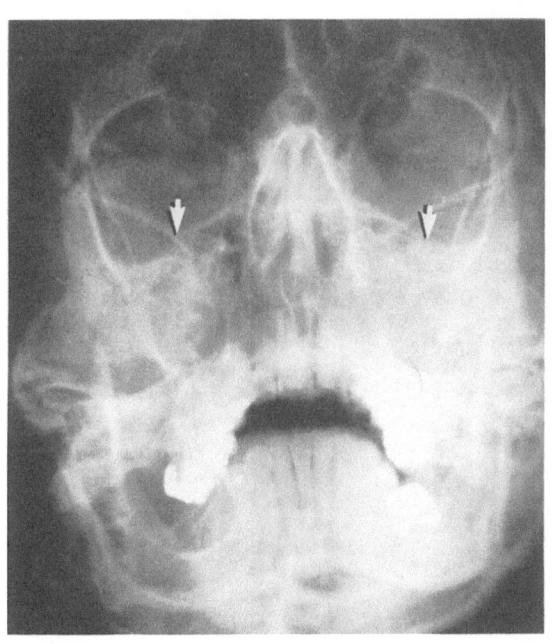

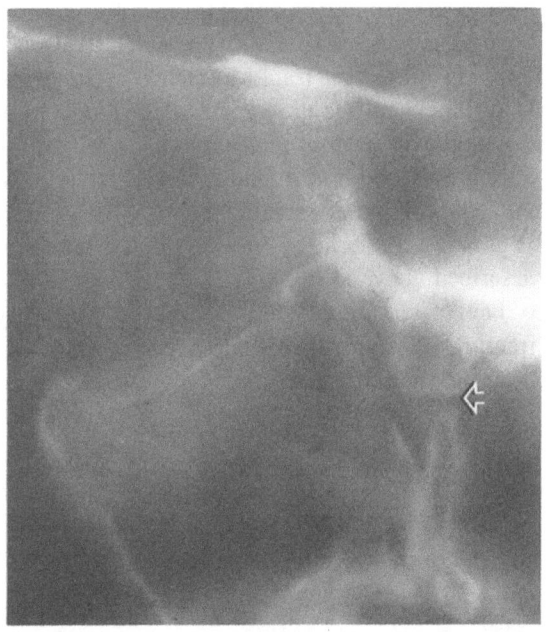

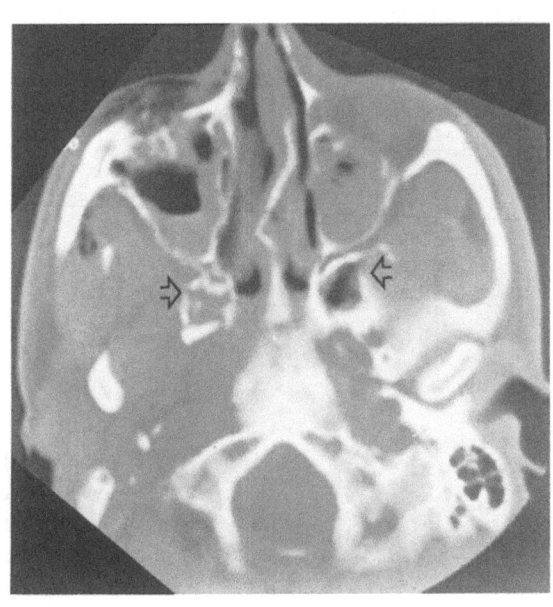

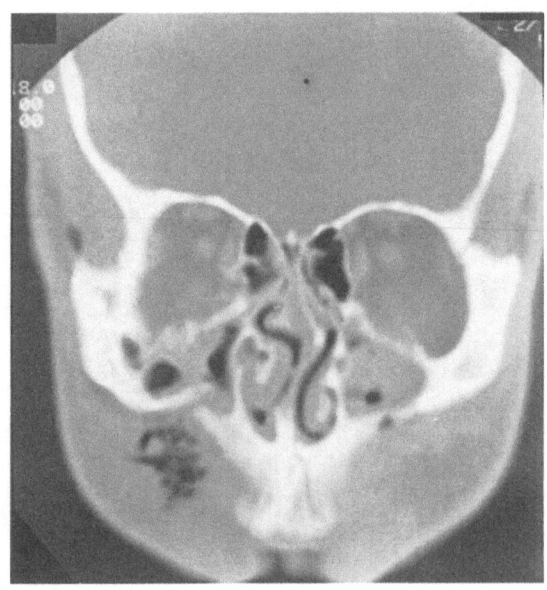

and is a transverse maxillary fracture that separates the palate from the body of the maxillae and the nasal septum (Fig. 16.15). Malocclusion, epistaxis, and subcutaneous emphysema are the most prominent clinical characteristics (15). Radiologically, in addition to the fracture sites, bilateral opaque maxillary sinuses are present.

LeFort types II and III are transverse, symmetric orbitomaxillary fractures. In LeFort II, the facial skeleton below the zygoma is separated from the cranial skeleton. (Fig. 16.16). The fracture is termed a pyramidal fracture of the maxilla, because the fracture has a pyramidal shape when viewed anteriorly. The fracture also involves the nasal bones, frontal process of the maxilla, lacrimal bone, zygomatic maxillary suture, and lateral walls of the maxillae. The fracture extends to the pterygoid plates and the pterygomaxillary fossa. Rupture of the medial canthal tendons bilaterally cause telecanthus, and disruption of the normal lacrimal sac relations may result in tearing. The LeFort II is a severe form of the nasoorbital fractures described above.

The Waters projection is optimal for maxillary fractures. Posteroanterior and lateral views sometimes are helpful, but tomography often is neces-

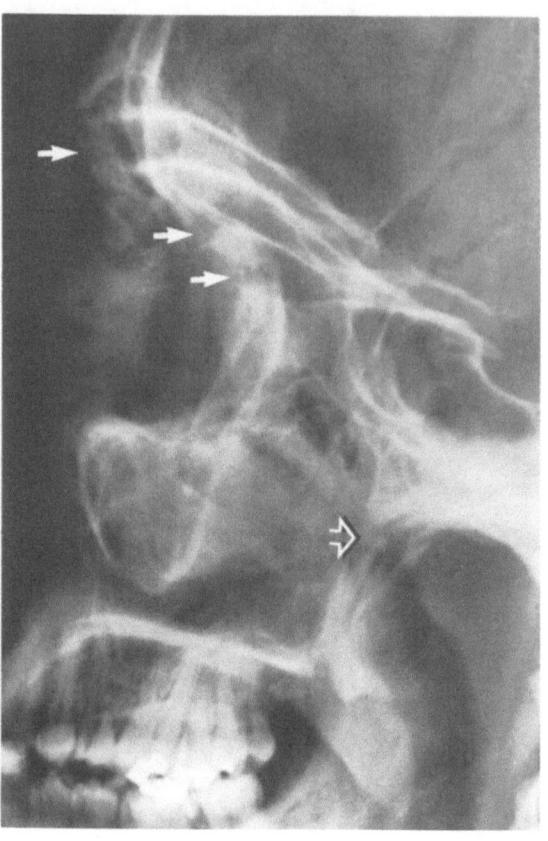

A

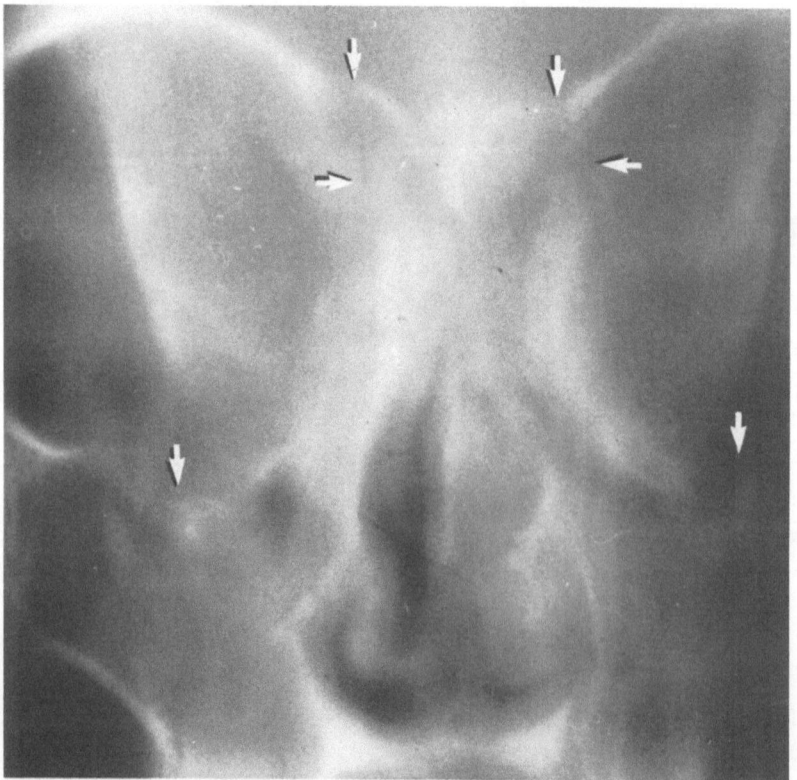

B

Figure 16.17. LeFort III. Plain lateral x-ray films (**A**) and complex motion tomography (**B**) in anteroposterior projection.

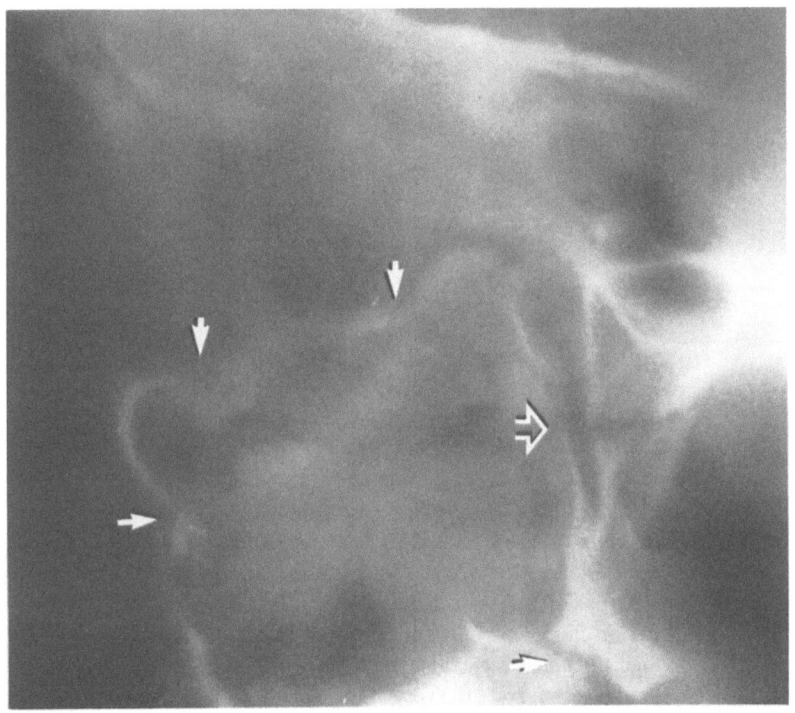

C

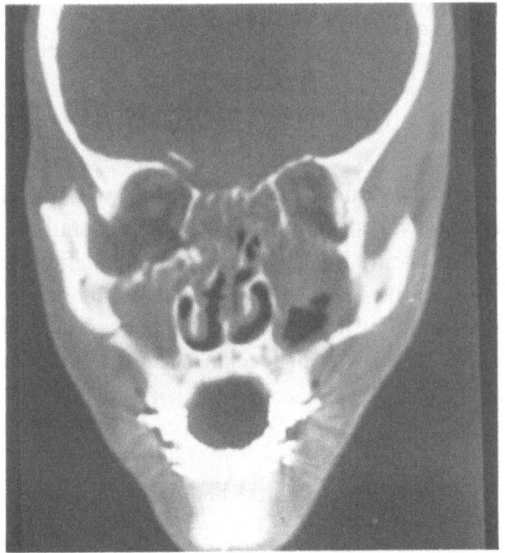

D

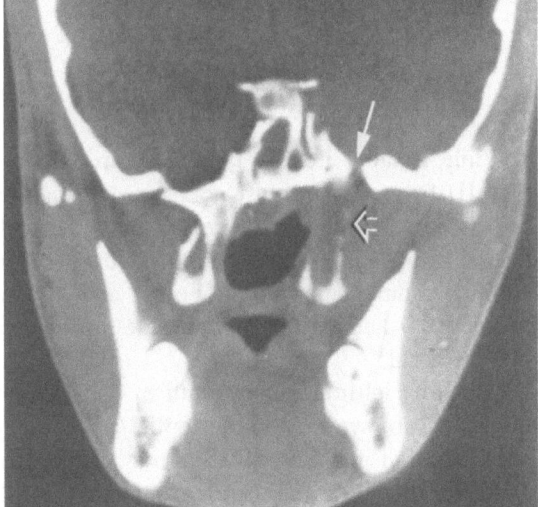

E

Figure 16.17 C. Lateral projection (complex motion tomography). **D, E.** Coronal CT scans are shown. Multiple bilateral fractures involving the maxillary antrum, medial wall of the orbits, and the zygomatic frontal suture (arrows) are shown. The fracture extends posteriorly to involve the pterygoid plates (open arrows).

sary to demonstrate all the fracture sites (Fig. 16.1B). The CT scan is increasingly relied on in the evaluation of these fractures due to the clarity of both contrast and spacial resolution.

In LeFort type III, the middle third of the facial skeleton is completely separated from the base of the skull. The fracture extends from the nasofrontal suture to involve the lacrimal bones and lamina papyracea, the floor of the orbit, and the zygomaticofrontal suture and zygomatic arches (Fig. 16.17). For this reason, tearing may occur as a consequence of LeFort III.

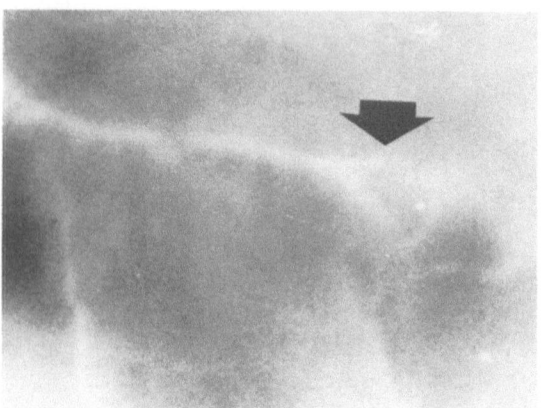

A

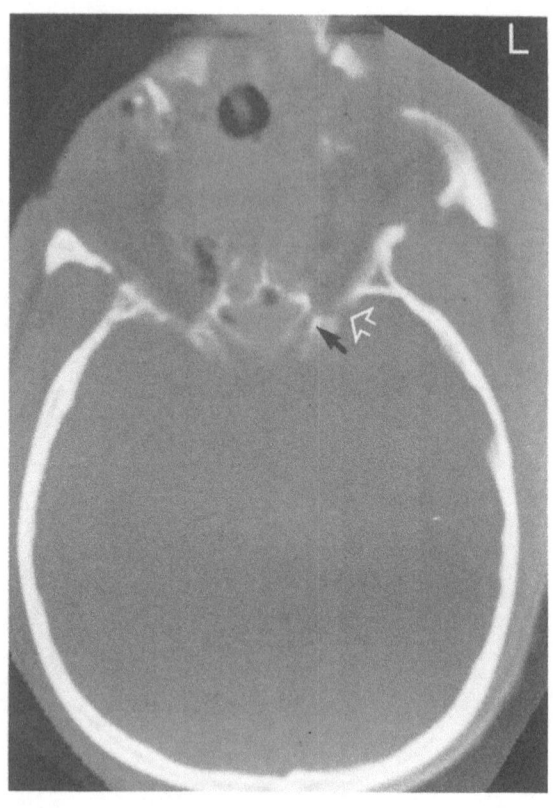

B

Figure 16.18. Fracture of the superior orbital fissure and optic canal. **A.** Orbital complex motion tomography done in the Rheese position. Displaced comminuted fracture of the optic canal (arrow) is seen, along with complete loss of vision in the eye after the trauma. **B.** Another case. An axial CT scan demonstrates a fractured left anterior clinoid process (open arrow), with an anterior medial-rotated segment compromising the optic nerve canal (arrow). Note the very extensive facial fractures in this 28 year old man. The patient had a blind left eye with good vision in the right eye on recovery.

While isolated LeFort type I is rare, LeFort type III fractures are more common and may be associated with other fractures, including tripod, frontal sinus, and/or nasoorbital fractures (3). In addition, combinations of LeFort I and II and of LeFort II and III on opposite sides of the face may occur (1).

Maxillofacial injury may result in the superior orbital fissure syndrome or in optic canal injury with loss of vision. Loss of vision may result from a nonpenetrating injury to the optic nerve with or without a demonstrable fracture (Fig. 16.18).

Gunshot Injuries and Orbital Foreign Bodies

The CT scan is of tremendous value in analyzing gunshot injuries to the head and orbit. Both orbital soft-tissue injury and bullet fragments are evident and can be localized (Fig. 16.19). Although intraocular structures probably were best studied by ocular ultrasonography, the CT scan and MRI may show considerable intraocular detail—such as a dislocated lens or intraocular hemorrhage (Fig. 16.20). Associated fractures of the orbit and intracranial injuries also can be examined. For further discussion of foreign bodies, see Chapters 4, 7, and 8.

Following trauma, superimposed infection may cause ophthalmologic symptoms. (Fig. 16.21)

Associated intraorbital hemorrhage may be assessed by the orbital CT scan. Surgical evacuation or decompression of an orbit for hemorrhage is not performed unless compromise of the optic nerve circulation is documented.

Orbital emphysema usually is secondary to fracture of the paranasal cavities; mainly the ethmoidal, maxillary, and frontal sinuses. Orbitopalpebral and palpebral emphysema are due to fracture of the lacrimal bone anterior to the tarsoorbital fascia, with rupture of the lacrimal sac (12). Both varieties are well visualized on the CT scan and have been extensively illustrated in this chapter.

Figure 16.19. Metallic foreign bodies. **A, B.** Intraorbital bullet fragment at the orbital apex on the optic nerve (arrowheads) is shown. Perforation of the affected eye globe (small arrows) is also seen. **C.** The bullet fragment is seen at the orbital apex adjacent to the optic nerve in another case (arrowhead). An intraocular hemorrhage is seen in the right eye (small arrows).

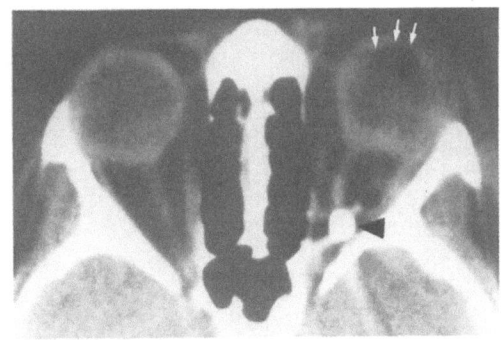

A

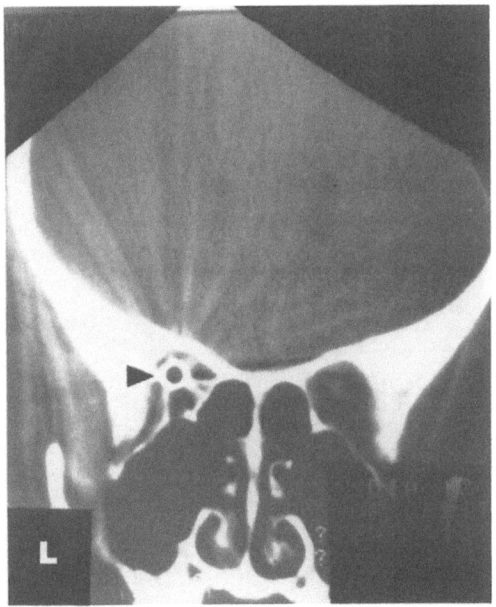

B

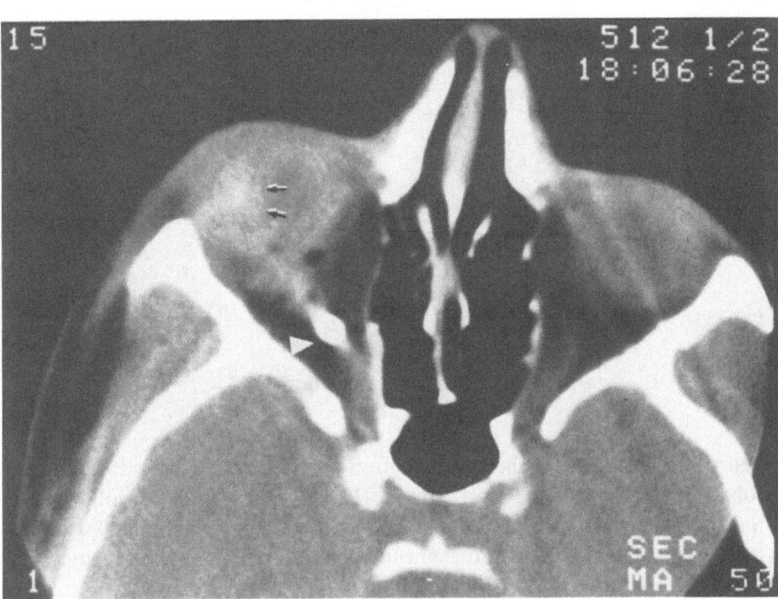

C

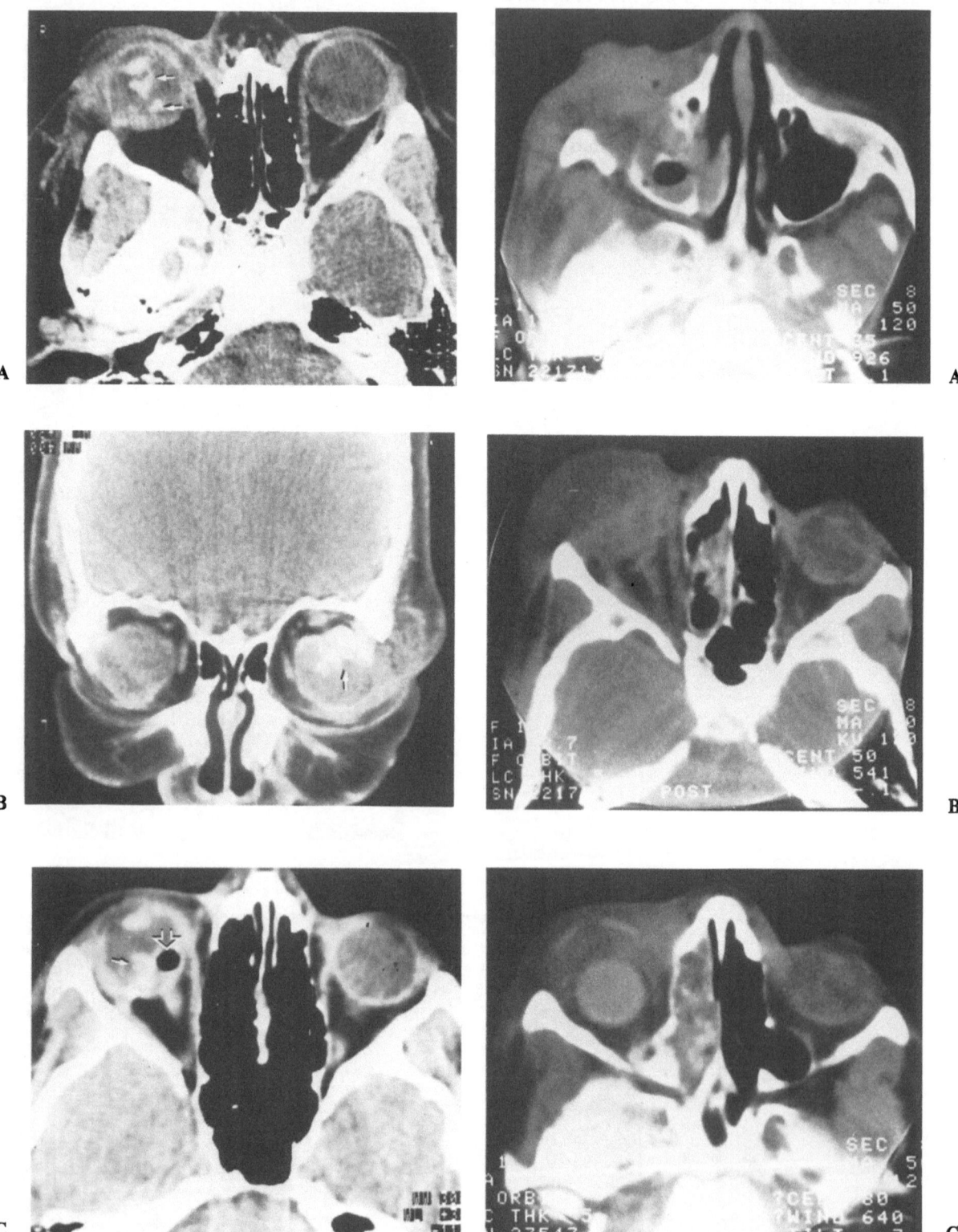

Figure 16.20. Intraocular hemorrhage from penetrating globe injury. Axial (**A, C**) and coronal (**B**) CT scans showing posttraumatic intraocular hemorrhages (arrows). Air within the globe documenting perforation is also seen (open arrow).

Figure 16.21. Infection after trauma. **A, B.** Intraocular abscess following facial trauma involving the maxillary and ethmoid sinuses. **C.** Postsurgical status after drainage of the abscess and enucleation of the eye. A prosthesis is in place.

References

1. Arger PH: Fractures of the orbit, in (ed): Arger PH *Orbit Roentgenology.* New York, John Wiley & Sons, 1977, pp 56–66.

2. Berkowitz RA, Putterman AM, Patel DB: Prolapse of the globe into the maxillary sinus after orbital floor fracture. *Am J Ophthalmol* 91:253–257, 1981.

3. Brant-Zawadek M, Pitts LH: CT of maxillofacial injury, in Federle MP, Brant-Zawadek M (eds): *Computed Tomography in the Evaluation of Trauma.* Baltimore, Williams & Wilkins, 1982, pp 60–96.

4. Converse JM, Smith B: Symposium: Midfacial fractures, nasoorbital fractures. *Trans Am Acad Ophthalmol Otolaryngol* 67:622–634, 1963.

5. Dodick JM, Galin MA, Kwitko M: Medial wall fracture of the orbit. *Can J Ophthalmol* 4:377–378, 1969.

6. Dodick JM, Galin MA, Littleton JT, et al: Concomitant medial wall fracture and blowout fracture of the orbit. *Arch Ophthalmol* 85:273–276, 1971.

7. Edwards WC, Ridley RW: Blowout fracture of medial orbital wall. *Am J Ophthalmol* 65:248–249, 1968.

8. Fischbein FI, Lesko WS: Blowout fracture of the medial orbital wall. *Arch Ophthalmol* 81:162–163, 1969.

9. Flanagan JC, McLachlan DL, Shannon GM: Orbital roof fractures. *Ophthalmology* 87:325–329, 1980.

10. Grove A, Tadmor R, Momose K, et al: Computerized tomography for evaluation of fractures and foreign bodies of the orbit, in Junk W (ed): *Proceedings of the 3rd International Symposium on Orbital Disorders. Amsterdam, September 5–7, 1977.* Orbital Centre of the Amsterdam University Eye Hospital, The Hague, The Netherlands, 1978, pp 130–139.

11. Jones IS: Symposium: Midfacial fractures x-ray findings. *Trans Am Acad Ophthalmol Otolaryngol* 67:635–642, 1963.

12. Lombardi G: *Radiology in Neuroophthalmology.* Baltimore, Williams & Wilkins, 1967, pp 100–101.

13. Mauriello JA, Flanagan JC: Unusual late complications of orbital floor implant (in preparation).

14. Miller GR, Glaser JS: The retraction syndrome and trauma. *Arch Ophthalmol* 76:662–663, 1966.

15. Mclachlan DL, Flanagan JC, Shannon GM: Complications of orbital roof fractures. *Ophthalomology* 89:1274–1278, 1982.

16. Schultz RC: Fractures of the Upper Third of the Face in *Facial Injuries.* Chicago, Year Book Medical Publishers, 1970, pp 126–169.

17. Shannon GM: Orbital Fractures Today in Guibor P (ed): *Orbital Fractures Today in Oculoplastic Surgery and Trauma.* New York, Stratton Intercontinental Medical Book Corporation, 1976, pp 89–96.

18. Smith B, Regan W: Blowout fracture of the orbit. *Am J Ophthalmol* 44:733–739, 1957.

19. Smith B, Grove A, Guibor P: Fractures of the orbit, in Duane TD (ed): *Clinical Ophthalmology.* Philadelphia, Harper & Row, 1982, vol 2, pp 1–48.

20. Soll DB, Poley BJ: Trapdoor variety of blowout fracture of the orbital floor. *Am J Ophthalmol* 60:269–272, 1965.

21. Zizmor J, Noyek AM: Radiographic diagnosis of orbital fractures, in Aston SJ, Hornblass A, Meltzer MA, et al (eds): *Third International Symposium of Plastic and Restructive Surgery of the Eye and Adnexa.* Baltimore, Williams & Wilkins, 1982, pp 66–85.

17
Radiation Therapy for Malignant Intraocular Tumors

Luther W. Brady, Jerry A. Shields, James J. Augsburger, John L. Day,
Arnold M. Markoe, Joseph R. Castro, and Herman D. Swit

There is a wide role for radiation therapy in the management of malignant tumors of the eye. Some investigators state that all primary intraocular malignant tumors, with the exception of retinoblastoma, are best treated by surgical techniques. They point out that the reason to irradiate the eye in patients with such lesions would be to preserve vision. These investigators further state that irradiation to cancerocidal levels may produce an iridocyclitis, resulting in an imbalance between aqueous production and absorption ending in glaucoma. In the past, definitive radiation therapy was pursued only if the lesion was located in the posterior half of the globe. However, with the advent of contemporary innovative techniques of radiation therapy, reassessment of this position indicates that there are specific circumstances under which malignant tumors of the eye can be treated successfully.

In the United States in 1985, the American Cancer Society anticipates that there will be 1,800 new cases of primary malignant tumors of the eye (3). The most common primary malignant tumor of the eye is malignant melanoma of the choroid, which comprises about 75% of all primary malignant tumors of the eye (Table 17.1). The second most common primary malignant tumor of the eye is retinoblastoma, which accounts for about 20% of the cases. The remaining 5% of primary malignant tumors of the eye include epithelial tumors of the uvea, connective tissue and other mesenchymal tumors, hematopoietic tumors, and meningiomas of the optic nerve. In autopsy series, metastatic tumors to the eye—arising most often as secondaries from the breast, lung, or as a part of a lymphomatous or leukemic process—are the most common malignant tumor of the eye. With

the advent of more effective means of treating malignant tumors (using surgery, radiation therapy, and chemotherapy), more patients are surviving to have unusual secondary sites of metastases, such as those occurring in the eye. Therefore, the incidence of metastatic disease to the eye will become more common as more effective treatment techniques result in greater long-term survival.

Posterior Uveal Melanomas

Ophthalmologists have been familiar with posterior uveal melanomas for many years, but there still remains considerable controversy regarding the best approach to diagnosis and treatment. Current data remain confusing, since most information comes from individual case reports or small series of cases, with authors advocating the methods of treatment that each uses (1, 2, 8, 15–17, 28, 29, 30, 31–33).

New techniques for diagnosis and management of choroidal melanoma offer exciting prospects for an improvement in prognosis. In the past, the diagnosis often has been made by direct ophthalmoscopy alone, and errors resulting in unnecessary enucleation were frequent (26). Recent studies have shown that the use of new techniques, such as indirect ophthalmoscopy, fluorescein angiography, ultrasonography, and the P32 test, can reduce the incidence of diagnostic error substantially (25). Computed tomography (CT) as well as magnetic resonance imaging (MRI) may offer even greater accuracy in diagnosis of ocular melanomas while simultaneously assisting in determination of the extent of the tumor.

Melanomas located in the anterior uvea usually

Table 17.1. Malignant intraocular tumors

Primary	Incidence	Secondary
Pigmented tumors	~75%	Metastatic
Retinoblastoma and other neuroectodermal		Lung
tumors of the retina	~20%	Breast
Epithelial—uvea	<1%	Lymphoma
Connective tissue and other mesenchymal		Leukemia
tumors	<1%	
Hematopoietic	<1%	
Meningioma	Rare	

are detected earlier than those located posteriorly, and they may be removed either by iridectomy or by iridocyclectomy. Histologic confirmation of the diagnosis is obtained. However, lesions of the posterior uvea are not readily accessible to biopsy procedures, and the clinical diagnosis occasionally may be difficult. Imaging studies are necessary to arrive at a diagnosis in those circumstances. If there remains a degree of uncertainty as to the diagnosis, a conservative approach with a period of careful observation may be indicated.

The traditional treatment program pursued in the past for posterior uveal melanomas has been enucleation of the eye. Zimmerman, et al have recently challenged the actual benefits of enucleation (33, 34). As a result, there has been increased interest in alternative forms of treatment for this condition. In selected instances, authorities have advocated periodic observation (12), photocoagulation (10, 30), ^{60}Co plaque therapy (10, 24), proton beam irradiation (14), helium ion beam irradiation (5), ^{125}I episcleral plaques (21, 24), ^{192}Ir plaques (24), and ^{106}Ru plaques (19). Depending on the clinical circumstances, a patient with a posterior uveal melanoma is managed by periodic observation, photocoagulation for very small tumors, radionuclide plaque treatment, local resection, or enucleation. Most patients whose tumors show unequivocal signs of progressive growth are managed by one of these forms of active treatment, rather than by simple observation.

In the interval from May 26, 1976 through July 31, 1983, 560 patients had been managed using ^{60}Co plaques, ^{125}I episcleral plaques, and ^{192}Ir episcleral plaques. This was a joint cooperative clinical study carried out by the Oncology Service at the Wills Eye Hospital and the Department of Radiation Oncology at the Hahnemann University Hospital. The first 100 patients treated have been analyzed. The ^{60}Co plaque therapy was carried out

in a uniform fashion for all 100 patients. The presurgical clinical estimation of the basal size of the tumor and the A-scan ultrasonographic measurement of tumor thickness were used to select the proper size of the plaque to be used in the individual patient. Computer programs were designed to determine the appropriate duration of plaque application required to deliver at least 8,000 rads (100 rads = 1 Gray) to the tumor apex, but not to exceed 45,000 rads to the tumor base—knowing the activity of the particular plaque to be used in a given case. The precise position of the melanoma was identified and the locations of the margins of the tumor were marked at surgery on the overlying sclera with surface diathermy. The plaque was secured to the sclera with nonabsorbable sutures, and the conjunctiva was closed. After the plaque had remained in position for the predetermined number of hours, it was removed under local anesthesia.

Treated patients were reexamined at 3- to 6-month intervals. The follow-up examinations included complete routine ocular re-examination, indirect ophthalmoscopy, fundus drawings, 45° and wide-angle fundus photographs, A- and B-scan ultrasonography, and fluorescein angiography.

The tabulation of data included the tumor response, visual acuity results, complications, and mortality. The 100 patients ranged in age from 29–83 years, with a mean age of 60 years. Forty-seven patients were men and 53 were women. The tumor involved the right eye in 48 patients and the left eye in 52 patients. Seven of the tumors were classified as small, 41 as medium, and 52 as large.

The mean tumor dimensions before and after treatment were determined for the small, medium, and large melanomas (Table 17.2). It is apparent that the greater change occurred in tumor thickness, rather than in basal dimension. At the time

Table 17.2. Pretreatment and posttreatment tumor dimensions for 100 posterior uveal melanomas managed by cobalt plaque radiotherapy

Tumor size		Pretreatment mean tumor dimensions	Posttreatment mean tumor dimensions	Reduction in tumor volume (%)
Category	No.			
Small	7	7.6 × 6.6 × 2.3 mm (115.4 mm³)	7.1 × 6.1 × 1.0 mm (43.3 mm³)	62.5
Medium	41	9.6 × 8.0 × 4.2 mm (322.6 mm³)	9.4 × 7.8 × 2.7 mm (198.0 mm³)	38.6
Large	52	11.8 × 10.2 × 7.3 mm (878.6 mm³)	10.5 × 9.1 × 4.4 mm (420.4 mm³)	52.0

of the most recent follow-up, 96 of 100 treated tumors had shown a decrease in thickness following treatment; one had shown no change in thickness, and only three melanomas continued to increase in thickness following the treatment program. Two of the latter were subsequently managed by enucleation, and the third was managed by reapplication of the ^{60}Co plaque. Regression of the tumor in each instance was documented with wide-angle photography and A-scan ultrasonography.

Analysis of this group of patients revealed four distinctive patterns of tumor regression. The type I regression pattern was defined as minimal, if any, apparent change in size or appearance of the tumor following treatment. Tumors that exhibited this regression pattern generally were relatively small tumors with pretreatment clinical features suggesting chronicity or relative dormancy, such as extensive retinal pigment epithelial disruption or pigment clumping on the tumor surface.

The type II regression pattern was defined as a prominent decrease in tumor size without any appreciable exudative or hemorrhagic complications. Most of the tumors that exhibited this regression pattern originally were rather large, mushroom-shaped amelanotic tumors that had broken through Bruch's membrane. These tumors generally developed both irregular furrowing on their vitreal surfaces and whitish discoloration of the overlying retinal pigment epithelium as early signs of regression. Associated nonrhegmatogenous retinal detachments usually diminished or resolved within 6 weeks after the treatment. In many cases, all that remained of the original tumor after 3 or more years of follow-up was a plaque-like fibrotic pigmented scar. Fluorescein angiography of the regressed tumors generally revealed marked obliteration of both the choroidal and retinal vessels in the field of the radiation treatment.

The type III regression pattern was defined as marked shrinkage of the tumor, accompanied by a rather prominent exudative response. This regressive pattern was most commonly observed in eyes that had an extensive nonrhegmatogenous retinal detachment accompanying a moderate-to-intense melanotic nodular tumor. An exudative reaction generally developed first around the base of the tumor 6 months or more following the plaque treatment. The retinal and intraretinal exudative response generally increased in extent over the next 1–2 years before gradually resolving.

The type IV regression pattern was defined as mild-to-marked intravitreal or subretinal bleeding accompanying tumor shrinkage. This regression pattern generally occurred in patients with rather large, partially necrotic tumors that had already bled, to some extent, into the vitreous and subretinal spaces prior to treatment. A few eyes with relatively small, but fast-growing, tumors also developed this regression pattern.

Of the first 100 patients treated with ^{60}Co plaque treatment, 97 exhibited satisfactory local tumor control, which was defined as at least a slight tumor shrinkage and no subsequent tumor growth. Of the 97 eyes exhibiting a satisfactory local tumor response, the relative proportions of each of the 4 regression patterns at the 2 year post-treatment follow-up were as follows: type I regression, 10% of patients; type II regression, 60% of patients; type III regression, 21% of patients; and type IV regression, 10% of patients.

A number of factors influence the final visual outcome, including the size and location of the tumor and the extent of retinal detachment prior to plaque treatment. Most patients who exhibited type I or type II regression patterns retained relatively good vision in the duration of follow-up, unless the tumor was located less than 4–5 mm from the optic disc and/or fovea. In contrast, patients who exhibited type III or type IV regression patterns generally fared much worse visually, particularly if the subretinal exudates or subretinal hemorrhage involved the fovea region. Our preliminary results suggest that the long-term survival rates are likely to be highest in those patients with type I regression and lowest in those patients with rapid tumor shrinkage following plaque therapy.

Visual results of cobalt plaque radiotherapy on the eyes of 77 patients with posterior uveal melanoma in one eye and pretreatment visual acuity of 20/25 or better in both eyes were analyzed using actuarial methods. (Table 17.3) The study demonstrated that eyes receiving a radiation dose in excess of 5,000 rad to the fovea and/or optic disc commonly lose a substantial amount of vision within 2 to 3 years. It also showed that eyes treated by cobalt plaque radiotherapy for a large posterior uveal melanoma are more likely to suffer profound visual loss than those treated for a medium or small melanoma. The predominant cause of severe visual loss in these patients appeared to be foveal radiation retinopathy.

About 40% of the patients treated have developed complications thus far. Table 17.4 outlines the complications of radiation therapy that have been observed in those 100 patients during the 2–5-year follow-up period.

Follow-up has been obtained in all 100 patients. Only 3 of the 100 treated patients have died from metastatic melanoma during the full range of follow-up (Table 17.5). There were no deaths among the seven patients with small melanomas, one death among the 41 patients with medium-sized melanomas (2.4%), and two deaths among the 32 patients with large-sized melanomas (3.8%). The interval from the time of plaque application to death was 14 months for the one patient with a medium-sized melanoma; the mean was 9.7 months for the two patients with large-sized melanomas. Two patients died of causes unrelated to the melanoma, and neither had clinical nor laboratory evidence of metastatic melanoma. All of the remaining 95 patients are alive, with no evidence of metastases at the time that these data were tabulated.

In view of the recent controversy regarding enucleation as a form of therapy for posterior uveal melanomas, there has been an increasing interest in alternative forms of treatment. The ideal alternative treatment would be one that would: 1) destroy or inactivate the neoplasm; 2) maintain useful vision in the involved eye; 3) have few adverse side effects; and, most importantly; 4) provide the patient with a favorable prognosis for life. Since choroidal melanomas are relatively uncommon and the alternative therapies have not been widely used, no one has previously acquired a large series of validly matched patients to determine statistically how these methods compare to enucleation with regard to mortality rates. These investigators have assessed the relative survival rates of groups

Table 17.4. Complications of cobalt plaque therapy of 100 posterior uveal melanomas

Radiation tumor vasculopathy	18 }	30
Radiation retinopathy	12 }	
(with radiation papillopathy)	5	
Intravitreal hemorrhage	11	
Radiation cataract	7	
Punctal occlusion/epiphora	3	
Radiation anterior uveitis	2	
Scleral necrosis/thinning	2	
Persistent diplopia	2	

Table 17.3. Visual acuity results in 100 patients with posterior uveal melanoma treated with cobalt plaque radiotherapy

Initial visual acuity	No.	6/5–6/7.5	6/9–6/12	6/15–6/30	6/60–HM
6/5–6/7.5	37	19	7	7	4
6/9–6/12	26	6	11	6	3
6/15–6/30	25	2	4	5	14
6/60–HM	12	0	1	2	9
Total	100	27	23	20	30

Visual acuities recorded in meters.
HM, hand motions.

Table 17.5. Mortality data on 100 patients with posterior uveal melanoma managed by cobalt plaque radiotherapy

Tumor size		Metastatic melanoma	Death from all causes	Death from metastatic melanoma	Mean interval from plaque application to melanoma death
Category	No.				
Small	7	0	0	0	—
Medium	41	1	2	1 (2.4%)	14.0 Mo
Large	52	2	3	2 (3.8%)	9.7 Mo
Total	100	3	5	3	—

of patients matched for individual parameters, including age, sex, and size of tumor and treated by enucleation or cobalt plaque therapy.

The second major consideration is the effect of the ⁶⁰Co plaque radiotherapy on visual acuity in the involved eye. Preliminary data suggest that many patients who have good visual acuity at the time of the plaque application maintain useful vision during 1–5-year follow-up periods. This has been confirmed by MacFaul (20), who followed the patients treated by Stallard (27). Since we are currently treating larger melanomas with ⁶⁰Co plaque therapy, it is most likely that the long-term visual outcome will be somewhat poorer. However, if the long-term survival rate proves to be more favorable with radiotherapy than with enucleation, any result in visual loss seems acceptable.

In summary, ⁶⁰Co plaque therapy appears to be a reasonable alternative to enucleation in selected patients with posterior uveal melanoma. Some radiation complications are probably unavoidable, but this method of treatment appears to offer the patient a 5-year systemic prognosis as good as that following enucleation and at least the possibility of preservation of useful vision.

Treatment of Choroidal Melanomas by Fractionated Proton Beam Radiation Therapy

Since 1975, the Massachusetts General Hospital, the Massachusetts Eye and Ear Infirmary, and the Harvard Cyclotron Laboratory have pursued evaluation of the efficacy of fractionated proton beam irradiation in treating choroidal melanomas (14). The basic concept was to achieve a uniform distribution of radiation dose that was closely confined to the choroidal melanoma, thus permitting a very high dose delivered to the tumor with a high probability for tumor control. The physical characteristics of dose absorption of the proton beam make this an attractive modality for investigating the treatment of small, discrete, and well-localized lesions (13).

To date, the group has treated 245 patients definitively by using this radiation technique for choroidal melanoma. The diagnosis has been established in the previously described fashion. Also, the technical details of the treatment include the placement of small tantalum rings sutured onto the sclera around the perimeter of the lesion, which is determined by transillumination of the eye. Then the three-dimensional relationships between the tumor, the tantalum rings, and the normal anatomic structures of the eye are established based on detailed fundus drawings made at the time of pre-treatment examination, fundus photographs, and on ultrasonography. The general treatment plan has been to allow 1.5-mm margins around the visible tumor for microscopic extensions of the tumor, positional errors, and uncertainty about the position of clips relative to the tumor. The radiation dosages are given in five equal treatment fractions over a period of 8–10 days, with total doses ranging between 46–100 CGE. (CGE represents cobalt Gray [1 Gray = 100 rads] equivalents; they are obtained by multiplying the physical dose expressed in Gray by 1.10—the RBE factor.) Pre-treatment radiographs are used to achieve alignment of the beam in relation to the tumor. Closed-circuit television views the eye with fluoroscopic monitoring of the rings, assuring that the alignment is maintained.

The status of those patients followed for 6 months or more is presented in Table 17.6. Of the 95 patients treated by that time, six had small tumors; 50 patients had tumors that were greater than 15 mm in diameter and more than 5 mm

Table 17.6. Status of patients 6–89 months after proton beam therapy of choroidal melanoma[a]

No. patients	Mean follow-up (months)	Tumor size (mm)	Local control	Uncertain	Distant metastasis
7	29	Small 10 × 2	7	0	0
65	27	Medium 10–15 × 2–5	64	0	1
83	19	Large 15 × 5–10	81	2	5
13	—	Extra large 20 × 10	13	0	1

[a] Analysis, 3/83.

in height, which were termed large. At present, there are two marginal failures and one local failure in the entire experience. Five patients have developed distant metastases, all of whom had large tumors. Three patients have had enucleation (all of whom had large tumors), and the enucleation was performed because of persistent, unresolved retinal detachment. Table 17.7 presents the data in relation to the patient material, with 16 demonstrating reduction in visual acuity. The patients who demonstrated vitreous hemorrhage, rubeosis, or radiation retinopathy had large tumors. There were six patients who had macular edema. These patients had tumors abutting or overlapping the macula. Sixteen patients developed cataracts, which are an expected complication of the proton beam treatment; and several patients have had uncomplicated extractions of the cataracts.

In conclusion, these results are extremely attractive, in that major morbidity and mortality have not been encountered. The small- and medium-sized tumors have been treated without major complications and with good preservation of vision. There has been difficulty in obtaining proper resolution of retinal detachment in some patients who have had extensive tumors. Unfortunately, the follow-up interval for most patients treated by protons is still rather short.

High-Dose Radiotherapy: Helium Ion Treatment for Ocular Melanoma

In the last decade, beams of heavy-charged particles, such as proton and helium nuclei, have become available for clinical radiotherapy trials. Because of the Bragg peak effect and the extremely sharp penumbra of these beams, a high uniform dose can be delivered to a tumor while nearby structures receive an insignificant dose. At the distal edge of the Bragg peak, the dose falls from 90% to 10% in a 7-mm distance. Laterally, the fall-off is very sharp, going from 90% to 10% in 1 mm. Optimal use of this excellent localization of dose in the region of the Bragg peak requires extremely careful and accurate tumor localization, treatment planning, patient immobilization, and treatment verification. Having accomplished all this, charged-particle radiotherapy offers the possibility of irradiating ocular melanomas as close as 3 mm from the disc or macula and yet preserving useful vision. These techniques are currently being tested in clinical trials conducted at the Harvard Cyclotron using a proton beam and the Berkeley Laboratories using a helium ion beam derived from a 184-inch synchrocyclotron.

The group at the University of California at San Francisco and the Lawrence Berkeley Labora-

Table 17.7. Status of normal tissue in 100 patients at 6–78 months after proton beam therapy for choroidal melanoma[a]

	No. patients
Visual acuity	16
Vitreous hemorrhage	2[b]
Rubeosis	4[b]
Radiation retinopathy	2[b]
Macula edema	6
Cataract	16

[a] Analysis, 1/82.
[b] In patients with large tumors.

tory have treated patients with ocular melanoma over a 5-year period. The clinical results from the helium ion beam at the Lawrence Berkeley Laboratory have been promising (4, 6, 7).

In the interval from January 1, 1978 through December 31, 1982, 96 patients with ocular melanoma received helium ion radiotherapy at the Lawrence Berkeley Laboratory. Seventy-five of these patients had a 3 month or greater follow-up. All of the patients were evaluated in the ocular oncology unit at the University of California at San Francisco. The work-up was carried out in the usual fashion, with the diagnosis being established by the standard method of evaluation using noninvasive techniques. Patients accepted for the helium ion therapy program: 1) had a growing lesion less than 14 mm in diameter and less than 7 mm in height; 2) had a small stable lesion, with the patient electing to have this therapy; and 3) refused to have enucleation regardless of the size or status of the lesion.

After having been accepted for the protocol, the patients had four or more 2-mm in diameter tantalum rings sutured to the sclera to mark the borders of the base of the tumor. The base of the tumor was localized by transillumination of the globe and indirect ophthalmoscopy. The patient, after having recovered from the surgical procedures, had a custom-molded polystyrene head holder made for immobilization and underwent a simulation session to obtain x-ray films for treatment planning. The program was then planned using a computer-derived program.

Once the treatment plan had been finalized, the treatment was delivered in five fractions, usually in an eight-day interval. A tumor dose of 70 to 80 Gray equivalents was given. For this fraction size, the RBE in the helium Bragg peak is 1.3 in relation to ^{60}Co. Twenty patients received a tumor dose of 70 Gray equivalents. Several local tumor failures occurred in this group. Subsequently, the dose was increased to 80 Gray equivalents for the remaining 55 patients.

The 75 patients ranged in age from 25–81 years, with a mean age of 60 years. There were equal numbers of men and women. There were three small tumors (less than 10 mm in diameter and less than 3 mm in thickness), 24 medium-sized tumors (10–15 mm in diameter and 3–5 mm in thickness), and 48 large tumors (greater than 15 mm in diameter or greater than 5 mm in thickness). All of the patients were evaluated 6 weeks after completion of the treatment program and every 3–4 months thereafter.

The results indicate a high local tumor control, with no metastases posttreatment and with a low incidence of serious morbidity. The mean follow-up time has been 18 months. Table 17.8 summarizes the local control from the two dose groups.

It is important to note that all five of the local failures have been salvaged. Four have been salvaged by enucleation and one by reirradiation with a helium ion beam. All five have no current evidences of tumor. None of the patients have developed distant metastatic disease following treatment.

The data obtained by ultrasound measurements following the treatment program indicate that the height remains stable for 6–8 months following treatment; then a slow shrinkage of the tumor begins. The time of onset of tumor shrinkage has been variable, ranging from 1–24 months.

Posttreatment complications are summarized in Table 17.9. Serious complications have been uncommon, although five patients have developed glaucoma in the irradiated eye; all five had tumors that were large. The most common side effect was a self-limited radiation reaction in the eyelid, which occurred when it was impossible to com-

Table 17.8. Local control in patients with choroidal melanoma treated with helium ion beam[a]

Dose	70 Gy E	80 Gy E
Number of patients	20	55
Local failure	4	1
Mean follow-up	30 mo	14 mo
All failures salvaged and no evidence of disease (NED)		

[a] 1983.

Table 17.9. Posttreatment complications in patients with choroidal melanoma treated with helium ion beam

Skin reaction in lid and/or lash loss	54
Radiation vasculopathy involving optic disc or macula	11
Cataract	6
Neovascular glaucoma	5
Punctal occlusion	4
Dry eye	2
Vitreous hemorrhage	2

pletely retract the eyelid away from the helium ion beam. This usually was accompanied by permanent loss of eyelashes in the region. Six patients had other sequelae from eyelid irradiation—two had dry eyes and four required treatment for stenosed tear ducts. Eleven patients developed radiation vasculopathy involving the macula and/or the optic disc. In all cases, the macula or disc was included in the high-dose region due to the proximity of the tumor to those structures. Six patients developed cataracts, with decreased visual acuity in three patients. Two patients have had vitreous hemorrhages—one in the immediate postsurgical period and one about 18 months following treatment.

Good visual acuity generally has been preserved in those patients with tumors more than 4 mm away from the disc and macula and with good vision prior to treatment. Table 17.10 summarizes the visual acuities for 42 patients with 1 year or more of follow-up and with the treated eye still in place. Causes suggested for poor vision (20/200 or worse) in the remaining third of the patients are given in Table 17.11. The most common cause

of poor vision is radiation vasculopathy of the macula or optic disc due to deliberate inclusion in the treatment volume when treating nearby tumors.

Six eyes have been enucleated and examined histologically—four for tumor recurrence, one because of severe pain in the glaucomatous blind eye, and one in a patient who resided in a rural area several thousand miles from the University of California at San Francisco. In the latter instance, the ophthalmologist became concerned because of pain in the eye and opacification of the lens, which made tumor follow-up difficult. Therefore, the eye was removed.

In conclusion, helium ion radiotherapy is an extremely promising treatment modality for ocular melanoma. The preliminary posttreatment follow-up data shows 93% of the patients without a relapse; all of the patients who relapsed have been salvaged with a second treatment, usually enucleation. No patients have developed metastases thus far after treatment, but follow-up is still relatively short. Visual acuity generally has been preserved if the tumor is more than 4 mm away from the disc and the macula. Normal tissue morbidity has been mild, although five patients have developed a neovascular glaucoma.

Table 17.10. Ocular melanoma: visual acuity in 42 patients followed ≥ 1 year treated with helium ion beam

Visual acuity	Number of patients
20/20–20/50	19
20/50–20/100	10
20/100–20/200	4
20/200–20/400	3
Count fingers at 6 ft	4
Perceives hand motion	2
Blind	1

Table 17.11. Ocular melanoma: reasons for poor vision (worse than 20/100) in helium-ion beam patients

Radiation vasculopathy involving optic disc or macula	7
Pretreatment retinal detachment	2
Cataract	1
Macular exudate of uncertain etiology	1
Macular degeneration of uncertain etiology	1
Senile macular degeneration predating treatment	1
Unknown	1

Other Therapies

Other therapeutic modalities have the potential for further benefit. Chemotherapy has not been given a clinical trial for treatment of primary malignant melanomas of the choroid. One report of bilateral metastatic melanoma to the iris reported a response to treatment with 1,3 Bis-(2-chlorethyl)-1 Nitrosourea (BCNU). A number of other chemotherapeutic agents are being used alone or in various combinations to treat systemic melanoma, but these have not been used in the treatment of ocular melanomas.

Immunotherapy of systemic melanomas is being investigated actively. Little has been done to evaluate its effectiveness for primary intraocular melanomas. DTIC (Bacillus Calmette-Guerin) vaccine has been used in some centers for the treatment of disseminated malignant melanomas, but its role in therapy for primary ocular melanomas is unknown. Monoclonal antibody therapies are currently being developed.

Conclusion

When managing patients with uveal melanomas, the use of the newer imaging techniques (ultrasonography, CT scanning, and possibly MRI) are essential in the diagnosis, treatment planning, and follow-up.

The best mode of treatment for patients with actively growing uveal melanomas is open to discussion. With enucleation of the globe, the 5-year survival rate (lesions less than 10 mm in diameter and 3 mm in elevation) probably is greater than 90%. However, at present, there is little evidence to indicate that this method of treatment alters the incidence of distant metastases. Thus, methods that preserve the globe and possibly useful vision are being studied. The promising results of the newer radiation therapy techniques (radioactive plaques, proton beams, and helium ions) indicate a need for continued evaluation and comparison of modes of therapy. The roles of immunotherapy need to be studied.

Precancerous Melanosis

Precancerous melanosis is a lesion in which malignant cells remain localized and intraepithelial in character. They extend horizontally and produce a widespread pigmented area over the conjunctiva, both over the globe and the undersurface of the eyelids. In general, no treatment is necessary at this stage of the disease. Malignant transformation can occur even after attempts at therapy are made. Treatment is reserved for the malignant area when it is positively demonstrated.

Cancerous Melanosis

Cancerous melanosis is a disease that invades the subepithelial tissue, and it may produce one or more malignant melanomas. Treatment programs can be pursued by using gamma radiation from tantalum-182 or from radium or cobalt plaques. In general, 3,000 rads in 5 days with a 1-week rest interval followed by 3,000 rads in 5 days may be used, or a continuous treatment program delivering 4,000–5,000 rads to the conjunctiva. As advocated in most instances, the entire conjunctiva surface must be included. Small areas of disease can be treated by using a ^{90}Sr plaque.

Conjunctival Melanomas

Conjunctival melanomas are epithelial in origin; they arise from the normal epithelium or (commonly) from a preexisting nevus or precancerous melanosis. Histologically, invasion of the epithelium by the melanoma is an important diagnostic point, as it does not occur in benign nevi. These conjunctival melanomas have a 5-year survival in the range of 20–25%. They usually occur near the limbus and often are unrelated to cancerous melanosis. Beta irradiation using ^{90}Sr plaques delivering 2,000–2,500 rads in a single dose at weekly intervals (from a total of 9,000–12,000 rads) has been used with good effect. These tumors usually are more localized than the cancerous melanosis, especially when occuring near the limbus.

Retinoblastoma

Retinoblastoma is the most common intraocular malignancy of childhood. The general statistics, epidemiology, genetics, and other aspects of this tumor are well described. Although the clinical features may vary, most children present with a white pupillary reflex (leukocoria), strabismus, or a fundus mass noted on eye examination. A number of benign conditions resemble retinoblastoma clinically by producing leukocoria, strabismus, or a fundal mass. For example, of 136 children referred to the oncology unit at the Willis Eye Hospital between 1974–1978 with conditions suspected of being possible retinoblastomas, 60 had retinoblastoma and 76 had lesions that simulated retinoblastoma.

Retinoblastoma can usually be diagnosed clinically on the basis of ophthalmic examination and appropriate ancillary studies. A detailed history, including a careful family history, should be taken prior to examination of all children with retinoblastoma. Children with retinoblastoma usually do not have a history of an evident ocular abnormality at birth. They typically develop strabismus or leukocoria in the interval between 6 months and 2 years of age. Most children will have a normal physical examination, although there occasionally may be other genetic syndromes. Most children present with no evidence of metastases at the time of the initial examination. External ocular examination, slit lamp biomicroscopy and indirect ophthalmoscopy, as well as radiologic examinations, ultrasonography, and CT scans, all contribute to the diagnosis and determination of the extent of the disease. Aqueous enzymes and cytologic examination of intraocular needle aspirates also may distinguish retinoblastoma from other disease entities involving the eye.

When retinoblastoma is found in both eyes, it is often markedly asymetric. In such cases, the treatment program that has generally been pursued includes enucleation of the worse eye and photocoagulation, cryotherapy or radiation therapy to the other eye. The radiation therapy to the remaining eye should be done in such a way as to encompass all of the tumor identified in the clinical examination, sparing the normal structures. Spread of the tumor beyond the globe occurs mainly by direct extension via the optic nerve. This pathway permits extension into the subarachnoid space, and access to the brain and spinal cord. Spread also may occur through emissary veins to the orbital tissues. Multiple foci of origin are common. Failure to adequately include all of the potential extension of the tumor may allow for subsequent recurrence. Other treatment techniques (coagulation, chemotherapy, and so on) often are added to maximize the potential for long-term control in the remaining eye. Radiation therapy can be employed primarily for both eyes if both have symmetric but potentially controllable disease and some chance for retention of useful vision. Bilateral treatment has been carried out by various investigators, including Shidnia et al (23) with no increase in the death rate and with a definite increase in the proportion of useful eyes.

Another treatment technique that can be used in selected cases is radioactive plaque therapy. The lesion should be localized and not involve the optic disc, with a maximum diameter not greater than 10–15 mm. The surface applicator must be accurately fixed over the lesion. The dose to the anterior portion of the eye must be low. This treatment technique has been carried out in 12 patients in a joint venture between the Department of Radiation Oncology at the Hahnemann University and the Oncology Service of Wills Eye Hospital. The most common retinal changes as a consequence of the radiation therapy are obliteration of retinal capillaries, retinal exudates, retinal detachment, and retinal hemorrhage (Brady, L.W., personal communication).

Metastatic Intraocular Tumors

Historically, metastatic cancer to the eye has been considered a rare disease. However, recent studies have suggested that metastatic disease is the most common intraocular malignancy. Ocular structures affected by metastatic disease include the globe, orbit, adnexa, optic nerve, extraocular muscles, and conjunctiva. The intraocular structures involved include the choroid, iris, ciliary body, and (rarely) the retina. The predilection in adults is for the uveal tract, with the choroid being the favorite site. While choroidal metastases most commonly arise from the breast and lung, other sites include skin melanoma, colon, stomach, esophagus, pancreas, and kidney. Twenty percent of patients present with bilateral disease. Metastases from the breast show a higher percentage of bilaterality than other primary sites. Multiple lesions within one or both eyes are evident in about 20% of cases.

Observation of small lesions may be the appropriate treatment program, since about 50% of metastatic lesions to the eye do not progress during the period of observation if the patient is on effective chemotherapy regimens. Stabilization and/or regression of metastatic intraocular tumors can be seen in response to systemically administered chemotherapy and, rarely, as a spontaneous phenomenon in some untreated patients. However, our recommendation is that radiation therapy should be initiated promptly if the macula or disc are involved or the vision is seriously impaired. In general, enucleation is not indicated unless the affected eye becomes blind and painful.

In a combined cooperative effort between the Department of Radiation Oncology at the Hahnemann University and the Oncology Service of the Wills Eye Hospital, individuals were selected for radiation therapy after evaluation with a careful history, slit lamp examination, and indirect ophthalmoscopy. Fluorescein angiography, ultrasonography, and occasionally other diagnostic techniques were often employed to help substantiate the clinical diagnosis. In the assessment of patients with metastatic disease in the eye, it is important to separate those individuals with no active systemic disease from those with active systemic disease. The former category of patients (those with active disease only in the eye) should be treated aggressively, with the potential expectation that long-term survival will result. On the other hand, those who have metastatic disease to the eye with active systemic disease should be treated more conservatively.

The technique for the radiation therapy program used involves either right-angled wedge fields using megavoltage techniques or direct lateral fields posterior to the lens using megavoltage techniques. In general, the radiation dosage was 3,000 rads in 3 weeks as the tumor-dose minimum for those patients who had both metastatic disease involving the eye and active systemic metastatic disease; or, 5,600 rads in 5.5 weeks as a tumor-dose minimum for those patients with metastatic disease to the eye with no active systemic disease. In the series from the Hahnemann University, 47 patients were evaluated, 11 of whom were male and 36 female. In the Wills Eye Hospital series, 17 of 70 patients were male and 53 female. The average age was 49.7 years. Table 17.12 indicates the primary source of metastases in both series. The dominant site was for lesions arising from the breast, with a second most common site being the lung. Tumors were defined as being metachronous when the primary lesion had been successfully controlled. Also, months or years had elapsed between the occurrence of the primary tumor and the development of a solitary focus within the choroid of the eye (72.3% of cases). These patients would be treated aggressively by radiation therapy to the eye, with a potential expectation for long-term survival. Precocious metastases represented those lesions appearing as the first sign of cancer (15.1% of cases). At that point, there were no detectable evidences of a hidden primary source, and these patients also were treated aggressively for expected potential long-term survival. Synchronous metastases representing solitary metastatic lesions occurred simultaneously with a de-

fined primary neoplasm (4.2% of cases). In 8.4% of the cases, these parameters were unknown.

In the Hahnemann University series, 58 eyes in 47 patients were treated by radiation therapy techniques. In the Wills Eye Hospital series of 70 patients, 35 of 83 eyes were treated by radiation therapy techniques, 36 of 83 eyes by observation, 11 of 83 eyes by enucleation, and one eye was treated by iridocyclectomy. This reflects the different referral patterns to the two departments.

The median survival after treatment in all patients was 8.5 months; 88.9% of all patients demonstrated a positive objective response to the radiation therapy programs being pursued. The median survival from time of diagnosis was 8 months in those patients with metastases from the breast, 3.3 months with those having metastases from the lung, and 4 months with those having metastases from other sites. No significant complications were encountered as a consequence of the radiation therapy.

Ocular metastases often simulate other better-known ophthalmic entities, and the diagnosis at referral was correct in only 38% of the cases seen. Appreciation of the clinical features, knowledge of the differential diagnosis, and use of modern diagnostic modalities should allow the physician to make the correct diagnosis in almost all instances. With earlier diagnosis and prompt treatment of uveal metastases, the visual morbidity may be reduced. Radiation therapy techniques using external beam sources can result in dramatic resolution of the tumor, return of vision, and prevention of serious complications for untreated tumor progression.

Soft-Tissue Sarcomas of Childhood

The soft-tissue sarcomas of childhood provide an excellent example of progress resulting from the integration of surgery, radiation therapy, and chemotherapy management. These tumors may arise at any site in the child, but the most frequent areas of origin are the head and neck region, the pelvis, and in or adjacent to the genitourinary system. In the head and neck group, soft-tissue sarcomas arising in the orbit represent a very common site; they are the most frequently occurring malignant orbital tumors in childhood. Originally, orbital sarcomas were treated by the ophthalmologist with the help of the radiation oncologist. More

Table 17.12. Malignant intraocular tumors: metastatic-primary tumor site

	HMCH	WEH
Breast	23	45
Lymphoma/Leukemia	9	—
Lung	8	10
Gastrointestinal	—	3
Other	7	12
Total	47	70

HMCH, Hahnemann University Hospital, Philadelphia, PA; WEH, Wills Eye Hospital, Philadelphia, PA.

appropriate, however, is a treatment comprised of an integrated program of management using the ophthalmologist, the radiation oncologist, and the medical oncologist.

When an orbital sarcoma is identified early in the history and appears to be limited to the orbital structures, it is associated with a better potential for survival than sarcomas in other sites of origin treated by surgery alone.

Treatment failure usually is manifested as a local intraorbital recurrence, and it may be salvageable by further aggressive local treatment. These tumors infrequently disseminate to more distant sites. Lederman (18) provided the foundations for appropriate integrated programs of management using surgery and radiation therapy. He developed guidelines for the radiation dosage and technique. Sagerman (22) suggested that higher radiation dosages were necessary. A minimum tumor dose of 5,000 rads (maximum 6,000 rads) should be delivered to the volume of interest using megavoltage equipment in 5–7 weeks. Ninety percent of the first 33 consecutive patients treated by radiation therapy alone achieved local tumor control. Although all of these tumors were classified as group III with gross residual disease, only a biopsy procedure to establish the histologic diagnosis had been performed in these patients with orbital rhabdomyosarcoma. Sixty-seven percent of the children who were treated remained alive and healthy for periods of 5–13 years after the treatment program had been completed.

All long-term survivors demonstrated late radiation effects ranging from minimal change to phthisis bulbi requiring enucleation (two cases). In general, the late effects correlated with age (worse in the younger child), the volume treated (more with a larger volume), the radiation dosage (more with a higher dose), and whether or not the eyelids were open or closed at the time of treatment. All patients treated developed cataracts that varied in severity, but generally permitted good vision. Also, they had hypoplasia of the orbital bones. No radiation-induced cancers had been observed in patients treated at the time of the last follow-up visit.

More recently, Donaldson, et al (9) added prolonged multidrug chemotherapy to high-dose radiation therapy programs to improve the cure rate in childhood sarcomas arising in the head and neck region. This has been associated with an improved survival rate compared with historic controls.

Many other groups are pursuing similar programs that integrate surgery, radiation therapy, and chemotherapy in the management of sarcomas involving the orbit. These combined integrated programs of management have resulted in marked improvement in the prognosis, with better long-term survival of the patient. A direct consequence of the better survival is greater concern for the late effects of each treatment mode on the quality of survival in cases in children (11).

The late effects of surgical resection and radiation therapy are relatively well defined compared to those with chemotherapy. Efforts have been made to rely more aggressively on chemotherapeutic management reducing the scope of resection or reducing the radiation therapy program. These studies have not yet produced sufficient results to resolve the question of how much of which therapy provides the best survival rate and the best functional result. It is the opinion of many investigators that surgery and radiation therapy are necessary to achieve tumor sterilization. Orbital irradiation may be chosen with a reasonable chance of preserving vision as opposed to pursuing a radical surgical exenterative procedure with loss of vision.

Malignant Lymphoma

The most common lymphomatous disease process involving the intraocular structures is diffuse histiocytic lymphoma. Other lymphomatous tumors involving the intraocular structures are very rare. There are major problems in differentiating between malignant intraocular lymphoma and benign reactive lymphoid hyperplasia. It occurs most commonly in older patients; and, it is most often unilateral on initial presentation, frequently involving the second eye within weeks to months after the initial diagnosis. The clinical features are quite variable, depending on whether the vitreous, retina, optic nerve, or choroid are involved. Symptoms may proceed with progression of disease, giving rise to central nervous system symptoms. The most common complaints are those of painless blurred vision. Most commonly, diffuse histiocytic lymphoma involves the posterior segment of the globe, but there may be extensive iris involvement. The lesion may be limited to the intraocular structures, but it may extend to involve the periocular structures as well.

Those patients with orbital involvement can have the diagnosis of histiocytic lymphoma established by a biopsy procedure. However, in those patients with intraocular involvement, the differential diagnosis may be difficult, including amelanotic melanoma, metastatic carcinoma, choroidal hemangioma, reactive lymphoid hyperplasia, and disseminated choroiditis from any cause.

In the past, diffuse histiocytic lymphoma usually was diagnosed after the eye had been enucleated for suspected melanoma or intratactable glaucoma. With the increased use of vitreous biopsy techniques, the diagnosis is now made more frequently by a fine-needle aspiration biopsy procedure or iridectomy.

After the diagnosis has been established, local radiation therapy is the treatment of choice. It can result in dramatic resolution of the involved tumor. In general, the treatment program is carried out by using right-angled wedge fields directed toward the entire orbit and angled in such a way as to avoid the opposite eye, delivering between 1,500–3,000 rads in 1.5–3 weeks as the tumor-dose minimum by using megavoltage radiation therapy equipment.

The treatment prognosis is excellent. Patients with diminished vision may see no major improvement in vision following completion of treatment. Longer survival rates have been reported in those patients who are treated aggressively by local radiotherapy supplemented with systemic administration of chemotherapy. Intraocular involvement with other lymphomatous disease (such as non-Hodgkin's lymphoma, Hodgkin's disease, and Burkitt's lymphoma) are rare. In general, the diagnosis should be established by biopsy procedure and the treatment program should be pursued in a manner prescribed for the treatment of diffuse histiocytic lymphoma.

Mycosis fungoides occasionally is reported to involve the intraocular structures. Again, local radiation therapy is an effective means for management of this particular problem.

Leukemias

Although leukemia does not occur primarily in the eye and the adnexa, these structures are involved as part of the systemic disease process in about 50% of all cases of leukemia. Ocular changes are more frequent in the acute leukemias, such as myelogenous, acute lymphatic, and monocystic leukemia.

Treatment of this particular involvement of the intraocular and orbital structures is by local radiation therapy. Between 1,500–3,000 rads delivered in 1.5–3 weeks cause prompt dramatic improvement and complete regression in the area irradiated. Again, right-angled wedge fields are appropriate by using megavoltage equipment that rotate the fields in such a way that the opposite eye is excluded from the treatment field. However, many patients will have bilateral orbital involvement from the very beginning. The prognosis for vision is good, and the prognosis for life is dependent on the basic histologic cell type of the leukemia, the type of disease, and the aggressiveness of the disease process.

Complications with Radiation Therapy

Complications from radiation therapy used in the treatment of malignant tumors of the eye may be acute, subacute, and chronic. The acute complications of treatment may involve the conjunctiva, where the changes will be similar to those seen in mucous membranes of the oral cavity. There may be injection, mucositis, confluent mucositis. Recovery proceeds even after higher doses of radiation have been delivered. It may take 5–8 weeks for a complete recovery. Acute changes involving the cornea may be injection, edema, superficial punctate keratitis, and ulceration. Higher-dose treatment may progress to ulceration and perforation. Acute changes involving the retina are primarily those of edema. Panophthalmitis rarely is seen in contemporary treatment of malignant tumors of the eye. When it does occur, it presents with signs and symptoms of severe pain, iridocyclitis, and secondary glaucoma.

Subacute changes due to radiation therapy may involve the conjunctiva, the cornea, the iris, and the ciliary body as well as the retina. Those changes involving the conjunctiva may be telangiectasia, secondary open-angle glaucoma, or secondary cosmetic problems with epilation of eyelashes. Corneal changes may be vascularization with a subsequent scar. Damage to the lacrimal gland may cause secondary drying and loss of corneal clarity. The subacute effects involving the iris and ciliary body may produce iridocyclitis and glaucoma, which occur more commonly when the entire globe is irradiated (tumor doses above 5,000 rads in 5 weeks). Subacute changes in the retina may be perimacular exudates or petechial hemorrhage. Chronic changes as a consequence of radiation therapy may involve the conjunctiva, cornea, iris and ciliary body, or retina. Conjunctival changes may be atrophy of the eyelids occurring with radionuclide implants of the lids or deformity of the lids. Entropion or extropion may result in keratinization, which may affect the cornea. Corneal changes would be those of keratinization and scarring, with a decrease in corneal sensitivity or anesthesia, as well as possible vascular opacification. Chronic changes involving the iris and ciliary body may result in glaucoma. This change occurring in the retina may appear as early as 10 months after completion of a radiation therapy program or 2–3 years later; it may consist of retinal hemorrhage, retinal exudates, retinal vascular occlusions, or vitreous hemorrhage. Punctal obstruction may occur, giving rise to epiphora. Scleral thinning may occur.

Complications that are specific to the use of radionuclide plaques for choroidal melanomas would include perimacular exudates, petechial retinal hemorrhage, vitreous hemorrhage, lens opacities, partial scleral sloughing, glaucoma, superficial punctate keratitis, arterial occlusions with neovascularization, disturbances of pigment epithelium, and changes related to the lacrimal gland and lacrimal duct.

Cataracts following brachytherapy seldom occur with dosages less than 2,000 rads. At 3,000 rads, there may be peripheral deterioration and cataract formation. With external radiation therapy, a single dose of 200 rads and, more commonly, 500–1,000 rads have been shown to cause cataracts. More than two thirds of the cases that received 900 rads have developed progressive cataract formation—all of which can be treated by surgical resection at periods well beyond completion of the radiation therapy program: 1 year or more. The sclera is resistant to dosages of radiation, and it may tolerate 40,000–45,000 rads delivered in 7–10 days without significant difficulty.

Summary

The eye is a complex organ made up of eyelids, extraocular structures, and intraocular structures. There is a wide diversity of roles for radiation therapy for malignant tumors of the eye.

With the advent of contemporary innovative techniques for radiation therapy, it has assumed an important place in the management of malignant tumors of the eye by virtue of its successful long-term control for many tumors involving the eye.

References

1. Abramson DH, Ellsworth RM, Tretter P, et al. Treatment of bilateral groups I through III retinoblastoma with bilateral radiation. *Arch Ophthalmol* 1981; 99:1761–1762.

2. Abramson DH, Ellsworth RM, Tretter P, et al. Simultaneous bilateral radiation for advanced bilateral retinoblastoma. *Arch Ophthalmol* 1981; 99:1763–1766.

3. Abramson DH, Notterman RB, Ellsworth RM, et al. Retinoblastoma treated in infants in the first six months of life. *Arch Ophthalmol* 1983; 101:1362–1366.

3A. Arneson K, Normes M: Malignant melanomas of the choroidal as related to coexistent benign nevus. *Acta Ophthalmol* 53:139–152, 1975.

3B. Ashton N, Wybar K: Primary tumors of the iris. *Ophthalmologica* 151:97–113, 1966.

3C. *Cancer Facts and Figures,* 1985. New York, American Cancer Society, 1985.

4. Char DH, Castro JR: Helium ion therapy for choroidal melanoma. *Arch Ophthalmol* 100:935, 1982.

5. Char DH, Castro JR, Quivey JM: Helium ion charged particle therapy for choroidal melanoma. *Ophthalmology* 87:565–570, 1982.

6. Char DH, Saunders WM: Helium ion therapy for choroidal melanoma. *Ophthalmology* (in press, 1985).

7. Char DN, Stone RD, Irvine AR: Diagnostic modalities in choroidal melanoma: Sensitivity, specificity, and reproducibility. *Am J Ophthalmol* 89:223, 1980.

7A. Creuss AF, Augsburger JJ, Shields JA, Donoso LA, Amsel J: Visual results following cobalt plaque radiotherapy for posterior uveal melanomas. *Ophthal* 91:131–136, 1984.

8. del Regato JA, Spjut HJ: Cancer of the eye, in *Cancer-Diagnosis Treatment, Prognosis,* ed 5. St Louis, CV Mosby, 1977.

9. Donaldson SS, Castro JR, Wilbur JR, et al: Rhabdomyosarcoma of head and neck in children. *Cancer* 31:26–35, 1973.

10. Ellsworth RM: Cobalt plaques for melanomas of the choroid, in Jakobiec FA (ed): *Ocular and Adnexal Tumors.* Birmingham, Aesculapius, 1978, pp 76–79.

11. Evans AE, Brand W, de Lorimier A, et al: Results

in children with local and regional neuroblastoma managed with and without vincristine, cyclophosphamide and imidazolecarboxamide: A report from the Children's Cancer Study Group. *Am J Clin Oncol* 7:No.(1):3–8, 1984.

12. Gass JDM: Observation of suspected choroidal and ciliary body melanomas for evidence of growth prior to enucleation. *Ophthalmology* 87:523–528, 1980.

13. Gragoudas ES, Goitein M, Verhey L, et al: Proton beam irradiation: An alternative to enucleation for intraocular melanomas. *Ophthalmology* 87(6):571–581, 1980.

14. Gragoudas ES, Goitein M, Verhey L: Proton beam irradiation: An alternative to enucleation for intraocular melanomas. *Ophthalmology* 87:571–581, 1980.

15. Jay B: Current development in ophthalmology: A follow-up of limbal melanomata. *Proc R Soc Med* 57:497–500, 1964.

16. Keller AZ: Histology, survivorship and related factors in the epidemiology of eye cancer. *Am J Epidemiol* 97:386–393, 1973.

17. Lederman M: Discussion of pigmented tumors of the conjunctiva, in Boniuk M (ed): *Ocular and Adnexal Tumors: New and Controversial Aspects.* St Louis, CV Mosby, 1964, pp 24–28.

18. Lederman M: Radiotherapy in treatment of orbital tumors. *Br J Ophthalmol* 40:592–610, 1956.

19. Lommatzsch P: Treatment of choroidal melanomas with 106Ru/106Rh beta-ray applicators. *Surv Ophthalmol* 19:85–100, 1974.

19A. Lommatzsch PK. Experience with beta-irradiation (106Ru/106Rh) of patients suffering from retinoblastoma: report on 33 patients. *Jpn J Ophthalmol* 1978; 22:424–430.

20. MacFaul PA: Local radiotherapy in the treatment of malignant melanoma of the choroid. *Trans Ophthalmol Soc UK* 97:421–427, 1977.

21. Packer S, Rotman M: Radiotherapy of choroidal melanoma with Iodine-125. *Ophthalmology* 87:582–590, 1980.

22. Sagerman RH, Tretter P, Ellsworth RM: The treatment of orbital rhabdomyosarcoma of children with primary radiation therapy. *Am J Roentgenol* 114:31–34, 1972.

22A. Sealey R, Buret E, Cleminshaw H, et al. Progress in the use of iodine therapy for tumors of the eye. *Br J Ophthalmol* 1980; 53:1052–1060.

23. Shidnia H, Hornback NB, Helveston EM, et al: Treatment results of retinoblastoma at Indiana University Hospitals. *Cancer* 40:2917–2922, 1977.

24. Shields JA, Augsburger JJ, Brady LW, et al: Cobalt plaque therapy of posterior uveal melanomas. *Ophthalmology* 89:1201–1207, 1982.

25. Shields JA, McDonald PR: Improvement in the diagnosis of posterior uveal melanomas. *Trans Am Ophthalmol Soc* 71:194–211, 1973; *Arch Ophthalmol* 91:259–264, 1974.

26. Shields JA, Zimmerman LE: Lesions simulating malignant melanoma of the posterior uvea. *Arch Ophthalmol* 89:466–471, 1973.

27. Stallard HB: Radiotherapy for malignant melanoma of the choroid. *Br J Ophthalmol* 50:14–155, 1966.

28. Stallard HB: The treatment of retinoblastoma. *Ophthalmologica* 151:214–230, 1966.

29. Starr HJ, Zimmerman LE: Extrascleral extension and orbital recurrences of malignant melanomas of the choroid and ciliary body. *Int Ophthalmol Clin* 2:369–385, 1962.

30. Vogel MH: Treatment of malignant choroidal melanomas with photocoagulation. Evaluation of 10-year follow-up data. *Am J Ophthalmol* 74:1–11, 1972.

31. Winter FC: Iridocyclectomy for malignant melanomas of the iris and ciliary body, in Boniuk M (ed): *Ocular and Adnexal Tumors: New and Controversial Aspects.* St Louis, CV Mosby, 1964, pp 341–352.

32. Winter FC: Surgical excision of tumors of the ciliary body and iris. *Arch Ophthalmol* 70:19–29, 1963.

33. Zimmerman LE, McLean IW: An evaluation of enucleation in the management of uveal melanomas. *Am J Ophthalmol* 87:741–760, 1979.

34. Zimmerman LE, McLean IW, Foster WD: Does enucleation of an eye containing a malignant melanoma prevent or accelerate the dissemination of tumor cells? *Br J Ophthalmol* 62:420–425, 1978.

Index

Aarskog syndrome, 140
Abscess
    orbital
        CT diagnosis of, 34, 315
        ultrasonography of, 316
    subperiosteal, 313
Acrocephalopolysyndactyly, 163
Acrocephalosyndactyly, 159–161
    type 3, 163
Adenoma, pituitary, 243–246,
        261
    clinical presentation of, 243–
        244
    diagnosis of, 244, 246
Adult
    epiphora in, 88–90
    orbital disorders associated
        with exophthalmos in,
        190
Aicardi syndrome, 127
Albers-Schoenberg disease, 177,
        180
Amniotic band syndrome, 151
Amputation neuroma, 207
Anencephaly, 152–153
Aneurysm
    carotid, magnetic resonance
        imaging of, 113
    carotid-cavernous, 261
    causing visual defects, 259
Angiography, carotid, 71–73
Angiomatosis, encephalotrige-
        minal, 172
Angiomatous tumor, ultrasound
        detection of, 66
Annulus of Zinn, 40
Anophthalmos, 125–126
Apert syndrome, 159–161
Arachnoid cyst, 257
Armendares syndrome, 164
A-scan ultrasonography, 57

Aspergillosis, 285
Astrocytoma, involving visual
        pathways, 251
Ataxia-telangiectasia, 176
Axial projection, of orbit, 7–8
Axial section, for orbital CT, 19

Bacterium(a), involved in orbital
        infections, 316
Baller-Gerold syndrome, 163
Bartholin syndrome, 148
Basal cell carcinoma, 227
    CT scanning of, 303
Basal cell nevus syndrome, 140–
        141
Base projection, of orbit, 7–8
BBB syndrome, 141, 143
Berant syndrome, 164
Berman locator, for foreign
        body localization, 95
Binder syndrome, 131
Biometry, with ultrasound, 68
1,3 Bis-(2-chlorethyl)-1 Nitro-
        sourea (BCNU), for ma-
        lignant melanoma, 350
Bixler syndrome, 143
Blow-out fracture, 323–327
    cause of, 323
    clinical signs of, 324–325
    CT scanning of, 51, 325–326
    "impure", 324
    "pure", 324
    surgical intervention in, 326–
        327
Bone
    effect of orbital lesion on, CT
        diagnosis of, 34
    neoplastic or infectious inva-
        sion of, MRI of, 108, 110
"Bone-free" techniques, in for-
        eign body localization, 93

Bone lesion, 261
Bonnet-Lechaume-Blanc syn-
        drome, 176–177
Bourneville-Pringle syndrome,
        171–172
Brachial arch syndrome, 151
Brachycephaly, 155, 158
Branchio-skeleto-genital syn-
        drome, 141
Breast carcinoma, metastatic to
        orbit, 233
Broad thumb-hallux syndrome,
        144
Brown's syndrome, 42–43, 45
    acquired, 43–45
    congenital, 43
B-scan ultrasonography, 57
    in orbital cellulitis, 316
Buphthalmos, 130

Caldwell projection, of orbit, 2–
        3
Cancerous melanosis, 351
Canthomeatal line (CM), 7
Capillary hemangioma, 210
Carotid aneurysm, magnetic
        resonance imaging of,
        113
Carotid angiography
    and diagnosis of orbital le-
        sions, 71–73
    indications for, 73
    technique of, 71
Carotid artery, external, 73
Carotid-cavernous aneurysm,
        261
Carotid-cavernous-fistula, 215
Carpenter syndrome, 163
"Cat-eye syndrome," 148
Cavernous hemangioma, 208–
        210

Cavernous sinus(es), 260–261
    and orbital cellulitis, 316, 318
    tumors of, 261, 263
Cebocephaly, 123–125
Cellulitis
    intraconal, 313
    orbital, 283, 310
        B-scan ultrasonography in,
            316
        preseptal, 311
        stages of, 311–318
        untreated, 316–318
    ultrasound detection of, 67
Cerebral gigantism, 141
Cerebrohepatorenal syndrome,
    141
Cerebro-oculo-facio-skeletal
    syndrome, 127–128
Chalazion, 308
Chemosis, 309
Chemotherapy, for malignant
    melanomas, 350
Chiasmatic cistern, 243
Child(ren)
    optic nerve gliomas in, 204
    orbital disorders associated
        with exophthalmos in,
        189–190
    retinoblastoma in, 351–352
    ultrasound detection of, 63
Chondroid tumor, 263
Chordoma, 261, 263
Choristoma, 217, 220–222
Choroid, detached, ultrasound
    detection of, 60
Choroidal melanoma, proton
    beam radiotherapy for,
    347–348
Choroiditis, 309
Chromosomal aberrations, 146–
    149
Chromosome 13q-syndrome,
    149
Chromosome 13r-syndrome, 149
Chromosome 18p-syndrome,
    149
Chromosome 18q-syndrome,
    149
Chromosome 22q+, 148
Chromosome deletion 4p-syn-
    drome, 148–149
Chromosome deletion 5p-syn-
    drome, 149
Cloverleaf skull, 158
Coats' disease, 229, 231
Cobalt plaque radiotherapy, for
    ureal melanomas, 346

Coffin-Lowry syndrome, 141
Colobomatous microphthalmos,
    127
Computed tomography (CT)
    in Brown's syndrome, 43
    in diagnosis of blow-out frac-
        tures, 325–326
    in diagnosis of optic nerve
        gliomas, 205–206
    in evaluation of diseased or-
        bits, 303–306
        findings in, 305–306
        technique of, 303–305
    in foreign body localization,
        95–96
    in Graves' disease, 195–198
    in ocular motility disorders,
        39–53
    of orbit, 19–36
    of orbital anatomy, 19–20, 24–
        29
    of orbital pathology, 29–36
    of paraorbital pathology, 281–
        301
Congenital abnormalities, 115–
    180
    chromosomal aberrations,
        146–149
    craniofacial clefts, 149–152
    of development and patholo-
        gy, 116–117
    diagnostic imaging techniques
        of, 120–121
    of embryology and develop-
        ment, 115–116
    of globe, 122–130
    of interorbital distance, 130–
        146
    of lacrimal drainage system,
        121–122
    miscellaneous, 177–180
    of skull, 152–164
Congenital tumor, 253, 257
Conjunctiva, infections of, 308–
    309
Conjunctival melanoma, 351
Contrast imaging, orbital inves-
    tigation by, 71–78
Contrast medium(a), for orbital
    CT, 19
Contrast techniques, orbital in-
    vestigation by, 71–78
Cornea, 309
    magnetic resonance imaging
        of, 104
Coronal section, for orbital CT,
    19

Craniocarpotarsal dysplasia,
    144–145
Craniodiaphyseal dysplasia, 140
Craniofacial clefts, congenital
    abnormalities of, 149–152
Craniofacial dysostosis, 158–159
Craniofacial microsomia, 151
Craniofrontonasal dysplasia,
    133, 135
Craniometaphyseal dysplasia,
    137, 140
Craniopharyngioma, involving
    visual pathways, 248, 250
Craniostenosis, bilateral prema-
    ture, 155, 158
Craniosynostosis, 153–164
    with dwarfism and retinitis
        pigmentosa, 164
    and fibular aplasia, 163
    with hypoplasia and hypertri-
        chosis, 163
    and radial aplasia, 163
    and radioulnar synostosis,
        163–164
    with syndactyly and obesity,
        163
Craniosynostosis syndrome, 45
Craniotelencephalic dysplasia,
    131
Cri-du-chat syndrome, 149
Crouzon's syndrome, 45, 158–
    159
Cryptophthalmos syndrome,
    126–127
Cyalume, in lacrimal drainage
    system studies, 84
Cyclopia, 123
Cyst
    arachnoid, 257
    dermoid, 220–222, 257, 293–
        295
    developmental orbital, CT as-
        sessment of, 293–295
    epidermoid, 253, 257, 293–
        295
    hematic, CT assessment of,
        291–293
    hydatid, CT diagnosis of, 34
Cystic tumor, ultrasound detec-
    tion of, 65

Dacryocystitis, 309
Dacryocystography
    distention, 85
    intubation, 85
    radionuclide, 83–84
deGrouchy syndrome, 149

Dermoid cyst, 220–222, 257, 293–295
   CT diagnosis of, 34
Diagnostic imaging, of congenital abnormalities, 120–121
Doppler ultrasound, 56
Double elevator palsy, 45
Down syndrome, 148
Dubowitz syndrome, 141
Dysplasia
   craniocarpotarsal, 144–145
   craniodiaphyseal, 140
   craniofrontonasal, 133, 135
   craniometaphyseal, 137, 140
   craniotelencephalic, 131
   fibrous, 177
   maxillonasal, 131
   Streeter, 151
Dysthyroid exophthalmos, see Graves' disease

Echoes, ultrasound, 56
Edema
   of eyelid, 283
   preseptal, 311
   sud-Tenon's, 67
Edwards syndrome, 148
Elsahy-Waters syndrome, 141
Embryo, development of, congenital abnormalities in, 115–116
Embryonic tumor, 253, 257
Empty sella, 259
Encephalocele
   anterior, 145
   basal type of, 145–146
Encephalotrigeminal angiomatosis, 172
Endocrine ocular myopathy, 45
Enophthalmos, posttraumatic, factors in, 324
Epidermoid cyst, 253, 257, 293–295
Epiloia, 171–172
Epiphora, 81; see also Tearing
   in adults, 88–90
   in infant, 87–88
Epithelial malignancy, magnetic resonance imaging of, 108
Esotropia, 39
Ethmocephaly, 123
Ethmoid fracture, 328
Ethmoid sinus infection, 283
Exophthalmos
   causes of, 63
   definition of, 189

dysthyroid, see Graves' disease
   evaluation of, 189–192
   orbital disorders associated with, 189–190
Exotropia, 39
Extraconal neoplasms, 295
   magnetic resonance imaging of, 108, 110
Extraconal (EC) space
   orbital, 20
   structures in, 29
Extraocular muscle(s)
   anatomy of, 40–42
   CT scanning of, 24–25
Extraorbital infection, 319–320
Eye
   magnetic resonance imaging of, 99–113
   measurement of, ultrasound techniques in, 68
   normal, magnetic resonance imaging of, 102–104
   ultrasonography of, 55–68
Eyeball, see Globe
Eye changes, in Graves' disease
   class 0, 193
   class 1 and 2, 193–194
   class 3, 194
   class 4, 194–195
   class 5, 195
   class 6, 195
Eyelid
   edema of, 283
   infections of, 308
   lower, fistula in, 311
   upper, abscess-producing fistula in, 311
Eye motility disturbance, causes of, 39–40

Face, basal cell carcinoma of, 303
Facial clefting syndrome, 143
Facial-digital-genital syndrome, 140
Facial trauma, 320
Fetal face syndrome, 135–137
Fibrous dysplasia, 177
Fibrous histiocytoma, 222–223
Fistula, of eyelids, 311
Focal dermal hypoplasia, 128
Focal mass lesion, magnetic resonance imaging of, 110
Foreign body(ies)
   gunshot injury, and retention of, 320

localization of, 93–97
   Berman locator in, 95
   computed tomography in, 95–96
   radiographic studies in, 93–94
   ultrasound in, 61, 95
Fracture
   blow-out, 51, 323–327
   combined, 330–338
   ethmoidal, 328
   lateral wall, 330
   LeFort, 334, 336–338
   medial wall, 327–328
   nasoorbital, 333–334
   orbital roof, 329–330
   tripod or tripartite, 331, 333
Franceschetti-Zwalen-Klein syndrome, 151–152
Freeman-Sheldon syndrome, 144–145
Frontal vein, contrast imaging using, 73–74
   complications of, 75
Frontodigital syndrome, 131
Frontonasal dysplasia malformation complex, 131–133
Fungus(i), involved in orbital infection, 307–308

Germinoma, involving visual pathways, 253
Glaucoma, congenital, 130
Glioma
   involving visual pathways, 250–252
   optic nerve, 204–207
      CT scanning of, 205–206
      magnetic resonance imaging of, 206
      pathologic patterns of, 204
   ultrasound detection of, 65
Globe
   congenital abnormalities of, 122–130
   CT scan of, 20
Goldenhar syndrome, 151
Goltz syndrome, 128
Gorlin-Chaudhry-Moss syndrome, 163
Gorlin syndrome, 140–141
Granulomatous disease, 257–258
Graves' disease, 192–198
   B-scan ultrasonography in, 198
   classification of stages in, 193–195

Graves' disease (*cont.*)
  CT scanning in, 195–198
  definition of, 192
  evaluation of, 192–198
  ultrasound detection of, 67–68
Graves' orbitopathy, 30
Greig syndrome, 131
G1 trisomy syndrome, 148

Hallermann-Streiff syndrome,
      128, 130
Hamartoma, hypothalamic, 257
Head
  rhomboid-shaped, 154–155
  squamous cell carcinoma of,
      303
Helium ion treatment, for ocular
      melanoma, 348–350
Hemangiolymphangioma, 180
Hemangioma, 180
  capillary, 210
  cavernous, 208–210
  symptoms of, 281
  ultrasound detection of, 63,
      66
Hemangiopericytoma, 214–215
Hematic cyst, CT assessment
      of, 291–293
Hematoma, subperiosteal orbit-
      al, CT assessment of,
      290–293
Hemifacial microsomia, 151
Hemorrhage
  subretinal, ultrasound detec-
      tion of, 63
  vitreous, 62–63
Herpes simplex, infection with,
      307
Herpes zoster, infection with,
      307
Heterotropia, 39
Histiocytoma, fibrous, 222–223
HMC syndrome, 143
Holoprosencephaly, 122–123
Hordeolum, 308
Hydatid cyst, CT diagnosis of,
      34
Hypertelorism, 143
  orbital, 131–146
Hypertelorism-hypospadias syn-
      drome, 141, 143
Hypertropia, 39
Hypoplasia, focal dermal, 128
Hypotelorism, orbital, 131
Hypothalamic hamartoma, 257
Hypotropia, 39

Immunotherapy, of systemic
      melanomas, 350
Infant epiphora in, 87–88
Infection
  of conjunctiva, 308–309
  of cornea, 309
  of eyelid, 308
  of lacrimal drainage system,
      309–310
  orbital, 307–321
    direction of spread and
      clinical correlation, 310–
      311
  of paranasal sinuses, 310
  of sclera, 309
  of uveal tract, 309
Inflammation
  of intraconal space, 313
  orbital, 233–235
Inflammatory-congestive dis-
      ease, orbital, ultrasound
      detection of, 66–68
Inflammatory pseudotumor, ul-
      trasound detection of, 67
Injury, gunshot, 338
Innervation, reciprocal, Sher-
      rington law of, 42
Interorbital distance, congenital
      abnormalities of, 130–146
Interzygomatic line, 20
Intraconal (IC) space
  inflammation of, 313
  orbital, 20
  pathology of, magnetic reso-
      nance imaging of, 110
  structures in, 24
Intraocular tumor
  metastatic, 352–353
    radiotherapy for, 353
  with orbital extension, 229–
      232
  radiotherapy for, 343–356
  ultrasound detection of, 61–63
Intravenous contrast medium(a),
      for orbital CT, 19
Isotope studies, of lacrimal
      drainage system, 83–84

Jones tests, 82–83

Kleeblattschadel anomaly, 158
Knapp procedure, reverse, 51

Lacrimal drainage system, 81–90
  anatomy of, 81–82
  clinical aspects of, 86–90

congenital abnormalities of,
      121–122
  evaluation techniques
    experimental studies, 84
    isotope studies, 83–84
    Jones tests, 82–83
    radiologic studies, 84–86
    taste test, 83
  infections of, 309–310
  physiology of, 82
Lacrimal duct, anatomy of, 81
Lacrimal gland
  CT scanning of, 29
  tumor of, 215, 217, 295–296
    benign mixed, 215, 217
    malignant mixed, 217
Lacrimal sac, anatomy of, 81
Lamina papyracea, CT scanning
      of, 29
Larsen syndrome, 143
Lateral view, of orbit, 4–5
Lateral wall fracture, 330
LeFort fracture, 334–335
Lens, magnetic resonance imag-
      ing of, 104
Lenz microphthalmia syndrome, 130
Leopard syndrome, 143
Lesion(s)
  bone, 261
  focal mass, magnetic reso-
      nance imaging of, 110
  involving visual pathways,
      239–278
  metastatic, 257
  orbital, *see* Orbital lesion(s)
  paraseller, 260–263
  vascular, shape of, 30
Leukemia, treatment of, 355
Levator palpebrae muscle, CT
      scanning of, 25
Limbal ring, in foreign body lo-
      calization, 94
Lipiodol, in lacrimal drainage
      system studies, 84
Lipoma, 222
Liposarcoma, 222
Louis-Bar syndrome, 176
Lowry syndrome, 163
Lymphangioma, 180, 213–214
  ultrasound detection of, 66
Lymphoma, 235
  lymphocytic, magnetic reso-
      nance imaging of, 108
  malignant, 354–355
    radiation therapy for, 355
  ultrasound detection of, 65, 66

Macrodacryocystography, 85

Maculopathy, disciform, ultrasound detection of, 63

Magnetic resonance imaging (MRI)
  basic principles of, 99–102
  in diagnosis of optic nerve gliomas, 206
  of eye and orbit, 99–113
  of ocular pathology, 105–108
  of optic nerve, 110–111
  of orbital apex, 111–113
  of orbit pathology, 108–110
  surface coil imaging, 102

"Male Turner syndrome," 143–144

Mandibulofacial dysostosis, with epibulbar dermoids, 151

Marble bone disease, 177, 180

Maxillonasal dysplasia, 131

Meckel syndrome, 130

Medial wall fracture, 327–328
  CT scan of, 328
  signs of, 327

Median cleft face syndrome, 131–133

Meglumine iothalamate, used in orbital venography, 74

Melanoma
  choroidal, proton beam radiotherapy for, 347–348
  conjunctival, 351
  magnetic resonance imaging of, 105–106
  malignant, 231–232
    chemotherapy for, 350
    ultrasound detection of, 62
  ocular, high dose radiotherapy for, 348–350
  systemic, immunotherapy of, 350
  uveal, 343–347
    cobalt plaque radiotherapy for, 346

Melanosis
  cancerous, treatment of, 351
  precancerous, 351

Meningioma, 201–204, 261
  CT assessment of, 299–301
  involving visual pathways, 246–247
  optic nerve sheath
    clinical manifestations of, 202

involving visual pathways, 246–247
  treatment of, 202–203
  sphenoid ridge, 203–204, 299
  ultrasound detection of, 65, 66

Meningocephalocele, 145

Mesenchymal tumor, 222–225

Metallic markers, in foreign body localization, 94

Metastatic disease, 232–233, 296–298

Metastatic lesions, involving visual pathways, 257

Metastatic tumor, ultrasound detection of, 63

Metopic suture, premature closure of, 158

Meyer's loop, 263

Microphthalmos, 127

Microtia, 143

Mongoloidism, 148

Motility disorders, ocular, see Ocular motility disorders

Mucocele, 225–227, 319
  clinical features of, 288–289
  CT diagnosis of, 34, 289
  etiology of, 287
  radiographic characteristics of, 289
  sinus of origin of, 287–289
  sphenoid sinus, 263

Mucopyocele, 319–320

Mucormycosis, 320
  pathology of, 284–285
  radiographic findings of, 285

Multidirectional tomography, of orbit, 8

Multiple lentigines syndrome, 143

Multiple nevois basal cell carcinoma syndrome, 140–141

Myopathy, endocrine ocular, 45

Nanophthalmos, 127

Nasolacrimal apparatus
  congenital abnormalities of, 122
  obstruction of, 309

Nasolacrimal duct, anatomy of, 81

Nasoorbital fracture, 333–334

Nasopharynx, malignant tumors of, 263

Neck, squamous cell carcinoma of, 303

Neurilemmoma, 207–208

Neurofibroma, 207–208

Neurofibromatosis, 167, 169–171

Neurogenic tumors, of peripheral nerve origin, 207–208

Neuroma, 261
  amputation, 207

Noonan syndrome, 143–144

Norrie disease, 130

Oblique muscle, CT scanning of, 25

Ocular melanoma, high dose radiotherapy for, 348–350

Ocular motility disorders
  causes of, 39–40
  conclusions, 51
  evaluation of, CT scanning in, 39–53
  traumatic, 45, 51

Ocular muscle
  imbalance of, 39
  nerve supply to, pathologic process involving, 40

Ocular myopathy, endocrine, 45

Ocular pathology, magnetic resonance imaging of, 105–108

Oculo-auriculo-vertebral syndrome, 151

Oculodentodigital syndrome, 130

OPD syndrome, 144

Ophthalmic artery
  CT scanning of, 24
  radiographic appearance of, 71–72

Ophthalmic vein
  CT scanning of, 24
  inferior, anatomy of, 76
  superior, 75–76

Opitz syndrome, 141, 143

Optic canal
  anatomy of, 1–2
  Rhese view of, 5, 7
  tomgraphy of, 9

Optic chiasm
  lesions of, visual field deficit in, 243
  and parachiasmal area, 240, 242–243

Optic chiasma, lesions of, visual field defect in, 243

Optic nerve
  CT scanning of, 20
  gliomas of
    CT scanning of, 205–206
    magnetic resonance imaging
      of, 206
    pathologic patterns of, 204
  magnetic resonance imaging
    of, 110–111
  surface coil imaging of, 111
  tumors of, involving visual
    pathways, 239–240
Optic nerve sheath, meningiomas of
  clinical manifestations of, 202
  treatment of, 202–203
Optic nerve/sheath, 20
Orbit
  anatomy of, 1–2
    normal CT scanning of, 19–
      20, 24–29
    spread of infection and,
      282–283
  basal and squamous cell tu-
    mors of, 303–306
  base or axial projection of, 7–
    8
  blow-out fracture of, see
    Blow-out fracture
  Caldwell projection of, 2–3
  and complications of sinus
    diseases, 283–287
  computed tomography of, 19–
    36
    technique for, 19
  diagnostic ultrasonography of,
    63–68
  infection of, 307–321
    direction of spread and
      clinical correlation, 310–
      311
    postsurgical, 318
  inflammations of, 233–235
  inflammatory-congestive
    diseases of, ultrasound
    detection of, 66–68
  investigation of, by contrast
    techniques and, 71–78
  lateral view of, 4–5
  magnetic resonance imaging
    of, 99–113
  metastasis to, 232–233
  multidirectional tomography
    of, 8–17
  normal
    magnetic resonance imaging
      of, 102–104

  ultrasonography of, 63–65
  plain film radiography and
    polytomography of, 1–17
  Rhese view of, 5–7
  routine examination of, 2–8
  trauma to, 323–340
    CT assessment of, 289
    investigation of, 323
    subperiosteal hemartoma
      following, 290–291
    ultrasonography of, 55–68
    vascular anomalies of, ultra-
      sound detection of, 68
  Water's projection of, 3–4
Orbit canal, Rhese view of, 5–7
Orbit pathology, magnetic resonance imaging of, 108–
  110
Orbital abscess, CT scanning of,
  315–316
Orbital apex, magnetic resonance imaging of, 111–
  113
Orbital cellulitis, see Cellulitis,
  orbital
Orbital cyst, developmental, CT
  assessment of, 293–295
Orbital disease
  associated with exophthal-
    mos, 189–190
  evaluation of, 190–192
Orbital fissure
  inferior, anatomy of, 1
  superior, 1
    CT scanning of, 29
Orbital floor fracture, proptosis
  following, 326–327
Orbital hypertelorism, 131–146
Orbital hypotelorism, 131
Orbital lesion(s)
  characteristics of, 30
  cystic, 34
  location of, 30
  shape of, 30
Orbital metastasis, CT assessment of, 296–298
Orbital pathology, CT diagnosis
  of, 29–36
Orbital pseudotumor, 233–235,
  318–319
  magnetic resonance imaging
    of, 110
Orbital roof fracture, 329–330
  clinical signs of, 329
Orbital tumor(s), 201–236
  secondary, 225–228
  symptoms of, 281–282

  ultrasound detection of, 65–66
  vascular, 208–215
Orbital varix, 215
Orbital venography, 73–76
  anatomy indicated by, 75–76
  indication for, 76
  pathology indicated by, 76
  technique of, 73–75
Orbital wall, periostitis of, 313
Osteopetrosis, 177, 180
Otocephalia, 125
Otopalatodigital syndrome, 144

Palsy, double elevator, 45
Paranasal sinus, infections of,
  310
Paraorbital pathology
  anatomic considerations, 282–
  283
  computed tomography of,
    281–301
Paraorbital tumor, CT assess-
  ment of, 295–296
Parasellar lesion, 260–263
Parinaud's syndrome, 266
Patau syndrome, 148
Periostitis, 31
  of orbital wall, 313
Pfeiffer syndrome, 161
Phakomatosis, 165–177
Pinealoma, 266
Pituitary adenoma, 243–246, 261
Plagiocephaly, 154–155
Polytomography of orbit, 1–17
Precancerous melanosis, 351
Proptosis
  definition of, 189
  following orbital floor frac-
    ture, 326–327
Pseudoexophthalmos, 189
Pseudotumor(s)
  inflammatory, ultrasound de-
    tection of, 67
  orbital, 233–235, 318–319
    magnetic resonance imaging
      of, 110
  sclerosing, ultrasound detec-
    tion of, 66
Punctum(a), congenital abnor-
  malities of, 121–122

Radiation therapy
  cobalt plaque, for uveal
    melanomas, 346
  complications with, 355–356
    high dose, for ocular melano-
      mas, 348–350

for malignant intraocular tumors, 343–356
for malignant lymphomas, 355
proton beam, for choroidal melanomas, 347–348
for soft-tissue sarcomas, 354
Radiographic studies, in foreign body localization, 93–95
Radiography, plain film, of orbit, 1–17
Radiologic studies, of lacrimal drainage system, 84–86
Radionuclide dacryocystography, 83–84
Rectus muscle(s)
anatomy of, 40
CT scanning of, 25
Retina, detached, ultrasound detection of, 59–60
Retinoblastoma, 229, 231, 351–352
magnetic resonance imaging of, 106–107
treatment of, 352
ultrasound detection of, 63
Rhabdomyosarcoma, 223–225
differential diagnosis of, 224–225
histologic types of, 223–224
orbital, 224
Rhese view, of orbit, 5, 7
Rhinocerebral mycotic infection, 284–285
Rhomboid-shaped head, 154–155
Robinow-Silverman-Smith syndrome, 135–137
Rubinstein-Taybi syndrome, 144

Saethre-Chotzen syndrome, 163
Sarcoma
soft-tissue, in children, 353–354
radiotherapy for, 354
ultrasound detection of, 65–66
Scalp, basal cell carcinoma of, 303
Schwannoma, 208
Sclera, 309
magnetic resonance imaging of, 104
Scleritis, 309
Sclerosing pseudotumor, ultrasound detection of, 66
Sclerosis, tuberous, 171–172
Sclerosteosis, 140

Sella turcica, 242–243
enlargement of, 259
Sherrington law, of reciprocal innervation, 42
Sinus disease, orbital complications of, 283–287
Sinus malignancy, 227
Sinus of Maier, 81
Skull
base of, lesions of, 260–263
cloverleaf, 158
congenital abnormalities of, 152–164
Soft tissue, passage of sound beams through, 55–56
Sotos syndrome, 141
Sphenoidal fissure, 29
Sphenoid ridge, meningiomas of, 203–204, 299
Sphenoid sinus mucocele, 263
Squamous cell carcinoma
CT scanning of, 303
of sinus, 227
Squint, 39
Strabismus
nonconcomitant, 39–40
CT scanning in, 42–53
nonparetic, 39
Streeter dysplasia, 151
Sturge-Weber syndrome, 172
Sty, 308
Subarachnoid space, 20
Subperiosteal orbital hematoma, CT assessment of, 290–293
Sud-Tenon's edema, 67
Summitt syndrome, 163
Superior oblique tendon sheath syndrome, see Brown's syndrome
Suprasellar tumor, and tumor-like lesions, 243–259
Surface coil imaging, 102
of optic nerve, 111
Swelling, periorbital, 311
Symptomatic sequences, diagnostic value of, 281
Synophthalmia, 123

Taste test, 83
Taybi syndrome, 144
Tearing
excessive, 81
physiology of, 82
Tendon of Lockwood, 40
Tendon of Zinn, 40
Teratoma, 220

Thyroid myopathy, 45
Thyroid ophthalmopathy, see Graves' disease
Tissue, soft, passage of sound beams through, 55–56
Tolosa-Hunt syndrome, 76
magnetic resonance imaging of, 113
Tomography
computed, see Computed tomography (CT)
multidirectional, 8–17
of optic canal, 9
Trauma
facial, 320
orbital, 323–340
CT assessment of, 289
investigation of, 323
Treacher-Collins syndrome, 151–152
Trigoncephaly, 158
Tripartite fracture, 331, 333
Tripod fracture, 331, 333
Trisomy 13, 148
Trisomy 18, 148
Trisomy 21, 148
Trisomy D1, 148
Trisomy E, 148
Tuberous sclerosis, 171–172
Tumor(s); see also specific types
congenital, 253, 257
cystic, ultrasound detection of, 65
embryonic, 253, 257
intraocular
with orbital extension, 229–232
radiotherapy for, 343–356
ultrasound detection of, 61–63
lacrimal gland, 215, 217
mesenchymal, 222–225
metastatic, ultrasound detection of, 63
optic nerve, 239–240
orbital, see Orbital tumor(s)
paraorbital, CT assessment of, 295–296
regression of, patterns of, 345
solid, ultrasound detection of, 65–66
suprasellar, 243–259

Ulcer, bacterial corneal, 309
Ullrich syndrome, 143–144

Ultrasonography
  A-scan, 57
  B-scan, 57
    in Graves' disease, 198
    in orbital cellulitis, 316
  biometry with, 68
  diagnostic
    equipment and techniques, 56–57
    historical aspects of, 55
    technical factors, 55–56
  of eye and orbit, 55–68
  in foreign body localization, 95
  ocular diagnosis by, 59–63
  orbital diagnosis by, 63–68
  physical basis of, 55
  water immersion technique, 57
Ultrasound
  definition of, 55
  Doppler, 56
Ultrasound signals, 55, 56
Uveal melanoma, 343–347

Uveal tract, 309
Uveitis, 309

Valve of Hasner, 82
Valve of Krause, 81
Varix (varices), orbital, 215
Vascular anomalies, orbital, ultrasound detection of, 68
Vascular lesion
  causing visual defects, 259–260
  shape of, 30
Vascular malformations, 215
Vascular orbital tumor, 208–215
Vein, nonopacification of, 76
Venography, orbital, 73–76
Virus(es), involved in orbital infections, 307
Visual acuity, of cobalt plaque radiotherapy, for uveal melanomas, 346
Visual pathways
  lesions involving, 239–278
  posterior, lesions of, 263–278

Vitreous, magnetic resonance imaging of, 103–104
Vitreous cavity, abnormalities of, ultrasound detection of, 60–61
Vitreous hemorrhage, ultrasound detection of, 62–63
von Hippel-Lindau syndrome, 172, 176
von Recklinghausen neurofibromatosis, 167, 169–171

Water immersion technique, of ultrasonography, 57
Water's projection, of orbit, 3–4
Whistling face syndrome, 144–145
Wolf syndrome, 148–149
Wyburn-Mason syndrome, 176–177

Zellweger syndrome, 141
Zinn, annulus of, 40